Essential Human Development

Essential Human Development

Edited by

Samuel Webster
PhD, FHEA
Senior Lecturer in Anatomy & Embryology
Swansea University Medical School
Swansea, UK

Geraint Morris
MB, BCh, FRCPCH
Consultant Neonatologist and Clinical Director,
Children's Services
Singleton Hospital
Swansea, UK

Euan Kevelighan
FRCOG, FAcadMed, DipMed Ed
All Wales Head of School & Associate Dean for Obstetrics and Gynaecology
Honorary Associate Professor, Swansea University Medical School
Honorary Secretary of Welsh Obstetrics and Gynaecology Society
Swansea, UK

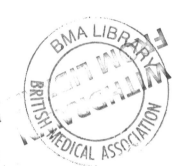
WILEY Blackwell

Registered Office(s)
John Wiley & Sons, Inc., 111 River Street, Hoboken, NJ 07030, USA
John Wiley & Sons Ltd, The Atrium, Southern Gate, Chichester, West Sussex, PO19 8SQ, UK

Editorial Office
9600 Garsington Road, Oxford, OX4 2DQ, UK

For details of our global editorial offices, customer services, and more information about Wiley products visit us at www.wiley.com.

Wiley also publishes its books in a variety of electronic formats and by print-on-demand. Some content that appears in standard print versions of this book may not be available in other formats.

Library of Congress Cataloging-in-Publication Data
Names: Webster, Samuel, 1974- editor. | Morris, Geraint, editor. |
    Kevelighan, Euan, editor.
Title: Essential human development / edited by Samuel Webster, Geraint
    Morris, Euan Kevelighan.
Description: Hoboken, NJ : John Wiley & Sons, 2018. | Includes index. |
    Identifiers: LCCN 2017022080 (print) | LCCN 2017037734 (ebook) | ISBN
    9781118528600 (pdf) | ISBN 9781118528617 (epub) | ISBN 9781118528624 (pbk.)
Subjects: LCSH: Life cycle, Human. | Developmental biology. | Embryology,
    Human.
Classification: LCC QP83.8 (ebook) | LCC QP83.8 .E87 2018 (print) | DDC
    571.8--dc23
LC record available at https://lccn.loc.gov/2017022080 9781118528624

Cover image: © Nicholas Eveleigh/Gettyimages
Cover design by Wiley

Set in 10/12 pt AGaramondPro-Regular by Thomson Digital, Noida, India
Printed and bound in Singapore by Markono Print Media Pte Ltd

1   2018

Contents

List of Contributors

Rebecca Balfour, MB BCh MRCPCH
Specialty Doctor, Community Child Health
Singleton Hospital
Swansea, UK

Marion Beard, MB BS
Consultant Obstetrician & Gynaecologist
Cardiff and Vale University Health Board
Cardiff, UK

Dana Beasley, State Examination Medicine MRCPCH
Consultant Paediatrician
Morriston Hospital
Swansea, UK

Christopher Bidder, BMedSci BM BS MRCPCH
Consultant Paediatrician with Special Interest in
Diabetes and Endocrinology
Morriston Hospital
Swansea, UK

Aisling Carroll-Downey, MB BCh
Belfast City Hospital
Belfast Health and Social Care Trust
Belfast, County Antrim, Northern Ireland

Benjamin Chisholme, MB BCh, BSc (Hons), DRCOG, MRCGP
General Practitioner
Llynfi Surgery
Maesteg
Wales, UK

Jennifer Davies-Oliveira, MB BCh
Speciality Registrar in Obstetrics & Gynaecology
Cardiff and Vale University Health Board
Cardiff , UK

Maitreyee Deshpande, MB BS
Specialty Registrar in Obstetrics & Gynaecology
Cardiff and Vale University Health Board
Cardiff, UK

Jamie Evans, MB BCh MRCPCH
Specialty Registrar, Neonatal Medicine
University Hospital of Wales
Cardiff, Wales, UK

Ruth Frazer, MB BCh
Consultant in Contraception and Sexual Health
Morriston Hospital
Swansea, UK

Nitin Goel, MBBS MD FRCPCH
Consultant Neonatologist
Singleton Hospital
Swansea, UK

Fran Hodge, MB BS
Consultant Obstetrician & Gynaecologist
Morriston Hospital
Swansea, UK

Sharif Ismail, MB BS
Consultant Obstetrician & Gynaecologist
Brighton and Sussex University Hospitals NHS Trust
Sussex, UK

Nisha Kadwadkar, MB BS
Consultant Obstetrician & Gynaecologist
Lancaster Hospital
Lancaster, UK

Euan Kevelighan, FRCOG FAcadMed DipMed Ed
All Wales Head of School & Associate Dean for Obstetrics
and Gynaecology
Honorary Associate Professor, Swansea University
Medical School
Honorary Secretary of Welsh Obstetrics and
Gynaecology Society
Swansea, UK

Aleksandra Komarzyniec-Pyzik, MD Poland, FRSH Dip
Specialty Doctor Obstetrics & Gynaecology
Nevill Hall Hospital
Aneurin Bevan University Health Board
Abergavenny, UK

Franz Majoko, MB BS[†]
Consultant Obstetrician & Gynaecologist
Formerly of Morriston Hospital
Swansea, UK

Colm McAlinden, MD MB BCh BSc (Hons) MSc, PhD MRCOphth
Consultant Neonatologist
University Hospital of Wales
Cardiff, UK

† Recently deceased.

Geraint Morris, MB BCh FRCPCH
Consultant Neonatologist and Clinical Director, Children's Services
Singleton Hospital
Swansea, UK

Ian Morris, MB BS (Hons) MRCPCH
Consultant Neonatologist
University Hospital of Wales
Cardiff, UK

Marsham Moselhi, MB BS
Consultant Obstetrician & Gynaecologist
Morriston Hospital
Swansea, UK

Deepa Balachandran Nair, MB BS
Registrar in Obstetrics and Gynaecology
Morriston Hospital
Swansea, UK

Manju Nair, MB BS
Consultant Obstetrician & Gynaecologist
Morriston Hospital
Swansea, UK

Cerys Scarr, MB BS
Consultant Obstetrician & Gynaecologist
Royal Gwent Hospital
Newport, UK

Lakshmipriya Selvarajan, MBBS MRCPCH
Specialty Registrar, Paediatric Gastroenterology
Birmingham Children's Hospital
Birmingham, UK

Catrin Simpson, MB BCh BSc (hons) MRCPCH
Consultant Community Paediatrician
Cardiff and Vale University Health Board
Cardiff, UK

Gurpreet Singh Kalra, MB BS
Consultant Gynaecologist
Morriston Hospital
Swansea, UK

Alan Treharne, MB BS
Specialty Registrar, Obstetrics and Gynaecology
St Georges Hospital Medical School
Cardiff, UK

Surekha Tuohy, MB BS MRCPCH
Consultant Community Paediatrician
Singleton Hospital
Swansea, UK

Pramodh Vallabhaneni, MB BS MRCPCH Dip Medical Education
Consultant Paediatrician
Morriston Hospital
Swansea, UK

Sophie Walker MB BS
Clinical Research Fellow
Queen Mary University of London
London, UK

Samuel Webster, PhD FHEA
Senior Lecturer in Anatomy & Embryology
Swansea University Medical School
Swansea, UK

Shabeena Webster, MBBCh MRCPCH Dip Paed Neurodis
Specialty Registrar, Community Paediatrics
Llandough Hospital
Cardiff, UK

Cathy White, MB BS FRCP FRCPCH
Consultant Paediatric Neurologist
Morriston Hospital
Swansea, UK

Bethan Williams, MB BCh MRCPCH
Consultant Community Paediatrician
Cardiff and Vale University Health Board
Cardiff, UK

Toni Williams, MB BCh MRCPCH
Consultant Paediatrician
Glangwili Hospital
Carmarthen, UK

Kinza Younas, MB BS
Consultant Obstetrician & Gynaecologist
Morriston Hospital
Swansea, UK

Preface

Medical education is forever expanding as our understanding of medicine and the human body broadens. Books become larger, thicker and are continually updated. This book combines subject areas associated with biological human development for the undergraduate student new to these fields and for the postgraduate looking for a resource to refer to. Chapter authors and editors have selected topics and focused study upon areas chosen for their importance and likely occurrence. This has created a single resource to help inform the reader and prepare them for clinical work.

The book is organised around the human life cycle, beginning with fertilisation and embryological topics, continuing through obstetric medicine, then neonatal care and child health, and ultimately leading into further fertility and gynaecological medicine.

Each chapter begins with a hypothetical clinical case. Each case relates to important aspect(s) of the chapter, intending that the reader considers the problems posed while reading. Every chapter concludes with more information about the case derived from the results of investigations or treatments, and discusses what has occurred and how the person may be treated, and may also discuss likely effects on that person's future.

Topics within the chapter have been organised into chunks, limiting the size of each section and making searching for information easier and faster. Chapters include key information points that summarise the main ideas discussed, and each chapter has an online collection of single best answer (SBA or multiple choice) and extended matching questions (EMQs) to test the reader's understanding. Some of the questions may extend outside the written chapter.

In this way we have aimed to produce a helpful, informative and more concise resource for a wide range of associated topics. This blending of subjects and disciplines matches many modern medical curricula.

Samuel Webster
Geraint Morris
Euan Kevelighan

How to use your textbook

Features contained within your textbook

Every chapter begins with the **learning outcomes** to the topic.

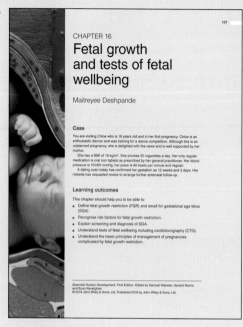

117

CHAPTER 16

Fetal growth and tests of fetal wellbeing

Maitreyee Deshpande

Case

You are visiting Chloe who is 18 years old and in her first pregnancy. Chloe is an enthusiastic dancer and was training for a dance competition. Although this is an unplanned pregnancy, she is delighted with the news and is well supported by her mother.

She has a BMI of 19 kg/m². She smokes 20 cigarettes a day. Her only regular medication is oral iron tablets as prescribed by her general practitioner. Her blood pressure is 100/60 mmHg, her pulse is 86 beats per minute and regular. A dating scan today has confirmed her gestation as 12 weeks and 3 days. Her midwife has requested review to arrange further antenatal follow-up.

Learning outcomes

This chapter should help you to be able to:

- Define fetal growth restriction (FGR) and small for gestational age fetus (SGA).
- Recognise risk factors for fetal growth restriction.
- Explain screening and diagnosis of SGA.
- Understand tests of fetal wellbeing including cardiotocography (CTG).
- Understand the basic principles of management of pregnancies complicated by fetal growth restriction.

Essential Human Development, First Edition. Edited by Samuel Webster, Geraint Morris and Euan Kevelighan.
© 2018 John Wiley & Sons, Ltd. Published 2018 by John Wiley & Sons, Ltd.

▼ **Case studies** give further insight into real-life patient scenarios.

Case

A 36-year-old man, Mr Bandar, presents to you with his 35-year-old wife in your primary care clinic and they describe their difficulty in trying to conceive. They have been engaging in approximately weekly, unprotected intercourse for 2 years without successful conception. Mr Bandar has no history of hernia, orchitis, erectile dysfunction, undescended testes, diabetes, smoking, or recreational drug use. He estimates that he drinks around 5–6 units of alcohol per week and jogs regularly twice a week. His body mass index (BMI) is within the normal range. He suffered testicular torsion of his left testicle at the age of 19, probably as a result of an incident during rugby training. He had mumps as a young child for a short period and recovered well.

Clinical case

Investigations

After taking a full medical history from Mr and Mrs Bandar, you ask Mr Bandar to provide a semen sample for analysis. When discussing the couple's sexual history it becomes clear that Mr Bandar does not have any impotence issues, but he has developed some stress while trying to conceive.

Mr Bandar's semen sample has a volume of 2.3 mL with a concentration of 15 million spermatozoa per mL. The spermatozoa have grade c motility with 30% observed motility. Ten percent have abnormal morphology. Semen pH is measured as pH 7.4.

Mr Bandar has asthenozoospermia (reduced sperm motility). All other factors are normal.

Case conclusion

A repeat semen sample is requested from Mr Bandar and tested. The results are similar to the first sample. He is educated about factors that affect normal sperm development, and Mr and Mrs Bandar attend counselling to reduce their stress related to trying to conceive. One year later they have still failed to conceive and begin considering in vitro fertilisation methods of conception.

SUMMARY

Key learning points

- Antenatal care is a framework that aims to identify variations from the normal course of pregnancy to allow early intervention. Establishing a rapport with the woman and her family means that she is then empowered to participate in achieving the best pregnancy outcome.
- The team involved in care may be community-based by midwives and the general practitioner or have additional consultant-led aspects. In the case of pre-existing or emerging medical, surgical or psychiatric problems, urgent referral to and shared care with other secondary care specialties is the norm.
- The basic clinical skills of communication, history and examination are fundamental in identifying risk factors so that investigation and management can be timely.

Systematic review at points throughout the pregnancy will lead to earlier intervention where this is required, and is the basis of a risk-reduction model of preventative healthcare. In women with health problems a clear plan should be jointly arrived at by community and hospital based teams together with the woman and her family.

Although based on the generic principles of physical examination, it takes time and experience to gain facility with the obstetric examination. Abdominal palpation is a practical clinical skill that involves creativity in visualising the fetus. Time with the mother taking a careful history and learning gentle but informative examination skills will be well spent.

◀ **Key learning points** give a summary of the topics covered in a chapter.

Your textbook is full of **illustrations and tables**.

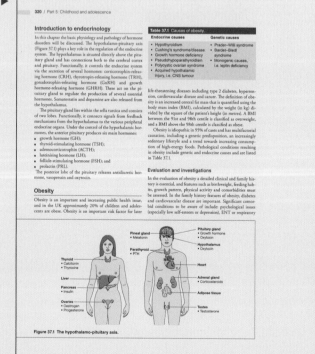

320 / Part 5: Childhood and adolescence

Introduction to endocrinology

In this chapter the basic physiology and pathology of hormone disorders will be discussed. The hypothalamo-pituitary axis (Figure 37.1) plays a key role in the regulation of the endocrine system. The hypothalamus is situated directly above the pituitary gland and has connections both to the cerebral cortex and pituitary. Functionally, it controls the endocrine system via the secretion of several hormones: corticotrophin-releasing hormone (CRH), thyrotropin-releasing hormone (TRH), gonadotrophin-releasing hormone (GnRH) and growth hormone-releasing hormone (GHRH). These act on the pituitary gland to regulate the production of several essential hormones. Somatostatin and dopamine are also released from the hypothalamus.

The pituitary gland lies within the sella turcica and consists of two lobes. Functionally, it connects signals from feedback mechanisms from the hypothalamus to the various peripheral endocrine organs. Under the control of the hypothalamic hormones, the anterior pituitary produces six main hormones:

- growth hormone (GH);
- thyroid-stimulating hormone (TSH);
- adrenocorticotrophin (ACTH);
- luteinising hormone (LH);
- follicle-stimulating hormone (FSH); and
- prolactin (PRL).

The posterior lobe of the pituitary releases antidiuretic hormone, vasopressin and oxytocin.

Obesity

Obesity is an important and increasing public health issue, and in the UK approximately 20% of children and adolescents are obese. Obesity is an important risk factor for later life-threatening diseases including type 2 diabetes, hypertension, cardiovascular disease and cancer. The definition of obesity is an increased central fat mass that is quantified using the body mass index (BMI), calculated by the weight (in kg) divided by the square of the patient's height (in metres). A BMI between the 91st and 98th centile is classified as overweight, and a BMI above the 98th centile is classified as obese.

Obesity is idiopathic in 95% of cases and has multifactorial causation, including a genetic predisposition, an increasingly sedentary lifestyle and a trend towards increasing consumption of high-energy foods. Pathological conditions resulting in obesity include genetic and endocrine causes and are listed in Table 37.1.

Evaluation and investigations

In the evaluation of obesity a detailed clinical and family history is essential, and features such as birthweight, feeding habits, growth pattern, physical activity and comorbidities must be assessed. In the family history features of obesity, diabetes and cardiovascular disease are important. Significant comorbid conditions to be aware of include: psychological issues (especially low self-esteem or depression), ENT or respiratory

Table 37.1 Causes of obesity.

Endocrine causes	Genetic causes
• Hypothyroidism	• Prader–Willi syndrome
• Cushing's syndrome/disease	• Bardet–Biedl
• Growth hormone deficiency	syndrome
• Pseudohypoparathyroidism	• Monogenic causes,
• Polycystic ovarian syndrome	i.e. leptin deficiency
• Acquired hypothalamic	
injury, i.e. CNS tumour	

pathology (such as obstructive sleep apnoea), orthopaedic problems (slipped femoral epiphysis or osteoarthritis) and metabolic issues (principally impaired glucose tolerance or type 2 diabetes, hypertension and polycystic ovarian syndrome).

The investigation of obesity may include an oral glucose tolerance test (OGTT), a thyroid function test, a liver function test, determination of cortisol levels and a fasting lipid profile.

The management of obesity is difficult, but is best done through a multidisciplinary approach based on making significant changes to the patient's nutritional intake and lifestyle. Behaviour modifications and family therapy have also shown positive effects whilst medication and bariatric surgery are rarely required.

Diabetes mellitus

The incidence of diabetes has increased steadily and has a prevalence of around two cases per 1000 children. Diabetes in children is almost exclusively insulin-dependent (type 1) diabetes although the rate of non-insulin-dependent (type 2) is increasing due to the increasing rates of childhood obesity.

- Insulin-dependent (type 1) diabetes: This is an autoimmune disorder characterised by T-cell-mediated destruction and progressive loss of pancreatic B cells resulting in insulin deficiency.
- Non-insulin-dependent (type 2) diabetes: This is a multifactorial condition in which the balance between insulin secretion and insulin sensitivity is impaired, with a relative insulin insufficiency unable to overcome an underlying high tissue insulin resistance (Figure 37.2).

Insulin-dependent (type 1) diabetes

Aetiology

Type 1 diabetes is thought to be caused by the interaction of genetic predisposition and environmental precipitants. The co-twins of children with type 1 diabetes and children whose parents have type 1 diabetes all have an increased risk of the disease. Studies have shown an association between human leucocyte antigen (HLA) classes DR3 or DR4 and an increased risk of developing type 1 diabetes.

Pathophysiology

Insulin-dependent diabetes is a chronic autoimmune condition characterised by the development of autoantibodies against specific pancreatic B cell antigens. This causes T-cell activation, inflammation and pancreatic B cell destruction resulting in the characteristic insulin deficiency.

Clinical features

Diabetes is uncommon before the age of 1 year and reaches a peak incidence between 12 and 13 years, more commonly occurring at the onset of puberty. The clinical features include

Chapter 37: Metabolic and endocrine disorders / 321

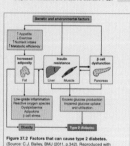

Figure 37.2 Factors that can cause type 2 diabetes. (Source: C.J. Bailey, BMJ (2011, p.342). Reproduced with permission of BMJ Publishing Ltd.)

polyuria, polydipsia and weight loss. Less common presenting features include skin infection, typically with *Candida*, and other persistent infections.

Uncommonly, children can present with the life-threatening complication of diabetic ketoacidosis (DKA). The symptoms of DKA include vomiting, dehydration, abdominal pain, a characteristic smell of ketones on the breath and hyperventilation due to acidosis. If untreated, continued deterioration leads to hypovolaemic shock, drowsiness and coma, which can be fatal.

Diagnosis of diabetes

A typical history and single blood glucose level measurement above 11.1 mmol/L will establish a diagnosis without the need of additional investigations such as an oral glucose tolerance test in childhood.

A blood glucose level greater than 11.1 mmol/L taken 2 hours after an oral glucose tolerance test, glycosuria and ketonuria, or a fasting blood glucose of greater than 7.0 mmol/L are also diagnostic indicators. Raised glycosylated haemoglobin (Hb A1C) levels can also be a helpful marker of persistently raised glucose levels.

Initial management

Most children who present as a new case of diabetes will be clinically stable, are able to eat and drink, and can be managed

Figure 37.1 The hypothalamo-pituitary axis.

 The website icon indicates that you can find accompanying self-assessment resources on the book's companion website.

About the companion website

Don't forget to visit the companion website for this book:

www.wileyessential.com/humandevelopment

There you will find valuable material designed to enhance your learning, including:

- Multiple choice questions (MCQs)
- Extended matching questions (EMQs)

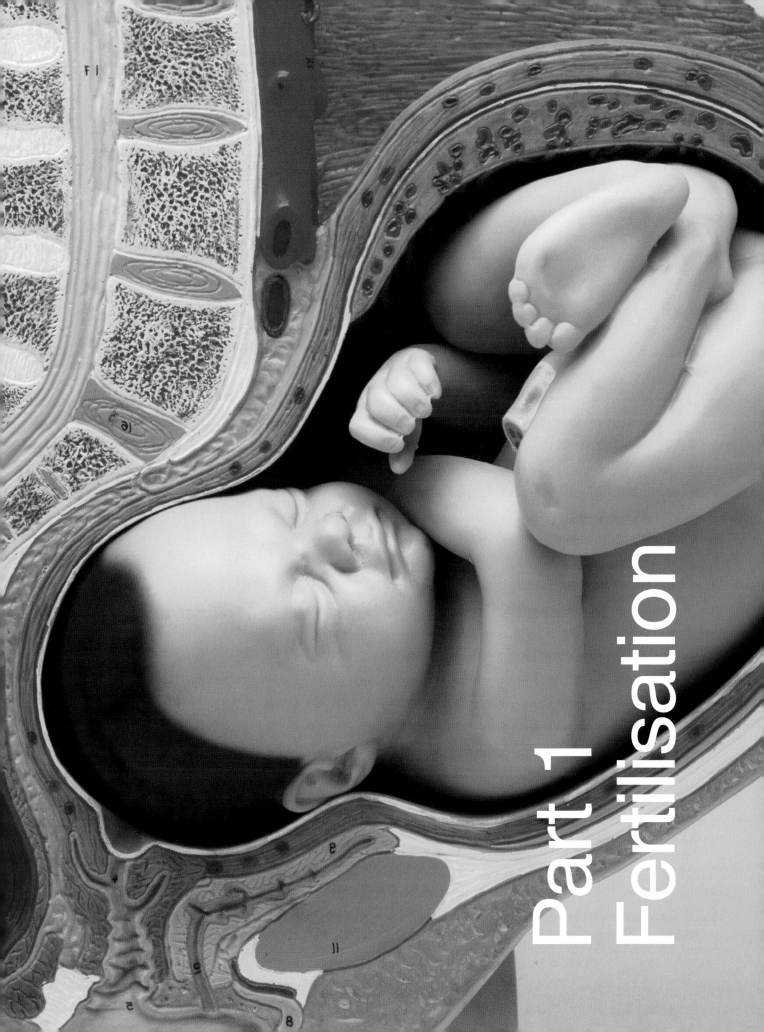

Part 1
Fertilisation

CHAPTER 1
Principles of development

Sam Webster

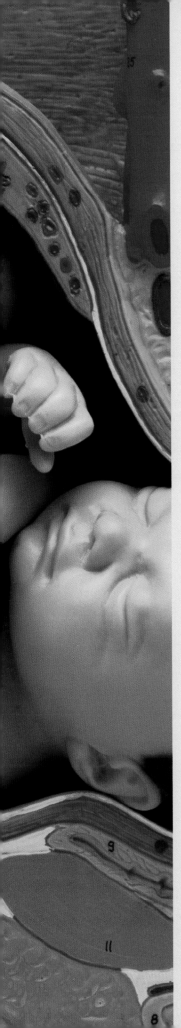

Case

Jamie is a 4-month-old boy presenting with disparity between limb length, trunk length and cranial circumference. His height is under the fourth percentile, his weight is under the fourth percentile and his head circumference is above the 97th percentile. Motor development milestones are delayed. Jamie's mother and father have typical heights (168 cm and 176 cm respectively).

Learning outcomes

- You should be able to recognise the stages of cell division in mitosis and meiosis.
- You should be able to describe the basic principles of growth and differentiation.

Essential Human Development, First Edition. Edited by Samuel Webster, Geraint Morris and Euan Kevelighan.
© 2018 John Wiley & Sons, Ltd. Published 2018 by John Wiley & Sons, Ltd.

Chromosomes

As a basis of biology cell theory is a crucial part of understanding development. Complex organisms grow from a single cell. The cell is the fundamental unit of structure in the organism, and new cells are formed from existing cells. All structure, function and organisation relates to the unit of the cell. In development we consider how the cells of the gametes merge to form a cell with a new genetic composition, the division of that cell to form new cells, and how those cells become organised, form shapes and tissues of multiple differentiated cell types.

DNA is stored in chromatin form within the nuclei of cells, and RNA is present in the cytoplasm. When cells divide the chromosomes are duplicated and the daughter cells gain exact copies of the DNA of the parent cell (hopefully, if the replication and error checking mechanisms work correctly).

Somatic cells contain 23 pairs of chromosomes including 22 pairs of autosomes and one pair of sex chromosomes (Figure 1.1). Each chromosome is an organised package of DNA.

In a homologous pair of chromosomes the same genes are encoded on each chromosome but the genes may occur as slightly different versions. One chromosome has been inherited from the father, and the other from the mother. For example, the gene for head hair pigment colour will occur on both chromosomes of a homologous pair, but one copy may encode for blonde hair and the other for brown. These copies are alleles, and the dominant pigment allele will be represented in the phenotype of the individual. This is a simplified example, and many hair pigments are at play in determining a person's final hair colour, accounting for the wide variation of natural shades that occurs. The mixing up of alleles across

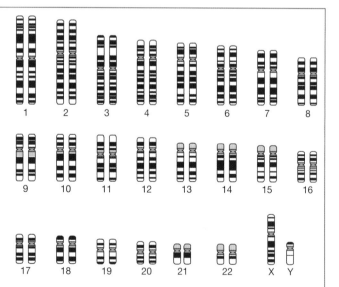

Figure 1.1 Human karyotype. (Source: S. Webster and R. de Wreede (2016) *Embryology at a Glance*, 2nd edn. Reproduced with permission of John Wiley & Sons, Ltd.)

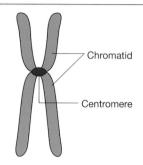

Figure 1.2 The structure of a chromosome. (Source: S. Webster and R. de Wreede (2016) *Embryology at a Glance*, 2nd edn. Reproduced with permission of John Wiley & Sons, Ltd.)

homologous chromosomes during cell division is an important part of the genetic diversity advantage given by sexual reproduction over asexual reproduction.

If a cell has two copies of each kind of chromosome (e.g. one copy from the mother and one copy from the mother) it is said to be diploid. If it only had one copy it would be haploid.

We can also describe a cell by the number of copies (n) of each unique double-stranded length of chromosomal DNA. Chromosomal DNA inherited from the mother is different to chromosomal DNA inherited from the father. In a pair of chromosomes the genes are the same but the alleles are different. A haploid cell has only one copy of each kind of chromosome so it is described as $1n$. Somatic cells are normally diploid, and during part of the cell cycle only have one DNA strand for each kind of chromosome so are described as $2n$. They have two copies of each kind of chromosome (one from the mother and one from the father). When a cell copies its DNA in preparation for cell division it will have four copies of each kind of chromosome and be described as $4n$.

If the DNA strand of a chromosome is duplicated its two duplicates are joined together at the centromere forming the familiar X shape of most chromosomes (Figure 1.2). Each of the two duplicates is a sister chromatid.

Mitosis

Mitosis is the process by which cells divide and increase in number in eukaryotic organisms. The result of mitosis is two daughter cells that contain the same genetic information. Mitosis is the method by which cells repair tissues, it is one way in which growth can occur, and it is how cells lost through normal processes are replaced. Some cells are very good at proliferating by mitosis, such as epidermal keratinocytes, which are lost daily as flakes of skin, and some cells are very poor at mitotic division, such as neurones of the central nervous system, which are expected to survive for the lifetime of the organism (although it is not yet clearly understood how long neurones live, but they are not naturally replaced after brain

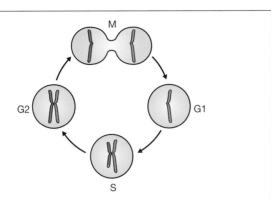

Figure 1.3 The cell cycle. (Source: S. Webster and R. de Wreede (2016) *Embryology at a Glance*, 2nd edn. Reproduced with permission of John Wiley & Sons, Ltd.)

do not divide are considered to have left the cell cycle. The stages of the cell cycle are gap 1 (G1), synthesis (S), gap 2 (G2) and mitosis (M). The stages of G1, S and G2 are also known collectively as interphase. A cell's DNA is duplicated during S phase, adding a sister chromatid to the existing chromatid. A cell that no longer divides can be described as existing within a G0 phase.

When a cell begins mitosis its chromosomes become condensed and form their recognisable X shapes during the first phase of mitosis, called prophase (Figure 1.4). At this stage it is diploid (4*n*). Centrioles are cylindrical structures that have a number of functions within eukaryotic cells, and during mitosis they arrange and separate DNA. During prophase the centrioles move to opposite ends of the cell.

In the next stage, prometaphase, the nuclear membrane breaks down and disappears releasing the DNA into the cytoplasm. Microtubules link the centromeres of the chromosomes to the centrioles, and during metaphase the chromosomes begin to move, pulled by the microtubules to line up along the middle of the cell.

The centromeres are cut in the telophase step, splitting each chromosome into its separate, genetically identical chromatids.

damage). Mitosis is a major mechanism of growth in the embryo and fetus.

Cell division is a step within the cell cycle (Figure 1.3). The cell cycle describes a series of carefully controlled events in the life of cell that take part in cell division, and cells that

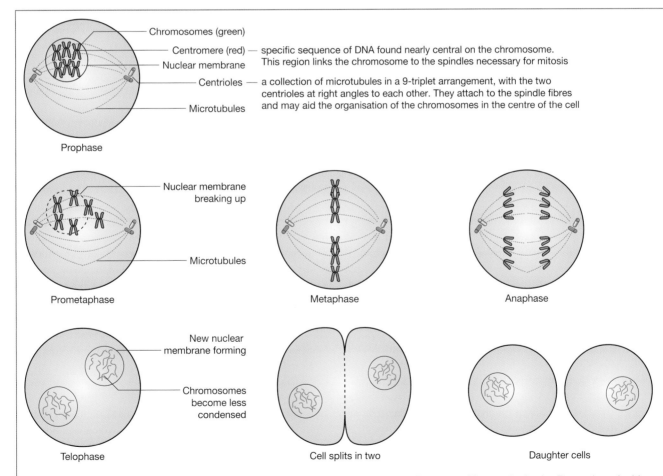

Figure 1.4 Mitosis. (Source: S. Webster and R. de Wreede (2016) *Embryology at a Glance*, 2nd edn. Reproduced with permission of John Wiley & Sons, Ltd.)

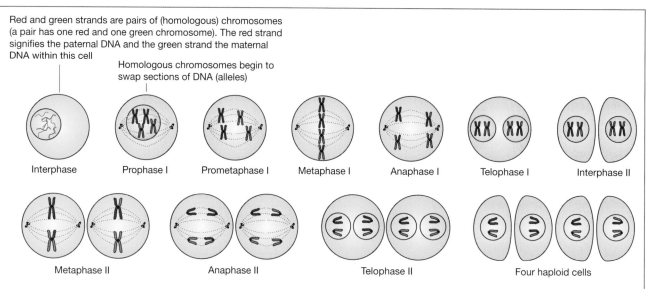

Red and green strands are pairs of (homologous) chromosomes (a pair has one red and one green chromosome). The red strand signifies the paternal DNA and the green strand the maternal DNA within this cell

Homologous chromosomes begin to swap sections of DNA (alleles)

Interphase Prophase I Prometaphase I Metaphase I Anaphase I Telophase I Interphase II

Metaphase II Anaphase II Telophase II Four haploid cells

Figure 1.5 Meiosis. (Source: S. Webster and R. de Wreede (2016) *Embryology at a Glance*, 2nd edn. Reproduced with permission of John Wiley & Sons, Ltd.)

One of each pair of chromatids is pulled to opposite ends of the cell by microtubules and the centrioles.

In telophase the chromatids reach the ends of the cell, begin to lengthen again and are no longer visible under a light microscope. Two new nuclear membranes begin to form around the chromatid DNA to create two nuclei. Cytokinesis follows during which a ring of actin filaments appears around the midline of the cell and shrinks, splitting the cell into two. Mitosis is complete, and the two cells return to the G1 phase. During the G1 phase each cell has a full, diploid complement of DNA but only one copy of each chromosome (2n).

Meiosis

Meiosis is a specialised method of cell division in eukaryotes that produces gamete cells. The primary function of meiosis is to produce cells with a haploid (n) complement of chromosomes. Somatic cells have two homologous copies of each chromosome (diploid) and gametes have one copy of each chromosome (haploid, n). When the male and female gametes combine during fertilisation the resulting cell has a restored, diploid complement of 23 pairs of chromosomes.

Meiosis is similar to mitosis, but differs in a couple of ways. Cell division occurs twice during a full cycle of meiosis, producing four daughter cells from one cell. Alleles of homologous chromosomes are randomly exchanged between those chromosomes during a process known as homologous recombination. Cells produced as a result of meiosis will have all of the genes of the parent cells (hopefully in the same locations within chromosomes as the parent cells if the process occurs accurately) but with a random allocation of the alleles of those genes. This genetic variability is an important advantage of

sexual reproduction over asexual reproduction. If, for example, the original diploid cell contained the allele for a blue iris on one chromosome and the allele for a green iris on the homologous chromosome, any cell formed as a result of meiosis could contain either allele. Alleles of the genes on the same chromosome may or may not be carried across with the allele for iris colour, as homologous recombination maintains the order of genes but alleles may be swapped around.

During S phase the cell's DNA is duplicated. The two parts of meiosis are described as meiosis I and meiosis II. Prophase I begins with homologous recombination of DNA across homologous chromosomes before the chromosomes shorten, thicken and become condensed (Figure 1.5). The centrioles move to either end of the cell and microtubules are extended, beginning to form the mitotic spindle. The cell at this stage has a diploid (4n) complement of DNA. Metaphase I follows, with the chromosomes aligning themselves along the midline of the cell. During anaphase I pairs of homologous chromosomes split up, with one chromosome of each pair pulled to either end of the cell by the mitotic spindle. Each chromosome at this stage is made up of a pair of identical sister chromatids joined together at the centromere. With telophase I , two new nuclear membranes form around the chromosomes that have collected at either end of the cell, forming two nuclei. An actin ring appears around the middle of the cell and constricts, splitting the cell into two daughter cells by cytokinesis. The cells resulting from meiosis I are haploid (2n). They have 23 chromosomes and each chromosome has two chromatids. The chromosomes are not paired at this stage.

In the second part of meiosis the cell goes through division again, beginning with prophase II. The cell's DNA is not duplicated between meiosis I and meiosis II, so it enters

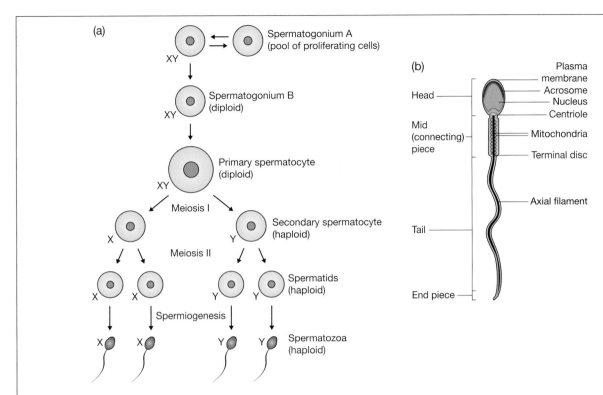

Figure 1.6 Spermatogenesis. (Source: S. Webster and R. de Wreede (2016) *Embryology at a Glance*, 2nd edn. Reproduced with permission of John Wiley & Sons, Ltd.)

the second part with the haploid (2*n*) complement of chromosomes. Again the chromosomes are in a condensed, thickened configuration and the centrioles move to either end of the cell. In prometaphase II the nuclear membranes break down and microtubules link the chromosomes to the centrioles. The chromosomes become aligned along the middle of the cell during metaphase II, and then the chromosomes are split during anaphase II. The chromosomes are divided into their two sister chromatids, which are each pulled towards opposite ends of the cell. In telophase II the chromatids reach the ends of the cell and nuclear membranes begin to form around them, forming two nuclei. Cytokinesis forms an actin ring around the middle of the cell that contracts and splits the cell into two.

At the end of meiosis four cells have been produced from one, and each cell has 23 unpaired chromosomes. Each cell is haploid (*n*).

Spermatogenesis

Spermatogenesis describes the development of haploid spermatozoa from germ cells in the testes. The germ cells of the seminiferous tubules are diploid spermatogonia (typically 2*n* before they duplicate their DNA to 4*n* for cell division) with a full complement of chromosomes, including X and Y

sex chromosomes. Spermatogonia maintain their numbers throughout life by mitotic division.

Spermatogenesis comprises two stages: spermatocytogenesis and spermiogenesis. A type A spermatogonium cell from the pool of proliferating cells will enter the process of maturation, becoming a type B spermatogonium B cell (Figure 1.6). Groups of type B spermatogonia cells begin spermatocytogenesis in synchrony, eventually producing large numbers of mature spermatozoa. Type B spermatogonia cells are linked to one another at this stage by cytoplasmic bridges and divide mitotically, increasing their numbers and becoming primary spermatocytes.

Primary spermatocytes enter the first round of meiotic division (meiosis I). One diploid (4*n*) primary spermatocyte becomes two haploid (2*n*) secondary spermatocytes, and a secondary spermatocyte may contain either an X or a Y sex chromosome as part of their complement of 23 chromosomes. During this first round of meiosis homologous recombination of chromosomes occurs.

Secondary spermatocytes divide again through the stages of meiosis II. The resulting cells are spermatids (haploid, *n*) and four spermatids are derived from one primary spermatocyte. There are 23 unpaired chromosomes within each cell at the end of meiosis II. The spermatid stage marks the end of spermatocytogenesis.

The spermatid changes shape, lengthening and forming a rounded head and an elongated tail during the process of spermiogenesis. The tail is packed with mitochondria, the cell loses cytoplasm, and the head contains the nucleus. An acrosome layer of specialised enzymes that will enable penetration of an ovum forms around the head of the cell. With these changes the spermatid becomes a spermatozoon.

These processes of spermatogenesis take around 64 days to produce spermatozoa from spermatogonia A cells, and the spermatozoa remain inactive as they are passed to the epididymis. They continue to mature over a seven-day period within the epididymis, at which point they become motile and ready for fertilisation.

Oogenesis

Oogenesis describes the development of haploid oocytes, within follicles, from germ cells in the ovaries. Female germ cells are diploid and contain a pair of X sex chromosomes. They divide mitotically to produce a large number of oogonia, which will enter meiosis (Figure 1.7).

Oogonia begin meiosis I during the 12th week of fetal development. The cell at this stage is known as the primary oocyte, and becomes surrounded by a thin layer of squamous epithelial cells to form a primordial follicle. The primary oocyte only passes through meiosis as far as prophase I with homologous recombination and condensation of the chromosomes (diploid, $4n$). The primary oocyte is held, paused in this state. It will only continue its development if it is released from the ovary by ovulation.

Millions of primordial follicles are formed during the first trimester but many degenerate leaving around 400 000 follicles at birth. When puberty begins some of the paused primary oocytes continue their development. Each month a few primordial follicles change. The primary oocyte within becomes larger and the follicular cells become cuboidal. The follicular layer thickens to form a primary follicle. The follicle becomes a secondary follicle when more than one layer of follicle cells has developed. The granulosa cells of the follicle and the oocyte create a layer of glycoproteins on the surface of the oocyte. This layer is the zona pellucida and has important functions during fertilisation (see also Chapter 4).

Although during any particular monthly cycle a number of follicles begin to develop further only one continues leaving the others to degenerate. It is not clear how one follicle is chosen over the others. In the follicle that survives the number of layers of follicular cells continues to increase, and the follicle becomes an antral follicle when it has more than five layers of cells. An antrum appears as a space between the layers of granulosa cells, and this structure becomes the cumulus oophorus.

The follicle is embedded within an ovary, and has been growing and becoming a more prominent structure. The cells of the ovary around the follicle now respond to the follicle's development by differentiating to build two layers of theca interna and theca externa. The follicle is considered to be a mature vesicular follicle (or Graafian follicle). In response to luteinising hormone (LH), thecal cells produce androgens, which are converted into oestrogen. Oestrogens cause repair and thickening of the endometrial lining of the uterus between days 5 and 14 of the menstrual cycle, preparing the endometrium to receive a blastocyst (see Chapter 4).

Only now, in response to spikes in LH and follicle-stimulating hormone (FSH), does the oocyte resume meiosis I and continue in its stalled processes of cell division. At the end of meiosis I the cell divides into a large secondary oocyte (haploid, $2n$) and a small polar body (haploid, $2n$). The oocyte retains most of its mass and cellular components and the polar body acts as a vessel for the removed chromosomal material. The oocyte is now a haploid cell and the polar body degenerates.

The secondary oocyte enters meiosis II but stalls again, during metaphase II. It will only continue to divide if it is fertilised by a spermatozoon. If this occurs the cell becomes the definitive oocyte (haploid, n, if considered on its own and ignoring the spermatozoon) and produces a second polar body (haploid, n)

If you do the maths and assume that ovulation begins with puberty at around age 11, and ends with menopause at around age 55, at 12 ovulations per year for 44 years only 528 primary oocytes (in this scenario) will continue their development. In truth, only if an oocyte is fertilised by a spermatozoon will it complete meiosis (see Chapter 4), so of the millions of oogonia originally produced only a few are likely to survive.

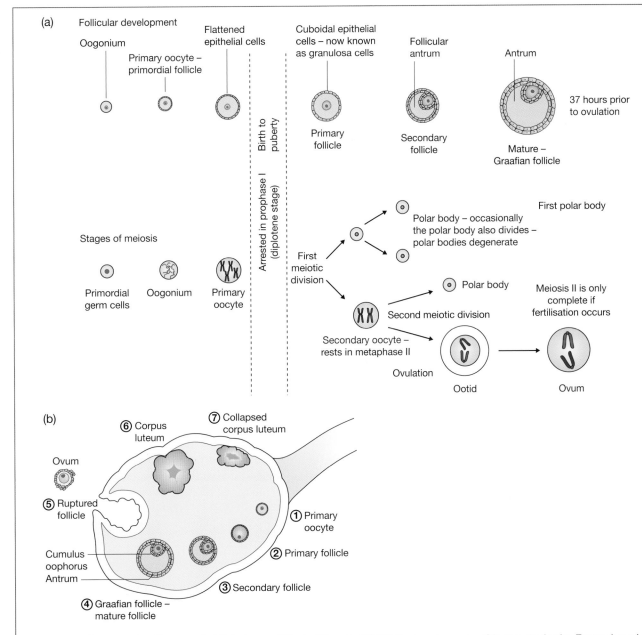

Figure 1.7 Oogenesis. (Source: S. Webster and R. de Wreede (2016) *Embryology at a Glance*, 2nd edn. Reproduced with permission of John Wiley & Sons, Ltd.)

Growth

Biological growth may be defined as an increase in the mass or size of a tissue or organism, and is a key process of development. Growth can occur through three mechanisms: an increase in cell number, an increase in cell size, or an increase in extracellular material.

Cellular proliferation, that is, an increase in cell number through mitotic cell division, is the most common method of achieving growth. The cells of many adult tissues are also able to proliferate, often as part of a repair mechanism in response to injury. Some adult tissues are very good at cellular proliferation, and some are very poor. Stem cells are an important source of cell renewal in tissues that lose cells constantly, such as the epidermis of the skin and the epithelium of the gut.

Cellular hypertrophy describes an increase in cell size, and is a normal part of the endochondral ossification process, for example, in which chondrocytes lay down a cartilaginous precursor that is modified by hypertrophic chondrocytes and replaced by bone. In adult tissues skeletal muscle responds to the repeated loading of weight training with hypertrophy.

Cells of connective tissues secrete and surround themselves with the extracellular matrix that forms much of the tissue. Chondrocytes and osteocytes increase the amount of matrix in response to loading, increasing the size of the tissue by accretion.

Differentiation

Embryological multipotent cells have the potential to form the wide range of cells needed to build the structures and tissues of the embryo. The process of an embryonic stem cell becoming a specialised, determined, mature cell type is differentiation. The differentiated cell type is stable, meaning that cells formed as a result of mitotic division are typically of the same cell type. Differentiated cells do not normally change cell type, but it is possible to take some mature cells and direct them to dedifferentiate and return to a stem-cell-like state in the laboratory. Adult stem cells also exist and are partly differentiated and able to produce a limited number of cell types, often relevant to the tissue in which they reside.

Signalling

A signal produced by a cell or group of cells is able to influence another cell or group of cells that have receptors for that signal. This is an important concept in embryological development, and much of contemporary research investigates what signals are involved and how they affect cells during development.

Hormones are an example of a signal in adult physiology, and often act in a system-wide manner by passing through the circulatory system from a local source to cells elsewhere in the body. In the embryo the signals may remain attached to the secretory cell or be released to diffuse through the tissue. The distances involved are very small.

Cells respond to the signals in different ways, by differentiating, migrating, proliferating, changing shape, or entering apoptosis, for example.

Organisation

The first shape that the embryo forms after the embryoblast ball of cells is a flat sheet. The sheet appears to be a uniform, oval plate of cells, and to the eye it would be difficult to guess which end will be the head or the tail, and which side is left and right, yet the cells by this point are organised and will respond to one another to form the structures, cell types, and tissues appropriate to the region they are within and the phase of development.

Cells are aware of their location within the embryo. One way in which this can occur is by the diffusion of signalling molecules synthesised by one group of cells across the tissue, and a variable response to the concentration of that signal by cells with appropriate receptors. The cells may respond differently depending upon whether the concentration of the molecule is high, low or somewhere in between.

Morphogens acting as signals in this way are a fundamental part of development. If this signalling is interfered with it can have profound effects and may prevent the embryo from continuing to develop or cause a congenital abnormality.

Morphogenesis

The formation of shape during development is morphogenesis. Cells are able to change their shape, extend processes to pull themselves along and migrate, and a tissue may grow in size. These are all processes that occur during development to cause cells to form shapes and structures. The flat sheets of the germ layers roll up in the very early stages of development, forming tubes and spaces, for example.

Summary

Clinical case

Investigations and treatments

Jamie is displaying characteristic features of achondroplasia. He has disproportionate short stature, macrocephaly (large cranium), megaloencephaly (large brain), frontal bossing (a prominent forehead), a low nasal bridge, and some facial features are underdeveloped. Jamie has a long trunk and shortened limbs. He has limited elbow extension and forearm supination.

The diagnosis can be further confirmed by radiology and genetic analysis. Radiological investigations will give further insight into specific aspects of Jamie's condition. Jamie will have hypermobile joints and display genu varum (bowed legs). His hearing should be assessed regularly as children with achondroplasia are more likely to develop middle ear infections. Children with achondroplasia are also more likely to have obstructive sleep apnoea.

Case conclusions

There is no cure for achondroplasia, and Jamie may develop a number of issues as he grows. It is typically caused by a mutation in the *FGFR3* gene that encodes a fibroblast growth factor receptor important in bone and brain growth and development. The mutation is inherited in an autosomal dominant pattern, and only one copy of the defective gene will cause achondroplasia. If two copies of the gene are inherited the developmental defects are likely to be severe enough to cause death, as the thoracic cage is too poorly developed for effective respiration.

In most cases of achondroplasia both parents are of normal height and are not carriers of a defective *FGFR3* gene. The cause of achondroplasia in these cases is a spontaneous mutation of the gene.

It is likely that Jamie will develop normal intelligence although developmental milestones will be delayed.

Milestones and growth charts for children with achondroplasia can be used to track Jamie's development and growth. He should have a normal lifespan and live independently when he becomes an adult. He may develop spinal and joint problems, or respiratory and cardiovascular difficulties during his development or later in life.

Key learning points

- An understanding of spermatogenesis and oogenesis helps explain many causes of subfertility.
- Men are able to produce new gametes throughout life, but a woman's ova are all produced before birth and are suspended partway through meiosis until each is selected during an ovulatory cycle. The decision to have children later in life has effects on fertility and on the risk of occurrence of some congenital genetic conditions.
- The processes of growth are relevant to embryonic development, fetal growth, childhood development and adolescence. In adults processes of repair are similar.

 Now visit **www.wileyessential.com/humandevelopment** to test yourself on this chapter.

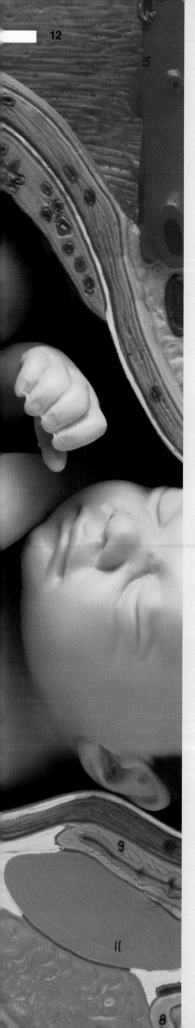

CHAPTER 2
The female reproductive system

Sam Webster

Case

A 39-year-old woman and her 36-year-old husband present to you in your primary care clinic describing their inability to conceive despite regular, unprotected intercourse for 2 years. You find out that Mrs Amble has a regular 28-day menstrual cycle, that she has never been pregnant, they both have a good understanding of the timings of ovulation and the fertility period, neither smoke nor take recreational drugs, and both drink alcohol occasionally in moderation. Mrs Amble is of normal weight for height and her blood pressure is within the normal range. Mr Amble has never had abdominal or pelvic surgery. She had her appendix removed when she was 15 years old. Neither have a history of urinary tract infections or any sexually transmitted disease, nor diabetes mellitus or thyroid problems. The husband had mumps as a child, and has worked as an electrical engineer for 15 years. Mrs Amble works as a school teacher.

Learning outcomes

- You should be able to recognise the anatomical structures of the female reproductive system and pelvis.
- You should be able to describe the physiology of the menstrual cycle.

Essential Human Development, First Edition. Edited by Samuel Webster, Geraint Morris and Euan Kevelighan
© 2018 John Wiley & Sons, Ltd. Published 2018 by John Wiley & Sons, Ltd.

Anatomy

Bones of the pelvis

The pelvis forms initially as three separate bones on either side, joined by cartilage. The three bones are the ilium, the ischium and the pubis (Figure 2.1). Endochondral ossification converts the cartilage into bone, and the bones are joined to become the continuous curved bowl of the pelvis with foramina and bony protuberances to which muscles attach. The acetabulum of the hip joint is formed by all three bones, and articulates with the head of the femur. The hip bones of either side are joined anteriorly by the midline pubic symphysis and posteriorly to the bones of the sacrum (Figure 2.2).

The ilium forms the curved, anteriorly concave, fan-shaped superior part of the pelvis. The superior rim of the ilium is the iliac crest, terminating at the anterior superior iliac spine (ASIS) and the posterior superior iliac spine, both of which are palpable landmarks. The smooth, fan-shaped part of the ilium is the ala (or wing), and the narrower section inferior to this is the body. The anteromedial surface of the ilium here is the iliac fossa. The ilium articulates with the sacrum posteromedially

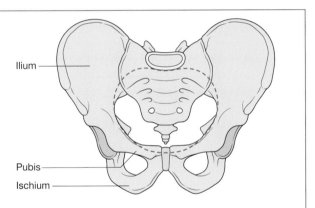

Figure 2.1. The neonatal bony pelvis.

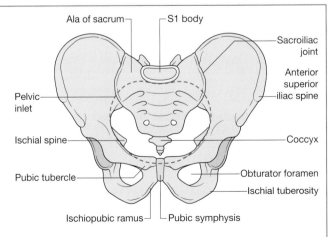

Figure 2.2. The adult bony pelvis.

at the sacroiliac joint – a weight-bearing joint with irregular, interlocking surfaces that is partly synovial and partly syndesmosis, supported by sacroiliac ligaments. The sacrum projects anteriorly at the level of the sacroiliac and lumbosacral joints as the sacral promontory.

The ischium sits posteriorly and inferiorly, and its body contributes to the acetabulum. It has a ramus that projects anteriorly to meet the inferior ramus of the pubis, which together with the the superior ramus of the pubis, the body of the pubis and the body of the ischium, forms the obturator foramen. The ischial tuberosity is a large, bony protuberance projecting posteriorly and inferiorly, providing an attachment site for the hamstring muscles. A smaller posteromedial protuberance from the body of the ischium is the ischial spine, an attachment point for ligaments of the pelvis. Superior to this, between the ischial spine and the sacroiliac joint, is the greater sciatic notch. Inferiorly, between the ischial spine and the ischial tuberosity, is the lesser sciatic notch.

The pubis is the anterior part of the bony pelvis, with a body anteriormost and two rami projecting posteriorly to the acetabulum (the superior pubic ramus) and the ischium (the inferior pubic ramus). The anterior part of the body of the pubis is thickened as the pubic crest.

Ligaments

A number of strong ligaments are involved in supporting the sacrum and the sacroiliac joints, particularly when high loads are applied to the vertebral column that would encourage the superior part of the sacrum to rotate anteriorly. The sacroiliac joints lie posterior to the loading axis of the vertebral column when landing heavily (e.g., after a parachute jump) or when lifting a heavy load in, or to, a standing position.

The sacrotuberous ligament runs from the inferior lateral sacrum and posterior ilium between the posterior superior and posterior inferior iliac spines to the ischial tuberosity (Figure 2.3). This anchor prevents the inferior sacrum from rotating posteriorly. Similarly, the sacrospinous ligament running between the inferior lateral sacrum and the ischial spine also acts as a support and an anchor to the sacroiliac joint. With the addition of this ligament the greater and lesser sciatic foramina are formed superiorly and inferiorly to the sacrospinous ligament, respectively. Sacroiliac ligaments play key roles in the transfer of weight from the axial skeleton to the lower appendicular skeleton, partly by locking together the irregular articulating surfaces of the sacroiliac joint, and partly by supporting the bony structures to transfer load under tension.

Pelvic inlet and outlet

The pelvic inlet describes the superior pelvic aperture, formed by the superior edge of the pubic symphysis, the superior ramus of the pubis, the arcuate line of the ilium, the anterior

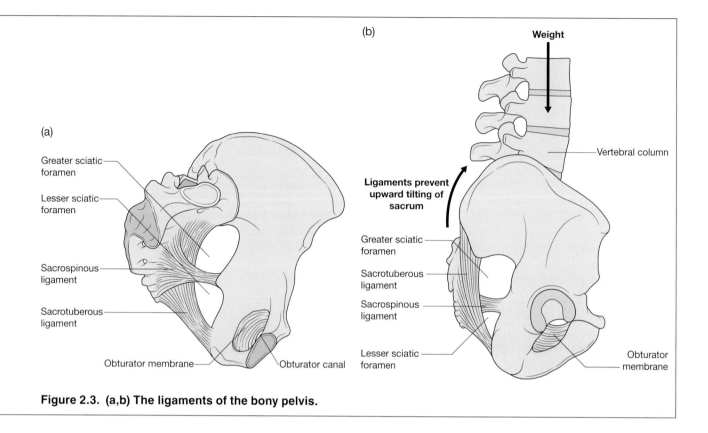

Figure 2.3. (a,b) The ligaments of the bony pelvis.

border of the ala, the posterior border of the pubic crest and the sacral promontory. The pelvic outlet describes the inferior pelvic aperture, and is bounded by the inferior edge of the pubic symphysis, the inferior ramus of the pubis, the ischial tuberosity, the sacrotuberous ligament and the inferior end of the coccyx.

The pelvic cavity is divided into the greater pelvis and lesser pelvis. The greater pelvis is superior to the pelvic inlet and bounded by the abdominal wall, the ala of the ilium, and the L5 and S1 vertebrae. The lesser pelvis is the space between the pelvic inlet and the pelvic outlet, with the bones of the sacrum and coccyx forming the posterior wall. The levator ani muscle group forming the pelvic diaphragm closes this space inferiorly.

The shape of the pelvis varies between and within sexes. For the female pelvis this can affect childbirth. The shapes of the pelvis are classified as android, gynecoid, anthropoid and platypelloid (Figure 2.4). The gynecoid is the most common female pelvis shape, and the pelvic inlet is a wide, well-rounded oval. Women with an android pelvis have a pelvic inlet that is narrower transversely and deeper anteroposteriorly, and may have more difficulty with a vaginal fetal delivery.

The obstetrical conjugate describes the distance between the pubic symphysis and the middle of the sacral promontory within the lesser pelvis, and is the narrowest fixed distance through which the fetal head passes during vaginal delivery. Non-fixed narrowings of the pelvis are able to widen with

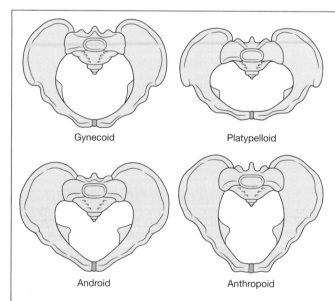

Figure 2.4 Android, gynecoid, anthropoid and platypelloid shapes of the pelvis.

relaxation of the pelvic ligaments in response to increased levels of sex hormones and the hormone relaxin.

The obstetrical conjugate should be at least 11 cm. It can be measured radiographically but not during vaginal examination because of the position of the urinary bladder. It can be

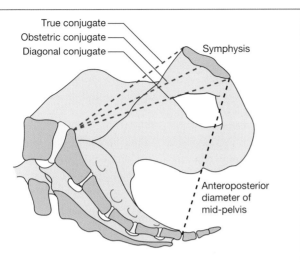

Figure 2.5. A "how to measure" illustration showing the obstetrical and diagonal conjugates.

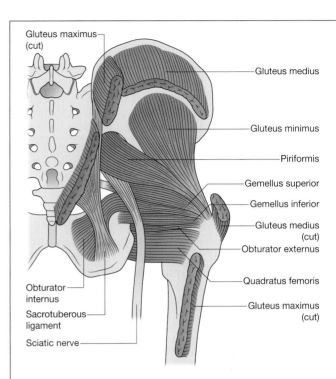

Figure 2.6. Muscles of the hip joint within the pelvis.

estimated from the diagonal conjugate, which is the distance between the inferior edge of the pubis and the lower sacrum at the level of the ischial spines, and is 1.5 to 2 cm shorter than the obstetric conjugate (Figure 2.5).

The pelvic floor

The walls of the pelvic cavity are formed by muscles of the hip joint (Figure 2.6). The obturator foramen is covered by the obturator membrane, which is covered by the obturator internus muscle that forms much of the lateral pelvic wall and passes

out through the lesser sciatic foramen to insert into the greater trochanter of the femur. The piriformis muscle runs from the superior part of the sacrum through the greater sciatic foramen to form the posterolateral wall, and also inserts into the greater trochanter.

 Clinical notes 2.1 Fractures

Pelvic fractures
High-impact insults to the pelvis, such as from high-speed motorcycle collisions or crush injuries, can fracture the ring of pelvic bones and cause traumatic injuries to the viscera within. Anteroposterior and lateral compression forces often fracture pubic rami, alae of the ilium, the acetabula and the sacroiliac joints or the sacrum. Multiple fractures are likely and ligament attachment sites may suffer avulsion fractures. A heavy landing on to one foot can force the head of the femur through the acetabulum. Pubic rami fractures can rupture the urinary bladder and urethra, and blood vessels and nerves in this region can be damaged.

Osteoporosis, femoral neck fracture
Older people with osteoporosis are at risk of low-energy pelvic fractures from simple falls or when loading the pelvis descending stairs. Female patients are particularly at risk, but most pelvic fractures in this group are classified

as stable injuries and treatment strategies focus on pain management and mobilisation. Transverse fractures of the pubic rami caused by weakened bone unable to withstand normal loading forces pose a risk to the urinary bladder, urethra and nearby blood vessels and nerves. Lateral compression fractures are more likely to cause haemorrhage in older patients than in younger patients.

Hamstring avulsion
The hamstring muscles biceps femoris, semitendinosus and semimembranosus run from the ischial tuberosity to attachment sites in the lower limb. Eccentric overload through muscle contraction with rapid hip flexion and knee extension can cause these muscles to tear, for example when sprinting or hurdling, but occasionally the bony origin site will fracture instead. This avulsion fracture is often misdiagnosed as a simple "hamstring pull" but should be considered for surgical treatment.

Levator ani

The bowl-shaped floor of the pelvic cavity is formed by a group of curved, flat muscles grouped together as the levator ani and coccygeus (or ischiococcygeus) muscles, known as the pelvic diaphragm. This group of muscles also forms the roof of the perineum.

The coccygeus muscle passes from the ischial spine and the sacrospinous ligament to the inferior sacrum and coccyx. The levator ani muscle group comprises the puborectalis, pubococcygeus and iliococcygeus muscles, and with the coccygeus muscles are suspended between the walls of the lesser pelvis to function as a support to the pelvic viscera. Contraction of these muscles is an important aspect of support when resisting increases in intra-abdominal pressure during coughing, sneezing or fixation of the trunk during heavy lifting. The fascia covering the obturator internus muscles thickens as a tendinous arch and provides an attachment site of part of the pelvic diaphragm.

The puborectalis muscle is the most medial part of levator ani and runs from the pubis bone posteriorly to sling around the rectum, as suggested by its name. This anatomy allows the puborectalis muscle to pull an anterior kink into the rectum, an important mechanism of faecal continence (Figure 2.7).

The pubococcygeus muscle lies laterally to puborectalis, passing from the body of the pubis to the coccyx and the pubococcygeus muscle of the opposite side, forming a midline raphe. This raphe is part of the anococcygeal body running between the anus and the coccyx.

The most lateral and thinnest part of levator ani is the iliococcygeus muscle, passing from the ischial spine and the tendinous arch of the obturator fascia and inserting into the anococcygeal body.

Three apertures in the pelvic diaphragm allow passage of the urethra, vagina and anal canal in the female pelvis. The levator ani must relax for urination and defecation to occur, and the pelvic floor drops with relaxation. With the restoration of normal, tonic contraction of levator ani the pelvic floor rises again.

Internal reproductive organs

Bladder and urethra

The urinary bladder is the most anterior organ in the pelvis, lying partially superior and posterior to the body of the pubis. It is fixed only by its inferior neck with the pubovesical ligament in the female pelvis, and the lateral ligaments of the bladder. The vagina lies against the posterior wall of the bladder, and the uterus sits superiorly upon the empty bladder, anteflexed at the cervix (Figure 2.8). The urethra passes inferiorly from the internal urethral orifice of the bladder, through the external urethral sphincter and the perineal membrane to

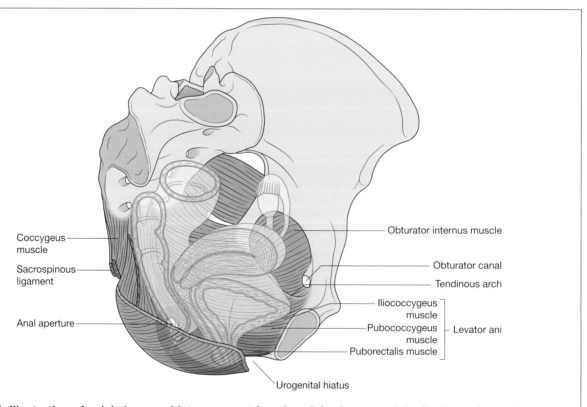

Coccygeus muscle

Sacrospinous ligament

Anal aperture

Obturator internus muscle

Obturator canal

Tendinous arch

Iliococcygeus muscle

Pubococcygeus muscle — Levator ani

Puborectalis muscle

Urogenital hiatus

Figure 2.7. Illustration of pelvic bones with transparent female pelvic viscera and the levator ani muscles.

Clinical notes 2.2 Vaginal prolapse

If the levator ani muscle becomes stretched and weakened, for example by childbirth, its ability to support internal structures is diminished. With straining and raised intra-abdominal pressure the anterior wall of the vagina and the bladder may be pushed into the vagina (cystocoele). A urethra and bladder pushed into the anterior vaginal wall is termed a cystourethrocoele and is the most common type of genitourinary prolapse. Damage to the levator ani may also cause urinary stress incontinence (the leaking of urine with raised intra-abdominal pressure).

If the supporting muscles of the posterior pelvic floor and perineum weaken the rectum may prolapse into the vagina (rectocoele). With menopause and the consequent fall in circulating oestrogen the pelvic floor muscles weaken, and become less supportive, increasing the risk of prolapse and the probability of urinary or faecal incontinence. Pelvic floor exercises designed to maintain the strength and tone of the pelvic diaphragm muscles are an important preventative measure, particularly with increasing age or after childbirth.

open at the external urethral orifice in the vestibule between the labia minora. The female urethra is typically 4 cm long.

Vagina

The vagina is a distensible, muscular tube, lined with a mucosal epithelium. It is around 8 cm long and opens externally at the vaginal orifice in the vestibule. The superior end of the vagina meets the cervix of the uterus. The cervix holds the vagina open, but the rest of the tube is normally closed into a cross-sectional "H" shape when relaxed. The vagina lies anterior to the rectum, and is surrounded and supported by a number of muscles in addition to the levator ani, including

pubovaginalis, the external urethral sphincter, the urethrovaginal sphincter, and bulbospongiosus.

The vaginal and internal pudendal arteries supply blood to the middle and inferior parts of the vagina, and the superior part receives branches from the uterine arteries. These arteries are all branches of the internal iliac arteries. Vaginal venous plexuses surround the sides of the vagina and drain blood into the uterine veins, and anastomose with the rectal and vesical venous plexuses. Lymphatic vessels typically follow the venous routes to internal iliac lymph nodes, common iliac and para-aortic lymph nodes.

The innervation of the vagina is a mix of visceral and somatic. The major superior length (approximately three-quarters) of

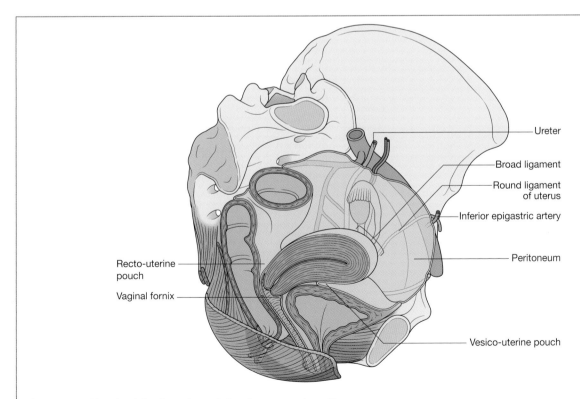

Figure 2.8. Hemipelvis, female, pelvic viscera and peritoneum.

the vagina has sympathetic, parasympathetic and visceral afferent fibres that pass through the uterovaginal plexus, part of the inferior hypogastric plexus found around the uterine artery within the layers of the broad ligament. Parasympathetic innervation arises in S2–S4 nuclei. Somatic innervation and sensitivity to touch is limited to the inferior quarter of the length of the vagina via the deep perineal nerve, a branch of the pudendal nerve.

The vagina meets the uterus at the cervix – the narrow, tubular opening of the uterus. The external os of the uterus projects into the upper vagina, and a recess surrounding the cervix within the vagina is termed the vaginal fornix (see Figure 2.8). The cervical canal opens within the uterus as the internal os, linking the vagina with the uterine cavity. The uterus, cervix and vagina comprise the birth canal.

Uterus

The uterus is a thick, hollow, muscular organ, lined internally with a specialised mucous layer termed the endometrium (Figure 2.9). The uterus is able to change size considerably during pregnancy, and a muscular myometrium layer contracts forcefully to expel the fetus during childbirth. The outermost surface of the uterus is covered by a connective tissue layer of perimetrium. The uterine tubes link the ovaries to the uterus and enter laterally.

The uterus is supported within the lesser pelvis by a number of ligaments. The round ligament of the uterus runs from the uterus at the site where the uterine tubes join, and passes through the inguinal canal to the labia majora. This

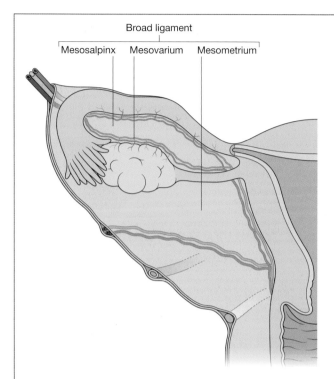

Figure 2.10. The broad ligament in cross-section.

ligament is a remnant of the embryonic gubernaculum, a structure that guides the descent of the gonad from the abdomen and into the pelvis. An ovarian ligament runs between the uterus near the site of the uterine tube and the ovary. It is continued laterally as the suspensory ligament of the ovary, which is actually a collection of ovarian vessels and nerves passing from the pelvic brim to the ovary beneath the peritoneum. The peritoneum is draped upon the pelvic structures in such a way as to form a folded sheet here, rather than a true, supportive ligamentous structure. The peritoneal covering continues inferiorly, covering the round ligament, the uterine tube and the ligament of the ovary, and meeting itself to form a folded, two-layered mesentery. This is the broad ligament, and it aids in supporting the uterus (Figure 2.10).

The uterus is supported by the bladder upon which it lies and the pelvic diaphragm beneath that, but also by the ligaments described. This support is important when the intra-abdominal pressure is raised, and the cervix is further supported by transverse cervical (cardinal) ligaments between the cervix and the lateral pelvic walls at the ischial spines, and the uterosacral ligaments passing posterosuperiorly around the rectum to the middle of the sacrum.

Uterine tubes

The uterine tubes (Fallopian tubes or oviducts) run from the uterine horns posterolaterally within the mesosalpinx to curve

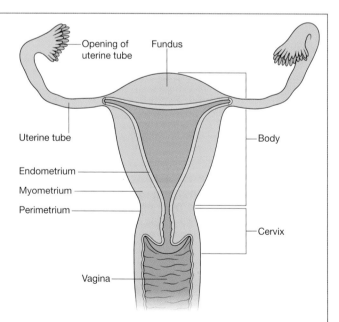

Figure 2.9. The parts and layers of the uterus, uterine tubes and ovaries.

Clinical notes 2.3 Uterine tube obstruction

The uterine tubes are shaped a little like a Greek wind instrument similar to a trumpet and called a salpinx, because of their flared infundibular ends. Pathologies and procedures associated with the uterine tubes often use this word. Salpingitis is an inflammation of the uterine tubes and can cause uterine tube obstruction, as can pelvic inflammatory disease (PID) and endometriosis.

An obstruction here will affect fertility. Other infections, appendicitis, peritonitis, adhesions or complications of abdominal surgery can affect tubal patency or distort the path of the uterine tube, pulling it away from the ovary. Around 20–25% of female infertility is caused by uterine tube problems.

The surgical removal of a uterine tube is a salpingectomy.

around and open near the ovaries (see Figure 2.9). Their positions, with the ovaries, are somewhat variable. The distal infundibulum of the uterine tube surrounds a part of the ovary with finger-like processes of fimbriae, and the muscular tube itself is lined with a mucosal columnar ciliated epithelium. With ovulation the ovum passes into the uterine tube at the infundibulum and is transported towards the uterus. Sperm passes into the uterine tube from the opposite direction and fertilisation occurs here, before the fertilised egg continues on to implant into the uterus.

Ovaries

The almond-sized ovary is suspended in the lesser pelvis within the mesovarium of the broad ligament. It is attached to the lateral pelvic wall by the suspensory ligament of the ovary and to the uterus by the ovarian ligament. The ovaries produce oocytes and reproductive hormones and are the sites of maturation of oocytes into mature follicles. With ovulation an ovum is released from the follicle into the peritoneum, and is usually caught by the fimbriae of the uterine tube.

The ovaries are supplied with blood by the ovarian arteries, which are lateral branches from the abdominal aorta, indicating the original site of gonad development in the embryo and the route of the gonads' subsequent descent into the pelvis. The ovarian arteries pass along the posterior abdominal wall and lie anterior to the iliac vessels at the pelvic brim, running to the ovaries within the suspensory ligament of the ovary. They continue from the ovaries to the uterine tubes and uterus, anastomosing with the uterine arteries and creating a collateral circulation from abdominal and pelvic blood vessels.

A pampiniform plexus of veins drains blood from the ovary and becomes a single ovarian vein on either side that runs with the ovarian artery into the abdomen. Veins of the uterine tube drain to the ovarian and uterine veins. The left ovarian vein typically drains into the left renal vein because of the right-sided nature of the caval system. The right ovarian vein drains into the inferior vena cava at a similar level. The lymphatic drainage of the ovary follows the venous vessels to reach abdominal lumbar (para-aortic) lymph nodes directly .

Visceral afferent fibres that carry pain sensations from the regions of the vagina and cervix inferior to the pelvic pain line

follow the paths of the parasympathetic fibres to the S2–S4 levels of the spinal cord. Visceral afferent fibres carrying pain sensations from the the regions of the uterus (the intraperitoneal fundus and body of the uterus), uterine tubes and ovaries superior to the pelvic pain line follow the routes of the sympathetic fibres back to the lower thoracic and upper lumbar regions of the spinal cord.

External genitalia

The perineum describes the space inferior to the pelvic diaphragm, and is also used when referring to the region of skin between the medial thighs, the gluteal folds and the mons pubis. The compartment of the perineum lies between the pelvic diaphragm and the skin, and is bounded anteriorly by the pubis bone, laterally by the ischial tuberosities, and posteriorly by the sacrotuberous ligaments, the sacrum and the coccyx (Figure 2.11). A flat sheet of perineal membrane (fascia) lies between the left and right ischiopubic rami, terminating with an abrupt posterior edge found running transversely between the vagina and anus. The urethra and vagina pass through the perineal membrane; the anal canal does not. The perineal membrane divides the perineum into superficial and deep perineal pouches. Many structures of the external genitalia lie within the perineum.

The perineal body is a fibromuscular mass that lies deep to the skin between the anal canal and the perineal membrane. It is an attachment site for perineal membrane, the rectovaginal septum, the bulbospongiosus muscle, the external anal sphincter, the superficial and deep transverse perineal muscles, the levator ani, the external urethral sphincter and other local muscular and connective tissues. Damage to the perineal body will weaken the pelvic diaphragm.

The superficial perineal pouch contains the clitoris, the bulb of the vestibule, the bulbospongiosus muscle, the greater vestibular glands and the superficial transverse perineal muscles. Deep perineal branches of the internal pudendal artery and vein, and of the pudendal nerve pass from the deep perineal pouch through the superficial perineal pouch to supply the external genitalia (also termed pudendum or vulva).

The clitoris is an erectile organ with a crus either side of the midline, two corpora cavernosa, a root and a body. The glans of the clitoris projects most superficially and extends towards

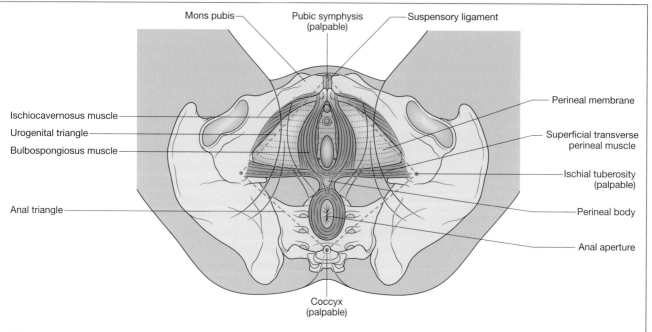

Figure 2.11. Illustration of the location of the perineum in relation to pelvic bones and skin.

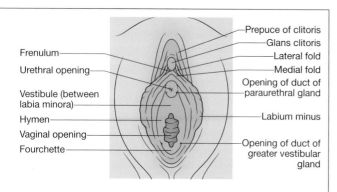

Figure 2.12. Illustration of the female external genitalia.

the vestibule (Figure 2.12). The clitoris becomes turgid in response to parasympathetic innervation, filling with blood as a result of local arterial vasodilation and inhibited venous return. The clitoris is highly innervated by fibres of the dorsal nerve of the clitoris.

The vestibule is surrounded laterally by the labia minora, and the swellings of the labia majora. The labia minora also contain erectile tissue, are hairless and well innervated by somatic sensory fibres. The labia minora converge anteriorly to form the prepuce of the clitoris. Within the vestibule the urethra and vagina open externally. The ducts of the greater and lesser vestibular glands (also known as Bartholin and Skene glands, respectively) open within the vestibule and secrete mucus in response to sexual arousal.

The anterior pudendum is innervated by the anterior labial nerves branching from the ilioinguinal and genitofemoral nerves that arise from L1–L2 spinal nerves. The posterior pudendum is innervated by the pudendal nerve and the perineal branch of the posterior femoral cutaneous nerve.

Pituitary gland

The pituitary gland is a key part of the reproductive system. The hormones it secretes regulate other organs and hormone production elsewhere in the body, including the ovaries (Figure 2.13).

The pituitary gland sits within a hollowed out region of the sphenoid bone in the skull, called the sella turcica. It is

Clinical notes 2.4 Urinary tract infection

The female urethra is short, and colonies of microorganisms at the opening of the urethra can pass to the bladder and cause cystitis (bladder infection) more easily than in the male pelvis. The opening of the female urethra is near the opening of the anus, increasing the chance of bacteria from the digestive tract attaching to the urethra. Frequent sexual intercourse is also a risk factor for urethral infection. Infection may pass up the ureters to the kidneys (pyelonephritis). Recurrent urinary tract infections (UTIs) after an initial infection are common, and with menopause the risk of developing a UTI increases.

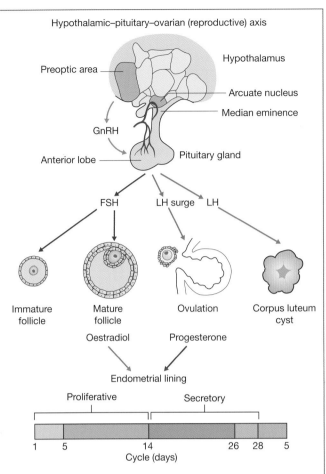

Hypothalamic–pituitary–ovarian (reproductive) axis

Figure 2.13. **The hypothalamic-pituitary-ovary (HPO) axis and feedback loops–oestrogen, progesterone, gonadotrophin-releasing hormone (GnRH), follicle-stimulating hormone (FSH) and luteinising hormone (LH).**

The anterior pituitary appears more glandular histologically than the posterior part, and cells here produce luteinising hormone (LH), follicle-stimulating hormone (FSH), thyroid-stimulating hormone (TSH), growth hormone (GH), prolactin and adrenocorticotrophic hormone (ACTH). FSH encourages development of the ovarian follicle and stimulates oestradiol and progesterone synthesis. LH induces ovulation. TSH, GH and prolactin are involved in growth and metabolic regulation, whereas ACTH acts upon the adrenal glands to stimulate the release of corticosteroids.

The concept of the hypothalamic-pituitary-ovary (HPO) axis and the cyclical actions of the hormonal feedback loops between these organs is crucial to normal function.

Physiology

Menstrual cycle

A fertilised ovum is passed to the uterus to implant into the endometrial wall. For successful implantation and subsequent development of the embryonic and extra-embryonic tissues the endometrium makes certain preparations. The endometrial lining undergoes a series of changes that cycle through approximately 4-week periods. There are three main stages: the proliferative (or follicular) phase, the secretory (luteal or progestational) phase, and the menstrual phase (Figure 2.14).

Proliferative phase

The proliferative phase describes the thickening of the endometrium between days 5 and 13 of the cycle, giving an increase in vascularisation as spiral arteries lengthen and glandular structures are renewed. In the ovary a few follicles begin to mature.

These changes are initiated by FSH secreted by the anterior part of the pituitary gland. FSH stimulates the development of the follicles, and their follicular (or granulosa) cells secrete oestrogen, in turn stimulating growth of the endometrium and myometrium. One of the (now Graafian) follicles in the ovary becomes dominant late in the proliferative phase. On day 13 the pituitary gland releases a surge of LH, inducing the ovary to release the ovum of the dominant follicle around day 14.

The empty follicle continues to produce oestrogen, which at high levels induces FSH and LH production by the pituitary

directly connected to the brain via the infundibular stalk and the hypothalamus. The posterior part of the pituitary gland receives axons from the hypothalamus and releases oxytocin and vasopressin. Oxytocin causes contraction of the myometrial muscles of the uterus and the myoepithelial cells of the mammary glands. Vasopressin acts upon the kidneys to increase water reabsorption and raise blood pressure.

 Clinical notes 2.5 Hyperprolactinaemia

Levels of prolactin are normally low other than during pregnancy and breastfeeding. If a tumour of prolactin-secreting cells (lactotrophs) of the pituitary gland develops, or if the dopamine from the hypothalamus that normally inhibits the secretion of prolactin is unable to reach these cells, levels of prolactin can rise. In women this can cause galactorrhoea (abnormal milk secretion from the breasts), oligomenorrhoea (abnormally infrequent menstrual periods), amenorrhoea (absence of menstrual periods) and reduced libido. If a pituitary tumour becomes enlarged it may affect vision (as the optic chiasma lies superior to it) or cause headaches. Men may suffer from erectile dysfunction.

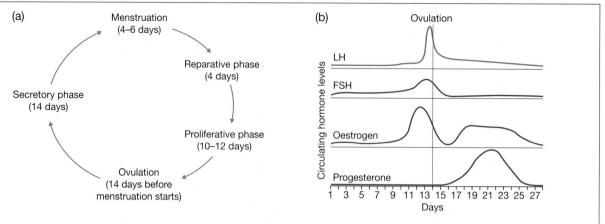

Figure 2.14. The phases of the menstrual cycle and the levels of circulating hormones. (Source: S. Webster and R. de Wreede (2012) *Embryology at a Glance*. Reproduced with permission of John Wiley & Sons, Ltd.)

gland, further reinforcing oestrogen production and its effects upon the endometrium.

Secretory phase

The dominant follicle continues to mature and becomes the corpus luteum, a structure that produces progesterone and oestrogen. The endometrium continues to develop, thicken and increase in vascularity. Progesterone maintains the developing endometrium and increases uterine gland secretions, but also inhibits gonadotrophin-releasing hormone (GnRH) secretion by the hypothalamus as levels of progesterone rise during this phase. With decreasing GnRH levels the pituitary gland reduces its secretions of LH and FSH.

By around day 28 of the cycle the corpus luteum degenerates because of a lack of LH and FSH stimulation and becomes the corpus albicans.

Menstrual phase

Decreasing levels of oestrogen and progesterone are followed by ischaemia of the endometrium towards the end of the secretory phase as endothelin and thromboxane cause vasoconstriction of its spiral arteries. The apoptosing endometrium and blood are shed during menstruation. Menstruation is described as beginning on day 0 of the cycle, and continuing to day 4.

With reduced circulating oestrogen and progesterone levels the hypothalamus increases production of GnRH, stimulating FSH synthesis by the pituitary gland and restarting the cycle.

GnRH synthesis is inhibited by high levels of oestrogen, but stimulated by low levels. GnRH is released in pulses, and the frequency of pulses determines their effect on the pituitary cells. Low-frequency pulses cause FSH release, and high-frequency pulses cause LH release (Figure 2.14).

 Clinical notes 2.6 Polycystic ovary syndrome

Polycystic ovaries contain a number of small cysts that develop from follicles but have been arrested at an antral stage. High levels of LH or insulin may induce abnormally raised levels of androgen synthesis by the ovaries in polycystic ovary syndrome (PCOS) causing oligomenorrhoea or amenorrhoea, infertility due to ovulation failure, increase in weight, acne and hirsutism.

SUMMARY

Clinical case

Investigations

After taking a full medical history from the couple you perform a pelvic examination with bimanual palpation upon Mrs Amble.

You ask Mrs Amble to attend the phlebotomy clinic on day 21 of her menstrual cycle for progesterone analysis, as her cycle has a fairly consistent length of 28 to 30 days.

Progesterone levels will indicate whether ovulation has occurred, and it will be helpful to repeat this for three cycles. If Mrs Amble is anovulatory you will subsequently assess GnRH and oestrogen levels to assess hypothalamic-pituitary dysfunction or failure, and ovarian failure.

If you were concerned about the function of Mrs Amble's pituitary gland you might investigate blood prolactin levels. Likewise you might consider assessing the function of Mrs Amble's thyroid gland.

Results

The results of the pelvic exam revealed no areas of tenderness, indications of infection or abnormalities of the vagina, cervix, uterus or ovaries. You found no unusual masses.

Blood progesterone levels for the 3 months at day 21 were measured as 16 ng/mL, 18 ng/mL and 15 ng/mL.

As Mrs Amble is ovulating regularly but finding it difficult to conceive you refer her to a secondary care fertility clinic. The consultant arranges a hysterosalpingogram to assess Mrs Amble's uterine tube patency using X-ray fluoroscopy and a contrast material passed into the uterus via the vagina.

The shapes of the uterus and left uterine tube are normal, but the right uterine tube is narrowed and only allows a little of the contrast material to pass beyond the middle of the ampulla.

Treatments

The results of the investigations are discussed with Mrs Amble. She is ovulating normally, and one uterine tube is narrowed but the other is patent. This may be linked to the abdominal surgery she received as a child when she had an appendicectomy as Mrs Amble has never shown symptoms of endometriosis or pelvic inflammatory disease.

The results of Mr Amble's investigations indicate that Mr Amble's fertility is good.

Mr and Mrs Amble are advised that they should be able to conceive naturally and you discuss with them contemporary guidance and normal patterns of conception. You advise regular sexual intercourse (two to three times per week) throughout Mrs Amble's cycle, and to consider that stress can affect libido and the relationship. They are aware that with increasing age fertility rates can decrease.

Case conclusions

Six months after their final consultation Mrs Amble becomes pregnant naturally. The couple comment to you that the results of the consultations and investigations gave them confidence that "everything was working normally", which removed some of the stress of trying to conceive. Nine months later Mrs Amble gives birth to her first baby, a 3.5kg boy.

Key learning points

- The musculoskeletal anatomy of the female pelvis is an important part of normal function, and can change with age and childbirth. Parts of pelvic anatomy and the female reproductive system should not be considered in isolation but should be associated with these musculoskeletal structures.

- The physiology of the menstrual cycle is a core component of normal reproductive function and relates to a number of areas of development, fertility and pregnancy.

 Now visit **www.wileyessential.com/humandevelopment** to test yourself on this chapter.

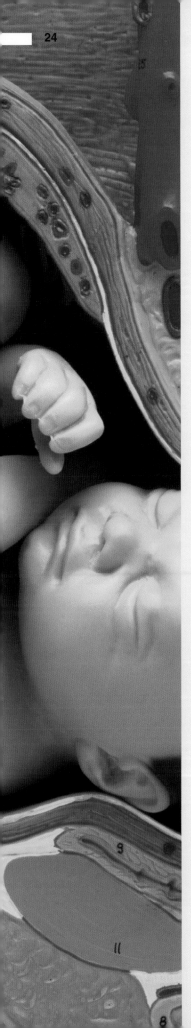

CHAPTER 3
The male reproductive system

Sam Webster

Case

A 36-year-old man, Mr Bandar, presents to you with his 35-year-old wife in your primary care clinic and they describe their difficulty in trying to conceive. They have been engaging in approximately weekly, unprotected intercourse for 2 years without successful conception. Mr Bandar has no history of hernia, orchitis, erectile dysfunction, undescended testes, diabetes, smoking, or recreational drug use. He estimates that he drinks around 5–6 units of alcohol per week and jogs regularly twice a week. His body mass index (BMI) is within the normal range. He suffered testicular torsion of his left testicle at the age of 19, probably as a result of an incident during rugby training. He had mumps as a young child for a short period and recovered well.

Learning outcomes

- You should be able to recognise structures of the anterior abdominal wall involved in forming the inguinal canal.
- You should be able to recognise the structures and normal functions of the male reproductive system.
- You should be able to describe the process of spermatogenesis and the maturation of spermatozoa.

Essential Human Development, First Edition. Edited by Samuel Webster, Geraint Morris and Euan Kevelighan
© 2018 John Wiley & Sons, Ltd. Published 2018 by John Wiley & Sons, Ltd.

Anatomy

Bones of the pelvis

The osteology of the pelvis is discussed in Chapter 2 with the female pelvis. Android and anthropoid shaped pelvises are the most common male pelvis shapes. The subpubic angle formed by the left and right inferior pubic rami meeting at the symphysis pubis is narrower (more acute) in the male pelvis, and the tips of the ischial tuberosities are closer together than is typically seen in the female pelvis. The bones of the male pelvis are thicker and heavier, the pelvic inlet is narrower and heart-shaped, and the pelvic outlet is smaller. The male pelvis above the pelvic brim (also known as the pelvis major, the greater pelvis or the false pelvis) is taller than in the female. The lesser pelvis (the pelvis below the pelvic brim, also known as the pelvis minor or the true pelvis) is narrower and deeper than the wide and shallow female lesser pelvis. These differences cause the obturator foramen in the male pelvis to be round, but oval or triangular in the female pelvis. The female adaptations are necessary for natural childbirth of a fetus with a large head.

Anterior abdominal wall and the inguinal canal

Layers of muscles and fascia linking the ribs and pelvic bones form the anterior and lateral abdominal walls. Fat and parietal peritoneum underlie these layers, and fat and skin cover them superficially. The walls are able to contract and distend, enabling an increase in intra-abdominal pressure or the accommodation of fat, ingested food, or pathology (or pregnancy in the female abdomen). The muscles of the abdominal wall are important contributors to the stability of the pelvis and spine when lifting heavy loads.

Anteriorly two strips of the flat rectus abdominis muscle pass vertically from the pubic symphysis and pubic crest to the xiphoid process and costal cartilages of ribs 5 to 7. Most of the muscle is broad and relatively thin, but it thickens and narrows inferiorly. Each strip of muscle is separated into three or four sections by tendinous intersections. The two strips of muscle are surrounded by the rectus sheath, and joined in the midline by the linea alba. These sheets and thickenings of connective tissues are created by the anterior continuations of the aponeuroses of the muscles of the anterolateral walls of the abdomen.

The deepest layer of muscle of the anterolateral wall of the abdomen is the transversus abdominis muscle, which runs from the 7th to 12th costal cartilages, the thoracolumbar fascia, the iliac crest, and the lateral third of the inguinal ligament to pass anteriorly into the pubis and pectineal line as the conjoint tendon and into the linea alba. Most of the fibres of the transversus abdominis muscle run transversely and the remainder run in an inferomedial direction, making the muscle effective at compressing the abdomen and pulling the anterior wall towards the spine. Deep to the transversus abdominis muscle lie layers of transversalis fascia, extraperitoneal fat, and parietal peritoneum.

The internal oblique muscle layer lies superficial to the transversus abdominis muscle. It runs from the thoracolumbar fascia, the anterior two-thirds of the iliac crest, and the lateral third of the inguinal ligament to the inferior borders of ribs 10–12, the linea alba and the pubis as the conjoint tendon. The external oblique muscle layer lies superficial to this layer, arising from the 5th to 12th ribs and inserting into the linea alba, pubic tubercle and anterior part of the iliac crest. The fibres of the internal oblique muscle run in a medial and superior direction, and most fibres of the external oblique muscle run in a medial and inferior direction.

The three layers of transversus abdominis, internal oblique and external oblique muscles form the anterolateral walls of the abdomen and pass their aponeuroses medially to surround the rectus abdominis muscle (as the rectus sheath), forming the anterior abdominal wall. The anterolateral muscles are involved in flexing and rotating the trunk, and the rectus abdominis muscle contributes to pelvic stability and trunk flexion. As a group the muscles support the contents of the abdomen and can increase intra-abdominal pressure, working with the diaphragm and muscles of the thorax during breathing movements, or when expelling air forcefully.

The inferior aponeurosis of the external oblique muscle has a free edge running between the anterior superior iliac spine and the pubic tubercle. This is the inguinal ligament, deep to which run the femoral vessels and nerves. This free edge curls underneath itself posteriorly, becoming a partial tube-like structure and forming part of the inguinal canal. A medial V-shaped gap between muscle fibres of the external oblique inserting into the pubic tubercle (lateral crus) and the pubic crest (medial crus) allows an anterior opening for the inguinal canal, called the superficial (or external) inguinal ring.

To form a complete inguinal canal the other walls of the canal are built from other layers of the abdominal wall. The transversalis fascia (the fascia layer between the parietal peritoneum and the transversus abdominis muscle) forms the posterior wall along with parts of the internal oblique and transversus abdominis muscles where they merge as aponeuroses medially. Aponeurotic parts of the internal oblique and transversus abdominis muscles also form much of the roof of the inguinal canal.

The inguinal canal is roughly 4 cm long and conveys through the abdominal wall the ilioinguinal nerve, blood vessels, lymphatic structures, the ductus deferens in males (much of these are contained within the spermatic cord) and the round ligament of the uterus in females. Its opening within the pelvis is called the deep (or internal) inguinal ring, and is found about halfway along the inguinal ligament a little superior to it.

Normally with increased intra-abdominal pressure the contraction of the external oblique muscle brings the floor of the inguinal canal towards the roof, and pulls on the lateral and medial crura of the superficial inguinal ring. Contraction of the internal oblique and transversus abdominis muscles and the increased pressure within the abdomen push the anterior

Clinical notes 3.1 Inguinal hernia

The inguinal canal presents a weakness in the structure of the anterior abdominal wall. It is larger in the male abdominal wall than in the female, and men are at greater risk of an inguinal hernia. Herniation of the intestine and parietal peritoneum through the inguinal canal can either form a direct or an indirect hernia.

A direct hernia passes into the inguinal canal outside the spermatic cord, and often passes only partway along the inguinal canal. It is often lateral to the cord, is unlikely to enter the scrotum, and forms as a result of a weakness in the anterior abdominal wall, leading to this type of hernia, also known as an acquired hernia. A direct hernia can be palpated by pressing a finger into the superficial inguinal ring, or at the inguinal triangle where the inguinal canal meets the lateral margin of the rectus sheath, by

asking the patient to cough or bear down. With the cough a direct hernia will be felt as it is pushed out of the abdominal cavity.

An indirect hernia is also known as a congenital hernia, and is more common. During development the testes descend into the scrotum led by the gubernaculum and an outpouching of the parietal peritoneum called the processus vaginalis. Normally this peritoneal layer fuses with itself and becomes the tunica vaginalis layer covering of the testis. If this fails to occur the peritoneum may remain continuous with the contents of the scrotum, or the peritoneum may extend through the inguinal canal. Herniated intestine passes within the spermatic cord through the inguinal canal and into the scrotum (or in females, into the labium majus).

and posterior walls of the inguinal canal together and also pull the roof of parts of the canal inferiorly. The canal is constricted and the anterior abdominal wall is strengthened in this way.

The scrotum hangs from the region of the superficial inguinal ring and contains the testes. It is a sac comprising layers of skin and dartos fascia. The dartos fascia is continuous with the membranous layers of subcutaneous tissue of the abdomen (Scarpa fascia) and of the perineum (Colles fascia). The layer contains smooth muscle fibres and is attached to the skin, causing the wrinkled surface appearance. A midline scrotal septum separates the left and right testes.

The spermatic cord links the testes to the abdomen, and is made up of layers of the anterior abdominal wall that form a canal through which blood vessels, nerves, lymphatic vessels and the ductus deferens pass between the scrotum and the abdomen. The testes are suspended by their spermatic cords within the scrotum.

The spermatic cord begins at the deep inguinal ring as layers of internal spermatic fascia (from the transversalis fascia), cremasteric fascia (from the fascia of the internal oblique muscle), and external spermatic fascia (from the fascia of the aponeurosis of the external oblique muscle). The cremasteric fascia contains cremaster muscle innervated by genital branches of the genitofemoral nerve, and is able to lift the testes superiorly within the scrotum in response to cold.

Testes

The male gonads are held outside the pelvis in the scrotum, and produce spermatozoa and androgens. They are primarily composed of germ cells and supporting Sertoli cells that form a tubular network, and surrounding interstitial Leydig cells. Spermatozoa form in the walls of the seminiferous tubules, through which they eventually are able to leave the testes.

Spermatogenesis, the process that forms new spermatozoa, works most effectively at a temperature a few degrees lower than body core temperature.

The normal adult testis has a volume of between 12 and 20 mL and is encapsulated by a thick, tough layer of tunica albuginea. Septa extend from the tunica albuginea into the testis dividing it up into around 300 small lobules.

Seminiferous tubules are convoluted loops of 150–200 μm diameter tube that empty into straight tubuli recti that pass into the rete testis within the connective tissue mediastinum testis. Through this route sperm leave the seminiferous tubules and pass into the head of the epididymis; a single coiled tube that descends along the surface of the testis and becomes the ductus deferens.

Seminiferous tubules are lined with seminiferous epithelium comprising spermatogonia and Sertoli cells (Figure 3.1). Sertoli cells synthesise a number of hormones with local and peripheral actions including oestradiol, inhibin, activin, transferrin and anti-Müllerian hormone during fetal development. The tubules are supported by a tunica propria of collagen, contractile myofibroblasts and a basal lamina.

A loose connective tissue with blood vessels, lymphocytes and Leydig cells lies between the seminiferous tubules. Leydig cells synthesise testosterone, androstenedione and dehydroepiandrosterone (DHEA) in response to luteinising hormone (LH) secretions from the pituitary gland.

The functions of the testes therefore are to produce sperm and androgens. The functions of the remainder of the male reproductive system are largely to facilitate passage of the spermatozoa from the testes to the female reproductive tract and to ensure their survival therein.

The testes initially form in the mesoderm of the posterior abdominal wall of the embryo during the 5th and 6th weeks of development. The intermediate mesoderm of the gonadal

Clinical notes 3.2 Testicular cancer

Most testicular tumours develop from the germinal epithelium of a seminiferous tubule (seminoma) or from a germ cell (non-seminomatous germ cell tumour). Testicular tumours have a low incidence but are the most common cancer in men aged between 15 and 44 years old. They are typically discovered as a small lump on the testis, and the patient may complain of a testicular ache. Because

of the testes' descent from the abdomen during development metastatic cells may spread to para-aortic lymph nodes. Treatment initially includes orchiectomy (removal of the affected testis) with the option of a prosthetic testis, followed with radiotherapy or chemotherapy if required. Removing one testis does not normally affect fertility, and the effectiveness of treatment is greater than 95%.

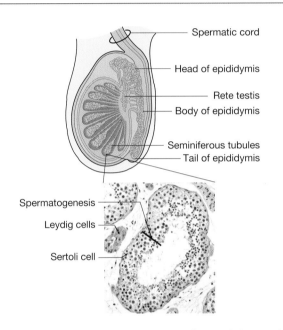

Figure 3.1. Gross anatomy and histology of the testis.

ridge forms Leydig cells as mesodermal epithelium in this region forms primitive sex cords that later become the tubes of the seminiferous tubules and the rete testis (Figure 3.2). Germ cells from the extra-embryonic endoderm of the yolk sac migrate to the gonadal ridge and invade the mesoderm. Reciprocal interactions between the germ cells and the mesoderm-derived cells ensure continued development of the gonads. The germ cells will become the early cells of spermatogenesis, the spermatogonia.

The testes move towards the scrotum guided by embryonic mesenchymal gubernacula. Each gubernaculum passes from the inferior pole of a testis to a labioscrotal fold (the future scrotum) and guides the testis through the layers of the anterior abdominal wall and into the developing scrotum as the embryo lengthens. The blood vessels follow this path.

Each testis has a testicular artery that begins as a lateral branch of the abdominal aorta just inferior to the renal artery, indicating the organ's embryonic site of origin. The testicular arteries run retroperitoneally to the deep inguinal rings, crossing the ureters and internal iliac arteries, to pass through the inguinal canal into the scrotum (Figure 3.3). The testicular veins begin as a pampiniform plexus of veins arising from each testis and surrounding the testicular arteries. Each plexus

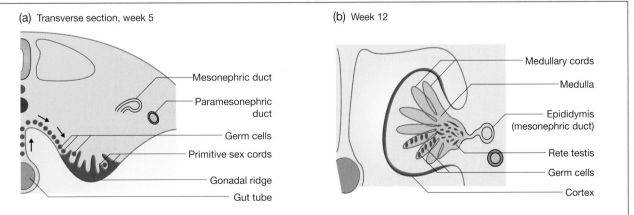

Figure 3.2. In the 5th week of development germ cells migrate from the yolk sac to the gonadal ridge in the mesoderm. At 12 weeks many of the structures of the testis have formed. (Source: S. Webster and R. de Wreede (2012) *Embryology at a Glance.* Reproduced with permission of John Wiley & Sons, Ltd.)

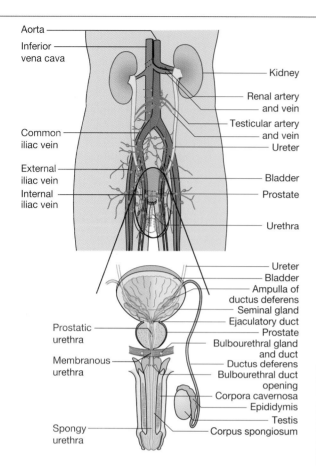

Figure 3.3. Illustration of the posterior abdominal wall and testes showing the testicular arteries, veins and lymphatic drainage to pre-aortic lymph nodes.

becomes a single testicular vein that passes with the testicular artery to the posterior abdominal wall. The left testicular vein drains into the left renal vein and the right testicular vein commonly drains into the inferior vena cava. The pampiniform plexus of veins helps regulate the temperature of the testis.

The pathway of lymphatic drainage of the testes follows the route of the blood vessels to reach pre-aortic (lumbar, para-aortic) lymph nodes in the posterior abdomen (see Figure 3.3). The scrotum by contrast receives blood vessels from external and internal pudendal arteries, and innervation from branches of the ilioinguinal, genitofemoral, pudendal and posterior cutaneous femoral nerves. Lymphatic drainage from the scrotum is to superficial inguinal lymph nodes.

Ductus deferens and glands

The epididymis empties into the ductus deferens (or vas deferens). The ductus deferens passes within the spermatic cord through the inguinal canal into the pelvis, and along the lateral pelvic wall, medial to the ureter and posterior to the bladder. It ends as a widened section called the ampulla of the ductus deferens that joins with the duct of the seminal vesicle to form the ejaculatory duct. During ejaculation spermatozoa are carried within the ductus deferens to the ejaculatory duct within the prostate gland, which links the ductus deferens to the urethra. The ductus deferens is a muscular tube, and a peristaltic wave pushes the spermatozoa into the urethra during ejaculation. A vasectomy cuts and ligates the ductus deferentia for the purpose of male sterilisation.

The seminal vesicles are a pair of glands posterior to the base of the bladder and superior to the prostate gland that extend laterally for 5–7 cm (see Figure 3.3). They secrete an alkaline solution containing fructose, vitamin C, prostaglandins and proteins and contribute about half of the volume of the ejaculate. Fructose provides energy for the spermatozoa, and the alkaline pH helps neutralize the acidic environment of the female reproductive tract and extend the survival time of spermatozoa. The secretory cells of the seminal vesicles are surrounded by elastic and smooth muscle fibres, and during ejaculation the secreted fluid is forced into the ejaculatory ducts and the urethra.

The prostate gland lies inferior to the base of the bladder and anterior to the rectum, and surrounds the urethra, which runs through it (see Figure 3.3). The ejaculatory ducts open into the urethra within the prostate gland. The latter is about the size of a walnut, and the epithelial secretory cells produce an alkaline fluid, contributing to around half of the volume of the semen ejaculate. Smooth muscle fibres force the prostatic fluid into the prostatic urethra through multiple ducts during ejaculation. The prostate gland is surrounded by a thick fibromuscular connective tissue. Synthesis by cells within the seminal vesicles and prostate gland is regulated by androgens.

The prostate gland produces prostate-specific antigen (PSA), a glycoprotein that thins semen and cervical mucus allowing sperm to travel within the female reproductive tract more easily. PSA levels are elevated in prostatic cancers and can be used as a marker for diagnosis and treatment.

🔍 Clinical notes 3.3 Testicular torsion

Testicular torsion may present with the sudden onset of severe pain in one testis, extreme tenderness, scrotal swelling on one side, and possibly nausea or vomiting. The spermatic cord is twisted, compressing the testicular artery and pampiniform plexus of veins, causing the development of testicular ischaemia. It is more likely to occur if the testis is not held in place by connective tissues within the scrotum. Urgent surgery to repair the torsion is required. After 6 hours of testicular torsion there is a high probability of the testis becoming non-functional. It is likely to atrophy and will need to be removed.

Clinical notes 3.4 Prostatic hypertrophy

Benign prostatic hyperplasia is a condition of the prostate common in older men involving epithelial and stromal proliferation. As the prostate gland enlarges it may constrict the urethra and affect the sphincter at the base of the bladder, as the gland is restricted from external expansion by its fibromuscular covering. Symptoms typically include increased urinary frequency, urinary urgency, difficulty initiating urination, a weak urine stream, difficulty in completely emptying the bladder and the loss of small amounts of urine (dribbling). Diagnosis is made by digital rectal examination of the prostate gland to assess size and shape. Urinalysis, urine culture, assessment of prostate-specific antigen, ultrasonography and endoscopy of the lower urinary tract may be helpful.

Benign prostatic hypertrophy often does not need treatment and may be managed with lifestyle changes. Treatments include surgical resection or the use of finasteride or dutasteride, drugs that block the effects of dihydrotestosterone (DHT). Alpha blockers can be helpful in relaxing bladder musculature and aid in relief of lower urinary tract symptoms.

The paired bulbourethral glands (or Cowper's glands) are found at the base of the penis, lateral and posterior to the urethra. They are small, pea-sized glands and produce a small volume of pre-ejaculate fluid that lubricates the urethra and buffers any lingering acidic urine within the membranous and spongy parts of the urethra.

Penis

The penis is made up primarily of three tubes of erectile tissue surrounded by fibrous capsules: two corpora cavernosa forming the dorsal part and one corpus spongiosum ventrally (see Figure 3.3). Anatomically the penis is considered erect when describing the anatomical position. The root of the penis is attached to the pelvis by ischiocavernosus and bulbospongiosus muscles, the bulb of the penis and the crura. Each corpus cavernosum extends posteriorly as a crus and attaches to the medial surface of the ischiopubic ramus. The bulb of the penis describes an expanded posterior end of the corpus spongiosum within the perineum. Deep fascia blends with the deep fascia of the penis and forms a suspensory ligament of the penis.

The body of the penis hangs freely, and the corpus spongiosum expands distally to form the glans penis. The urethra runs within the penis and opens externally at the distal tip of the glans. The skin covering the penis extends as a double folded layer that partially covers the glans as the prepuce (or foreskin) attached ventrally at the frenulum of the prepuce.

The nerves of the penis are derived from branches of the pudendal nerve (with spinal roots of S2–S4), and the main nerve is the dorsal nerve of the penis. Parasympathetic innervation arises in S2–S4 nuclei and passes to the penis from the prostatic nerve plexus. Branches of the internal pudendal artery supply blood to the penis, and blood is drained by a venous plexus that forms the deep dorsal vein of the penis.

Embryology

The development of the male reproductive system is linked to that of the renal system, and up to week 7 the development of the male and female systems is identical; this is the indifferent stage. Mesonephric (Wolffian) and paramesonephric (Müllerian) ducts develop in the mesoderm of the posterior wall of the embryo and descend into the future pelvis. A gonadal ridge forms in the posterior wall of the embryo and the surface epithelial cells proliferate and extend into the mesoderm beneath and form sex cords. Neighbouring mesenchyme is induced to differentiate and become Leydig cells. The cells of the male embryo contain the *SRY* gene (sex-determining gene of the Y chromosome), triggering the development of the testis-specific cells and degeneration of the paramesonephric ducts.

The sex cords become the tubes of the seminiferous tubules and the rete testis, and link with the mesonephric ducts, which will become the epididymis, the ductus deferens and the ejaculatory duct. The seminal vesicles grow from the ductus deferens whereas the prostate gland develops from budding growths of the urethra.

The external genitalia develop from common structures on the surface of the embryo from week 9 (Figure 3.4). An anterior genital tubercle becomes the penis, labioscrotal swellings on either side of the midline are joined to form the scrotum, and the urethra extends along the ventral surface of the penis initially as groove. The female embryo's clitoris is larger than the male embryo's penis for much of this developmental period, so determining the sex of a fetus by ultrasonography is best performed at a 20-week scan or later if necessary. Further development includes the closure of the urethral groove until the urethra opens at the distal end of the penis only, accounting for the midline raphe.

 Clinical notes 3.5 Hypospadias

If the urethral groove of the developing penis does not close normally, the urethra opens externally on the ventral surface. This may occur at any point along the body of the penis but is most common towards the glans. Often the abnormality is minor and treatment is not necessary, but surgery using skin from the prepuce can extend the urethra to the glans if needed.

Clinical notes 3.6 Cryptorchidism

The most common abnormality of male reproductive system development is the failure of one or both testes to descend to their adult locations in the scrotum. An undescended testis may remain at any point along its route of descent from the posterior abdominal wall at the level of the kidneys to the inguinal canal, or elsewhere within the body not on that path. Men with an undescended testis are more susceptible to reduced fertility, testicular cancer, testicular torsion, and inguinal hernia. Orchiplexy surgery may be used to move the undescended testis to the scrotum and to prevent it from returning through the inguinal canal.

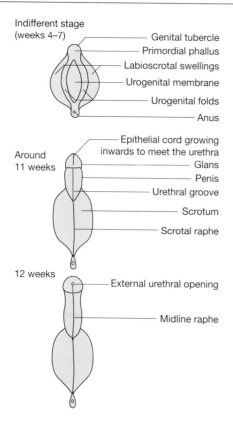

Figure 3.4. Development of the male external genitalia. (Source: S. Webster and R. de Wreede (2012) *Embryology at a Glance.* Reproduced with permission of John Wiley & Sons, Ltd.)

Physiology

Chapter 1 covers the processes of spermatogenesis.

Erection, emission and ejaculation

Erection and emission are controlled autonomically in response to physical and mental stimuli. Parasympathetic stimulation closes arteriovenous anastomoses within the penis and the bulbospongiosus and ischiocavernosus muscles contract, compressing the veins and inhibiting venous return from the penis. The corpora fill with blood and become turgid, and the penis becomes erect.

During emission the glandular secretions of the seminal vesicles and prostate gland are pushed into the prostatic urethra as sperm are delivered to the same region by the ductus deferens. Emission is initiated by the sympathetic nervous system (from the L1–L2 spinal level). Combined, the gland secretions and sperm continue onwards within the urethra and are expelled by ejaculation. The internal urethral sphincter to the bladder is closed, and the urethral and bulbospongiosus muscles contract.

After ejaculation sympathetic innervation dilates arteriovenous anastomoses within the penis, and the bulbospongiosus and ischiocavernosus muscles relax allowing blood to leave the penis. A latent period of variable length occurs after ejaculation during which a subsequent erection is not possible.

 Clinical notes 3.7 Erectile dysfunction

Failure of penile erection (impotence) is often caused by psychological factors. Higher brain centres are able to apply inhibitory or excitatory effects upon the autonomic innervation of the blood supply to the penis. Physical causes include cardiovascular disease such as atherosclerosis and can be treated with statins, lifestyle changes, or sildenafil (also sold as Viagra). Vacuum pumps that increase blood flow into the penis can also be effective. Damage to the parasympathetic nerves of the prostatic plexus or the cavernous nerves will also cause impotence.

Clinical case

Investigations

After taking a full medical history from Mr and Mrs Bandar, you ask Mr Bandar to provide a semen sample for analysis. When discussing the couple's sexual history it becomes clear that Mr Bandar does not have any impotence issues, but he has developed some stress while trying to conceive.

Mr Bandar's semen sample has a volume of 2.3 mL with a concentration of 15 million spermatozoa per mL. The spermatozoa have grade c motility with 30% observed motility. Ten percent have abnormal morphology. Semen pH is measured as pH 7.4.

Mr Bandar has asthenozoospermia (reduced sperm motility). All other factors are normal.

Case conclusion

A repeat semen sample is requested from Mr Bandar and tested. The results are similar to the first sample. He is educated about factors that affect normal sperm development, and Mr and Mrs Bandar attend counselling to reduce their stress related to trying to conceive. One year later they have still failed to conceive and begin considering in vitro fertilisation methods of conception.

Key learning points

- The anatomy of the anterior abdominal wall is an important part of male anatomy and is related to the reproductive system by the spermatic cord that passes through it. The inguinal canal is formed by a number of structures and is a weakness prone to herniation.
- Testicular development helps explain the anatomy of the adult links between the testes and structures of the posterior abdominal wall. This should be remembered in terms of blood supply and lymphatic drainage (and metastatic spread of tumours).

- The autonomic nervous system governs normal erection, emission and ejaculation. The parasympathetic nerve fibres of the vagus nerve do not descend into the pelvis, so parasympathetic neurones extend from parasympathetic nuclei in the spinal cord at the T12–L1 levels out through the S2–S4 spinal nerves. Sympathetic nerves descend into the pelvis with the sympathetic trunk, having left the spinal cord at upper lumbar levels. Bear this in mind when considering the effects of spinal injuries.

 Now visit **www.wileyessential.com/humandevelopment** to test yourself on this chapter.

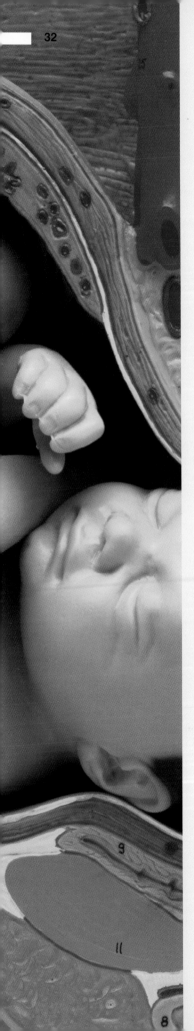

CHAPTER 4
Fertilisation

Sam Webster

Case

A 24-year-old woman, Miss Cooper, arrives at the accident and emergency department with severe lower abdominal pain and cramps, and nausea. The previous day Miss Cooper had noticed some spotting of blood vaginally. Her last menstrual period was approximately 6 weeks ago. She has not experienced this pain before and has not previously had a sexually transmitted disease. Her menstrual cycle is usually around 28 days long. Miss Cooper is in a long-term relationship with her boyfriend, but they have not been trying to conceive.

Learning outcomes

- You should be able to describe the normal movement of gametes required for fertilisation to occur, the location of fertilisation and ectopic pregnancy.

- You should be able to describe the process of fertilisation in terms of sperm meeting with ovum and combining genetic material.

Essential Human Development, First Edition. Edited by Samuel Webster, Geraint Morris and Euan Kevelighan

Anatomy

Ovulation occurs around 2 weeks before menstruation begins and the secondary oocyte (or ovum) released from the ovary is collected by the fimbriae at the opening of the uterine tube. If the ovum meets a spermatozoon within 24 hours it has a chance of becoming fertilised.

Spermatozoa are passed from the epididymis of each testis into the ductus deferens, and propelled by peristaltic contraction to the ampulla of the ductus. The seminal vesicles add their secretions to the spermatozoa and the fluid is pushed into the ejaculatory ducts and urethra within the prostate gland. The prostate gland adds prostatic fluid and the semen is pushed out through the urethra by ejaculation.

The ovum is moved towards the ampulla as spermatozoa deposited in the vagina find their way through the cervix and uterus towards the uterine tube. It is likely that spermatozoa can survive for up to 5 days in the female reproductive system, giving a longer window of opportunity for fertilisation than the 24-hour viability of the ovum would suggest. Unprotected sex days before ovulation may result in fertilisation.

Cell biology

Spermatozoa released into the female reproductive tract enter a final stage of maturation called capacitation. Mixing with the secretions of the glands of the male reproductive system, and probably in response to cues within the vagina, some of the glycoproteins and proteins of the spermatozoa's acrosomes are shed. The spermatozoa become hyperactive.

The ovum is surrounded by a layer of cumulus cells (the corona radiata) and a successful spermatozoon must break through this remnant of the follicle to reach the oocyte itself. The first layer of the oocyte that the spermatozoon meets is the zona pellucida (Figure 4.1), and the first spermatozoon to come into contact with this triggers an acrosome reaction.

The zona pellucida surrounds the plasma membrane of the ovum, and has functions during oogenesis, fertilisation and the early development of the blastocyst. There are a number of glycoproteins on its surface, and zona glycoprotein 3 (ZP3) is responsible for binding to proteins on the surface of capacitated spermatozoa in mammals. This mechanism allows for species-specific fertilisation only, and initiates the acrosome reaction.

The acrosomal cap of the head of the spermatozoon contains enzymes, such as hyaluronidase and acrosin. A small region of the ovum's plasma membrane is digested and penetrated at the binding point of the spermatozoon and the plasma membrane of the spermatozoon is modified and blended with that of the ovum. The contents of the head of the spermatozoon begin to enter the ovum.

This is the start of the process of fertilisation, and usually occurs within a uterine tube. Fertilisation takes around 24 hours to complete, so the notion of a definitive point in time of fertilisation is inappropriate.

As the head of the spermatozoon enters, the contents of cortical granules residing just beneath the surface of the plasma membrane of the ovum are released by exocytosis, causing the entire zona pellucida to alter the nature of its ZP2 and ZP3 binding proteins. As a result of this cortical reaction no other spermatozoa are able to bind with the ovum. Polyspermic fertilisation of an ovum is not viable.

The ovum at this stage is a secondary oocyte (see Chapter 1), paused partway through meiosis II. With the addition of the spermatozoon the cell is triggered to continue meiosis, splitting into two new cells as would be expected. One of the cells formed is termed the second polar body, and is merely a small sphere of plasma membrane, little cytoplasm and a haploid set of chromosomes (Figure 4.2).

🔍 Case box 4.1 Ectopic pregnancy

Fertilisation typically occurs within the uterine tube and the cells continue into the uterus to implant into the uterine wall. Sometimes this doesn't happen and implantation occurs somewhere else, such as the wall of the uterine tube. An ectopic pregnancy like this is not viable, can be life threatening and is often a medical emergency when symptoms present. If a tubal ectopic pregnancy is not removed it may lead to the death of the mother. An ectopic pregnancy may also occur in the cervix, the abdomen or an ovary. Ectopic pregnancy occurs at a rate of 11 per 1000 pregnancies.

The increasing size of the embryo is a primary danger with an ectopic pregnancy, but the invasion of the embryo and its supporting tissues into maternal organs poses a high risk of damaging vascular structures and causing internal haemorrhage. Early diagnosis and surgical intervention is important in reducing maternal mortality, although some ectopic pregnancies may end in miscarriage and resolve themselves.

Sometimes the mother may not yet realise she is pregnant as symptoms commonly develop between 4 and 8 weeks after the start of the last menstrual period. Symptoms include lower abdominal pain and vaginal bleeding, and may develop as further abdominal pain, pelvic pain, shoulder and lower back pain, cramping and pelvic tenderness. Symptoms may be similar to appendicitis, pelvic inflammatory disease and other urinary and pelvic disorders.

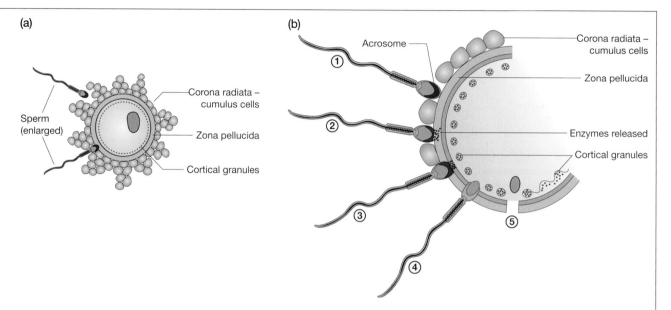

(a)

Sperm
(enlarged)

Corona radiata –
cumulus cells

Zona pellucida

Cortical granules

(b)

Acrosome

Corona radiata –
cumulus cells

Zona pellucida

Enzymes released

Cortical granules

Figure 4.1 Spermatozoon passing through cumulus cells and meeting zona pellucida. (Source: S. Webster and R. de Wreede (2012) *Embryology at a Glance*. Reproduced with permission of John Wiley & Sons, Ltd.)

The polar body is a discarded by-product of the process and the ovum becomes the definitive oocyte, maintaining most of its size.

The ovum now contains the DNA of the spermatozoon as the male pronucleus and the DNA of the ovum as the female pronucleus. The two haploid pronuclei shed their nuclear membranes, their DNA is duplicated and packed into condensed chromosomes, and maternal and paternal chromosomes are aligned at the cell's equator.

This cell represents a new, genetically unique individual with DNA from two parents and alleles mixed randomly during the homologous recombination of chromosomes in meiosis I of gamete formation (see Chapter 1). This is of key significance to sexual reproduction.

The cell is now a zygote, and has a diploid number of chromosomes (2*n*). The spermatozoon brought either an X or a Y 23rd sex chromosome, and the oocyte contained an X 23rd sex chromosome. An XY pair will produce a male embryo, and an XX pair will produce a female embryo.

Sister chromatids from each chromosome are pulled to opposite ends of the cell, mitosis continues and the cell is split into two. The zygote has begun to divide.

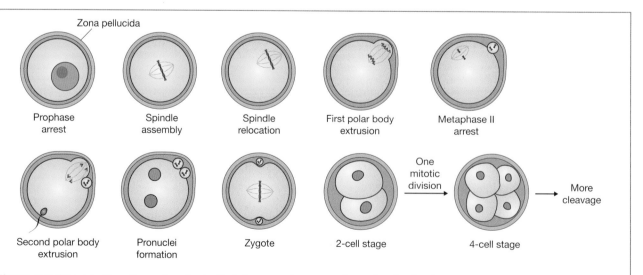

Zona pellucida

Prophase
arrest

Spindle
assembly

Spindle
relocation

First polar body
extrusion

Metaphase II
arrest

Second polar body
extrusion

Pronuclei
formation

Zygote

2-cell stage

One
mitotic
division

4-cell stage

More
cleavage

Figure 4.2 The continuation of meiosis II giving a mature oocyte and polar body; maternal and paternal DNAs meet, are duplicated and form a diploid cell: the zygote.

Case box 4.2 Timings

It is difficult to measure the date of ovulation in humans, although changing levels of luteinising hormone (LH) and follicle-stimulating hormone preceding ovulation can be good predictors (see Chapter 2). The date of the start of the last menstrual period is often recorded, and can be used to estimate the stage of gestation. The length of the menstrual cycle is variable but is on average 28 days. The second part of the cycle is most reliable in length, averaging 14 days between ovulation and the onset of menstruation. Nonetheless, given the variable nature of biology,

estimating the length of gestation as 40 weeks from the start of the last menstrual period (LMP) gives a fair indication of when birth may be expected (Figure 4.3).

While the length of gestation may be recorded as a number of weeks from the LMP fertilisation occurs around 2 weeks after the start of the LMP. Embryologically speaking fertilisation occurs at time point 0, but this date may be noted clinically as occurring at 2 weeks (or with the notation 2/40). There is a 2-week difference between clinical and embryological timings.

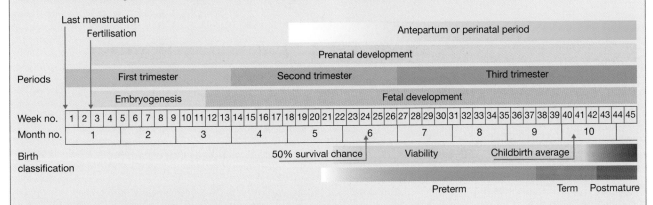

Figure 4.3 An illustration of the timings of the start of the last menstrual period, ovulation and fertilisation, and the gestation trimesters to predicted week of birth. (Source: S. Webster and R. de Wreede (2012) *Embryology at a Glance*. Reproduced with permission of John Wiley & Sons, Ltd.)

Physiology of fertilisation and the endometrium

With the implantation of the blastocyst into the endometrium (see Chapter 5) a number of physiological changes occur to prevent the usual continuation of the menstrual cycle and to maintain conditions appropriate for the development of the embryo and fetus. A number of maternal physiological changes occur in pregnancy to increase the efficiency of fetal growth. These will be discussed in Chapter 8.

The physiology of the menstrual cycle is described in Chapter 2. The ovaries, hypothalamus and pituitary gland respond to hormones and regulate their secretion, causing a monthly cycle of events.

Oestrogen in low plasma concentrations causes the secretion of the gonadotrophins follicle-stimulating hormone (FSH) and luteinising hormone (LH) to be reduced in response to gonadotrophin-releasing hormone (GnRH) released from the hypothalamus. High plasma concentrations of oestrogen cause increased secretions of LH and FSH in response to GnRH.

A high plasma concentration of progesterone when oestrogen is also present inhibits secretion of GnRH by the hypothalamus.

During the follicular phase (the first 2 weeks) of the menstrual cycle levels of plasma oestrogen rise, causing surges in

FSH and LH secretion late in the follicular phase (Figure 4.4). Progesterone levels are low. A few follicles containing oocytes are stimulated to develop, and around 2 weeks into the cycle one follicle becomes ready to be released and its granulosa cells develop LH receptors. The surge in LH causes ovulation, and the oocyte leaves the ovary while the granulosa cells remain.

The granulosa cells that are left in the ovary from that follicle develop further and begin to synthesise high levels of oestrogen and progesterone. The granulosa cells will survive as long as LH is present, even at the low levels that are found during the luteal phase (the second 2 weeks of the menstrual cycle). These cells form the corpus luteum.

The corpus luteum secretes large amounts of progesterone and oestrogen. The high levels of circulating progesterone inhibit GnRH secretion and subsequently also inhibit LH and FSH secretion, preventing the development of any other follicles during the luteal phase. The high levels of progesterone also act upon the cells of the endometrium, which has thickened during the follicular stage in response to oestrogen. During the luteal phase the endometrium develops further, as glands become larger, coiled, and filled with glycogen and enzymes, and the vascularity of the tissue increases as blood vessels lengthen and become coiled. Progesterone inhibits myometrial contractions.

Levels of progesterone peak midway through the luteal phase, but because progesterone inhibits secretion of the LH

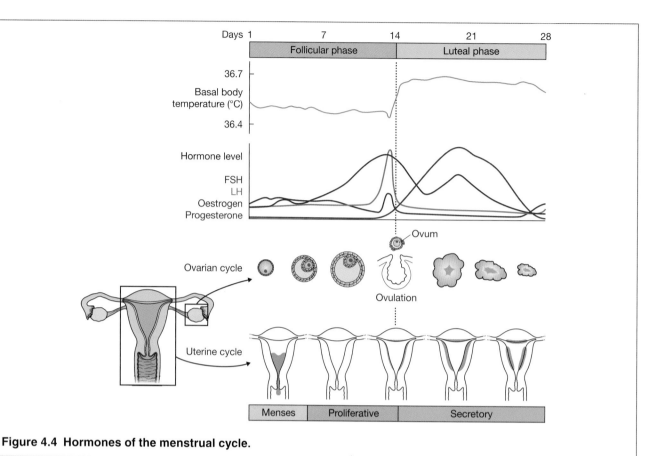

Figure 4.4 Hormones of the menstrual cycle.

that the corpus luteum needs to maintain itself, the corpus luteum begins to degenerate. The adaptations of the uterus to this point have occurred to prepare it for implantation of a blastocyst, and if this does not occur the corpus luteum degrades through a process of luteolysis, and levels of progesterone and oestrogen decrease. The corpus luteum becomes the corpus albicans and continues to exist within the ovary for a short period until it is resorbed.

The low levels of progesterone cause contraction of the blood vessels within the uterus, subsequently causing the superficial layer of the endometrium to disintegrate. The myometrium contracts, and much of the endometrium is lost during menstruation. A deep layer of endometrium persists, which will thicken again during the next cycle. After vascular constriction the arterioles dilate again, resulting in some blood loss.

With the loss of progesterone synthesis by the corpus luteum the hypothalamus increases secretion of GnRH, leading to FSH secretion by the pituitary gland and the start of the development of a new follicle.

If a blastocyst implants into the endometrium during the luteal phase the syncytiotrophoblast that forms (see Chapter 5) secretes human chorionic gonadotrophin (hCG), human placental lactogen (HPL) and progesterone. The corpus luteum will not degenerate in the presence of hCG, and continues to secrete progesterone and oestrogen, maintaining the endometrium and preventing menstruation. LH secretion by the pituitary gland decreases as hCG levels increase.

Summary

Clinical case

Investigations and treatments

Miss Cooper's symptoms could relate to a number of conditions, such as appendicitis, a urinary tract infection or disease, a spontaneous abortion, ovarian torsion, a ruptured ovarian cyst or salpingitis. A pregnancy test is a first step towards narrowing the diagnosis.

Miss Cooper gives a urine sample and agrees to a pregnancy test. A urine hCG (human chorionic gonadotrophin)

dip test is performed. The test returns a positive result, and is followed up by transvaginal ultrasonography that identifies the location of the pregnancy as being in the left uterine tube.

In this case laparoscopic surgery is advised for treatment to remove the ectopic pregnancy, and Miss Cooper is offered a salpingectomy (removal of the uterine tube; the term "salpinx" refers to the uterine tube) to reduce the risk of future ectopic pregnancies as she has no other risk factors for infertility. This information and decision making are discussed with Miss Cooper and her partner in a sensitive manner and they are given evidence-based information about these procedures and future considerations.

Case conclusions

Miss Cooper recovers well from surgery with no complications. Miss Cooper and her partner have some concerns about the ability to conceive in future, but still have no immediate plans to try for a baby.

Key learning points

- The cell biology of fertilisation, of sperm capacitation, the acrosomal reaction and other processes are important in normal fertility. If these processes do not occur then subfertility or infertility will occur. These processes are also important for the success of in vitro fertilisation techniques.

- The menstrual cycle prepares the endometrium of the uterus to receive a fertilised ovum. Implantation of the blastocyst causes physiological changes that maintain the endometrium, ensuring that it will support the development of the embryo.

 Now visit **www.wileyessential.com/humandevelopment** to test yourself on this chapter.

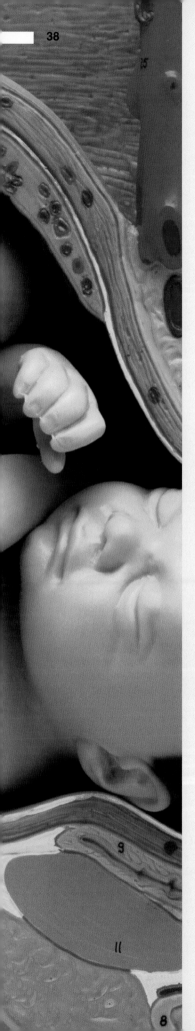

CHAPTER 5
Embryology: zygote to blastocyst

Sam Webster

Case

Mrs Davies attends the antenatal clinic for an ultrasound scan at approximately 12 weeks gestation. Mrs Davies is 26 years old, 166 cm tall, weighs 60 kg and has a BMI of 21.8. This is her first pregnancy after some difficulty conceiving and she was previously diagnosed with polycystic ovaries. Mrs Davies received clomifene citrate for six menstrual cycles to aid ovulation and fertilization. The aims of the scan are to measure the crown to rump length of the fetus to better determine gestational age and predict the estimated date of delivery, to check for major abnormalities, to find out if there is more than one fetus in the uterus, to check the positions of the fetus and the placenta, and to check that the fetus is growing normally. Mrs Davies has two fetuses within her uterus, and both appear to be growing equally and normally. Mr and Mrs Davies would like to know how and why twinning occurs.

Learning outcomes

- You should be able to describe the formation of the blastocyst from the zygote, and the parts of the blastocyst as it continues to develop.
- You should be able to describe the changes that occur in the endometrium in preparation for pregnancy.
- You should be able to describe the process of implantation and how the placenta and extra-embryonic sacs begin to form.

Essential Human Development, First Edition. Edited by Samuel Webster, Geraint Morris and Euan Kevelighan

Zygote

The zygote forms as a result of a spermatozoon combining with an ovum during fertilisation. The zygote is the simplest early form of the new individual and has a complete, diploid set of chromosomes. It begins to become more complex by dividing into new cells that will become more specialised and form structures and shapes.

Around 24 hours after fertilisation the zygote begins this division by mitosis, doubling the number of cells within the mass each time. The structure remains the same size and the cells become smaller with each division. This process is known as cleavage, and the cells of the zygote at this stage are called blastomeres (Figure 5.1).

The cells form a mass called the morula, derived from the Latin word for "mulberry", which this structure now resembles. The morula forms at around the 12-cell stage. The cells of the morula are already communicating with one another by sharing signalling molecules and are becoming organised. The cells of the morula will form not only the embryo but also the supporting structures, including part of the placenta.

The blastomeres in the middle of the morula become the embryoblast, or inner cell mass. These cells will directly form the embryo. The cells on the outside of the morula become the trophoblast or outer cell mass. These cells will become some of the supporting structures for the embryo.

Around 4 days after fertilisation the morula reaches the uterus, leaving the uterine tube. Within the uterus the cells of the trophoblast begin to pull luminal fluid from the uterine cavity into the centre of the morula, creating a fluid-filled space called the blastocoele, or blastocyst cavity. The ball of cells is now known as the blastocyst. The cells of the embryoblast are pushed towards one end of the blastocoele and become called the embryonic pole. The structure is no longer symmetrical.

By 5 days post-fertilisation the blastocyst has still not increased in size and remains within the zona pellucida of the ovum. At this stage the blastocyst squeezes itself out of the zona pellucida by "hatching" from it. By doing so the structure is now able to grow in size, and also to interact with the uterine wall.

Decidualisation

By this time the uterus has completed the proliferative phase of the menstrual cycle and has entered the secretory phase. The endometrium has thickened, coiled arteries within it have lengthened and the endometrial glands are well developed. An implantation window of about 4 days in duration begins 5 days after ovulation, during which time some of the uterine fluid is absorbed and the uterus flattens, bringing the blastocyst closer to the endometrium.

In the later part of the secretory phase the cells of the endometrium begin a process of decidualisation, preparing the tissue for implantation and continuing afterwards as part of the process of implantation and in the development of the placenta. The endometrium is often referred to as the decidua. Local immune cells are also affected and a uterine natural killer cell appears. With increasing levels of progesterone a layer of large, rounded or polygonal decidual cells develops on the endometrial surface from stromal fibroblasts, and they produce laminin and fibronectin, and accumulate glycogen. They secrete vascular endothelial growth factor (VEGF) and synthesise metalloproteinases. VEGF further encourages new blood capillary growth in the endometrium by angiogenesis.

> ### Clinical notes 5.1 Intrauterine contraceptive devices
>
> Devices implanted within the uterus can be used to prevent fertilisation. Copper is used as a localised spermicide, and devices that release a regulated dose of a progestogen hormone such as levonorgestrel will act locally in a paracrine manner to prevent fertilisation. This occurs through limiting endometrial development, thickening cervical mucus, reducing the lifespan of spermatozoa within the uterus and in some cases inhibiting ovulation. Hormonal intrauterine devices (IUDs) are also effective at reducing menstrual bleeding. They are a common, effective method of reversible contraception but have a limited lifespan and need to be replaced every 3–5 years.

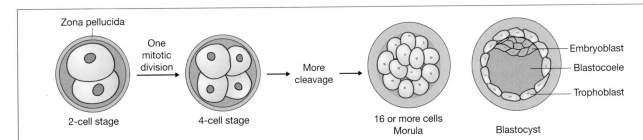

Figure 5.1 The zygote becomes a morula and then a blastocyst. (Source: S. Webster and R. de Wreede (2012) *Embryology at a Glance*. Reproduced with permission of John Wiley & Sons, Ltd.)

The blastocyst typically implants into the superior part of the uterus on either the anterior or posterior walls. The trophoblast cells contact the decidua, aided by the fibronectin and laminin on the surface of the decidua. This is the apposition phase. If the blastocyst does not initially adhere with the embryoblast cells closest to the decidua the blastocyst rotates until it is aligned in this way. Adhesion follows and the cells of the blastocyst begin to communicate with the cells of the decidua, beginning invasion of the uterine epithelium by the blastocyst's trophoblast cells.

Implantation usually begins by day 8 post-fertilisation. During implantation the cells of the embryoblast will form more complex shapes (see Chapter 7) at the same time as the cells of the trophoblast combine with the cells of the uterus to begin to construct supporting structures.

Implantation

The embryoblast differentiates into two flattened layers of cells lying on top of one another. This is the bilaminar disc, and the hypoblast layer is adjacent to the blastocyst cavity. A new cavity, the amniotic cavity, forms next to the epiblast layer (Figure 5.2). The cells of the epiblast will become the embryo, and the cells of the hypoblast will become extra-embryonic membranes such as the chorion and the yolk sac.

To this point the blastocyst has relied on the energy stored within its cells and nutrients within the uterine fluid. For it to grow it needs to get nutrients from the maternal blood, which it does by developing the placenta.

The cells of the trophoblast invade into the decidua and form two layers of cells: an inner cytotrophoblast layer and an outer syncytiotrophoblast layer. The cytotrophoblast cells are typical mononuclear cells, but the syncytiotrophoblast forms by groups of cells combining and losing parts of their plasma membranes. They become large, multinucleated cells. A similar process occurs during the development of skeletal muscle,

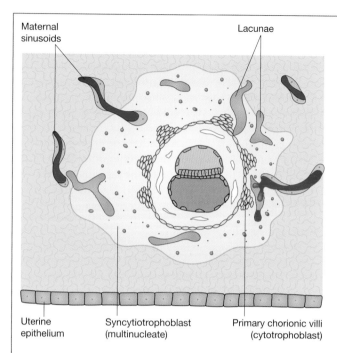

Figure 5.3 The syncytiotrophoblast expands into the maternal endometrium, modifying and eroding blood vessels that will fill the lacunae of the syncytiotrophoblast with blood. The cytotrophoblast extends cells into this and will receive blood vessels of the embryo in the future, laying the foundations of the placenta. (Source: S. Webster and R. de Wreede (2012) *Embryology at a Glance*. Reproduced with permission of John Wiley & Sons, Ltd.)

the cells of which are also multinucleated. The syncytiotrophoblast cells continue to penetrate into the endometrium.

The blastocyst becomes embedded within the endometrium, surrounded by the syncytiotrophoblast (Figure 5.3). The uterine epithelium closes over the entrance made by the blastocyst and at this stage a small "implantation bleed" may occur. Although blood loss is lighter than during the menstrual phase the timing of this bleed may coincide with the date of the expected start of the menstrual period. The mother may not yet realise that she is pregnant and note this as the start of a normal menstrual cycle. When using the date of her last menstrual period to predict gestational age and the estimated date of delivery this bleeding would make predictions 4 weeks late.

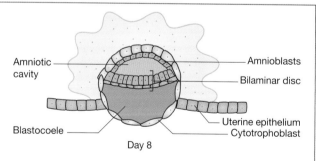

Figure 5.2 Implantation of the blastocyst into the endometrium. The embryoblast has formed a bilaminar disc of epiblast and hypoblast layers. The trophoblast develops cytotrophoblast and syncytiotrophoblast layers. (Source: S. Webster and R. de Wreede (2012) *Embryology at a Glance*. Reproduced with permission of John Wiley & Sons, Ltd.)

 Clinical notes 5.2 Miscarriage

It is thought that abnormalities in normal blastocyst development are common, and that most blastocysts do not implant into the uterus, showing no signs of pregnancy. The abnormalities are often genetic or chromosomal disorders.

An ultrasonography scan to measure the length of the fetus in the first 3 months of pregnancy will limit this error.

Placenta

Lacunae form within the syncytiotrophoblast as it grows inside the endometrium. It comes into contact with maternal endometrial blood vessels, which it erodes causing the lacunar spaces to fill with blood (known as sinusoids). With time the sinusoids will eventually all become interconnected, forming a single intervillous space lined by the syncytiotrophoblast. Cells of the cytotrophoblast modify the structures of maternal spiral arteries as they are recruited to the sinusoids, causing them to lose their smooth muscle layers.

Clumps of cells of the cytotrophoblast push into the syncytiotrophoblast forming primary trophoblast villi. More cells, either from the cytotrophoblast or the bilaminar disc, push into the villi forming hollow, tubular villi (the secondary villi). These extend into the maternal sinusoids and by the end of the third week capillaries form within the villi that will connect with the circulatory system of the embryo as it develops. These are now tertiary villi, and a system placing the blood of the embryo adjacent to the blood of the mother is forming. The cells that formed the villi disappear and the two circulatory systems are separated by the very thin remnant of the syncytiotrophoblast, allowing the exchange of gases, nutrients, waste metabolites, hormones and antibodies. More villi grow from the tertiary villi increasing the surface area of the structure.

Sacs of the embryo

An amniotic cavity forms within the blastocyst between the epiblast layer of the disc and the cytotrophoblast, lined with a thin epithelial layer of amniotic cells. The space on the other side of the bilaminar disc is the primitive yolk sac, or exocoelomic cavity, and is lined by an exocoelomic membrane probably created by cells from the hypoblast.

Between the amnion, exocoelomic membrane and the trophoblast a thickening of cells develops that becomes extra-embryonic mesoderm (see Figure 5.3). Cavities form within the extra-embryonic mesoderm, enlarge and join up.

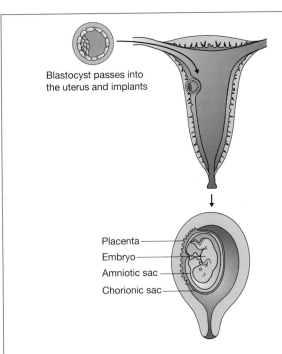

Figure 5.4. The embryo is surrounded by an amniotic sac and a chorionic sac. (Source: S. Webster and R. de Wreede (2012) *Embryology at a Glance*. Reproduced with permission of John Wiley & Sons, Ltd.)

The new, confluent cavity is the extra-embryonic coelom, and it leaves the mesoderm in two layers, an outer extra-embryonic somatic mesoderm layer lining the trophoblast and an inner extra-embryonic splanchnic mesoderm layer covering the yolk sac. The extra-embryonic somatic mesoderm combines with the trophoblast layers to become the chorion, the sac that envelops the fetus and separates her from the mother. The amniotic cavity will become the amniotic sac when the embryo folds and begins to develop shape (Figure 5.4).

As the trophoblast enlarges and invades the endometrium, the bilaminar disc of the embryo, the amniotic cavity and the yolk sac do not grow, but remain attached to the trophoblast by a connecting stalk that extend across the extra-embryonic coelom.

 Clinical notes 5.3 Twins

If two ova are released at ovulation and both are fertilised by different spermatozoa two blastocysts will implant into the uterus. The two fetuses will be genetically distinct from one another and the babies born will be non-identical twins, also known as dizygotic or fraternal twins. Each fetus will have its own amniotic sac, chorionic sac and placenta. The two placentas may be close enough to one another to merge, creating a potential for a link between the two circulatory systems.

It is also possible for the zygote to split into two, forming twin fetuses that are genetically identical. The cell mass of the embryoblast divides into two groups of cells. The babies born will be monozygotic, or identical twins. The stage at which the splitting of the zygote occurs affects the development of the supporting structures tat form with the embryo.

While dizygotic twins are dichorionic, monozygotic twins often share a placenta (they are monochorionic) but have separate amniotic sacs. This indicates that the blastocyst split sometime between 4 and 8 days after fertilisation. If splitting of the blastocyst occurs later than this, the fetuses will share a single amniotic sac too. The later the splitting occurs the greater the risk of failure to develop normally. Dizygotic twins have the lowest mortality risk. The risk of conjoined twins forming increases significantly if the blastocyst splits later than 12 days after fertilisation.

When monozygotic twins share a placenta the blood perfusion is commonly well balanced to each. Sometimes one twin receives a greater blood supply than the other leading to improved growth of one twin and restricted growth of the other.

Monozygotic twins are less common than dizygotic twins and both are more common if assisted reproduction techniques are used. Clomid (a brand name for clomifene citrate), for example, is a drug that blocks oestrogen receptors causing the pituitary gland to secrete more follicle-stimulating hormone (FSH). As a result more follicles mature in the ovary to be released, improving the chance of fertilisation.

Summary

Clinical case

Investigations and treatments

Multiple pregnancy is linked to increased risks of complications for mothers and babies, and needs more support and monitoring. At the first trimester ultrasound scan the chronicity of the fetuses should be determined by the number of placental masses or the shapes of the chorionic membrane to placental junction (described as a λ sign in dichorionic twins and a T sign in monochorionic twins) and the thickness of the membranes.

The growth of the fetuses should be monitored and compared by ultrasound scan from 20 weeks every 4 weeks to look for intrauterine growth restriction of either fetus. There is a higher incidence of anaemia in mothers with multiple pregnancies, and a full blood count should be performed at 20–24 weeks. Mrs Davies' twins are dichorionic with no obvious fetal abnormalities and both have biparietal diameters (the transverse diameter of the head) of 47 mm at 20 weeks, which is comparable to that of a typical singleton pregnancy. Mrs Davies is mildly anaemic with Hb of 10 g/dL.

The parents should be informed of the chance of premature labour and the risks, signs and symptoms, and the possible use of corticosteroids to aid fetal lung development in this case. Methods of delivering the twins should also be discussed.

Case conclusions

At 34 weeks Mrs Davies develops intermittent abdominal pain and is admitted with a diagnosis of preterm labour. She is given a tocolytic and corticosteroids, and labour is delayed. The presenting fetus is in a breech position so the twins are delivered by caesarean section 36 hours after admission. Twin 1 has an Apgar score of 7 and weighs 2.1 kg, and twin 2 has an Apgar score of 6 and weighs 1.9 kg. The twins are non-identical (dizygotic) as suggested by the ultrasound scan. Both twins receive continuous positive airway pressure (CPAP) after birth and are transferred to the neonatal intensive care unit (NICU). Mrs Davies recovers in the labour ward and visits the twins as soon as she is able. She leaves hospital 4 days after surgery and returns to NICU daily. The twins are cared for in NICU and progress well, leaving 2 weeks after birth.

Key learning points

- The zygote is the simplest form of the new organism and divides repeatedly to form a multicellular morula. From this it becomes a blastocyst, the innermost cells of which will become the embryo and the outer cells will contribute to the placenta.
- The phases of the menstrual cycle serve to prepare the endometrium of the uterus for implantation of the blastocyst. Decidualisation is the final step. If a blastocyst is present and implants the endometrium will persist and be further adapted to support the embryo. If there is no blastocyst the endometrium will be lost with menstruation.

 Now visit **www.wileyessential.com/humandevelopment** to test yourself on this chapter.

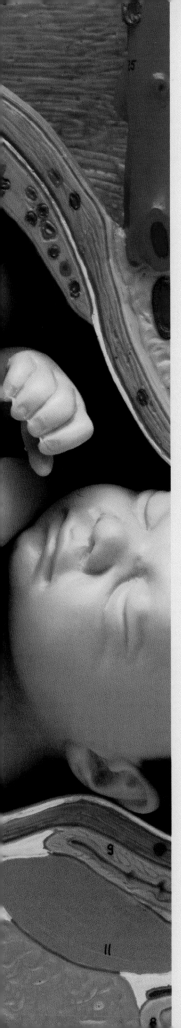

CHAPTER 6
Embryonic stem cells

Sam Webster

Case

Anna is 15 years old and has been feeling easily tired for a few months. She complains of occasional breathlessness and aching joints. Her parents comment that Anna has been unusually pale and generally unwell for some time, with regular minor illnesses such as coughs and colds that take longer than usual to clear. They are also worried about her low weight and some enlarged lymph nodes in Anna's neck. Anna has also suffered from some nosebleeds in recent months and bruises easily, although her parents had ascribed that to an effect of her pale skin.

Upon examination Anna has enlarged lymph nodes in her upper neck and axilla, and splenomegaly. An urgent blood count, erythrocyte sedimentation rate (ESR) and C-reactive protein analyses are requested.

Learning outcomes

- You should be able to describe what stem cells are and how they may be used in medicine.
- You should be able to introduce the main arguments for and against the use of embryonic stem cells in medicine.

Essential Human Development, First Edition. Edited by Samuel Webster, Geraint Morris and Euan Kevelighan
© 2018 John Wiley & Sons, Ltd. Published 2018 by John Wiley & Sons, Ltd.

Embryonic stem cells

During the very early stages of embryonic development the morula is made up of only a few cells. At its earliest stages any cell removed from the morula would have the potential to form any adult cell type if directed to differentiate appropriately (Figure 6.1). These cells are described as totipotent and can develop into cells of the embryoblast (inner cell mass) or the trophoblast, and subsequently cells of the embryo or cells of the cytotrophoblast or syncytiotrophoblast (see Chapter 5).

With the formation of the blastocyst the cells begin to become specialised, and cells of the embryoblast are described as pluripotent. These embryonic stem cells are capable of differentiating into cells of any of the three germ layers (ectoderm, mesoderm or endoderm).

In adult tissues some cells are able to develop into a restricted range of differentiated cells. These stem cells exist as pools of dividing cells that contribute to a cell population replacing those that are lost normally. Haematopoietic stem cells are an example of this type of cell that may be described as multipotent. They can form erythrocytes, reticulocytes, lymphocytes, macrophages, granulocytes and megakaryocytes naturally, but will not normally become cells of other adult tissue types.

Most adult tissues are primarily composed of terminally differentiated cells that are mitotically stable. Generally speaking, when they proliferate their daughter cells are of the same differentiated phenotype. For example, a fat cell will divide and only produce more fat cells.

Stem cells are important in replacing cells that are lost through normal bodily functions, such as keratinocytes from the surface of the skin's epidermis (Figure 6.2), epithelial cells lining the gut, red blood cells that have a limited life span, and satellite cells in skeletal muscle. Usage of the terms "progenitor" and "stem cell" often overlaps, but a progenitor cell can

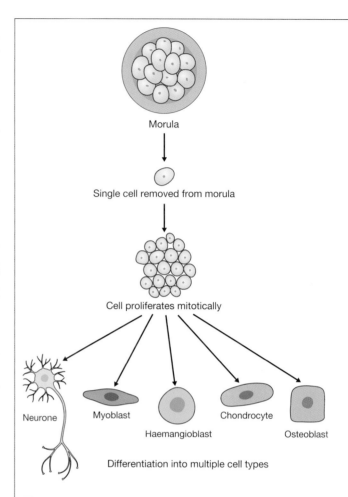

Figure 6.1. Illustration of a cell being removed from a morula, and then proliferating and differentiating into a range of different adult cell types.

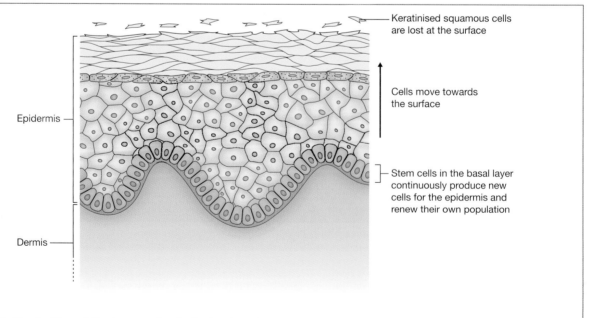

Figure 6.2. Illustration of the layers of cells in the dermis and epidermis.

be considered a cell that will normally only form one cell type, whereas an adult stem cell is able to produce a small range of different cell types. The primary function of both is to replace lost cells, and they are relatively inactive until required to produce new cells. Stem cells in the embryo form the complex tissues of the body and create the different cell types involved, but adult stem cells maintain those tissues.

Stem cells in medicine

With disease or injury tissues often suffer damage that the natural healing processes of the body are unable to repair. For example, severed nerves leave structures without innervation, causing sensory loss or muscular impairment. As nerves are made up primarily of the long axons of neurones the severance of these axons means that much of each cell remains intact but no longer reaches its target structures. There is no way for the neurones to reattach the severed ends of the axons appropriately (and tens of thousands may have been cut at once) and no way for the neurone to extend new axons out to the original targets. The damage is permanent and can cause significant quality of life changes. Severing the spinal cord is a similar issue.

Could embryonic stem cells be used in nerve regeneration? In fact, there are a number of processes that occur after nerve injury to inhibit regeneration. Work with embryonic stem cells in rats and mice suggests that stem cells aid nerve regeneration when directed appropriately (Figure 6.3).

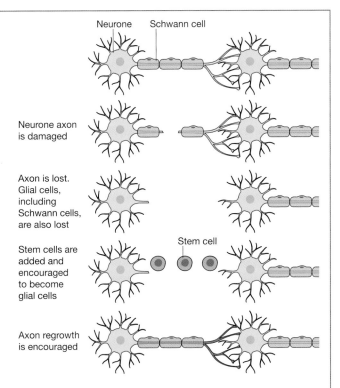

Figure 6.3. Illustration of a stem cell graft to a damaged peripheral nerve, stem cells differentiating to Schwann cells and encouraging axons to migrate.

In the central nervous system conditions such as Parkinson's disease have also attracted research into therapies using stem cells. Parkinson's is a progressive, degenerative disease, and neurones of the substantia nigra within the brain die for somewhat unclear reasons. Normally these neurones secrete dopamine and regulate other nerves involved in movement. With the loss of these neurones minor tremors appear in the patient's movements, followed by rigidity and a difficulty in initiating movements. Implanting stem cells into this region of the brain and encouraging them to differentiate appropriately is seen as a potential treatment for a debilitating disease in ageing populations and is an area of embryonic stem cell research.

Age-related macular degeneration is the most common cause of loss of vision in people over 50. A gradual loss of central vision occurs with breakdown of the retinal pigment epithelium (RPE), a layer of cells that nourish, support and protect the photoreceptors of the macula. Loss of cells within the macula follows. One form of the condition can be treated to slow or halt disease progression, but in most cases the loss of central vision is irreversible. Current research using embryonic stem cells is engineering replacement sheets of RPE and photoreceptors that are intended for delivery into the eye.

These are a few examples of how embryonic stem cells are being studied with the aim of treating currently incurable diseases. There are many more.

Embryonic stem cells are also being used in cancer research, as many of the abilities of tumour cells are similar to those of embryonic stem cells, such as immortality. Also, many tumours may be caused by stem cells that do not remain within the normal checks of the cell cycle and enter uncontrolled proliferation. It is likely that some cancer treatments are effective at destroying most of the cancer cells but fail to kill cancer stem cells. This may explain the recurrence of some cancers after many disease-free years. For these reasons stem cells are a target of cancer research, to better understand how cancers begin and how to treat them more effectively.

Embryonic stem cells can be taken from the zygote, morula or blastocyst stages of development, and could be taken from surplus embryos created by in vitro fertilisation (IVF) methods, which will not be implanted into the uterus. Embryonic stem cells can also be taken from existing cell lines maintained in laboratories.

Induced pluripotent stem cells (iPSCs) are adult cells taken from a range of tissues that have been genetically modified to act as pluripotent stem cells using genetic vectors injected into the cells by viruses. These cells act like embryonic stem cells, express typical stem cell markers and can be directed to differentiate into cell types of all three germ layers, but it is unclear if, or how iPSCs might differ from embryonic stem cells. Because of the viral method of modifying these cells they are not regarded as safe for use in humans. Creating iPSCs from a patient's own cells and subsequently using those iPSCs to repair tissues should overcome problems of rejecting grafted tissues from other sources.

Ethical arguments

The ethical debates around using embryonic stem cells focus on a conflict between two contradicting moral ideals: to alleviate human suffering, and to preserve human life.

Embryonic stem cells have the potential to treat currently incurable conditions, but when does life begin, and what is the moral status of the embryo?

There are a number of views on when life begins, and no single view has been accepted definitively. Some viewpoints are associated with religion and the concept of a soul, and some are based upon biological aspects of development. Historically our understanding of when life begins has changed, provoked by changes in our understanding of the biology of development.

Life could be described to begin when a spermatozoon and an ovum combine during fertilisation to form a new, genetically individual zygote. Arguments that support this view include the idea that development is a continual process from this point, and as an infant is a person in development a zygote will become a person and should have the same rights and respect. Arguments against this view are that the zygote needs to implant into the mother's uterus to survive, and will not continue to develop on its own. Many zygotes in nature do not implant and survive to birth, so something that has the potential to become a person should not be treated in the same ways as a person. Spermatozoa and oocytes have the potential to become a new individual but are generally not regarded in the same way. It is also argued that a very simple zygote or blastocyst does not have any of the psychological or emotional aspects that we associate with a person, and should not be treated in the same way.

Does the moral status of an embryo increase as the embryo develops, and are there definitive points in development that we might consider as thresholds? The blastocyst implants into the uterus on day 6. Gastrulation and the formation of the germ layers occur by day 18. There will be a point at which neural activity in the brain can be detected. There is a point at which movement of the fetus begins. There will be a point at which the fetus can survive without support, if born prematurely, for example. The counter argument to that point is that even full-term, newborn babies cannot survive alone. Arguments against a changing moral status with development include the idea that by doing this we are making arbitrary decisions about what qualifies as a person, or what is human. As our understanding of development changes will our definition change? It is arguable that if we are unsure of whether an embryo at a specific stage of development is a human life or not, we should not destroy it.

A further argument follows that we protect life and the freedoms of that life not because of society's point of view but because of the importance to the person involved. Life has a value to the embryo. Conversely, we feel differently about the end of a life depending upon the stage of the life lost. We expect death at the end of a long life. It is likely that more fertilised eggs are lost naturally than are implanted and continue to develop into people. Should we be concerned about using very early embryos in medicine if the loss of embryos is such a common, natural occurrence?

The cells of the zygote have the potential to become a person. Cloning technologies have developed the possibility of taking any somatic cell, and by injecting its nucleus into an ovum, forming an embryo and a cloned animal from that cell. This somatic-cell nuclear transfer (SCNT) technique was used to create Dolly, the cloned sheep. It is hoped that this method may be used to create custom stem cells matched to a patient's cells. It has not been performed with human cells to create a cloned person, but the potential exists. Does this mean that any somatic cell also has the capability to become a person, and should be treated with the same rights that are conferred to an embryonic stem cell? The counter argument says that somatic cells require outside interventions for this to be possible, but this is also true to a lesser extent for the embryo. The blastocyst cannot continue its development without implanting into a uterus and gaining all the support that the mother's tissues provide. Embryos created by IVF techniques need considerable external help to continue their development. Unused embryos created by IVF methods are a current source of embryonic stem cells. If it is impossible to consider trillions of somatic cells in each person with the same moral status as we might apply to the cells of the zygote, does a distinction between these cells exist?

Embryos created specifically for research would be created with the intention of destroying them. Embryos created by IVF procedures have the potential to be implanted into the mother's uterus and to become children. The two purposes are morally distinct. The destruction of surplus embryos after IVF treatment is a foreseeable consequence of procreation by IVF. Is there a moral distinction between the purposes for the creation of the embryos that are destroyed?

While arguments exist for and against the use of embryonic stem cells in medicine, both sides do ascribe a level of respect to the uses of human embryos. Proponents of embryonic stem cell research aim to alleviate human suffering, and generally do not wish to destroy embryos for purposes other than this.

Law

In the UK embryonic stem cell research is permitted subject to a licence from the Human Fertilisation and Embryology Authority (HFEA) for certain purposes, including developing knowledge of the causes of congenital disease, miscarriage, embryonic development and serious disease, and to improve infertility treatments. Across Europe different countries have different regulations relating to the use of embryonic stem cells in research. Most countries permit their use, but do not allow the production of human embryos specifically for research purposes.

In the USA there are no federal restrictions on embryonic stem cell research that is funded privately. New embryonic stem cell lines may not be created using government funding at a federal level, although individual states have passed laws that permit human embryonic stem cell research using state funds. It is permitted to use federal funds in research using approved existing human embryonic stem cell lines. States vary in their restrictions of human embryonic stem cell research, with some states permitting certain activities and others applying more restrictive laws.

Clinical case

Investigations and treatments

The results of Anna's blood tests show an RBC count of 8 g/dL and a leucocyte count of less than 10 000 cells/mm^3. A bone marrow aspirate shows high numbers of leukaemic blast cells. CT scans of her thorax, abdomen and pelvis find no discernible masses. Immunophenotyping confirms the diagnosis of acute B-lymphoblastic leukaemia (ALL) and cytogenetic analysis finds hypoploidy (fewer than 23 pairs of chromosomes).

Anna begins chemotherapy and undergoes induction, consolidation and maintenance phases to kill the leukaemia cells and prevent their return, but 18 months later the disease recurs. Anna repeats the chemotherapy treatment that again kills the ALL cells. Again, 18 months later the disease returns so Anna begins intensive high-dose chemotherapy and radiotherapy treatments to eradicate any cancerous cells, but much of Anna's bone marrow stem cell population is also destroyed. This treatment has a much higher probability of killing all of the cancerous lymphoblasts but for Anna to survive such an intensive treatment she will need a bone marrow stem cell transplant.

Anna's older sister is already on the bone marrow register and has a good tissue type match for Anna. The donor's bone marrow is collected and the bone marrow stem cells are isolated. At a later date they are transplanted into Anna's blood, from which they pass into bone marrow spaces, become embedded and slowly repopulate Anna's haematopoietic stem cell population. Anna is very unwell for a long period and is cared for carefully to avoid infection during this time. She responds to the graft well and there are no signs of rejection.

Case conclusions

It takes some months for Anna to recover from her treatment and regain weight. She recovers fully, and 5 years later remains in remission. Anna has left home, and has a full-time job and an active lifestyle. It is unlikely that she will be able to conceive naturally because of the high-dose chemotherapy treatment, but the bone marrow stem cell transplantation has allowed Anna and her doctors to treat an otherwise fatal disease.

SUMMARY

Key learning points

- Embryonic stem cells have the potential to be directed to form many different cell types, aiding regenerative medicine therapies.

- Embryonic stem cells currently have advantages over adult stem cells but there are ethical dilemmas concerning their use.

 Now visit **www.wileyessential.com/humandevelopment** to test yourself on this chapter.

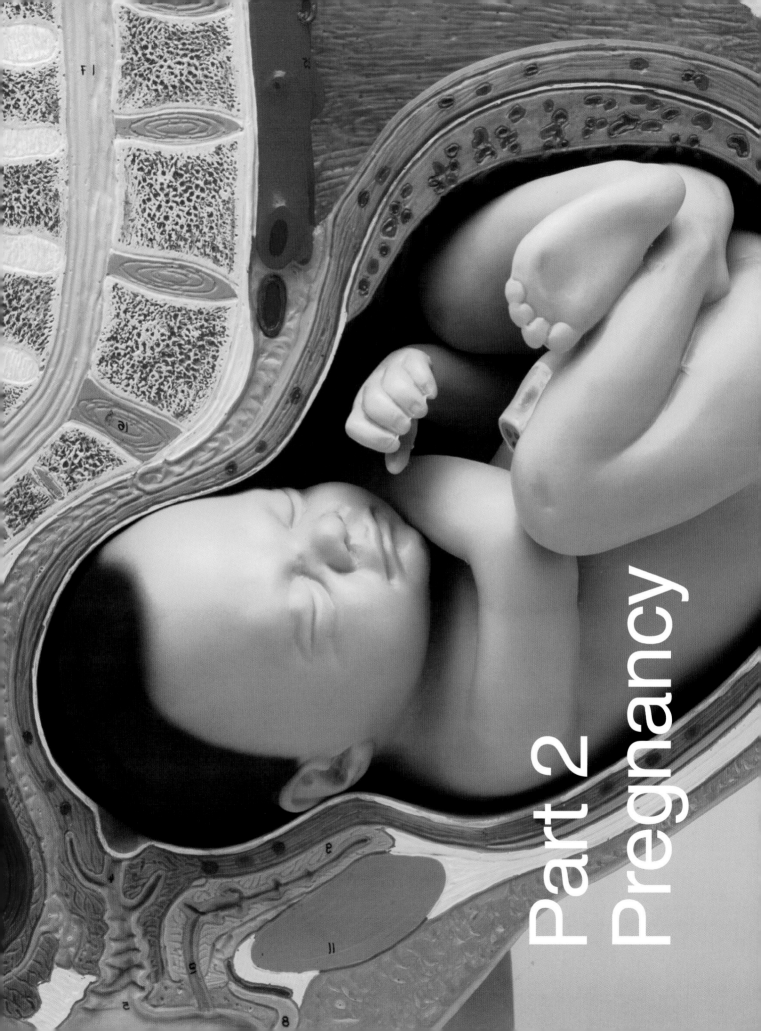

Part 2
Pregnancy

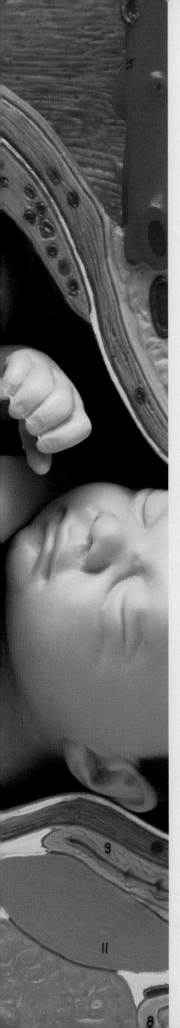

CHAPTER 7
Embryology

Sam Webster

Case

A 20-week antenatal ultrasound scan of a 39-year-old woman, Mrs Kinder, finds an anomaly in the lower back of the fetus. The femur length of the fetus is 32 mm and the biparietal diameter is 50 mm. Both measurements confirm that the fetus is in the 20th week of gestation, and the head size is likely to be normal. A second ultrasound scan is scheduled and confirms the presence of a posterior defect in the sacral vertebrae. The parents are informed of the probable diagnosis and discuss the likely effects upon the baby and available treatments.

Learning outcomes

- You should be able to describe the effects of female reproductive hormones upon organs and tissues during the menstrual cycle and first trimester of pregnancy.

- You should be able to describe how the systems of the body begin to form in the embryo.

Essential Human Development, First Edition. Edited by Samuel Webster, Geraint Morris and Euan Kevelighan
© 2018 John Wiley & Sons, Ltd. Published 2018 by John Wiley & Sons, Ltd.

Embryological development

As the very early embryo passes into the uterus and implants into the endometrium it has already begun to develop shape and form (Figure 7.1). The cells within have been communicating to one another for a few days, and have organised themselves to perform different functions. With time these cells will form all of the tissues and organs of the fetus and parts of the supporting structures that will link with the mother. The embryonic period occurs during the first 8 weeks of development.

Gastrulation

The implanted blastocyst comprises two sheets of cells layered together as epiblast and hypoblast, surrounded by a primitive amniotic cavity on the epiblast side and a yolk sac on the hypoblast side (see Chapter 5). On the 18th day of development the cells of the epiblast layer begin to migrate towards the midline in the caudal half of the sheet, forming a groove as they descend beneath the uppermost layer of cells. They push aside the hypoblast cells beneath and form two new layers. The three layers of the new sheets are the ectoderm, mesoderm and endoderm (Figure 7.2).

The ectoderm will become the outermost layer of the embryo, forming the epidermis of the skin and the nervous system. The endoderm creates epithelial cell layers lining internal surfaces of the body that are exposed to external substances, such as the gastrointestinal tract and the respiratory tracts of the lungs. The cells of the mesoderm contribute to many tissues of the body, including the musculoskeletal, renal, reproductive, cardiovascular and immune systems. Other cells of the blastocyst will contribute to structures that will support embryonic and fetal development such as the placenta.

Embryology of the gastrointestinal system

As the flat sheets of the embryo fold laterally and along its length, and roll up, the yolk sac shrinks and is pulled in. The endoderm layer becomes the innermost tube, and remains connected to the yolk sac via the vitelline duct (or stalk). The epithelium of the gastrointestinal tract and glandular parts of associated organs will develop from cells of the endoderm, and the mesoderm will contribute other parts of these tissues.

The ends of the early gut tube are sealed closed by membranes. The buccopharyngeal membrane at the future mouth breaks down in the fourth week of development, and the cloacal membrane ruptures in the seventh week to create the anal opening.

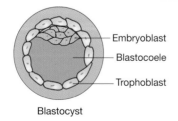

Figure 7.1. The parts of the blastocyst. (Source: S. Webster and R. de Wreede (2012) *Embryology at a Glance*. Reproduced with permission of John Wiley & Sons, Ltd.)

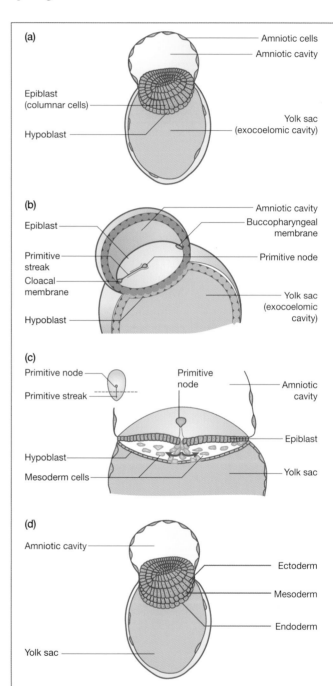

Figure 7.2. Gastrulation. (Source: S. Webster and R. de Wreede (2012) *Embryology at a Glance*. Reproduced with permission of John Wiley & Sons, Ltd.)

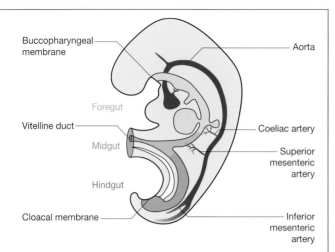

Buccopharyngeal
membrane

Aorta

Foregut

Vitelline duct

Coeliac artery

Midgut

Superior
mesenteric
artery

Hindgut

Cloacal membrane

Inferior
mesenteric
artery

Figure 7.3. Embryonic gut tube. (Source: S. Webster and R. de Wreede (2012) *Embryology at a Glance.* Reproduced with permission of John Wiley & Sons, Ltd.)

The region of the gastrointestinal tract connected to the yolk sac at this early stage is known as the midgut. The region between the mouth and the midgut is the foregut, and the remainder of the tube reaching to the anal opening is the hindgut (Figure 7.3). In the adult anatomy the foregut reaches to the duodenum at the point of the opening of the pancreatic duct and common bile duct. The length between this point and a point two-thirds of the way along the transverse colon is the midgut, and the remainder is the hindgut. As the early gut tube develops three arterial branches grow from the aorta to supply it with blood. The foregut receives the coeliac artery, the midgut receives the superior mesenteric artery, and the hindgut receives the inferior mesenteric artery. Branches of these arteries supply the same adult regions of the gastrointestinal tract and the organs that grow from the embryonic gut tube.

The foregut lengthens as the embryo grows, and the section of tube that forms the oesophagus becomes filled with proliferating epithelial cells. During the fetal period the tube will reopen and become lined with a squamous epithelium, and this process is similar in other lengths of the gastrointestinal tract. If this process fails to occur normally blockages may occur within the infant's bowel.

In the fourth week a section of foregut dilates, with the dorsal edge growing faster than the ventral part. The expanding section of tube rotates, bringing the left side around ventrally. This is the stomach, and the rotation explains the passing of the left vagus nerve to the anterior stomach. The rotation of the stomach pulls around the duodenum forming its characteristic C-shape.

Two buds of tissue grow from the embryonic duodenum in weeks 4 and 5 of development. The dorsal bud is larger than the ventral bud, and with the rotation of the stomach and duodenum both buds are brought together to form the

pancreas. Each bud develops its own duct that opens into the duodenum initially, and as the buds are brought together the ducts typically anastomose giving just one opening. Sometimes both openings persist and an accessory pancreatic duct is found in the adult. Exocrine and endocrine cells differentiate from endodermal cells, and insulin is secreted at 4 months of development.

The gut tube is suspended from the dorsal wall of the embryo by a dorsal mesentery, and at the level of the stomach a ventral mesentery extends to the ventral wall of the embryo too. Around this level the thorax will be separated from the abdominal cavity. The septum transversum is a sheet of mesoderm that will contribute to this by becoming parts of the diaphragm. An epithelial outgrowth pushes into the septum transversum and the cells proliferate, forming an early liver bud. As the liver bud grows it is connected to the duodenum by the bile duct. The gallbladder forms between the liver and the duodenum and is connected to the bile duct. The liver is a large part of the embryo and early fetus and is a major source of haematopoietic cells during the development of the cardiovascular system.

The midgut lengthens and coils, protruding into the umbilicus in the sixth week as it becomes too large for the abdomen to contain. As the abdominal cavity becomes larger the midgut is drawn back in, and rotates around 270° in an anticlockwise direction when viewed from an anterior perspective. This rotation drops the caecum into the lower right quadrant of the abdomen and sets up the anatomy of the large intestine "framing" the small intestine.

The hindgut ends in a cloacal cavity. The cloaca will form part of the bladder and urethra, as well as the rectum and anal canal. A urorectal septum of mesoderm grows within the cloaca during weeks 4 to 7, splitting the ventral and dorsal parts of the cloaca. When the septum reaches the cloacal membrane two spaces are formed: the urogenital sinus and the anorectal canal. The cloacal membrane ruptures in the seventh week. In this region the ectoderm-derived tissue covering the embryo meets the endoderm-derived lining of the gut tube, and the adult vasculature reflects this. The cephalic part of the anal canal is supplied with blood by branches from the inferior mesenteric artery, whereas the caudal part of the anal canal receives blood from branches of the internal iliac arteries.

Neuroembryology

With gastrulation and the formation of the germ layers a rod of cells formsw in the midline of the tissue sheets. This notochord signals to the cells of the overlying ectoderm, causing a thickened neural plate to form that is wider cranially. The neural plate dips inwards in the middle along its length, forming a neural groove. As the groove becomes deeper the dorsal parts of the neural folds are brought together and meet. The neural tube sinks beneath the ectoderm, and neural crest cells migrate away through the mesoderm (Figure 7.4). The neural tube will become the spinal cord along its length and the brain

(a)   **(b)**   **(c)** Neural crest cells migrate

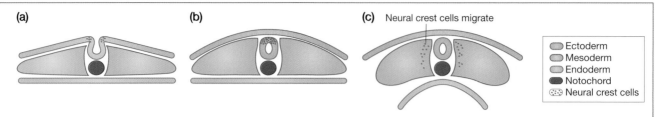

Ectoderm
Mesoderm
Endoderm
Notochord
Neural crest cells

Figure 7.4. Neurulation. (Source: S. Webster and R. de Wreede (2012) *Embryology at a Glance*. Reproduced with permission of John Wiley & Sons, Ltd.)

at its cephalic end. The neural crest cells will contribute to a wide range of tissues, including neurones of the peripheral nervous system.

The neural tube forms a closed tube initially in a central region along its length, leaving both ends open as neuropores. The closing of the neural tube extends cranially and caudally, eventually closing the neuropores. If the neural tube does not close normally the central nervous system will not develop normally. If the cranial neuropore does not close the brain will not develop, causing anencephaly. If the caudal neuropore fails to close the development of the spinal cord, its meninges, vertebral bones and peripheral nerves may be affected. In spina bifida occulta a small gap may be present in a vertebral bone in the L5–S1 region, and the change in signalling may be reflected by an unusual patch of dark hair on the back in this region. In spina bifida meningocoele a gap within and between vertebrae may be so large as to allow external protrusion of the meninges and spinal cord or spinal nerves (spina bifida meningomyelcoele) affecting innervation of the lower limbs and bladder and bowel continence.

Cardiovascular embryology

Embryonic cardiovascular cells appear in the mesoderm around the neural plate at the cranial end of the early embryo by vasculogenesis. Angioblasts collect together in the third week of development to form blood islands. As the embryo folds the blood islands at the cranial end are brought together to form a curved tube lined with endothelial cells. Myoblasts surround the tube, forming an early heart tube. A pair of dorsal aortae extend cranially.

In the fourth week the heart tube folds, bringing the early, single ventricle ventrally and taking the atrium dorsally. Veins draining into the heart at the sinus venosus contribute to the future right atrium. An initially paired, symmetrical venous system becomes right-sided within the fetus as veins on the left side degenerate and veins on the right side predominate, forming the inferior vena cava and superior vena cava.

The heart tube is divided into four chambers, splitting the original single flow route into two, each with its own atrium and ventricle (Figure 7.5). A number of processes occur during

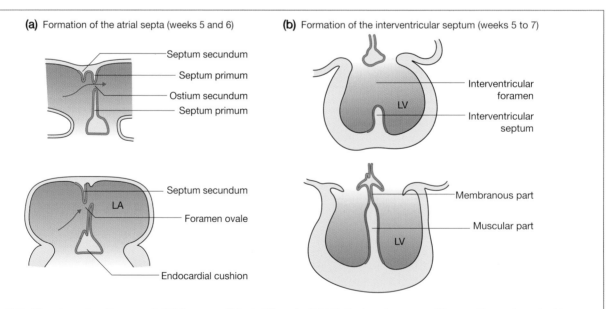

(a) Formation of the atrial septa (weeks 5 and 6)

Septum secundum
Septum primum
Ostium secundum
Septum primum

Septum secundum
LA
Foramen ovale

Endocardial cushion

(b) Formation of the interventricular septum (weeks 5 to 7)

LV
Interventricular foramen
Interventricular septum

Membranous part
Muscular part
LV

Figure 7.5. Heart septa. (Source: S. Webster and R. de Wreede (2012) *Embryology at a Glance*. Reproduced with permission of John Wiley & Sons, Ltd.)

the fifth week simultaneously, creating these divisions. The walls of the single atrioventricular canal thicken, creating two endocardial cushions opposite one another that push inwards, eventually meeting and creating two atrioventricular canals.

A muscular interventricular septum grows from the floor of the single ventricle towards the endocardial cushions, almost dividing the space in two. An interventricular foramen remains. The endocardial cushion extends inferiorly as a membranous part of the interventricular septum, completing the divide and leaving two ventricles.

In the roof of the atrium a curved sheet of tissue grows downwards as the septum primum, working towards the endocardial cushion. Before it reaches and joins with the endocardial cushion a section of the septum primum degenerates, and a hole (the ostium secundum) is formed. In this way the two atria remain connected. A second divider, the septum secundum, also grows from the roof of the atrium to the right of the septum primum. It grows part way towards the endocardial cushion, parallel to the septum primum. The flap valve of the foramen ovale is formed between the two atria, and the higher pressure of blood in the right atrium pushes open the flap of the septum primum and blood flows into the left atrium. If the pressure within the left atrium is higher than the right (as occurs after birth) the flap will be pushed back against the wall of the septum secundum and the valve is closed. Blood can only flow from the right side to the left.

With the atrium and the ventricle divided, the single outflow tract of the conus arteriosus and truncus arteriosus must also be split and connected to the appropriate ventricles. Two helical ridges of tissue appear in the wall of the conotruncal tube and they grow towards one another, splitting the tube in two. The aorta and pulmonary trunk are formed, and the inferior end of the conotruncal septum must meet the muscular interventricular septum in the right way to enable blood from the right ventricle to pass into the pulmonary trunk and blood from the left ventricle to pass into the aorta. The helical nature of the conotruncal septum accounts for the spiralling of the aorta and pulmonary trunk around one another as they ascend in adult anatomy.

Defects in the development of the septa that divide up the heart can occur congenitally, with a failure to correctly divide the primitive ventricle being the most common variant.

During the fetal period the developing lungs have a high resistance to blood flow, and the blood that would pass to the lungs in the newborn is redirected across the heart from the right side to the left side to avoid the lungs. Between the pulmonary trunk and the aorta a ductus arteriosus blood vessel connects the two, allowing blood from the pulmonary trunk to pass directly into the aorta and the systemic circulation, again avoiding the lungs.

Respiratory embryology

The lungs begin to form in the third and fourth weeks of development as a simple bud from the gut tube at the level of the oesophagus. The bud branches and branches again to support

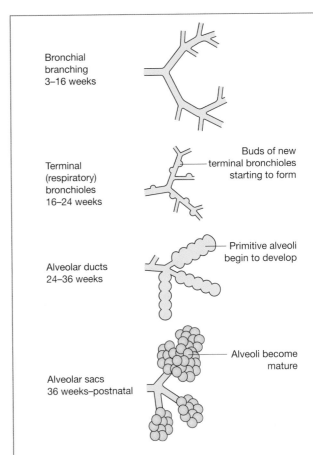

Figure 7.6. The embryonic respiratory tree. (Source: S. Webster and R. de Wreede (2012) *Embryology at a Glance*. Reproduced with permission of John Wiley & Sons, Ltd.)

the two-lobe and three-lobe arrangements of the left and right future lungs. As the respiratory tree is an outgrowth of the gut tube its epithelial lining will also be derived from the endodermal germ layer. Cells of the mesoderm will form other parts.

The first stage of embryonic lung development in weeks 3 to 5 sees the lung bud branch repeatedly (Figure 7.6). From six weeks onwards the branching continues and an extensive network of tubes develops. This stage is known as the pseudoglandular stage as histological sections of the lungs look more like a gland than lung tissue. Lung- and airway-specific cells differentiate creating ciliated epithelial cell-lined bronchi and type II alveolar cells (pneumocytes). Terminal bronchioles are formed by the end of this stage.

The canalicular stage begins in week 17, during which time tubes (canaliculi) extend from the terminal bronchioles and terminal sacs form around them. These are primitive alveoli, and the cells forming their walls become thinner, type I alveolar cells. Capillaries grow into the mesenchyme surrounding the primitive alveoli and the combined factors of the surface area available for gaseous exchange, blood supply and the thickness of the tissue between air and blood are important in determining whether an infant is capable of breathing unaided. Prematurely born infants often need respiratory support because the lungs are not sufficiently developed.

Late in the fetal period from 25 weeks to birth the lungs continue to develop by increasing the number of primitive alveolar sacs, increasing the capillarisation of the alveoli, and increasing the number of type II alveolar cells that produce surfactant – a phospholipoprotein that reduces fluid surface tension and prevents the walls of the alveoli sticking together. This is the saccular stage, and it overlaps with the alveolar stage.

In the final weeks before birth the alveoli increase in diameter and in number, and the type I alveolar cells form thinner alveolar walls. The primitive alveoli become mature alveoli with these changes, and the alveolar stage continues after birth into childhood. There are around 20 to 50 million alveoli in the lungs at birth, and around 400 million in the adult.

Musculoskeletal embryology

Cells of the mesoderm on either side of the midline collect together and clump, creating somitomeres, which become somites from around day 20. The first pair form in the head, and subsequent pairs form, pair by pair, extending towards the tail at a rate of about three pairs per day. The somites are visible on the surface of the embryo's back as paired swellings covered by ectoderm.

A space forms within each somite, and the cells of the somite begin to migrate to form dorsal and ventral groups (Figure 7.7). The cells of the ventral somite form the sclerotome, and will migrate to surround the notochord and neural tube, where they create the vertebral bones, the intervertebral discs, ribs and other connective tissues. The cells of the dorsal somite form a dermomyotome mass that splits into myotome and dermatome groups. The cells of the myotome will differentiate into myoblasts and migrate around

the wall of the embryo to form the skeletal muscle layers of the body wall and limbs. Some cells from the myotome will migrate dorsally a short distance to create the epaxial muscles of the back. Cells of the dermatome will migrate out under the ectoderm and form the dermis and subcutaneous layers of skin.

As cells migrate from somites around the body wall of the developing embryo axons of spinal nerves at the same level as the somite follow the cells, accounting for the dermatome and myotome patterns of innervation and segmentation seen in adult anatomy. The pattern within limbs is disrupted by the fusing of some early muscles, and by the bending and rotation of the limbs about joints.

Splanchnic mesoderm is found within the embryo at sites of organ formation. Smooth muscle, of the gastrointestinal tract for example, and the cardiac muscle of the heart is created by differentiation of splanchnic mesoderm cells.

Urogenital embryology

The development of the renal and reproductive systems is linked, and these systems share structures with the hindgut. Within the intermediate mesoderm, lateral to the aorta, three pairs of kidney structures appear, one after another. The first to form is the pronephros in the third week. This is a vestigial non-functional kidney in the neck of the early embryo that disappears just a week later.

In the fourth week two mesonephroi form attached to mesonephric (or Wolffian) ducts on either side. The mesonephric ducts run along the length of the dorsal embryo to open at the cloaca. Renal corpuscles form within each mesonephros and capillaries pass into the tissue, creating a functional kidney that produces urine from the sixth week onwards, but the whole structure soon starts to degenerate in the 7th to 10th weeks (Figure 7.8).

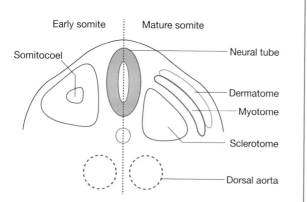

Figure 7.7. The cells of the somite. (Source: S. Webster and R. de Wreede (2012) *Embryology at a Glance*. Reproduced with permission of John Wiley & Sons, Ltd.)

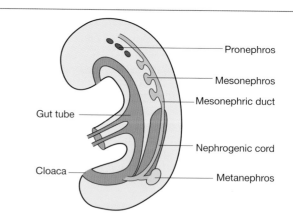

Figure 7.8. The embryonic kidneys. (Source: S. Webster and R. de Wreede (2012) *Embryology at a Glance*. Reproduced with permission of John Wiley & Sons, Ltd.)

The third and final kidney structures that form are the metanephroi. They begin to grow in the fifth week of development, overlapping with the functional existence of the mesonephroi. Each metanephros is also a bud from a mesonephric duct, but at the caudal end of the embryo. The bud induces the surrounding cells of the intermediate mesoderm to form a metanephric cap. The ureteric bud will form the urine collecting system, and the metanephric cap will form the nephrons of the kidney. The metanephros will continue as the adult kidney.

The original location of the metanephroi is very low within the caudal embryo, and as the fetus grows the kidneys ascend from the pelvis to the lumbar region. As the kidneys move, new blood vessels form, linking the kidneys to the aorta and inferior vena cava (or common iliac vessels), and the most inferior vessels degenerate. In some cases the earlier vessels remain, and an adult kidney may have more than one renal artery or vein as a result.

Paramesonephric (or Müllerian) ducts are found parallel and lateral to the mesonephric ducts in the intermediate mesoderm of the embryo (Figure 7.9). Up to week 7 both pairs of ducts exist together, but after this point one pair will degenerate.

In the male embryo the mesonephric ducts continue to develop and the paramesonephric ducts degenerate. In addition to their contributions to the renal system the mesonephric ducts will also create the tubes of the male reproductive system, including the efferent ductules and epididymis of each testis, the ductus (vas) deferens and the ejaculatory duct. The seminal vesicles will grow from the ductus deferens, but the prostate gland will form from the urethra, which it will surround.

The remainder of the testis will develop in the early lumbar region of the embryo, with epithelium covering the posterior wall of the internal abdominal cavity invaginating into the mesoderm to form sex cords, and the mesoderm differentiating into Leydig and Sertoli cells. The sex cords will form the tubes of the testis: the seminiferous tubules and the rete testis. Germ cells migrate into the early gonad region from the extra-embryonic endoderm of the yolk sac following the dorsal mesentery of the hindgut during weeks 5 and 6. By the fourth month of development the germ cells will form spermatogonia within the seminiferous tubules.

Lengths of ligamentous connective tissue (gubernaculum) pass from the inferior pole of each gonad to labioscrotal folds in the pelvis. As the fetus grows each testis is pulled inferiorly through layers of the abdominal wall that will become the inguinal canal to a final position within the scrotum. The adult vasculature and lymphatic drainage reflects this, passing to vessels within the abdomen.

Similar processes occur during formation of the ovaries in the female embryo. The mesonephric ducts degenerate and the paramesonephric ducts extend inferiorly and meet in the midline in the pelvis as a uterovaginal primordium. This structure lies adjacent to the early urogenital sinus as the paramesonephric tubercle and induces the development of two sinovaginal bulbs from the urogenital sinus. The paramesonephric ducts will form the uterine tubes, the uterovaginal primordium will become the uterus and superior part of the vagina, and the sinovaginal bulbs will contribute to inferior parts of the vagina.

The ovaries begin to form in a similar way to the testes, but the sex cords degenerate and form follicles around the germ cells that migrate in. The gubernaculum runs along the same course as in the male fetus but the ovaries descend only as far as the pelvis. The gubernaculum exists in the adult female pelvis as the round and ovarian ligaments.

External genitalia are formed from structures common to both sexes during the indifferent stage between weeks 4 and 7. An anterior genital tubercle develops into either a clitoris or a penis, and labioscrotal swellings become either labia or a scrotum. In the female fetus the urethra and vagina open at the urogenital membrane, but in the male fetus the midline remains intact as a scrotal raphe and a midline raphe of the penis. The urethra continues along the ventral surface of the penis as a groove that closes with time, leaving a single opening in the glans. It is difficult to detect a difference between male and female external genitalia through the fourth month of development as the clitoris is larger than the penis. It is more reliable to attempt to determine the sex of a fetus by ultrasound scanning from 20 weeks onwards.

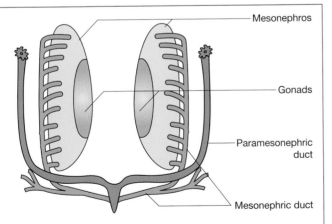

Mesonephros

Gonads

Paramesonephric duct

Mesonephric duct

Figure 7.9. The mesonephric and paramesonephric ducts during the indifferent stage. (Source: S. Webster and R. de Wreede (2012) *Embryology at a Glance*. Reproduced with permission of John Wiley & Sons, Ltd.)

Summary

Clinical case

Case investigations

The fetal sacral vertebrae defect has occurred because of a failure of the caudal neuropore to close normally. The cranial neuropore has closed, and the brain and upper central nervous system have developed normally.

The fetal anomaly ultrasound scan can detect a defect in a spina bifida case but the type of lesion and its size are assessed at birth. Mrs Kinder begins labour in her 37th week of gestation and gives birth to her baby normally. There is an opaque cyst protruding from baby Kinder's lower back, which is covered in an aseptic film.

Later, in the neonatal unit, the cyst is assessed and is found to contain meningeal layers, cerebrospinal fluid and a small amount of nervous tissue. The cyst is protruding from the sacrum, and is diagnosed as sacral spina bifida myelomeningocoele. Baby Kinder has surgery 36 hours later to remove the cyst, restore the herniating spinal nerves to the vertebral canal, and repair the tissues and skin overlying the lesion. The operation goes well.

In the 2 weeks following surgery baby Kinder develops hydrocephalus, and has a second operation to implant a shunt that drains cerebrospinal fluid into the peritoneal cavity.

Case conclusions

As baby Kinder develops she has difficulty with bladder continence, has minor bowel incontinence, and some lower limb weakness. Her legs have developed normally. Throughout her childhood she is supported by physiotherapists and urologists, and is able to walk unaided and manage her bladder and bowels effectively by the time she begins secondary school. She has some social difficulties in her teenage years and early adulthood, but performs well at school.

Mrs Kinder becomes pregnant again 3 years after the birth of baby Kinder, and is offered tests for high levels of maternal alpha-fetoprotein during the pregnancy as she has an increased risk of having a baby with spina bifida again. Mrs Kinder takes folic acid supplements prior to becoming pregnant and for the first trimester. Her second child develops normally and is born with no congenital defects.

Key learning points

- The development of the systems of the body helps describe and explain adult anatomy, and explains congenital defects and abnormalities.

- This chapter briefly describes the formation of a number of systems and the timings of these descriptions overlap. More detailed and expansive information can be found in books dedicated to this subject.

 Now visit **www.wileyessential.com/humandevelopment** to test yourself on this chapter.

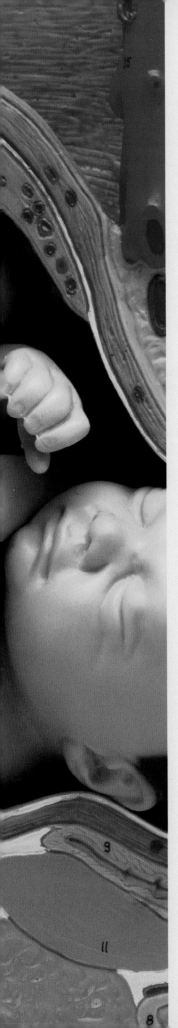

CHAPTER 8
Physiology of pregnancy

Sam Webster

Case

A 26-year-old woman, Jane, is 26 weeks pregnant with her first child. The pregnancy has been unremarkable so far; her blood pressure is 140/88 mmHg, heart rate is 78 bpm, and her before pregnancy BMI was 31 (weight 81 kg, height 1.62 m). Antenatal care has not highlighted any issues. Her father has type 2 diabetes, and her mother has a history of obesity and some developing osteoarthritis. Jane works in an office environment, does not exercise regularly, has never smoked, and has been becoming tired easily.

Jane is at risk of developing gestational diabetes mellitus (GDM) and will be screened for this as part of her antenatal care.

Learning outcomes

- You should be able to predict the physiological changes that occur during normal pregnancy and relate them to changes in various examinations, and blood and other test results.

Essential Human Development, First Edition. Edited by Samuel Webster, Geraint Morris and Euan Kevelighan

Systemic changes during pregnancy

Hormonal changes

With the implantation of the blastocyst into the endometrium of the uterus, the menstrual cycle (see Chapter 2) is ended and with it the cyclical changes in the levels of some circulating hormones. Progesterone levels remain high as the corpus luteum does not degenerate, and when the syncytiotrophoblast forms its cells produce progesterone, human placental lactogen (hPL) and human chorionic gonadotrophin (hCG). The developing placenta will be the main source of progesterone after around 2 months of gestation.

Levels of progesterone and oestrogen are high throughout pregnancy, and one effect of this is inhibition of gonadotrophin-releasing hormone (GnRH) secretion, causing low levels of follicle-stimulating hormone (FSH) and luteinising hormone (LH). No follicles develop in the ovaries during pregnancy, and ovulation does not occur (see also Chapter 2).

One form of oestrogen, oestriol, is present during pregnancy but cannot be made by the placenta on its own. The fetal adrenal cortex produces dehydroepiandrosterone sulphate (DHEA-S), which is converted to oestriol by the placenta. Oestriol can be detected in the blood, and its circulating levels can be used as a marker of fetal health.

The synthesis of other hormones also increases during pregnancy, including adrenocorticotrophic hormone (ACTH), thyroid-stimulating hormone (thyrotrophin), vasopressin, prolactin (from the pituitary gland), corticosteroids (from the adrenal glands), and triiodothyronine (T3) and thyroxine (T4) in the thyroid gland. The actions of prolactin are supplemented by hPL, causing many of the physiological changes observed during pregnancy. Growth hormone shares structural similarities with hPL. Levels of renin, erythropoietin, 1,25-dihydroxyvitamin D_3 (kidneys) and parathyroid hormone (parathyroid glands) are also elevated.

Reproductive system

High levels of progesterone and oestradiol affect the myometrium of the uterus, causing growth by hypertrophy and proliferation (hyperplasia). Later in pregnancy the size of the fetus stimulates growth of the uterus, partly by distension, and a fetus with restricted growth may be detected by abdominal palpation of the uterus and comparison of its size with the size expected for the gestational age. The uterus normally weighs around 50 g, but will increase in weight during pregnancy to around 1000 g by birth.

The uterus comprises three layers of muscular myometrium, and the superior part is more muscular than the inferior part. The outer layer is made up of smooth muscle fibres running longitudinally; the middle layer is much thicker and has fibres running in almost spiral fashion around the uterus; and the innermost layer's fibres run in transversely oriented circles (Figure 8.1). As the uterus becomes distended at full term the angles of the crossing muscle fibres are increased.

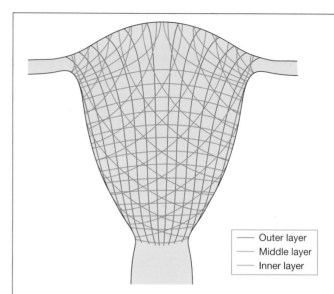

Figure 8.1. Diagram of the muscle fibre directions of the three layers of myometrium in the uterus.

- Outer layer
- Middle layer
- Inner layer

This effect is at its smallest at inferior regions, and incision for caesarean section is more suitable here. Anatomically, this region is between the site of attachment of the peritoneum of the rectovesical pouch and the internal cervical os.

Contraction of the interlaced muscle fibres of the myometrium causes occlusion of the blood vessels. Normally after the placenta has left the uterus muscular contraction closes the blood vessels, but if the placenta has formed in a lower part of the uterus the reduced muscular content of this region makes increased blood loss (postpartum haemorrhage) more likely.

The cells of the myometrium develop connections between one another as the myometrium grows. These connections enable synchronised muscular contractions through a rapidly spreading membrane depolarisation between smooth muscle cells. Painless contractions late in pregnancy are the first indications of this (Braxton Hicks contractions), and this system is later necessary for the coordinated contractions of labour.

During pregnancy the cervix changes, becoming softer and swollen as oestradiol acts on the columnar epithelium lining. Prostaglandins and local collagenase released from leucocytes break up some of the collagenous connective tissue of the cervix late in pregnancy, making it easier for the cervix to dilate during labour. Mucous glands in the cervix become enlarged and the blood supply is increased, which along with the changes to the epithelium make the cervix more prone to light bleeding from superficial damage.

Oestrogen also causes changes to the vagina, with thickening of the mucosa and muscle layers. The connective tissues become more distensible, enabling passage of the baby during birth. Desquamation of epithelial cells increases resulting in increased vaginal discharge during pregnancy.

Cardiovascular system

An increase in blood plasma volume occurs during pregnancy, and this is part of fluid retention that affects the mother's body as a whole. If, for example, the total weight gain during pregnancy is around 12 kg, 8 kg of that is likely to be due to total body water accretion. With an increasing plasma volume a number of physiological adaptations occur.

The volume of plasma increases by more than a litre over the gestation period, from around 2.6 L to 3.8 L (Figure 8.2). It is not clear how this occurs, but retention of sodium seems to be involved. There are decreases in plasma osmotic pressure and plasma oncotic pressure (or colloid osmotic pressure). The number of red blood cells increases to meet the increased oxygen demand of the placenta, but because of the increasing plasma volume the concentration of red blood cells actually drops. A haemoglobin concentration of 11 g/dL during the 36th week of pregnancy is normal, compared with the normal range of 11.5 to 16.5 g/dL in a non-pregnant woman.

Dietary iron is important for haemoglobin synthesis during pregnancy, and the gut adapts to absorb iron more effectively. Folic acid supplementation is also important during pregnancy; it is linked with reducing the incidence of macrocytic anaemia, but appears to be most beneficial during the early weeks of embryonic development in reducing the risks of neural tube defects (see Chapter 7) than later in pregnancy for increasing erythrocyte numbers. Vitamin B_{12} is important in erythrocyte formation but supplementation during pregnancy is generally not advised (and nor is folic acid supplementation after 12 weeks of pregnancy) unless anaemia is diagnosed, as dietary deficiency is rare.

The total number of white blood cells also increases, and even with the dilution effect of increasing plasma volume the white cell count increases to around 1×10^{10}/L (the normal reference range is 4–11 $\times 10^9$/L). The number of platelets increases, but there is usually a slight decrease in the platelet count.

Changes in coagulation cause a state of hypercoagulability during pregnancy that helps minimize blood loss when the placenta separates from the uterus. Levels of fibrinogen and thrombin rise, and inhibitors of fibrinolysis are produced, partly by the placenta. These changes are associated with an increase in the erythrocyte sedimentation rate (ESR). With hypercoagulability comes an increased risk of thromboembolism during pregnancy. Women with a history of thrombosis or thrombophilia should be considered as at greater risk.

Before an increase in blood volume develops, peripheral vasodilation occurs and an increase in heart rate is observed from around the fifth week of pregnancy. Stroke volume increases from the 13th or 14th week onwards, further increasing cardiac output. The combination of increased cardiac output and increased blood volume but decreased peripheral vascular resistance means that blood pressure falls. During most of the pregnancy arterial blood pressure drops slightly, and is expected to rise after 30 weeks. Diastolic blood pressure drops more than systolic blood pressure. High blood pressure during pregnancy is the most common cause for concern during pregnancy, and is associated with maternal and fetal morbidity and mortality (see Chapter 11).

The heart is pushed superiorly as pregnancy progresses and rotates anteriorly. With the increased cardiovascular load systolic murmurs are commonly heard, and diastolic murmurs occur in around 20% of pregnancies.

The increased blood flow is primarily for the benefit of the uterus and placenta, but flow is also increased to the kidneys, skin, mucous membranes, liver and breasts. Increased blood flow to the skin causes many pregnant women to feel warm and sweat more easily. Nasal congestion is more common and pregnant women may be more prone to nosebleeds.

Respiratory system

To meet the increased metabolic demands for oxygen the respiratory system adapts during pregnancy. Oxygen consumption increases by around 16%, but the partial pressure of arterial CO_2 decreases by 15–20% to improve the transfer of oxygen to (and carbon dioxide from) the fetus. This state of mild respiratory alkalosis occurs through progesterone causing hyperventilation, and levels of bicarbonate in the blood drop because of increased renal excretion to maintain pH.

Alveolar ventilation is increased, and the increase in cardiac output leads to increases in pulmonary blood flow. The tidal volume of the lungs also increases, by about 200 mL to 700 mL, with a decreased residual volume. Inspiratory capacity and vital capacity are increased, increasing ventilation by deepening respiration rather than by breathing more quickly. These changes are created by a superior displacement of the thoracic cage, with an increased transverse diameter. Diaphragmatic movement is increased. Dyspnoea is a common symptom of normal pregnancy, possibly because of these changes.

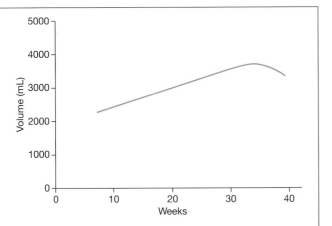

Figure 8.2. Graph showing the change in plasma volume over 40 weeks of pregnancy.

Gastrointestinal tract

An increase in appetite during pregnancy is associated with cravings for particular foods and aversion to others. Pica, an appetite for generally non-nutritive substances, can occur. Gastric acid secretion and gastric motility are decreased leading to delayed emptying, and the cardiac sphincter is relaxed increasing the probability of reflux oesophagitis and heartburn. High levels of progesterone cause these effects, and smooth muscle in the remainder of the gastrointestinal tract is similarly affected. Displacement of the cardiac sphincter into the thorax as a hiatus hernia is more likely during pregnancy.

Nausea in early pregnancy can cause the appearance of excess salivation (ptyalism) due to a reluctance to swallow, and the gums can become spongy and friable. Bleeding of the gums is more likely, as are gingivitis and periodontal disease.

With the reduction in gastrointestinal tract motility transit time is longer, increasing the likelihood of constipation as the colon absorbs more water. An increase in flatulence is also likely.

The effects on smooth muscle extend to the gallbladder, and emptying is decreased. This may lead to pruritus and gallstones, but a causative link has not been made. The liver is displaced superiorly and posteriorly as the uterus grows.

Renal

The urinary tract becomes dilated during pregnancy, also because of the effects of progesterone on smooth muscle. Prostaglandin E2 (PGE2) synthesis is increased during pregnancy and has been associated with these renal changes. Vasodilation increases the flow of blood to the kidneys and as a result the glomerular filtration rate is increased by about 50%, increasing the clearance of urea and creatinine from the blood, among other substances. Protein excretion in the urine increases to up to 0.3 g per day, and glycosuria may also occur as an expected consequence of pregnancy, as the glomerular filtration rate exceeds the reabsorption capacity of the kidneys. The normal ranges of substances examined in blood and urine analysis must be adapted to be specific for pregnancy.

As described above, during pregnancy there is a gradual increase in retained sodium and water, with most of the sodium taken up by fetal tissues. Levels of aldosterone rise (as do levels of renin and angiotensin II) and it acts on the distal tubules and collecting ducts of the nephrons to enable this retention. Blood pressure does not rise as it normally would be expected to do, largely because of the decrease in peripheral vascular resistance. Angiotensin II has a weakened action of vasoconstriction during pregnancy because of increased secretions of enzymes that degrade angiotensin (aminopeptidase A).

The changes to the urinary tract increase the risk of infection during pregnancy, and urinary tract infections (UTIs) are common (see also Chapter 12). The risk of developing pyelonephritis is also raised, often caused by untreated asymptomatic bacteriuria.

Metabolism

With pregnancy and the adaptations described above metabolic changes also occur. There is a gradual increase in the basal metabolic rate over the course of gestation. This change is variable, and is affected by activity levels and the pre-pregnancy body fat content. The metabolic change is minimal in the first trimester but increases thereafter to a requirement of roughly an extra 300 kcal/day in the third trimester. An increased protein intake of 6 g per day is recommended in the UK.

Activity of the thyroid gland remains generally normal in most pregnancies, with a decrease in thyroid-stimulating hormone (TSH) activity during the first trimester and subsequent increases in thyroxine and thyroid-binding globulin in the blood after 4 months accompanying the increasing basal metabolic rate.

Nutrition is important for a healthy pregnancy, and a poor intake of essential nutrients is associated with reduced fetal growth and increased risk of perinatal morbidity and mortality.

The resistance of the mother's cells to insulin rises and tolerance to glucose decreases, particularly in the second trimester, causing plasma glucose concentrations of 4.5–5.5 mmol/L after meals. The fetus uses glucose as its primary source of fuel, and glucose is actively transported across the placenta to the fetal blood supply. Fetal insulin production by the fetal pancreas increases use of glucose by relevant tissues.

Maternal hormones also affect carbohydrate metabolism. Progesterone increases insulin secretion, and cortisol increases conversion of liver glycogen to glucose. The effects of fasting are more pronounced during pregnancy. Oestrogen increases plasma cortisol levels. Blood sugar levels after meals remain higher for longer, encouraging fetal transfer of glucose. Insulin activity is antagonised by hPL, increasing glucose availability, and increases the synthesis of lipids. During the first two trimesters maternal fat storage increases, and in the third trimester hPL increases lipolysis.

Around an extra 0.5 kg of protein and 4 kg of fat are retained by the late stages of pregnancy. Most excess weight is lost during the 3 months postpartum.

Placenta

The formation of the placenta is described briefly in Chapter 5; it is fully formed by around week 12. It protects the fetus from the maternal immune system, and provides a site for gaseous exchange, nutrient transfer, and waste removal between the fetal and maternal circulatory systems. It produces human chorionic gonadotrophin during the first 2 months of pregnancy (maintaining the survival of the progesterone-producing corpus luteum in the ovary) and then synthesises progesterone from around 16 weeks. The placenta also synthesises oestrogens and hPL.

Maternal immunoglobulins can be transferred across the placenta, giving the fetus a passive immunity lasting for some months after birth. Most drugs, antibiotics and corticosteroids can pass across the placenta, as can some viruses and other pathogens, although the fetus is protected from most. Larger molecules, such as heparin, are unable to cross the placenta,

Placental insufficiency will cause intrauterine growth restriction of the fetus, and the placenta may adhere to the uterine wall in an unusually aggressive manner or in a location that may cause complications. These are covered in a number of other chapters.

Clinical case

Case investigations

Jane is given a 3-hour oral glucose tolerance test. She is not taking any medication. After fasting overnight, a venous blood sample is taken and then Jane is given 75 mg of glucose orally. Jane sits quietly and is not allowed to eat or drink. Subsequent blood samples are taken at 1, 2 and 3 hours after the baseline sample. Jane feels OK after the testing, and leaves the clinic to eat and then go back to work.

During pregnancy the mother's carbohydrate metabolism and insulin sensitivity are altered, raising blood glucose levels after eating to increase the effectiveness of glucose transport across the placenta to the fetus. Glucose levels are expected to remain raised for longer during pregnancy after eating. A post-fasting oral glucose tolerance test should show a decrease in blood glucose levels within defined margins over time after ingestion of glucose, but the levels are expected to be slightly higher in a pregnant woman and an appropriate reference range should be used (see also Chapter 12).

Case conclusions

Jane's venous blood glucose at baseline (after fasting) was 95 mg/dL (5.3 mmol/L). After 1 hour it was 170 mg/dL (9.4 mmol/L), at 2 hours it was 165 mg/dL (9.2 mmol/L), and at 3 hours it was 150 mg/dL (8.3 mmol/L).

The reference range indicates that Jane's glucose levels remain higher than normal, and that she has gestational diabetes. There are a number of complications associated with this, which Jane is advised of (see Chapter 12). Jane's diet is discussed, and exercise is suggested for initial conservative management over the following 2 weeks.

Two weeks later Jane's glucose management has not improved, and medical management is begun with metformin. A delivery plan is developed with Jane taking into account the risks associated with gestational diabetes.

Key learning points

- There are a number of physiological changes that occur during pregnancy that are normal and should be expected when analysing the results of investigations.

- Most systems of the body are affected by the elevated levels of hormones produced during pregnancy, causing a wide range of effects. After birth these changes typically revert back to the non-pregnant state.

 Now visit **www.wileyessential.com/humandevelopment** to test yourself on this chapter.

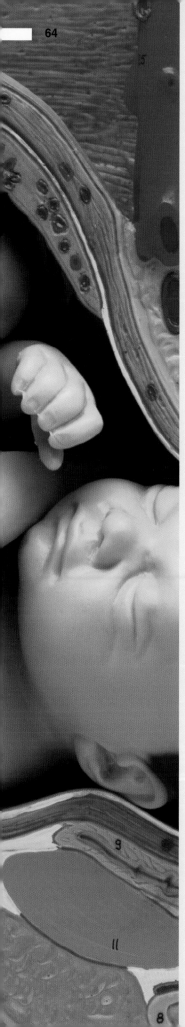

CHAPTER 9
Antenatal care

Marion Beard

Case

Mel attends the consultant Antenatal Clinic. The community midwife saw her at 10 weeks gestation and would like an opinion. Mel is 41 years old and in her first pregnancy. She is generally well, is not on any medication, but she has a raised BMI (37 kg/m^2). Her only visit to hospital was at the age of 23 when she had a hot, swollen leg shortly after commencing the combined oral contraceptive. She can't remember what the diagnosis was but she took tablets for a few months.

A dating scan today has confirmed her gestation as 12 weeks and 3 days.

On examination, Mel looks healthy, is pleased and surprised to be pregnant, but is concerned regarding the referral as she had heard that first-time mothers were low risk. She is still having some nausea related to early pregnancy although this is improving over the past couple of weeks. She has only vomited on two occasions and has a good appetite. She has recently quit smoking, with a ten-year pack history.

Her blood pressure is 132/82, her pulse is 86 and regular, and a soft systolic murmur is heard on auscultation.

Learning outcomes

This chapter should help you to be able to:

- List the goals of antenatal care.
- Recognise key risk factors affecting obstetric outcome.
- Explain the importance of communication and engagement in antenatal care.
- Describe the important aspects of obstetric history and examination.

Essential Human Development, First Edition. Edited by Samuel Webster, Geraint Morris and Euan Kevelighan

Assessment of risk

The fundamental purpose of modern antenatal care is to assess risk. The woman at low risk, and consequently likely to deliver normally, can be directed to midwifery-led care. Obstetric risk factors may predate the pregnancy or may emerge during its course. Consequently, the patient pathways for low- versus high-risk women are not rigidly in parallel, and a woman may move in either direction if there is an indication. The pattern of contact for antenatal care is reduced for the low-risk pregnancy so resources can be directed to the woman who has, or may develop, clinical features of concern.

The evidence supports assumption of normality in the absence of risk factors as these women are less likely to require medical attention. The cascade of intervention can be profound in obstetrics and may influence the quality of the experience of pregnancy and childbirth for the woman and her family, and more importantly may affect the optimum outcome of healthy mother/healthy baby. The potential for iatrogenic harm should always be balanced with the default risk aversion of the careful obstetric practitioner.

The basis of the assessment in early pregnancy is demographic information, the medical history and the clinical examination.

History

Symptoms of early pregnancy

The pregnant woman is in a normal physiological condition. This may nevertheless be new to her, so a range of non-specific symptoms may be worrying for the woman and her family, and reassurance is frequently required. Extreme tiredness and malaise, nausea and vomiting, and changes in taste and smell can be very debilitating and many women are concerned for the fetus. Treatment should be instigated if there is sustained loss of body mass or if the woman is vomiting clear fluids consistently. Dehydration of true hyperemesis gravidarum can cause metabolic derangement so rehydration, antiemetics and micronutrient supplementation may be required. An ultrasound scan is important in order to exclude multiple pregnancy or gestational trophoblastic disease (molar pregnancy). Many women will have days where they are unable to eat but this does not require medicalisation unless the woman is of very low prepregnancy weight (BMI < 18 kg/m^2).

Vague abdominal aches and pains do not require rigorous investigation unless persisting or escalating. Any vaginal bleeding should be considered a threatened miscarriage prior to viability.

Index pregnancy

Approximately one-third of pregnancies are reported to be unplanned. Preconceptual care such as consumption of folate and vitamin supplements (particularly vitamin D), optimisation of body mass and review of medicines is the ideal. If the pregnancy was not planned, was the unexpected welcomed? The diagnosis of pregnancy is life-changing for the mother and her immediate family, and ambivalence about a progressing pregnancy can be a major stressor.

A dating scan between 9 and 13 weeks gives a more accurate estimated date of delivery (EDD) than menstrual dating and allows planning of antenatal care.

Obstetric history

The total number of gestations including the current pregnancy is obtained. If ectopic pregnancy, miscarriages or terminations are reported, an enquiry as to the approximate gestation at which the pregnancy demised should be made. The doctor should be careful with terminology so as to minimise upset when taking a history of termination and miscarriage. Mid-trimester miscarriage and stillbirth need particularly sensitive communication, and records should be clearly marked for all professionals to be alert to past bereavement.

The detail of live births should be documented, with mode/gestation at delivery and detail of any complications. Be wary of assuming children are alive and well. Children with ongoing physical or mental challenges may give the woman anxiety that this was attributable to some aspect of that pregnancy or delivery. When discussing previous deliveries the woman will be more at ease if the child's name is used, including where there has been a stillbirth or neonatal death. Time spent on this aspect of the history is well spent as a first visit will set the tone for future consultations. Reassurance can be given if appropriate, myths and misunderstandings can be rectified, and the potential for problems in this pregnancy can be anticipated and discussed.

Gynaecological history

Most benign gynaecological conditions have no consequence for pregnancy, as there is obvious respite from menstrual symptoms and any subfertility has resolved.

Women with ovarian cysts and uterine abnormalities such as fibroids are inevitably anxious about the potential for effects on the pregnancy and delivery. In many cases watchful waiting is appropriate. Cysts, including teratomata (dermoids) to the ovary, can be monitored via ultrasound and any necessary surgery planned for the relative calm of the second trimester when miscarriage is very unlikely. Fibroids can, under the influence of oestrogen, rapidly outgrow their blood supply with consequent painful central necrotic change known as red degeneration. This should be in the differential for any

> **Tip 9.1** The SANDS 'teardrop' logo is placed on the outside of hand-held case notes so all UK healthcare staff handling notes are aware that the woman has suffered a stillbirth in a previous pregnancy. See www.uk-sands.org.

presentation with abdominal pain in pregnancy, particularly in the older mother.

Congenital abnormalities of the uterus can affect placentation. For example, the relatively avascular septum of the septate or subseptate uterus is less likely to sustain an early pregnancy than the lush environment of the bicornuate or unicornuate/didelphic uterus, although the latter are developmentally more extreme anomalies. The position of a viable fetus may be affected by the altered morphology of the single horn, with breech presentation and therefore risk of caesarean section delivery.

Any failed contraception needs discussion. In most cases this is due to user error with missed pills. LARC (long-acting reversible contraception) options such as intrauterine contraceptive devices (IUCDs), including the Mirena® intrauterine system (IUS), can cause consternation for the mother if pregnancy occurs and the coil is seen at dating scan. Although the pregnancy rate is low in IUCD/IUS users, 5–50% of these may be ectopic when conception occurs. Following discussion of the small risk of miscarriage, if less than 12 weeks gestation the device should be removed. If the woman requests that it be left in place, she needs to be aware that there is a small increased risk of midtrimester miscarriage. In general these pregnancies proceed normally but if there has not yet been a scan to confirm intrauterine pregnancy and the position of the device it should be requested.

Medical history

It is good practice to obtain the full medical record in early pregnancy to highlight important history. The Confidential Enquiry into Maternal Deaths, part of the rolling audit of maternal morbidity and mortality, has identified a need to make referral to any other specialty a priority for pregnant women. The long waiting list times for specialist assessment are not appropriate in pregnancy as the woman's condition may deteriorate. Good liaison between specialties is vital and all referrals for emerging conditions should be urgent. Key conditions that can be challenging in pregnancy are summarised in Table 9.1.

Medication taken currently and in the 3 months prior to conception should be identified for any that could be discontinued or changed to those with an established safety profile. Specific enquiry about any recent contraception should be made. Use of over-the-counter medicines and alternative/complementary substances including nutritional supplements also needs to be explored. The latter are unlikely to have evidence of safety.

A **systems review** during the history taking is a thorough but conversational means of eliciting any underlying illness. The woman's demeanour while telling her story is a key to understanding the impact of her health; what is important to the doctor may be almost forgotten by the patient, and ostensibly minor conditions may significantly affect the woman's quality of life.

Table 9.1 Pre-existing conditions that affect pregnancy.

Disorder/issue	Potential sequelae
Medical disorders	
Epilepsy	• Miscarriage • Teratogenicity
Obesity	• Stillbirth • Gestational diabetes • Dysfunctional labour
Gastrointestinal, e.g. coeliac, inflammatory bowel disease, post-bariatric surgery	• Pain • Malabsorption with fetal growth restriction
CVS, respiratory, renal, haematological	• Effects of medication on fetus • Augmentation of prothrombotic state
Psychiatric, endocrine	• Possible effects of medication on fetus • Postnatal exacerbation
Malignancy	• Challenges planning treatment • Progression
Surgical disorders	
Previous abdominopelvic surgery	Altered anatomy leading to: • Pain as pregnancy progresses • Dysfunctional labour
Ovarian masses/fibroids	• Pain as pregnancy progresses • Obstructed labour
Anorectal prolapse	Worsening of maternal condition
Lithiasis (urinary tract, biliary)	Worsening of maternal condition
Social issues	
Cigarette smoking >15/day	• Miscarriage • Fetal growth restriction, placental infarction/abruption • Venous thromboembolism
Alcohol consumption	• Teratogenicity • Poor nutritional status • Injury risk
Use of non-prescribed drugs	• Teratogenicity • Poor nutritional status • Drug-specific

A **family history** of the mother's first-degree relatives will alert to susceptibility to important disease such as diabetes or haemoglobinopathy. If a woman is without overt health conditions but has characteristics such as obesity or increased age, these may be independent risk factors, as can ethnic origin.

Obesity is becoming endemic to the UK. In some areas 40% of women present at booking in the obese range (BMI > 30 kg/m²), and there is year-on-year increase. As patients are young, the extent of potential health harms may not yet have emerged. Obesity presents challenges during antenatal, intrapartum and postpartum care, as excess body weight predisposes to fetal loss, growth disorder and anomaly, maternal hypertensive disorder, diabetes, and difficulties at delivery including postpartum haemorrhage. The obese mother is less likely to be sufficiently fit to allow labour to progress, and significant lower genital soft tissue mass in extreme morbid obesity (BMI > 40 kg/m^2) can obstruct vaginal delivery. If caesarean section delivery is required, this will be more complicated technically, the risk of haemorrhage is increased, and wound healing can be protracted. In the first meeting with a mother her understanding of healthy eating and drinking should be explored and she can be reassured that she need not increase her calorific intake.

The **older mother** (above 37 years) is also becoming more common, with social pressures on women to establish at work prior to starting a family. In 1974 the average age of first pregnancy in the UK was 24 and in 2010 it was 29; in several European countries the average age now exceeds 30. Medical conditions become more prevalent with age. Fitness and flexibility can decline and obesity is more common. Independently of these factors there is a small but consistent increased incidence of late stillbirth, thought to be a marker of the earlier decline in placental function in the older mother towards the due date.

The interactions of **lifestyle factors** such as cigarette smoking, poor (including excess) diet, use of 'street' drugs and alcohol consumption can present a complex mix of multiple risk. The context of poor social support and relative poverty can make tackling all of these in pregnancy seem insurmountable. The challenge for all healthcare professionals is to give uncomplicated, unbiased, evidence-based advice that may effect change in behaviour without causing alienation.

Examination and investigations

First trimester

Much healthcare provision is reactive, relying on the patient to present if symptoms become troublesome. In contrast, antenatal care is provided to apparently healthy people where the term 'patient' may be less appropriate. Young women may be entering their first experience of preventative healthcare since early childhood. Conditions such as cardiac or renal disease may be unmasked by routine investigation or examination as the mother's physiology adapts to a new circumstance.

As in all examination, the woman needs to know what to expect. Verbal consent and a brief outline of what you are doing helps to relax her. A simple commentary in the course of the examination is reassuring for the mother, and allows her to predict the sequence of the examination. The abdomen must be adequately exposed, so ask the woman to ease clothing up to the xiphisternum and down to just below the suprapubic skin crease. Use chaperones and curtaining to maintain privacy.

Observation will identify any pallor or skin phenomena such as the 'pregnancy mask' or melasma and nutritional level. The pigmented linea nigra or striae gravidarum may be present on the abdomen, and any scarring from surgery or trauma should be commented on (Figure 9.1). The clinical level of hydration is also important.

The early pregnancy, booking or late first trimester examination focuses on general health and early pregnancy problems. At the first visit the general examination will include height and weight, blood pressure and pulse, auscultation of the heart and lungs, and identification of any obvious physical, intellectual or communication difficulties that might affect access to care. While throughout pregnancy the priority is healthcare for the mother, fetal health is a consequence of good care, with the concept of having two patients predominating as term approaches.

The 'dating' scan may be the only imaging done unless there has been a history of early pregnancy problems such as bleeding or pain. Performed at 10–13 weeks, it is more accurate than menstrual dating (see Chapter 10).

Urinalysis and blood pressure measurement is a routine component of each antenatal visit, and 'booking bloods' act as a baseline to identify any progressive anaemia.

Second trimester

The principles of specific obstetric examination become routine after 12 weeks, when the uterus begins to rise from the bony pelvis. This will include assessment of the ascent of the uterus as pregnancy progresses. The 'hand on the tummy' gives information about the size and potential wellbeing of the fetus (Figure 9.2).

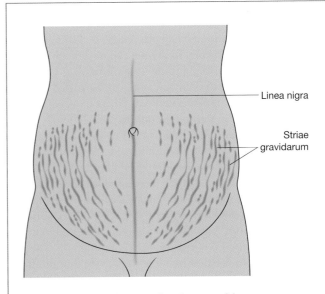

Linea nigra

Striae gravidarum

Figure 9.1 Linea nigra and striae gravidarum.

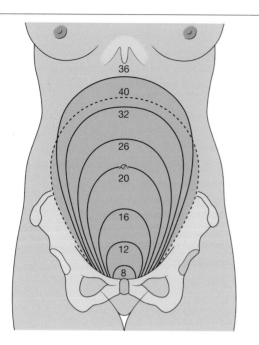

36
40
32
26
20
16
12
8

Figure 9.2 The changing fundal height with gestation.

A measurement of the distance in centimetres between the upper aspect of the symphysis pubis and the uterine fundus, the symphysis–pubis height (SFH), is a low-tech screening tool for fetal growth. From around 15 weeks, the fundus typically rises by around a centimetre a week. Correct technique increases the sensitivity of measurement, with the tape end anchored at the fixed point (the symphysis) and the tape depressed over the variable point (curve of the fundus) by the ulnar border of the other hand. Use the tape with measurements hidden so as not to influence your placement.

Auscultation of the fetal heart using a Pinard stethoscope or a hand-held ultrasound Doppler is done at visits over 16–20 weeks gestation. The tiny fetal heart can be difficult to locate at earlier gestations. Placental flow may be heard as a 'whooshing' sound, and from there the probe can be angled until the fetal heart sounds are directly heard. These have a distinctive clicking sound like a train on a railway track.

Fetal movements may be heard during auscultation, with a transient higher-pitched acoustic signal as fetal parts pass the probe. After 20 weeks, enquiry should be made during the examination as to whether the mother has felt any fetal movements. With primiparas, movements may not be experienced until 22 weeks, and the earliest is around 16 weeks in the experienced mother. As fetal movements are detected by cutaneous sensory nerves the obese woman is generally less aware of them due to the distance from the fetus to the skin surface.

At this point of the pregnancy, where early pregnancy symptoms have settled but the discomfort of late pregnancy has yet to arise, there may be a period of relative peace. Musculoskeletal pain arising from the softening and stretching of connective tissues may emerge. This has earlier onset in the multipara, becoming more problematic with each pregnancy, and is worsened in the obese woman, with the increased intra-abdominal mass impinging on pelvic and interspinous ligaments. These pains may be sharp and sudden in onset and require investigation to exclude more serious causes such as concealed placental abruption or surgical causes. To confirm this feature, pain on pressure to the symphysis or sacroiliac joints and on active and passive abduction of the legs suggests benign connective tissue softening. The term SPD (symphysis pubis dysfunction) describes only a part of this syndrome.

At 18–21 weeks a detailed ultrasound scan for fetal anomaly is offered. At this gestation the whole fetus is an appropriate size to survey the anatomy, including the brain, vertebrae, long bones of the limbs, craniofacial structures, the integrity of the abdominal wall, and the structure of the heart, lungs, liver, kidneys and bladder. Any serious anomaly not previously detected at early scan may trigger a referral to a regional Fetal Medicine Unit.

Third trimester

The general principles of communication, exposure, observation and palpation continue to apply in late pregnancy. With practice it is possible to focus history during examination, clarifying any changes in condition. A blood count is repeated to exclude anaemia and to confirm blood group.

Assessment of the normal growth of the fetus continues. The SFH remains the primary screen, with further investigation via ultrasound biometry if there is a discrepancy of more than 2 cm from the gestational age. In obesity this judgement can be difficult and ultrasound assessment is indicated to ensure that the fetus is within normal limits. The smaller fetus that is growing asymmetrically, where the abdominal circumference is growing less well than the head, or where the fetus is below the 10th centile for gestation, will need surveillance. These features may indicate a poorly functioning placenta from hypertensive disease or fetal compromise.

Slowed or negative change in SFH measurement late in pregnancy may be due to the fetal head moving into the bony pelvis. In primiparous women this engagement can occur from 36 weeks gestation. In multiparous women the fetal head frequently engages only at onset of labour.

Palpation of the fetus is more informative in the third trimester, with the presentation and axis becoming increasingly important from around 35 weeks.

Systematic palpation benefits from practice. Firm, confident movements with a sequence and flow are both informative for the clinician and comfortable for the mother. Superficial, perfunctory or unexpected moves can be unpleasant and can trigger uterine contraction. After measurement, finding the upper extent of the fetus at the fundus and defining it as either the rounder, ballotable head or the narrower, softer breech is the first step. Then, identification of the fetal back by locating a smoothly curved surface indicates the axis of fetal lie. This can be done using gentle movements fundus to symphysis alternating the flat of both hands. Palpating with both hands facing the woman's feet allows detection of the fetal head projecting above the symphysis pubis. This can be an uncomfortable manoeuvre and it is best to do it firmly once rather than indecisively a few times. Findings are described in notional fifths of the fetal head. For example, '3/5 palpable per abdomen' means that 3/5 of the fetal head can be felt in the abdomen. This suggests the head is not engaged as most of fetal head is still palpable in the abdomen. At 0/5, the head is well descended into the pelvis; this is more common in advanced labour. Excess or inadequate amniotic fluid may lead to difficulty in abdominal examination. Poorly defined landmarks or a mass of knobbly fetal parts may indicate poly- or oligohydramnios, respectively. The obese woman can be an ongoing challenge at examination, and if there is doubt about level of fluid or fetal presentation an ultrasound scan will help.

Musculoskeletal pain may emerge or worsen, at this point in pregnancy potentially involving intercostal connective tissue as the ribcage widens. As with abdominopelvic pain throughout, the more serious causes of chest and thoracic pain such as pneumonia, cardiac pain and pulmonary embolus need to be excluded. Pain on pressure to the sternum is suggestive of benign ligamentous pain.

The dependent oedema due to hypoproteinaemia of pregnancy can be a normal feature. Pitting oedema and puffiness extending to the face can be indicative of the worsening renal function of pre-eclampsia, and specific examination should always be made. If found the picture of hypertension, proteinuria and deranged biochemistry may emerge. Early detection of hypertensive disorder including pre-eclampsia allows timely surveillance, treatment and delivery if needed to reduce mortality and morbidity.

If the woman reports unusual loss *per vaginam*, either of discharge, fluid or bleeding, a sterile speculum examination may be be required. With consent and a chaperone, a lubricated cusco speculum is inserted to distend and retain the vaginal walls to visualise the ectocervix. Any discharge, blood or fluid should be swabbed for microscopy, culture and sensitivity. Pooling of quantities of clear, viscous fluid should raise the suspicion of rupture of the membranes. This is further supported if at a cough fluid emits from the cervical os. The cervix may be seen to be dilating in early labour.

If spontaneous labour does not proceed, a review post-EDD will allow planning of medical induction of labour. The risk of stillbirth rises after EDD + 14 days, so a combination of membrane sweeping and vaginal prostaglandin at 12 days is offered.

Clinical case

Case investigations

Mel's midwife has referred her due to the risk factors of age, weight and a history suggestive of venous thromboembolism.

Her surprise at the referral for obstetric opinion was acknowledged and she was counselled that she did not meet the criteria for midwifery-led care. Mel was invited to consider factors that she might be able to improve to reduce her risk. She seemed to have good understanding of the principles of healthy eating but had previously lacked motivation to moderate her portion sizes and to make lower-calorie choices. She was discouraged from dieting as such but was positive about the prospect of trying to maintain her weight, reassured that her baby would have adequate nutrition from her reserves, and planned to reduce her weight after the birth.

The medical record was reviewed, confirming a deep vein thrombosis to the leg 14 years previously, for which Mel was anticoagulated. At the time it was documented as likely to have had a hormonal trigger due to the preceding recent use of the combined oral contraceptive. Her current obesity and recent smoking history compounded the risk for oestrogen-provoked venous thromboembolism, and it was proposed that low molecular weight heparin injections as prophylaxis would reduce this.

Reassurance was given about her early pregnancy symptoms and she was told the cardiovascular findings, including the benign flow murmur from the hyperdynamic state, were normal.

Case conclusions

As the pregnancy progressed, Mel developed a moderate rise in blood pressure from 35 weeks. She did not have proteinuria and her liver and renal function remained normal. She was offered an induction of labour at her due date due to her age and she delivered a 3120 g baby boy at 40+1 weeks (i.e. 40 weeks + 1 day) with the assistance of forceps.

Key learning points

- Antenatal care is a framework that aims to identify variations from the normal course of pregnancy to allow early intervention. Establishing a rapport with the woman and her family means that she is then empowered to participate in achieving the best pregnancy outcome.
- The team involved in care may be community-based by midwives and the general practitioner or have additional consultant-led aspects. In the case of pre-existing or emerging medical, surgical or psychiatric problems, urgent referral to and shared care with other secondary care specialties is the norm.
- The basic clinical skills of communication, history and examination are fundamental in identifying risk factors so that investigation and management can be timely.

Systematic review at points throughout the pregnancy will lead to earlier intervention where this is required, and is the basis of a risk-reduction model of preventative healthcare. In women with health problems a clear plan should be jointly arrived at by community and hospital based teams together with the woman and her family.

Although based on the generic principles of physical examination, it takes time and experience to gain facility with the obstetric examination. Abdominal palpation is a practical clinical skill that involves creativity in visualising the fetus. Time with the mother taking a careful history and learning gentle but informative examination skills will be well spent.

 Now visit **www.wileyessential.com/humandevelopment** to test yourself on this chapter.

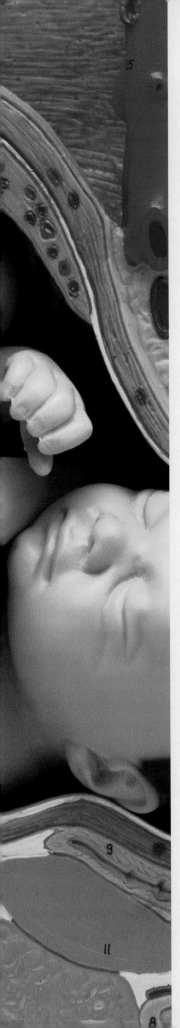

CHAPTER 10
Antenatal screening and prenatal diagnosis

Alan Treharne and Marsham Moselhi

Case

A 39-year-old patient, Mrs Jones, with an IVF pregnancy attends for her routine antenatal blood tests. She accepts the antenatal serum screening that is offered and the subsequent result gives a high risk of trisomy 21 at 1:15. She is counselled appropriately and an amniocentesis is planned and carried out at 18 weeks. When the fetal medicine specialist performs ultrasound prior to the amniocentesis, a congenital diaphragmatic hernia is suspected. The patient is informed about the finding and wishes to proceed with the amniocentesis.

Learning outcomes

- You should be able to discuss screening and diagnostic tests used in pregnancy.
- You should be able to discuss the common fetal abnormalities identified in the screening process.
- You should be able to discuss the maternal and fetal consequences of fetal infection.

Essential Human Development, First Edition. Edited by Samuel Webster, Geraint Morris and Euan Kevelighan
© 2018 John Wiley & Sons, Ltd. Published 2018 by John Wiley & Sons, Ltd.

Obstetric ultrasound screening for fetal anomaly

Obstetric ultrasound was pioneered during the 1960s and over the last few decades has gradually become deeply embedded in routine obstetric care. With advances in technology, and in particular image resolution, efforts have been made to advance fetal screening from the second trimester to the first trimester. Nevertheless, at present it is standard practice for low-risk pregnant women to be offered both a first- and second-trimester ultrasound examination.

In the UK the NHS Fetal Anomaly Screening Programme (FASP) was given responsibility by the National Screening Committee for the development of a national, quality assured obstetric ultrasound screening programme for England. In Wales this responsibility lies with Antenatal Screening Wales (ASW).

It is important that women are provided with adequate information so that they are able to make informed choices about their screening options. The objective of fetal anomaly screening is to identify fetal abnormalities. These abnormalities may be serious and could be incompatible with life or carry significant morbidity, and in this instance women may be able to make reproductive choices. In addition to this some anomalies may be suitable for antenatal intervention and some cases may benefit from delivery in specialist centres where early intervention may improve outcome. It is important therefore that following detection of an anomaly, which may be very traumatic for the patient, there is speedy access to skilled counselling.

Screening for fetal anomaly in this way results in a reduction of perinatal mortality rates as a consequence of termination of some affected pregnancies.

Although there is no clear evidence to link the use of ultrasound to any maternal or fetal hazards it is standard practice to limit the power of ultrasound used to the minimum required.

Depending on the nature of the anomaly, ultrasound will have varying rates for detection, and in situations where the woman has a very high body mass index or there is reduced or absent amniotic fluid, accurate ultrasound assessment may be difficult or even impossible.

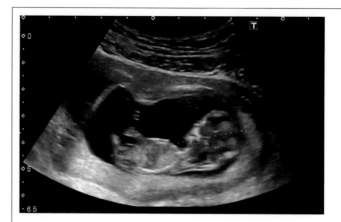

Figure 10.1 First-trimester ultrasound scan highlighting crown-to-rump length (CRL) measurement.

First-trimester ultrasound

Although ultrasound in the first trimester may be carried out at any point during the trimester, early scanning before 10 weeks will not be adequate for nuchal translucency (NT) screening (a crown–rump length between 45 and 84 mm is required) and may fail to identify some serious anomalies that can be identified more readily later (Figure 10.1). Many women will have had a scan done under 10 weeks if they have suffered from bleeding in early pregnancy, so it is important that a further scan is offered during the optimal window. First-trimester ultrasound serves a number of purposes including confirming fetal viability, providing dating information, and confirming and establishing chorionicity in multiple pregnancy. In addition measurement of nuchal translucency (the maximum thickness of the subcutaneous translucency between the skin and the soft tissue overlying the cervical spine) can contribute to aneuploidy screening and identify elevated risk of other conditions including fetal viral infection (e.g. parvovirus B19 infection) and cardiac anomalies. A measurement of NT of over 3.5 mm is considered an anomaly and should trigger further assessment and investigation. Large amounts of fluid in this area are known as cystic hygromas.

Ultrasound in the first trimester may identify other fetal structural anomalies such as some skeletal dysplasias, anterior abdominal wall defects (gastroschisis and omphalocoele) and major brain anomalies including anencephaly, encephalocoele and holoprosencephaly. With improving ultrasound resolution there is recognition that fetal echocardiography in the first trimester is feasible although at present this is not mainstream practice.

Identification of minor anomalies at this gestational stage can engender unnecessary anxiety for the mother, and some suspected anomalies may require follow-up ultrasound to enable a definitive diagnosis. However, there is no doubt that early identification of severe anomaly is beneficial for many parents and can allow the option of early termination of pregnancy.

Second-trimester ultrasound

The detailed fetal anomaly scan should take place between 18^{+0} weeks (i.e. 18 completed weeks of the pregnancy) and 20^{+6} weeks (i.e. 20 weeks + 6 days of the pregnancy). If this window is missed then the assessment should take place at the earliest opportunity, but the woman should be informed that optimal timing has been missed.

Although all women will be offered screening in this way it is important that the sonographer is aware of any risk factors for anomaly such as previous, personal or family history, drug or infection exposure or pre-existing medical conditions.

The anomaly scan is performed and reported in standardized fashion. Specific and reproducible views of the fetus are taken and ideally are stored digitally.

If an anomaly is suspected then a referral is arranged for review by an in-house consultant with fetal medicine experience, or a referral is made to the local fetal medicine unit. If the anomaly is confirmed then the patient is counselled and offered further investigation, treatment or termination of pregnancy depending on the nature of the anomaly.

Standard views include:

- Transverse section through the fetal head, which will provide information about the shape and size of the fetal skull and allow assessment of certain internal structures including the cavum septum pellucidum and the midline in addition to the cerebral ventricles and the cerebellum. In addition the fetal lips should be imaged.
- Sagittal and transverse views of the fetal spine.
- Longitudinal and transverse views of the fetal abdomen to display stomach, bladder, kidneys and the cord insertion.
- Transverse section through the fetal chest to display the fetal lungs, a four-chamber view of the heart and the major outflow tracts.
- The fetal limbs should be imaged down to the level of hands and feet.

The position of the placenta and an assessment of liquor volume will also be recorded for each patient.

CNS anomalies

Neural tube defects include anencephaly, encephalocoele and spina bifida. Anencephaly is usually identified at the 12-week scan when the cranial vault is noted to be absent. Spina bifida is more commonly identified at the 20-week scan when either the vertebral anomaly is identified or associated intracranial signs are picked up. Intracranial signs of spina bifida include a lemon-shaped skull and banana-shaped cerebellum, which occur as a result of herniation of the brainstem through the foramen magnum. Other CNS anomalies amenable to identification with ultrasound include ventriculomegaly (enlarged lateral cerebral ventricles) and microcephaly. These findings can have additional associations with genetic and chromosomal syndromes and may be secondary to viral infection such as cytomegalovirus. Holoprosencephaly (failure of midline cleavage) may occur in association with chromosomal and other anomalies. Although anencephaly is not compatible with life, other CNS anomalies carry uncertain prognosis and further investigation including karyotyping and MRI examination is often considered. Many patients choose not to continue with the pregnancy in the face of uncertainty.

Cardiac anomalies

Screening for cardiac anomalies includes a four-chamber view of the heart, which may identify such anomalies as hypoplastic left or right ventricles, septal defects and valve stenosis.

More recently imaging of the major outflow tracts to show their origin and crossover has been included in the screening programme and will help to identify such conditions as transposition of the great vessels. Pick up rates for major cardiac malformations remain variable and it is not unusual for these to be picked up incidentally in an ill neonate.

Thoracic anomalies

Examination of the fetal chest can reveal hydrothorax (pleural effusions), which may be a feature of hydrops or chylothorax. Diagnosis may be assisted by aspiration and analysis of the pleural fluid, and prognosis is dictated by the cause and severity of the problem and may be dependent on the degree of compromise of lung development (pulmonary hypoplasia). Occasionally prenatal treatment in the form of shunting may be helpful. Other chest pathology identifiable includes CCAML (congenital cystic adenomatoid lesion) and pulmonary sequestrations. These can appear as areas of increased echogenicity or cystic areas, and the prognosis largely depends on the size of the lesion and whether mediastinal shift results in cardiac compromise.

The finding of the stomach, bowel or liver within the fetal chest can reveal a congenital diaphragmatic hernia, which may be associated with chromosomal and other anomalies. Prognosis is largely dependent on whether associated pulmonary hypoplasia develops.

GI anomalies

Hernia type defects of the anterior abdominal wall include exomphalos (defect involving the umbilicus where the extruded organs are in a membraneous sac) and gastroschisis (paraumbilical defect where the organs are not surrounded by membrane). Karyotyping is usually offered for exomphalos. The prognosis for both is usually good in the absence of other anomalies. Women who have undergone serum screening for trisomy 21 and are noted to have elevated alpha-fetoprotein (AFP) levels may be offered an earlier ultrasound assessment of the fetus to exclude an anterior abdominal wall defect or an open neural tube defect as these anomalies are known to result in higher levels of alpha-fetoprotein.

Bowel atresias may be recognised by distended stomach and bowel proximal to the atresia and there may be associated polyhydramnios.

Fluid within the peritoneal cavity representing ascites may indicate hydrops, which has a vast and diverse aetiology including chromosomal and genetic anomalies, viral and cardiac causes in addition to fetal anaemia. The prognosis for hydrops is largely dependent on the underlying cause.

Urogenital anomalies

Renal anomalies are among the most frequent to be detected during screening. Obstruction to the collecting system may occur throughout the course of the ureter and will result in dilated proximal structures including the ureter itself and the renal pelvis. Obstruction of the urethra is most commonly secondary to posterior urethral valves in a male fetus and results in a distended bladder in addition to the proximal ureters and bilateral hydronephrosis. If the obstruction is complete oligohydramnios will result and this will lead to a risk of pulmonary hypoplasia.

Unilateral or bilateral renal agenesis or multicystic dysplastic kidneys (seen as multiple cysts of varying size within the kidney) are amenable to diagnosis by ultrasound, and where either condition is bilateral the prognosis is gloomy.

Skeletal dysplasias

Skeletal dysplasias are a large group of conditions characterised by abnormal bone and cartilage growth development that results in abnormal shape, size and proportion of the skeleton. It is important to differentiate lethal from non-lethal dysplasias, and referral to fetal medicine is usually appropriate.

Multiple anomalies

In the presence of multiple anomalies chromosomal and genetic causes should be considered and karyotyping offered.

Normal variants

Many examples of normal variants such as choroid plexus cysts and echogenic foci within the heart and a two vessel cord, which were previously considered to be soft markers for aneuploidy, should no longer be reported. Others including nuchal oedema (>6 mm), ventriculomegaly (atrial measurement >10 mm), echogenic bowel, short femur length (<5th centile), renal pelvis dilation (>7 mm) require reporting and consideration of further assessment.

Audit

Units should audit certain conditions for quality control. These conditions are anencephaly, bilateral renal agenesis, diaphragmatic hernia, gastroschisis and exomphalos, lethal skeletal dysplasias, open spina bifida, cleft lip and serious cardiac anomalies. Detection rates vary between 98% for anencephaly down to 50% for serious cardiac anomalies.

Screening for chromosomal anomalies

Multiple anomalies and some specified abnormalities that can be identified on ultrasound indicate a higher risk of aneuploidy and can trigger further investigation including karyotyping. However, some chromosomally abnormal babies, including those with Down syndrome, can appear normal at the time of the routine anomaly scan.

Considerable resources have been channelled into attempts to identify the fetus with trisomy 21 and these have developed from screening by maternal age (risk rising with advancing age) and previous history to more sophisticated methods.

Statistical analysis using maternal age combined with initially two hormone markers (double test) and more recently three (triple test) and now four hormone markers (the quad test) has been introduced. The quad test uses the hormones AFP, oestriol, beta-human chorionic gonadotrophin (BHCG) and inhibin A, and currently has a sensitivity of at least 75% with a 3% false positive test rate when used with a 1 in 150 cutoff.

The combined test uses measurement of the nuchal translucency and the levels of free b-HCG and pregnancy-associated plasma protein A (PAPP-A) to derive a risk for trisomy 21. This test currently has a detection rate of around 90% and a false positive rate of 2% when used with a cutoff of 1 in 150.

The combined test is recommended by the National Screening Committee to be the test of choice in the first trimester, and the quad test should be reserved for women who present too late for first-trimester screening.

Screen-positive women are then offered karyotyping by either chorionic villus sampling or amniocentesis.

Most recently cell-free fetal DNA screening has become available and is currently under review to determine whether it is appropriate to become the primary method of choice for screening. This method has a sensitivity in the region of 98% with a very low false positive rate. Although expensive the price is falling and in the future it is likely to supersede other methods of screening. In addition to a high degree of accuracy the test carries no risk as the analysis is performed on a maternal blood sample. It is likely also that in the interim it could perform a secondary screening role and reduce the number of women requiring invasive karyotyping after combined screening.

Invasive tests

If maternal or fetal screening indicates a fetus may be at risk of a given condition, tissue sampling is required for diagnostic purposes (Table 10.1). Obtaining fetal tissue requires invasive testing and this is most commonly done in the form of amniocentesis or chorionic villus sampling (CVS). If we assume 5% of women undergo invasive testing in pregnancy, in 2012 in the UK this would have resulted in 36 484 procedures. Early detection of these disorders not only allows for detailed planning of the pregnancy, but also allows an informed discussion regarding termination. Diagnostic testing is dependent on parental wishes and gestation. The risks of any procedure must be balanced against the benefits of any information gained and what decisions it will help make. Let us take the example of a high-risk trisomy 21 screening result – in some situations the risk of miscarriage may be unacceptable to some parents, despite the potential morbidity posed if diagnostic testing

Table 10.1 Antenatal diagnostic methods and targets.

	Examples	Diagnostic sample	Technique
Single gene defects	Cystic fibrosis	Amniotic fluid/placenta	Amniocentesis/CVS
Chromosomal problems	Trisomy 13/18/21, X0	Amniotic fluid/placenta	Amniocentesis/CVS
Infection	CMV, varicella	Amniotic fluid	Amniocentesis
Metabolic conditions	CAH, Tay–Sachs, G6PDD	Amniotic fluid/placenta	Amniocentesis/CVS
Fetal anaemia	PB19, aplastic crisis	Fetal blood	Cordocentesis
Fetal thrombocytopenia	ITP, von Willebrand	Fetal blood	Cordocentesis

CAH, congenital adrenal hyperplasia; CMV, cytomegalovirus; CVS, chorionic villus sampling; G6PDD, glucose 6-phosphate dehydrogenase deficiency; ITP, idiopathic thrombocytopenia; PB19, parvovirus B19.

proved positive (Table 10.2). Conversely, if for any reason parents would not continue a pregnancy in the result of a positive diagnostic test then the earlier the diagnosis, the fewer the complications of an early termination. Recently, non-invasive sampling of free fetal DNA in the maternal serum has become available.

Amniocentesis

Second-trimester diagnostic testing is commonly performed by amniocentesis (amniotic fluid obtained by *centesis* = the act of accessing a body cavity or organ with a needle in order obtain fluid). Common indications are listed in Table 10.3. The main concern of the parents is the risk of miscarriage with invasive testing, and while this is understandable, to the clinician there are many other significant risks and these are listed in Table 10.1. If a screening result indicates a high risk of fetal anomaly then amniocentesis should be offered. The procedure should be performed after 15 weeks. Amniocentesis performed prior to 15 weeks increases the incidence of fetal talipes, respiratory distress in the neonate and miscarriage. Third-trimester amniocentesis is also performed and is associated with a lower miscarriage rate but a higher incidence of blood staining of the collected sample.

Table 10.2 Antenatal screening risks.

	Gestation (weeks)	Tissue sample	Miscarriage rate
Amniocentesis	15+	Amniotic fluid	1%
CVS	11–13+6	Chorionic villi	2%
Cordocentesis	18–20+	Fetal blood	2–3%
FFDNA	10+	Fetal DNA in maternal blood	0%

CVS, chorionic villus sampling; FFDNA, free fetal DNA.

Procedure

This involves obtaining a 10–20 mL sample of amniotic fluid under aseptic conditions for molecular, cytogenetic or microbiological analysis.

Transabdominal aspiration (using a 20-gauge needle) under ultrasound guidance minimises blood staining of the sample and also reduces maternal (bowel) and fetal (body and cord) trauma.

Amniocentesis should not be performed without reviewing the results of serum and infection screening tests as well as any ultrasound scans performed. Written consent is required and the indications should be documented. Sepsis can be minimised by the use of aseptic techniques, and hepatitis B and C infections are not contraindications to amniocentesis. HIV infection is a relative contraindication but if the mother is receiving highly active antiretroviral therapy (HAART) and her viral load is suppressed, then amniocentesis may be permissible after discussion with the relevant specialists. Rhesus status

Table 10.3 Indications for amniocentesis.

- High-risk first or second trimester screening/raised nuchal translucency (NT)
- Suspected fetal infection (positive maternal IgM, no immunity)
- Structural anomaly/>two soft markers
- Severe IUGR (<3rd centile, especially if normal Doppler)
- Previous affected child
- Known parental translocation or autosomal dominant condition
- Parental carriers of autosomal recessive condition
- Sex determination
- Male fetus and X-linked inheritance
- Advanced maternal age
- Patient request

IUGR, intrauterine growth restriction.

should be checked and anti-D administered if appropriate to minimise the risk of sensitisation.

The wait for a result is usually around 2 weeks using standard laboratory techniques (cell culture). This causes considerable anxiety for the parents and with increasing gestation may make a termination procedure more complicated. Rapid results (within 48 hours) can be obtained using techniques such as FISH (fluorescence in-situ hybridisation) and QF-PCR (quantitative fluorescence polymerase chain reaction). Using specific gene probes or short tandem repeat (STR) probes faster results can be obtained. These tests are only suitable for the trisomies 13, 18 and 21 and monosomy X (Turner) as the identification of single gene defects still requires sample amplification (PCR). Similar techniques are used for the tissue samples obtained at CVS.

Chorionic villus sampling (CVS)

This invasive procedure is performed from 10 to 13^{+6} weeks gestation. It involves biopsy of the placental tissue via either the transcervical or transabdominal route. As it uses a larger bore needle, local anaesthetic is offered. It can detect chromosomal abnormalities and single gene defects, and the available genetic probes are continually increasing. Indications for use of CVS are shown in Table 10.4.

Done at an earlier gestational stage, CVS allows for earlier termination of a pregnancy than amniocentesis. The rare malformations associated with CVS include limb reduction defects and oromandibular defects. The precautions with regard to transmission of infection are the same as for amniocentesis. Serious complications include miscarriage, preterm premature rupture of membranes and sepsis. Anti-D prophylaxis is required for rhesus-negative mothers (Table 10.5).

There are three main sampling problems associated with CVS:

- maternal cell contamination;
- mosaicism;
- culture failure.

Interpreting the results

Any diagnostic test requested by a clinician must answer a clinical question or guide management for the procedural risks to be justifiable. A plan for the pregnancy, based on the results, must be made in conjunction with the parents. Their

Table 10.4 Indications for chorionic villus sampling (CVS).

- Abnormal serum screening results
- Raised nuchal translucency
- Ultrasound abnormality (e.g. cystic hygroma)
- Known parental gene defect (carriers or affected)
- Previous affected child
- Family history

Table 10.5 Complications of amniocentesis and chorionic villus sampling (CVS).

Maternal	Fetal
• Local pain • Infection (sepsis) • Preterm rupture of membranes • Preterm labour • Rhesus isoimmunisation	• Miscarriage/intrauterine fetal death • Malformations • Amniocentesis: talipes • CVS: limb reduction/hypoplasia/oromandibular defects • Prematurity • Respiratory distress syndrome in neonate • Infection – sepsis • Infection – vertical viral transmission

wishes must be respected at all times. Management plans may include the following:

1. Termination if the condition is lethal or carries considerable fetal morbidity.
2. Further investigation and monitoring.
3. Timing of delivery.
4. Multidisciplinary team planning.
5. Directed therapies.

Infection in pregnancy

The identification of infections in pregnancy relies on both screening (in the form of routine and high-risk antenatal screening) and clinical investigation in response to symptom presentation. Table 10.6 highlights the important bacterial and viral infections in pregnancy. Diagnosing infections early:

- reduces maternal morbidity and mortality;
- reduces congenital infection and thus fetal morbidity and mortality in utero;
- reduces vertical transmission at birth thus reducing neonatal infection and long-term consequences.

The effects on the fetus of infections in pregnancy depend on the infective agent, the gestation, previous exposure (maternal immunity) and the availability of specific treatments (to reduce infectivity, transfer and to treat fetal infection). Vertical transmission of infection (e.g. HIV or hepatitis) occurs from mother to fetus while in utero (transplacental) or at birth (vertical transmission; vaginal delivery and exposure to body fluids). Horizontal infections occur between members in the community, which can then pass vertically (e.g. varicella) to the fetus.

Screening for infection

All women in the UK who are pregnant are offered routine screening. This may include serum, urine and swab testing, and women have the right to refuse any or all of the tests offered. If this is the case, their ideas and concerns should be explored in detail and the reasons clearly documented in their notes. They should be offered further opportunities to participate in the screening programme, especially if they are thought of be high risk (e.g. known intravenous drug users or sex workers). They should be reassured that the results of any testing are confidential and will not be disclosed to third parties (with the exception of positive HIV tests, which may be disclosed to sexual partners at risk of continuing infection if the patient declines to inform them). Positive test results should be appropriately treated and the necessary multidisciplinary teams involved (e.g. neonatologists, infectious diseases). Table 10.6 shows a summary of fetal risks from maternal infections. Infections that are tested for routinely include:

1. **Urine tract infections.** A mid-stream urine (MSU) sample is sent at booking. Asymptomatic bacteriuria should be treated according to microbiological sensitivities. Even if asymptomatic, bacteriuria is associated with an increased incidence of pyelonephritis and hence preterm labour.

   Note: Group B streptococcus is not routinely screened for in pregnancy but if cultured the patient should receive prophylactic intrapartum antibiotics.

2. **HIV.** Women should be offered fourth generation (HIV antibody and p24 antigen) HIV testing in pregnancy. High-risk women should be offered repeat testing even if the initial testing is negative. If they continue to exhibit high-risk behaviours (intravenous drug abuse, unprotected intercourse with multiple partners, known HIV-positive partner without protected intercourse) testing should be repeated at 28 weeks and again in the third trimester. In addition to the standard first-trimester screening, HIV-positive women should also be offered testing for:
   - hepatitis C;
   - varicella immunity;
   - measles immunity;
   - *Toxoplasma*.

3. **Rubella.** Rubella infection in the non-immune can have multiple teratogenic effects in the baby (Table 10.7), especially if exposure occurs in the first trimester. Non-immune women should be vaccinated after birth. The MMR vaccine is a live vaccine and conception within a month of administration should be avoided.

   Measuring maternal IgM enables rubella diagnosis. A four-fold increase in antibody titres indicates infection, and a termination should be offered as an option in the first trimester. If it is declined a detailed anomaly scan and serial ultrasound scans for fetal growth are indicated.

4. **Hepatitis B.** Acute presentation of hepatitis may be with upper gastrointestinal symptoms such as nausea, vomiting, pain and jaundice or acute liver failure. The more chronic disease state may be complicated by liver cirrhosis and chronic liver failure.

There is no fetal syndrome but the vertical transmission at birth is a significant risk. To reduce the risk of vertical transmission no invasive procedures should be performed. The principles of preventing neonatal infection after birth include:
- administration of hepatitis B immunoglobulin (HBIG);
- vaccination;
- serological testing to confirm non-infection.

Partner testing and counselling is advised, as is testing of any siblings.

5. **Syphilis.** This disease has multiple stages of presentation:
   Primary stage: Primary chancre – painless ulcerated lesion that resolves in 6 weeks.
   Secondary stage: Widespread rash that may involve hands and back, mucous membranes and cause lymph node enlargement.
   Latent phase: No symptoms but positive serological testing.
   Tertiary stage: Not infective and may present as skin disease (gummatous disease), cardiovascular syphilis or neurosyphilis.

   In the infected fetus, presentation in the neonate may be with rash, jaundice, lympadenopathy and chorioretinitis.
   VDRL test: Venereal diseases reference laboratory tests for syphilis antibodies. Positive testing requires confirmatory testing by another method.

Infections not screened in routine antenatal care

Some infections do not meet the criteria to justify population-wide universal screening. However, they do cause fetal morbidity and mortality and should be diagnosed promptly to minimise these consequences. This relies on clinical acumen and will be suspected from a good history and examination.

1. **Herpes.** Herpes simplex virus type 1 and type 2 may present as a primary or recurrent infection in pregnancy. It is not screened for but a history of previous infection is enquired about at booking.

Primary herpes
- Presentation is characteristically with urinary retention and a vesicular rash.
- Is sexually transmitted.
- Serum IgG testing that is the same as the subtype isolated from a vaginal viral swab indicates recurrence rather than primary infection.
- Should be managed jointly with a genitourinary specialist.
- Aciclovir given to the mother can reduce the duration and intensity of the attack.
- Has a high risk of neonatal infection if the baby delivers vaginally (>40%).
- Within 6 weeks of delivery is an indication for caesarean section.
- If vaginal delivery is requested, no invasive procedures should be carried out on the fetus.

Table 10.6 Summary of infectious agents and associated fetal complications.

Infective agent	Type	Transmission to fetus	Maternal features	Risk factors for maternal infection	Congenital abnormalities	Diagnosis	Treatment
CMV	Herpes family DNA virus	Transplacental	Asymptomatic or flu-like illness	Contact with cat litter Contaminated foods	Jaundice Hepatomegaly Hepatitis Low platelets Splenomegaly Microcephaly Chorioretinitis Rash	Maternal antibodies Amniotic PCR	No fetal treatment Postnatal ganciclovir
Rubella	Virus	Transplacental	Rash Lymphadenopathy Arthritis May be asymptomatic	Respiratory secretion exposure	Deafness Cardiac malformations Cataracts Retinopathy Glaucoma	Maternal antibodies Maternal throat swabs (viral PCR) Ultrasound findings (fetal)	Termination in first trimester Postnatal vaccination (maternal)
Toxoplasma	Intracellular protozoan	Transplacental	Asymptomatic or flu-like illness	Contaminated, poorly cooked and washed food (meat and vegetables)	Intracranial calcifications Chorioretinitis Hydrocephalus	Maternal antibodies ELISA Amniotic PCR	Spiramycin Pyrimethamine Sulfadiazine
Listeriosis	Gram-positive bacilli	Transplacental	Flu-like symptoms Abdominal pain Diarrhoea Vomiting Conjunctivitis Pharyngitis	Contaminated foods	Nil Results in preterm labour, miscarriage, fetal death	Microbiological culture	Ampicillin Gentamicin
Varicella zoster		Herpes family	Transplacental	Vesicular rash Fever	Inhalation of infected respiratory droplets	Fetal varicella syndrome	Maternal antibodies Ultrasound Amniotic PCR

Disease	Organism	Transmission	Maternal features	Exposure	Fetal/neonatal effects	Investigations	Treatment
Parvovirus	DNA virus	Transplacental	Rash Arthralgia Anaemia/aplastic crisis	Contact with infected individuals	Pancytopenia Hydrops Anaemia IUD	Maternal antibodies PCR	Transfusion No drug treatment Conservative
Syphilis	Spirochaete (*Treponema pallidum*)	Transplacental Vertical	Depends on disease stage	Sexual transmission	Miscarriage IUD Deafness Bone defects	Maternal antibodies	Penicillin
Malaria	*Plasmodium* infection (protozoan)	Transplacental	Flu-like symptoms Jaundice Splenomegaly Hepatomegaly Pain Nausea/vomiting	Mosquito bites	Preterm labour Low birthweight IUD/stillbirth Congenital malaria	Blood films and microscopy	Antimalarials depending on gestation
HIV	Virus	Transplacental Vertical	Immunosuppression and consequences of medication toxicity	Blood and body fluid Contaminated needles	Virus infection only. No congenital syndrome.	HIV antibody tests P24 antigen	HAART
Hepatitis	Virus	Transplacental Vertical					
Herpes simplex	Virus	Transplacental Vertical	Primary and secondary infection associated with vaginal lesions and pain	Sexually transmitted	Risk of neonatal infection: • skin disease • local CNS disease • disseminated	Serum IgG Viral PCR from vaginal swab	Aciclovir orally

CMV, cytomegalovirus; ELISA, enzyme-linked immunosorbent assay; HAART, highly active antiretroviral therapy; IUD, intrauterine death; PCR, polymerase chain reaction.

Table 10.7 Rubella infection in the mother and fetus..

Maternal signs/symptoms	Fetal effects
• Asymptomatic • Rash • Lymphadenopathy • Joint pain • Pyrexia • Conjunctivitis • Loss of appetite	• Miscarriage • Sensorineural deafness • Eye defects (cataracts, microphthalmia, glaucoma) • Congenital heart defects (e.g. patent ductus arteriosis) • Hepatomegaly/splenomegaly • Thrombotic thrombocytopenic purpura (TTP) • Hydrops

Recurrent herpes

- Has a much lower rate of fetal infection at approximately 3%.
- Is not an indication for caesarean section; vaginal delivery is safer than with a primary attack.
- Suppressive aciclovir from 36 weeks may be given to reduce lesion appearance and hence reduce the risk of fetal transmission.

2. **Cytomegalovirus (CMV) and toxoplasmosis.** See Table 10.8.

Rashes in pregnancy

Generalized rashes, vesicular and non-vesicular, require immunological investigation and treatment based on the result. In pregnancy, measles, parvovirus B19 and rubella produce a generalised maculopapular rash as part of the systemic maternal infection. Diagnosis of the infectious agent is vital, as it will guide counselling on the fetal consequences and on necessary treatments. Varicella produces a vesicular rash and can be associated with profound fetal consequences.

1. **Measles (non-vesicular).** Measles should be a rare disease as infants are vaccinated as part of the MMR (measles, mumps, rubella) vaccine. Outbreaks have been seen in the UK following decreased uptake of the vaccine owing to unfounded concerns surrounding the vaccine. In non-immune adults the infection is often self-limiting with a rash and associated flu-like symptoms. In immunocompromised individuals infection can be fatal (Table 10.9).

Treatment is supportive with hydration, paracetamol (acetaminophen) and anti-inflammatory medications. Human normal immune immunoglobulin (HNIG) has been used to treat non-immune high-risk individuals following significant exposure. There is no fetal syndrome associated with measles infection. However, severe anaemia in the fetus may result in the development of hydrops fetalis and its resultant complications. Ultrasound follow-up is indicated to monitor for this, which usually occurs within 8 weeks of infection.

2. **Parvovirus B19 (non-vesicular).** This is a childhood infection, seen commonly in children of a young schooling age, and it is easily appreciated how pregnant women are exposed, and for a significant amount of time. The illness in adults is again a short-lived viral fever that presents with a rash (the characteristic slapped cheek syndrome) and mild joint pain. Infection can be confirmed by measuring rising titres of antibodies, and differentiating between IgG and IgM rises indicates a level of previous immunity. Caution should be taken in sickle-cell patients with parvovirus B19 as aplastic anaemia can be an acute complication in this group. Management is supportive.

Table 10.8 A comparison of cytomegalovirus (CMV) and toxoplasmosis infections.

	CMV	Toxoplasmosis
Infective agent	DNA virus	Protozoan
Route	Ingestion of contaminated foods	Body fluids
Fetal consequences	Microcephaly Jaundice, hepatosplenomegaly, low platelets Ventriculomegaly IUGR	Cerebral calcification Hydrocephalus Chorioretinitis
Maternal symptoms	Asymptomatic Flu-like symptoms	Asymptomatic Flu-like symptoms
Test	Maternal serum antibodies Amniocentesis Ultrasound follow-up	Maternal serum antibodies Amniocentesis Ultrasound follow-up
Treatment	No medical treatment Termination of infected fetus	Spiramycin Folinic acid Pyrimethamine Sulfadiazine

IUGR, intrauterine growth restriction.

Table 10.9 Complications of measles.

Common	Uncommon	Rare	Pregnancy related
Diarrhoea	Hepatitis	Blindness	Miscarriage
Vomiting	Meningitis	Cardiovascular complications	Stillbirth
Otitis media	Encephalitis	Subacute sclerosing panencephalitis (SSPE)	Intrauterine growth restriction (IUGR)
Pneumonia		Death	Preterm labour
Febrile convulsions			

3. **Varicella (chicken pox and shingles virus) – vesicular rash.** Primary varicella zoster infection in adults can be severe. A severe pneumonia resulting from it can be fatal. Key points in clinical management are:
   - Non-immune individuals should be given varicella zoster immunoglobulin (VZIG) within 72 hours of significant contact. It has no role once the rash has developed.
   - Admission to any part of the maternity unit should be avoided to avoid cross-contamination.
   - High-risk individuals may require admission for observation.
   - Aciclovir can be used to reduce the severity and intensity of the infection and is safe after 20 weeks gestation.
   - Neonates require a period of observation after delivery if the mother was recently infected.
   - Delivery may be delayed to confer passive immunity to the child.
   - VZIG may be given to the neonate if exposed and delivered to a non-immune mother.

A fetal syndrome is associated with varicella zoster, the fetal varicella syndrome (FVS). No documented case has been seen after 28 weeks gestation. This consists of:
   - limb defects including hypoplasia;
   - skin scarring in a dermatomal distribution;
   - deafness;
   - blindness;
   - cataracts;
   - chorioretinitis;
   - hydrocephalus;
   - microcephaly;
   - bladder sphincter dysfunction;
   - bowel sphincter dysfunction.

Fetal exposure and infection may be detected in variety of ways and include:
   - ultrasound follow-up looking for any of the above features;
   - amniocentesis;
   - cordocentesis.

Clinical case

Case investigations and discussion

The karyotype is normal and the hernia is again confirmed at the 20-week scan. The patient continues with the pregnancy and the remainder of her care is uncomplicated. Serial growth scans are normal and she is delivered vaginally after an induction of labour at 40 weeks in a tertiary centre.

Her baby is ventilated at birth and a nasogastric tube inserted to secure the airway and prevent aspiration. After a short period on intensive care, the infant undergoes surgery on day 3 and has a successful repair of the hernia.

Summary

Key learning points

- Antenatal care involves screening of the general population and further diagnostic testing of at-risk individuals.
- Fetal anomalies may be characteristically associated with specific genetic conditions or chromosomal problems.

- Maternal infection has fetal consequences, and these are dependent on the infectious agent and gestation of the fetus.
- Clinical judgement should guide investigation of maternal infection.

 Now visit **www.wileyessential.com/humandevelopment** to test yourself on this chapter.

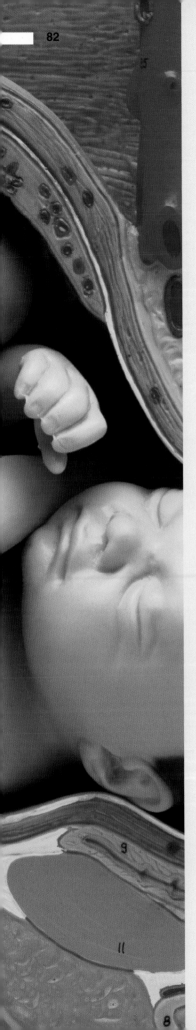

CHAPTER 11
Hypertensive disorders of pregnancy

Sharif Ismail

Case

A 30-year-old patient, Mrs Harris, presented with rupture of membranes at 37 weeks gestation. This was her second pregnancy, having earlier had an uneventful pregnancy ending in a normal vaginal delivery at term. At 35 weeks gestation, her blood pressure was noted to be 150/90 mmHg and she had no proteinuria. She was started on oral labetolol 200 mg twice daily but had to stop it because of headache. She was admitted to hospital for induction or augmentation of labour. Two hours after admission, she started to have abdominal pains, which were thought to be labour pains. Her pains were noted to be strong and frequent. The fetal heart was difficult to detect. The patient progressed to have a normal vaginal delivery but the baby was stillborn. There was a large retroplacental clot consistent with concealed placental abruption. After delivery, her blood pressure was 180/100 mmHg, she had ++++ protein in her urine and her reflexes were exaggerated.

Learning outcomes

- By the end of this chapter, you should be able to:
- Appreciate the risks associated with hypertension in pregnancy.
- Diagnose and assess patients with hypertension in pregnancy.
- Deliver essential and life-saving management of hypertension in pregnancy.
- Provide empathy to pregnant women and their families during a stressful time.

Essential Human Development, First Edition. Edited by Samuel Webster, Geraint Morris and Euan Kevelighan
© 2018 John Wiley & Sons, Ltd. Published 2018 by John Wiley & Sons, Ltd.

Introduction

Hypertension is one of the common and serious complications that can be encountered during pregnancy and delivery as well as after delivery. In the developed world, it is often detected early and pregnant mothers are kept under observation and provided with treatment, which enables management and delivery before serious complications develop. Nonetheless, rapid progression can still occur leading to serious complications, and the condition remains a leading cause of maternal mortality and morbidity. The situation is much worse in the developing world, where the lack of adequate antenatal care as well as limited uptake of services lead to late presentation often with serious complications and poor outcome.

The incidence of hypertension in pregnancy varies from country to country. In the UK, the estimated incidence is 10% (1:10 pregnancies). One-third of these will develop pre-eclampsia, which is hypertension in pregnancy associated with proteinuria. The rest will develop other types of pregnancy-induced hypertension.

Definitions

Hypertension in pregnancy includes a number of disorders; these have varied aetiologies, which may affect disease progression during pregnancy and its outcome after delivery (Table 11.1). Hypertension that appears for the first time in pregnancy tends to resolve with delivery whereas hypertension that antedates pregnancy may worsen during pregnancy and usually persists after delivery. The same applies to pre-existing renal disease, which predisposes to pre-eclampsia when hypertension develops.

Hypertension in pregnancy (gestational hypertension) is defined as a systolic blood pressure over 140 mmHg or a diastolic blood pressure over 90 mmHg at least on two occasions with a minimum of 4 hours interval after 20 weeks gestation. Reference to booking blood pressure should be noted, and a rise of 30 mmHg in systolic blood pressure or 15 mmHg in diastolic blood pressure over booking blood pressure is sufficient for making a diagnosis The diastolic blood pressure is taken at the fifth Korotkoff sound, which is total disappearance rather than muffling.

Proteinuria in pregnancy is defined as urinary protein concentration more than 300 mg/L during any 24-hour urine collection or more than 1 g/L in a random sample on two occasions at least 6 hours apart. The presence of "+" of protein on urine dipstick was formerly used for making the diagnosis, but automated reading is now recommended instead. Alternatively, a urine protein/creatinine ratio (PCR) of 30 mg/mmol or more can be used.

Oedema used to be the third of the pre-eclampsia triad (hypertension, proteinuria and oedema). It can be noted in the feet, ankles, fingers, face, sacrum and lower abdominal wall. However, it is very common in otherwise normal pregnancies, such that it is no longer considered a feature of pregnancy hypertension.

The combination of gestational hypertension and proteinuria marks the development of pre-eclampsia (gestational proteinuric hypertension). This is the case from the start in some patients, whereas either gestational hypertension or proteinuria may appear first followed by the other in some patients. The occurrence of tonic clonic convulsions (fits) on top of pre-eclampsia is known as eclampsia, hence the name pre-eclampsia for the presentation without fits. Eclampsia may manifest with fits without any prior features of pre-eclampsia, which often appears afterwards. This represents a variation in the disease course.

The development of proteinuria on top of pre-existing (essential) hypertension and the development of gestational hypertension on top of prior renal disease are known as superimposed pre-eclampsia. The occurrence of fits in these cases is known as superimposed eclampsia.

Risks of hypertension in pregnancy

The risks associated with hypertension in pregnancy vary according to the type and severity of the disease (Table 11.2). Mild gestational hypertension arising late in pregnancy bears hardly any risk to either the patient or her baby. On the other hand, the development of severe gestational proteinuric hypertension (pre-eclampsia) earlier in pregnancy may pose considerable risk to the life of the patient such that delivery becomes necessary even before fetal maturity. Hypertension carries the risk of cerebrovascular accident and heart failure. Renal damage may progress to renal failure. The development of HELLP (haemolysis, elevated liver enzymes and low platelets) syndrome may lead to hypoxia, liver damage and bleeding. Bleeding may lead to disseminated intravascular coagulopathy. Placental infarction can lead to intrauterine growth restriction and even intrauterine fetal death. Placental abruption is a recognised complication of pre-eclampsia and this can lead to fetal death as well as antepartum haemorrhage. The occurrence of eclamptic fits increases the risk to the mother, especially of hypoxia and injury. All these risk factors can lead to adult respiratory distress syndrome and increased risk of thromboembolism as well as maternal death. Early delivery may be required and this increases the risk of operative delivery for the mother and prematurity for the fetus. The risk to the mother does not end with delivery, as some may continue to suffer from hypertension and/or renal problems, and the disease might recur in a subsequent pregnancy.

Pathology of pre-eclampsia and eclampsia

The aetiology of gestational hypertension, proteinuria and proteinuric hypertension (pre-eclampsia) as well as eclampsia remains unknown. However, vasoconstriction affecting various

Table 11.1 Terms used in relation to hypertension in pregnancy.

Gestational hypertension
- Systolic blood pressure >140 mmHg on two separate occasions or a rise of 30 mmHg over booking systolic blood pressure at least 4 hours apart detected for the first time >20 weeks gestation
- Diastolic blood pressure >90 mmHg or a rise of 15 mmHg over booking systolic blood pressure on two separate occasions at least 4 hours apart detected for the first time >20 weeks gestation

Degree of hypertension
- Mild hypertension: <149/99 mmHg
- Moderate hypertension: <159/109 mmHg
- Severe hypertension: ≥160/110 mmHg

Significant proteinuria
- Urine protein ≥300 mg/L per 24 hours
- Urine protein >1 g/L in a random sample on two separate occasions at least 6 hours apart
- Urine protein/creatinine ratio (PCR) ≥30

Essential hypertension
- Pre-existing (essential/chronic) hypertension or hypertension diagnosed up to 20 weeks gestation

Chronic nephritis
- Pre-existing renal disease with proteinuria

Proteinuric gestational hypertension (pre-eclampsia)
- Gestational hypertension with significant proteinuria detected for the first time >20 weeks gestation

Severe pre-eclampsia
- Blood pressure ≥160/110 mmHg and/or
- Two features of severe disease including:
  - severe headache
  - visual disturbances
  - epigastric pain
  - vomiting
  - clonus (>three beats)
  - exaggerated (brisk) reflexes
  - epigastric tenderness
  - abnormal liver function tests
  - poor urine output
  - abnormal kidney function tests
  - falling platelets
  - HELLP syndrome (haemolysis, elevated liver enzymes and low platelets)

Fulminating pre-eclampsia
This term is used to describe cases where patient features deteriorate rapidly. This is a real risk in patients with pre-eclampsia; even patients with mild disease and those with controlled blood pressure for some time may suddenly develop symptoms of severe disease, and their physical signs as well as laboratory tests show dramatic changes over a short span of time

Eclampsia
- Development of tonic clonic convulsions (fits) on top of proteinuric gestational hypertension (pre-eclampsia)

organs, including the placenta, is a characteristic feature. This leads to hypertension and multiple organ damage as well as intrauterine growth restriction. Theories revolve around:

- Failure of the second wave of trophoblast invasion into the deciduas in early pregnancy. This leads to reduced placental blood flow and intrauterine growth restriction.

- Increased vasoconstriction, leading to hypertension. The vasoconstriction could be the result of:
  - disturbed prostaglandins balance with relative increase in thromboxane over prostacyclin;
  - decreased renal renin secretion;
  - decreased nitric oxide.

Table 11.2 Risks of hypertension in pregnancy.

Maternal risk
- Cerebrovascular accidents
- Heart failure
- Renal failure
- Liver failure
- Haemorrhage:
  - placental abruption
  - postpartum haemorrhage
- Disseminated intravascular coagulopathy
- Eclampsia:
  - hypoxia
  - injury
- Adult respiratory distress syndrome
- Thromboembolic disease
- Operative delivery
- Maternal death
- Long-term hypertension and/or renal impairment
- Recurrence in a future pregnancy

Fetal risk
- Intrauterine growth restriction/intrauterine fetal death
- Preterm labour

Other notable features of the disease include:
- Glomeruloendotheliosis leading to impaired glomerular filtration, with loss of albumin in urine.
- Platelet dysfunction.

The occurrence of hypertension in pregnancy depends on a number of factors that affect predisposition to the disease including:
- Hypertension:
  - pre-existing hypertension and/or renal disease;
  - previous pre-eclampsia;
  - hypertension on the combined oral contraceptive pill;
  - family history of pre-eclampsia.
- Increased placental tissue:
  - multiple pregnancy;
  - hydatidiform mole;
  - hydrops fetalis;
  - gestational diabetes.
- First pregnancy for any particular couple (primigravida or new partner).
- Pregnancy interval greater than 10 years.
- Body mass index greater than 30.
- Age ≥40 years.
- Antiphospholipid syndrome.
- Systemic lupus erythematosus.
- Thrombophilia.

Clinical picture

Symptoms

Pregnancy hypertension can be asymptomatic. Occasionally, patients may report facial puffiness or leg swelling, indicating oedema. However, if symptoms occur, they usually indicate severe disease and include:
- Headache (severe, persistent, not responding to simple analgesics).
- Flashing lights.
- Epigastric/right upper quadrant abdominal pain (liver oedema causing capsule stretch).
- Nausea and vomiting.

Signs

Pregnancy hypertension can be a disease of physical signs only, hence it is important to check the blood pressure properly even in asymptomatic pregnant women. This requires the use of an appropriately sized sphygmomanometer cuff. Patients with a high body mass index (BMI) will require a larger cuff to ensure accurate measurement. The cuff should be placed at the level of the heart and pregnant women should be either sitting or lying down to 45°. The diastolic reading should be at the level of total disappearance of the heartbeat, which is the fifth Korotkoff sound, rather than muffling. Oedema should be checked for in the face (puffiness), legs, lower abdomen and/or sacral area. Maternal weight should be obtained and excessive weight gain should be noted. Fundal height should be estimated to facilitate detection of a small-for-date baby.

In patients with features of pregnancy hypertension, signs of severe disease include:
- Tenderness in the epigastrium and/or right upper quadrant.
- Exaggerated reflexes.
- More than six beats of clonus.
- Papilloedema on ophthalmic examination.

Investigations

As proteinuria might be present without any symptoms or signs, urine dipstick should be carried out routinely in all patients. In patients with proteinuria, a midstream urine sample is obtained to exclude infection. A 24-hour protein in urine or protein/creatinine in urine ratio (PCR) is used to estimate the level of proteinuria.

Patients with gestational proteinuric hypertension (pre-eclampsia) require full blood count, clotting screen, urea and electrolytes, liver function tests and serum uric acid. Fetal monitoring (cardiotocography) and/or ultrasound examination is performed to check fetal growth and liquor volume. Young patients presenting with hypertension for the first time before or in early pregnancy (<20 weeks gestation) should be investigated to exclude an underlying cause such as coarctation of the aorta, renal artery stenosis, Cushing's syndrome or phaeochromocytoma,

Management

The management of pregnancy hypertension is usually covered by detailed guidelines and protocols in all maternity units. The actual management will depend on the type and severity of the disease as well as the stage of pregnancy.

Prevention

Daily low-dose aspirin (75 mg) from 12 weeks gestation until delivery has been shown to reduce the risk of developing pre-eclampsia in patients with a history of severe-onset pregnancy-induced hypertension in an earlier pregnancy. It is also advised in patients with more than one risk factor for developing pre-eclampsia, such as first pregnancy, age 40 years or older, pregnancy interval of more than 10 years, BMI of 35 kg/m² or more at first visit, family history of pre-eclampsia, and multiple pregnancy. Salt restriction, rest and low molecular weight heparin have not been shown to be effective preventive measures.

Pre-existing disease

Ideally, these patients should have been seen for pre-pregnancy counselling to ensure satisfactory blood pressure and/or renal disease management. This provides the opportunity to stop medication with teratogenic potential before pregnancy. The aim is to control blood pressure to avoid cerebrovascular accidents as well as end-organ (kidney and retina) damage. Antihypertensive medications that can be used during pregnancy include:

- Labetalol (alpha- and beta-blocker), but this should be avoided in patients with asthma.
- Alpha-methyldopa (centrally acting antihypertensive), but this should be stopped within 2 days of delivery due to the risk of postnatal depression.
- Nifedipine (calcium channel blocker), but this can cause headache.

Daily low-dose aspirin (75 mg) from 12 weeks gestation until delivery has been shown to reduce the risk of developing pre-eclampsia in patients with essential hypertension or renal disease.

These patients are at risk of developing pre-eclampsia and should therefore be regularly monitored, with blood pressure measurement, urinary protein check, fundal height estimation, fetal monitoring (cardiotocography) and fetal growth ultrasound scan. Patients should be counselled about symptoms suggestive of severe pre-eclampsia, so as to seek medical attention urgently.

Gestational hypertension

- Mild hypertension warrants regular observation, in the form of weekly check of blood pressure and urinary protein. Fundal height should be estimated, fetal monitoring (cardiotocography) should be carried out and fetal growth should be checked with ultrasound scans. Patients are at risk of developing pre-eclampsia and should therefore be counselled to seek medical attention urgently if they develop symptoms.
- Moderate hypertension requires treatment and patients should be monitored twice weekly; checking blood pressure and urinary protein. Fundal height should be estimated, fetal monitoring (cardiotocography) should be carried out and fetal growth should be checked with ultrasound scans. Oral antihypertensives can be used for control of blood pressure. Patients should be counselled to seek medical attention urgently if they develop symptoms of pre-eclampsia.
- Severe hypertension requires immediate admission for assessment, treatment and close inpatient monitoring for at least 24 hours. Antihypertensives are prescribed, as outlined above, and the dose is adjusted according to response. Intravenous treatment may be required, usually using labetalol or hydralazine. Sublingual nifedipine may also be required. With good control of blood pressure, patients can be discharged home on oral antihypertensives. Even after control of blood pressure, patients remain at risk of developing pre-eclampsia later in pregnancy and should be kept under regular observation. This observation includes frequent blood pressure measurements, urinary protein, fundal height, fetal monitoring (cardiotocography) and fetal growth ultrasound scans. Patients should also be counselled about symptoms suggesting severity, so as to seek medical attention urgently. Early delivery is sometimes required in these cases, particularly if the blood pressure is difficult to control or there is evidence of maternal and/or fetal compromise.

Pre-eclampsia

The appearance of proteinuria and hypertension together heralds multiple system involvement. This requires frequent assessment and monitoring. Observation includes blood pressure, urinary protein or protein creatinine ratio (PCR), fundal height, fetal monitoring (cardiotocography) and fetal growth on ultrasound scan. Blood tests include full blood count, clotting screen, liver function tests, urea and electrolytes, and serum uric acid. These tests may require repeating regularly, and the frequency will depend on the severity of the disease as well as its progression. Patients should be counselled about severity symptoms including headache, flashing lights and epigastric tenderness, and of the importance to inform medical staff if they occur.

Daily low-dose aspirin (75 mg) may help avoid worsening of the disease, in patients with risk factors, as outlined above.

Antihypertensives may be required, using the drugs outlined above. The aim is to keep blood pressure under control until 37 weeks gestation, when induction of labour can be organised, unless there is evidence of maternal or fetal compromise, when earlier delivery is warranted. Steroids are advised prior to 34 weeks gestation, to enhance fetal lung maturity. They are provided in the form of two intramuscular injections of 12 mg betamethasone or dexamethasone 24 hours apart. However, urgent delivery may be required occasionally such that there is no time to administer steroids or for them to work.

Severe pre-eclampsia

This requires immediate admission for assessment, close observation and inpatient treatment. Patients will need regular blood pressure monitoring, input/output fluid chart, daily fetal monitoring (cardiotocography) and 24-hour urinary protein estimation or protein/creatinine ratio (PCR) estimation. Intravenous access is established. Patients may need to be observed in a high-dependency unit. Blood pressure control may require intravenous medication using labetalol or hydralazine. Sublingual nifedipine may also be required.

If the disease can be controlled, then pregnancy can be allowed to progress and induction of labour can be considered at term (37 weeks gestation onwards). Oral antihypertensives are prescribed and patients can be discharged home, with at least twice-weekly checks of their blood pressure, urinary protein, fundal height, fetal monitoring (cardiotocography) and fetal growth ultrasound scans. Blood tests will be required at least once a week.

If the blood pressure cannot be adequately controlled, delivery may be required earlier (34 weeks gestation) or even urgently, usually through caesarean section. Administration of steroids to enhance fetal lung maturity prior to 34 weeks gestation is advised, but at times the urgency for delivery may not allow enough time for this. Once intravenous antihypertensives are required most patients require delivery and this is effected once blood pressure is stabilised, preferably with diastolic blood pressure maintained between 90 and 100 mmHg. Magnesium sulphate may be required in patients with cerebral symptoms to avoid eclamptic fits.

Eclampsia

Other causes of fits should be ruled out, including epilepsy, cerebral causes and hyperventilation.

The occurrence of an eclamptic fit tips the balance significantly against the continuation of pregnancy, even without immediately obvious deterioration in maternal condition.

Emergency management includes:
- Call for help.
- Airway (avoid aspiration and tongue biting and commence high-flow oxygen at 15 L/minute).
- Breathing (high-flow oxygen).
- Circulation (i.v. access for bloods, medication and i.v. fluids).
- Anticonvulsants (i.v. bolus dose of 4 g of $MgSO_4$ followed by a maintenance dose of 1 g/hour, titrated according to magnesium levels in the blood, for 24 hours after the last fit).

- Urinary catheter.
- Input/output fluid chart.
- Treatment of hypertension (usually intravenous, as outlined above).
- Consider delivery.

After controlling the situation and stabilising the patient, patients should be transferred to hospital, if they are not already admitted. They should be looked after in a high-dependency unit with close one-to-one monitoring of blood pressure, consciousness, reflexes, urinary output and proteinuria as well as fetal monitoring (cardiotocography). Sometimes, patients are so ill that they require ventilation and admission to an intensive care unit. Multidisciplinary patient management is essential with anaesthetic, obstetric and midwifery input to ensure optimal outcome. Regular 4–6-hourly blood investigations are performed and reviewed. A vaginal delivery is preferred, if feasible. The indications for a caesarean section include:
- Unfavourable cervix, as primigravidas are particularly at risk of pregnancy hypertension.
- Fetal distress or growth restriction.
- Other coincidental indications, such as breech presentation.

Care during delivery

Patients with pregnancy hypertension are high-risk patients who should deliver in hospital under consultant-led care. Regular monitoring of the blood pressure and the fetal heart is required. Epidural analgesia is recommended, as it facilitates controlling the blood pressure. Pethidine analgesia is not advised, as it is metabolised to norpethidine, which can have a convulsant effect. Antihypertensive medication is continued during delivery, and the patient is observed closely for symptoms and signs of fulminating pre-eclampsia. Oxytocin without ergometrine is used for the active management of the third stage of labour, as ergometrine causes vasoconstriction and therefore increases blood pressure.

Care after delivery

Patients with pregnancy hypertension usually improve after delivery, with drop of elevated blood pressure, increased urine output, decrease in oedema and improvement of abnormal blood tests. However, some patients deteriorate in the immediate period after delivery, hence the need for close observation for the first 24–48 hours. Patients may need to stay on antihypertensives, if their elevated blood pressure is slow to return to normal. Some patients may have long-term hypertension or renal dysfunction, and require follow-up and appropriate referral. Blood tests are repeated until they return to normal. Breastfeeding is not contraindicated, as long as the choice of antihypertensive(s) is taken into consideration. Patients are debriefed about events surrounding pregnancy and delivery, including any operative intervention. They are counselled about their care in a future pregnancy, including the risk of recurrence.

Clinical case

Case outcome

Mrs Harris had intravenous access established and blood samples were obtained for full blood count, group and save, clotting screen, urea and electrolytes, liver function tests and serum uric acid. She was transferred to the high-dependency unit on the labour ward and connected to automated blood pressure, heart rate and pulse-oximetry monitors, with observations recorded every 15 minutes. A self-retaining catheter was inserted and in/out fluid balance chart was started. Intravenous labetalol (antihypertensive) and prophylactic magnesium sulphate (anticonvulsant) infusions were started. The anaesthetic team was involved in her management. The family was supported during this difficult time, with the mother being so ill in addition to the loss of the baby.

The blood test results are shown in Table 11.3.

Mrs Harris had reduced urine output in the first 6 hours (20 mL/h) and was kept on 80 mL/h. This was followed by progressive diuresis. The patient's blood pressure remained stable. Her repeat blood tests improved next day and were all normal on the third postpartum day. Intravenous labetalol and magnesium sulphate were stopped after 24 hours and the patient was started on oral labetalol. The frequency of her observations was scaled down in the subsequent 24 hours and she was transferred after that to the postnatal ward. She was counselled about the events of her delivery. Her blood pressure stabilised and she required less and less labetalol until she finally came off it altogether on the fifth postpartum day. She was discharged home on the seventh postpartum day. She was followed up by the community midwife after discharge. She was counselled about the events during her pregnancy as well as the need for antenatal care in a subsequent pregnancy before discharge and seen again 6 weeks later in clinic.

Table 11.3 Blood test results for Mrs Harris.

Test	Result	Normal range for pregnancy
Haemoglobin	11 g/L	11–14 g/L
White cell count	7 × 10⁹/L	6–16 × 10⁹/L
Platelet	80 × 10⁹/L	150–400 × 10⁹/L
Prothrombin time	12 s	9.5–13.4 s
Activated partial thromboplastin time	40 s	30–45 s
Fibrinogen	4 g/L	2.4–6.2 g/L
International normalised ratio	1	0.9–1.2
Urea	4.0 mmol/L	2.4–4.3 mmol/L
Creatinine	95 mmol/L	34–82 mmol/L
Sodium	145 mmol/L	130–140 mmol/L
Potassium	3.5 mmol/L	3.3–4.1 mmol/L
Alanine transaminase	30 IU/L	6–32 IU/L
Gamma-glutamyl transaminase	41 IU/L	5–43 IU/L
Alkaline phosphatase	150 IU/L	30–300 IU/L
Bilirubin	10 mmol/L	3–14 mmol/L
Albumin	25 g/L	28–37 g/L
Serum uric acid	42 mmol/L	0.14–0.38 mmol/L

Key learning points

- Hypertension during pregnancy can be associated with serious risk to both mother and baby/babies.
- Being aware of the diagnostic criteria and alert to the risk factors should guide early detection and appropriate management of cases.
- Proper antenatal care is central to proper monitoring of patients and timely intervention by investigation(s), medical treatment and/or early delivery.
- Multidisciplinary team management may be required including obstetricians, midwives, neonatologists, anaesthetists and physicians. Care upon discharge from hospital is important and may involve the general practitioner in addition to the community midwife.
- Support to patients and families may be required during stressful times. Counselling is required in relation to future pregnancies.

 Now visit **www.wileyessential.com/humandevelopment** to test yourself on this chapter.

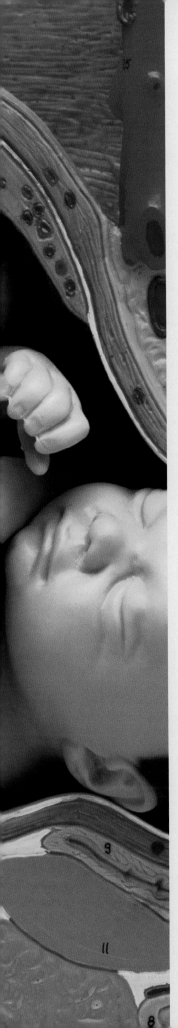

CHAPTER 12
Diseases
in pregnancy I

Alan Treharne and Cerys Scarr

Case

A 28-year-old type 1 insulin-dependent diabetic patient, Mary, presents to a pre-conception clinic. She has been using insulin since the age of 7 and her blood glucose measurements are very well controlled. Her renal function is normal and her retinal screening is up to date. A previous unplanned pregnancy was complicated by the diagnosis of a fetal neural tube defect, for which she had a termination at 22 weeks. She is advised to commence taking 5 mg of folic acid in this pregnancy. After stopping her contraception she conceives quickly and an early dating scan confirms viability. Her 20-week anomaly scan is normal and serial growth scans are also normal. She is seen two-weekly in the joint diabetic clinic and has an uneventful pregnancy. At 38 weeks she is induced and has a normal vaginal delivery. There are no neonatal complications. She returns to her pre-pregnancy insulin and after stopping breastfeeding at 6 months restarts a regular form of contraception.

Learning outcomes

- You should be able to describe the effects of diabetes during pregnancy and how gestational diabetes develops.

- You should be able to describe the management of blood glucose in a pregnant woman with diabetes.

- You should be able to describe the causes of rhesus disease and how to prevent it from occurring.

- You should be able to recognise high-risk infections, including HIV, that can affect pregnancy and describe how to test for and manage them.

Essential Human Development, First Edition. Edited by Samuel Webster, Geraint Morris and Euan Kevelighan
© 2018 John Wiley & Sons, Ltd. Published 2018 by John Wiley & Sons, Ltd.

Diabetes in pregnancy

Diabetes is the most common medical complication seen in pregnancy. It affects approximately 5% of all pregnancies, is associated with increased maternal and fetal morbidity, and is increasing in prevalence. It is important to distinguish between patients who have pre-existing type 1 or type 2 diabetes, and patients who develop diabetes in pregnancy (the gestational diabetics). Outcomes in both these groups are known to be worse, both for the mother and the baby.

Pre-existing diabetes

Pre-existing diabetes mellitus is associated with maternal and fetal complications (Table 12.1). These can be minimised by careful antenatal planning and pre-conceptual care (Table 12.2). Pre-conceptual care should be provided in a non-judgemental and supportive environment. This improves compliance. Contraception advice should be offered as early as possible.

Advice on diet, weight loss and exercise promotes improved glycaemic control. A BMI of <27 is ideal, but any significant weight loss pre-pregnancy can improve clinical outcomes. Even if a woman is morbidly obese, weight loss can reduce the technical challenges (invasive procedures, ultrasound image quality and delivery) often encountered in pregnancy.

High-dose folic acid at 5 mg/day is prescribed. Patients should be screened for evidence of end-organ damage. Renal screening should include measurement of protein in the urine and also serum creatinine or glomerular filtration rate (Table 12.3). Microvascular disease can also affect the eye and so dilated retinal assessment with digital imaging should be organised.

Medical management of blood glucose

Blood sugar levels should be maintained between 4 and 5.3 mmol/L before a meal and less than 7.8 mmol/L 1 hour, and less than 6.4 mmol/L 2 hours after a meal. Levels higher than this require active management to minimise complications.

The use of oral agents for the management of diabetes is increasing. The biguanide metformin is widely used in pregnancy. It does cross the placenta, but it not known to have any teratogenic effects. All other oral medications should be stopped as soon as possible. If blood glucose is not controlled on metformin then management with insulin should be commenced.

Insulin does not cross the placenta and should be continued if the patient was taking insulin pre-conceptually, or if measurements of blood glucose remain elevated despite treatment. Patients taking insulin should be educated about

Table 12.2 Considerations for conception in diabetic women.

Pre-conceptual care principle	Reason
Good contraception	Prevent unplanned pregnancy
Aim for BMI <27	Improved diabetic control
Renal assessment	Optimise BP and renal function
Retinal assessment	Identify deteriorating retinopathy
Folic acid supplements	Reduce incidence of neural tube defects
Aim HbA1C <6.1 % If >10% avoid pregnancy	Reduce teratogenic effects of hyperglycaemia
Discuss hypoglycaemia	Increased in early pregnancy as a result of nausea, poor diet, etc.
Multidisciplinary management	Reduce complications, increase patient support

BMI, body mass index; BP, blood pressure; Hb, haemoglobin.

Table 12.1 Complications of diabetes during pregnancy and labour.

Maternal complications	Complications for the fetus/neonate		
	First trimester	Second trimester	Third trimester/neonatal period
Weight gain	Miscarriage	Polyhydramnios	Macrosomia/accelerated growth
Pre-eclampsia	Renal agenesis	Accelerated growth	Polyhydramnios
Increased induction/ caesarean	Neural tube defects	Cardiomyopathy	Third trimester loss/stillbirth/ prematurity
Birth trauma	Sacral agenesis	Second trimester loss	Growth restriction
Increased type 2 diabetes in future	Duodenal atresia	Growth restriction	Shoulder dystocia/birth injury
Diabetic ketoacidosis/ hypoglycaemia	Structural cardiac defects	Second trimester loss/ stillbirth/prematurity	Respiratory distress
			Hypoglycaemia/abnormal biochemistry
			Future risk of diabetes

Note: some complications may exist as a progressive condition across trimesters, e.g. accelerated growth, and as such are not trimester specific.

Table 12.3 Renal testing in pregnancy.

Renal test	Value	Comment
Serum creatinine	>120 µmol/L	Refer to nephrologist
Glomerular filtration rate	<45/mL/minute/ 1.73 m²	Refer to nephrologist
Urine protein	>5 g/L	Refer to nephrologist = Nephrotic syndrome

hypoglycaemia and diabetic ketoacidosis (DKA), both of which can be medical emergencies.

Delivery

A delivery plan should be individualised for each woman. Induction of labour should be offered after 38 weeks, and caesarean section reserved for obstetric indications. The rationale is that this gestation time balances the risks of prematurity against the risks of macrosomia and sudden intrauterine death in the last 4 weeks. Caesarean section may be offered, after discussion, in those with an estimated fetal weight greater than 4.5 kg, but remember that only half of babies with a shoulder dystocia have an actual weight greater than 4.5 kg. Continuous fetal monitoring is advised. Blood glucose should be monitored and a sliding scale insulin infusion commenced if indicated (i.e. blood glucose is not controlled, or for all diabetics on insulin during pregnancy). Steroids for fetal lung maturation should not be offered routinely for all diabetics.

Implications of diabetes for the fetus

In 1952, Pederson described a model to explain how maternal diabetes and the resulting hyperglycaemia lead to fetal morbidity and mortality. While insulin does not cross the placenta, glucose does. Fetal serum glucose levels reach approximately 80% of maternal serum levels and this results in the fetal effects seen.

Fetal effects

1. **Serum glucose levels.** This unregulated hyperglycaemic state is responsible for the teratogenic effects listed in Table 12.1. This occurs in the first trimester during the period of organogenesis. Patients with pre-existing diabetes should have a detailed cardiac scan in order to confirm the normal anatomy of the four chambers and outflow tracts. Further investigations (such as a cardiac ECHO) may be indicated.
2. **Glucose levels remain elevated and a hyperinsulinaemic state results.** This acts as a growth factor resulting in macrosomia.
3. **Neural tube defects and sacral agenesis.** Associated with pre-existing diabetes.
4. **Growth restriction.** This may occur in patients with microvascular disease and so regular growth scans every 3–4 weeks are recommended from 28 weeks.

Neonatal complications

1. **Macrosomia.** The growth of the fetal head is normal. However, the altered metabolism redistributes fat to the upper abdomen disproportionately. The main risks are shoulder dystocia and relative cephalopelvic disproportion.
2. **Respiratory distress and transient tachypnoea of the newborn.** This results from a decrease in surfactant production as a result of intrauterine hyperglycaemia.
3. **Asphyxia,** as a result of either placental insufficiency (chronic) or intrapartum events (acute). This is a risk factor for subsequent development of hypoxic ischaemic encephalopathy and cerebral palsy.
4. **Polycythaemia, jaundice and hyperbilirubinaemia.** Chronic hypoxia and hyperinsulinaemia lead to increased erythropoiesis and polycythaemia. After delivery, due to fetal liver immaturity and increased red cell turnover, excess bilirubin is not rapidly cleared from the bloodstream resulting in jaundice. This can lead to kernicterus in the newborn.
5. **Hypoglycaemia.** The neonate after delivery has high insulin levels as a result of the intrauterine environment. After delivery, maternal glucose supply is abruptly removed and if the fetus does not feed soon after birth, or if feeding is insufficient, the high insulin levels and immature liver do not compensate rapidly enough, resulting in profound hypoglycaemia. Not all neonates of diabetics are macrosomic and some have growth restriction as a result of placental insufficiency. Hypoglycaemia may result because of insufficient glycogen stores.
6. **Hypocalcaemia.** Calcium and magnesium metabolism are closely related. The fetal parathyroid gland is not active until after delivery, and during the intrauterine period the fetus is dependent on maternal supplies via the placenta. A delay in parathyroid activity is seen in neonates of diabetic mothers resulting in low levels of parathyroid hormone.
7. **Birth trauma.** Clavicular fractures, nerve palsies and soft tissue damage are all increased.
8. **Long-term developmental delay.** This is multifactorial.

Mothers and babies should be monitored on a postnatal ward. If a baby develops complications then closer and more intensive monitoring should be instituted, with admission to the neonatal unit reserved for only the more unwell babies.

Gestational diabetes mellitus (GDM)

Unlike pre-existing diabetes, the effects of GDM do not become evident until the third trimester. If risk factors are present an oral glucose tolerance test (OGTT) should be requested at 24–28 weeks. It can be done earlier at 16–18 weeks should it be clinically indicated (e.g. in a mother with previous GDM). The pathological process is related to the relative insulin resistance seen in pregnancy. Patients with GDM have impaired fasting glucose metabolism following a 75-g glucose intake. In patients diagnosed with GDM the extra risk of congenital malformation is absent, as hyperglycaemia was unlikely to have existed during the critical first trimester. The exceptions to this rule are women who have pre-existing diabetes and have not been diagnosed prior to conception. This cohort of women will be hyperglycaemic in the critical period of organogenesis and are at increased risk of congenital malformations.

In the UK women are screened for GDM if they have one or more of these risk factors:

- BMI >30;
- baby >4.5 kg;
- previous GDM;
- first-degree relative with diabetes mellitus;
- ethnic origin South Asian, Black Caribbean or Middle Eastern.

After diagnosis a period of conservative management (diet alteration and exercise) can be trialled. If blood glucose measurements are not controlled within a 1–2-week period then medical management should be commenced. The protocols and agents used are the same as for pre-existing diabetes, and the same blood glucose target ranges are appropriate (Table 12.4). Gestational diabetics should be treated in the same way as a patient with pre-existing diabetes with respect to timing, mode of delivery and neonatal aftercare as they are at risk of the same third-trimester, intrapartum and neonatal complications.

After delivery, maternal glucose metabolism quickly returns to normal. A comprehensive plan for the management of GDM after delivery should be documented in the notes and may include the following:

- Stopping insulin or any oral hypoglycaemics.
- Involving the neonatologists.
- Monitoring blood glucose while in hospital.
- Postnatal investigation (offer an oral glucose tolerance test at 6 weeks).
- Discuss contraception.
- Counsel regarding risk reduction (changes to diet, weight loss, exercise).
- Discuss lifetime risk of developing type 2 diabetes and the importance of regular GP health checks.

Table 12.4 Blood glucose target ranges. The values in the table are for venous plasma samples. The diagnosis of gestational diabetes can be made if the venous plasma levels exceed the stated values following a 75-g oral glucose load.

	Blood glucose (mmol/L)
Fasting	≥5.6
2 hours	≥7.8

Rhesus disease

Rhesus disease is the result of an incompatibility between the blood types of the mother and the infant. Of the blood group antigens, rhesus status refers to the presence or absence of the D antigen. If the rhesus antigen (RhD) is present on the surfaces of erythrocytes in the fetus's blood it can trigger an immune response from a rhesus-negative mother. Anti-Rh antigens pass across the placenta and destroy fetal red blood cells. This is less likely to occur during the first pregnancy.

The disease actively present during pregnancy is called erythroblastosis fetalis or haemolytic disease of the fetus. The form of the disease affecting the newborn baby is subsequently called haemolytic disease of the newborn (HDN).

Pathology

The sensitivity of the maternal immune system to the RhD antigen can happen at any time during pregnancy, but is most likely to occur during delivery when the placenta is separating. It may also happen during an invasive diagnostic test, an abdominal injury, a miscarriage or an abortion.

In the first pregnancy of a Rh-negative mother with a Rh-positive fetus, the mother's immune system is most likely to recognise the Rh antigen in the fetal blood at birth, and is subsequently unable to affect it, so often the first baby is not affected by the haemolytic disease. In any subsequent pregnancy with a rhesus-positive baby the mother's immune system will have been sensitised to the RhD antigen, and will produce antibodies against it. The fetus's red blood cells are destroyed by the mother's alloantibodies. They are treated as 'foreign bodies'.

Signs of active rhesus disease

As rhesus disease affects the fetus, the mother will show few symptoms. Many mothers will complain of vaginal bleeding during pregnancy. Some of them will suffer from miscarriage or stillbirth.

With ultrasound scanning the fetus may show evidence of enlarged organs, fluid build-up (hydrops fetalis) or increased amniotic fluid. A Doppler ultrasound is more likely to detect changes, as the fetus will be anaemic (e.g. increased peak systolic velocity in the middle cerebral artery).

The newborn baby presents with signs of anaemia, sometimes with evidence of enlarged liver and spleen, and jaundice complicated by kernicterus.

Diagnostic test for rhesus disease

Blood group testing of the mother during standard antenatal testing will indicate the presence of the RhD antigen in the blood. If the mother is RhD positive, rhesus disease will not occur. If the mother is RhD negative her blood should also be tested for anti-D antibodies. The presence of anti-D antibodies in a pregnant woman with a RhD-negative blood group indicates a prior sensitisation event, and further testing of the fetal blood type and continued monitoring is indicated. Testing the father's blood type may help; if both the mother and father have RhD-negative blood types the fetus will also be RhD negative.

Rh antibody titre monitoring during the pregnancy can improve the outcome by aiding decision-making about delivery time. A low antibody titre (<1:4) is linked with a low possibility of acute complications. A raised titre (>1:15) has a high risk of haemolytic disease of the newborn.

Treatment

Treatment of rhesus disease depends upon the severity of the disease. More severe cases of erythroblastosis fetalis may require an intrauterine blood transfusion organised in a fetal medicine unit, or early delivery in uncontrolled cases. Newborn babies with haemolytic disease of the newborn might need phototherapy, a blood transfusion or intravenous immunoglobulin therapy.

Prophylaxis

By understanding the involvement of the D blood group antigen in rhesus disease we can prevent its development. Routine, early antenatal blood group testing of the mother's blood is recommended. If the mother is RhD negative and has not been sensitised to the RhD antigen she should be given anti-D immunoglobulin (also known as RhoGAM or RhIg) during potential periods of sensitisation. The anti-D immunoglobulin will destroy fetal red blood cells that come into contact with the mother's blood before cells of her immune system produce antibodies. Only a relatively small number of fetal erythrocytes will be affected. The prophylactic dose of anti-D is given at 28 weeks and within 72 hours of delivery, and after any bleeding or potential sensitising event. If the mother's immune system has been previously sensitised to the RhD antigen then anti-D will not prevent rhesus disease – it is like 'closing the stable door after the horse has bolted'.

Clinical case

Case investigations

Pre-conceptually good contraception is essential until all investigations are complete and blood glucose levels are well controlled. Results of Mary's maternal investigations were as follows:

- Urea: 2.4 mmol/L
- Creatinine 50 μmol/L
- No protein in urine. Normal albumin and protein/creatinine ratio
- BP 110/78 mmHg
- BMI 26
- HbA1C = 42 mmol/mol (6%)
- Fundoscopy: Normal. No evidence of retinopathy
- Neurological exam: Normal. No evidence of peripheral neuropathy

This patient's insulin regime was optimised to achieve excellent glycaemic control. High-dose pre-conceptual folic acid was commenced at 5 mg/day. An early dating scan was arranged to confirm viability and Mary's antenatal care was organised jointly between the obstetric and diabetic teams. There was further input from a diabetic nurse specialist and a dietician.

Her 20-week anomaly scan was normal and did not identify a neural tube defect, or sacral agenesis associated with diabetes, particularly when uncontrolled as in her history. Serial growth scans were organised, which demonstrated linear growth and calculated an estimated fetal weight of 3.6 kg at 38 weeks. There was no evidence of polyhydramnios at any stage of the pregnancy.

A medical induction of labour was arranged at 38 weeks gestation.

Case conclusions

The excellent maternal and fetal outcomes in this case are the result of fully optimised pre-conceptual, antenatal and intrapartum care. Pre-pregnancy planning in chronic diseases such as diabetes minimises the risks of complications. A multidisciplinary team approach is essential.

Key learning points

- Diabetes is an example of a chronic condition which requires pre-conceptual optimisation to minimise maternal and fetal complications

- Poorly controlled glycaemia can lead to fetal macrosomia and is associated with shoulder dystocia and potential maternal and fetal morbidity and mortality.
- Postnatal care should include good contraceptive advice.

 Now visit **www.wileyessential.com/humandevelopment** to test yourself on this chapter.

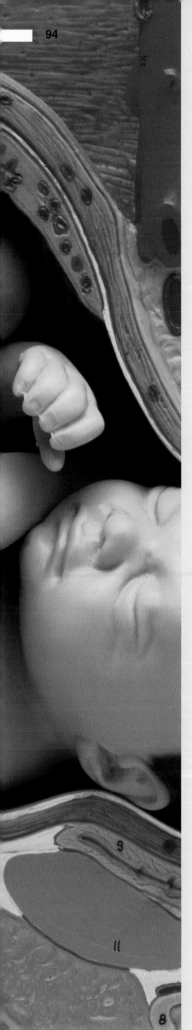

CHAPTER 13
Diseases in pregnancy II

Alan Treharne, Cerys Scarr and
Aleksandra Komarzyniec-Pyzik

Case

A 29-year-old, Jane, attends your antenatal clinic at 16 weeks for her consultant booking visit. In the course of the history it transpires that she has recently been referred to a rheumatologist for joint pain and a discoid rash. No formal diagnosis was made before she conceived. Over the same time period she was being investigated for recurrent miscarriages, but all her results, including an antiphospholipid screen were negative. At 32 weeks she was admitted as an emergency from the antenatal clinic where a recent growth scan had been performed as she was measuring small for her gestational age. The ultrasound scan had plotted the abdominal circumference below the fifth centile (customised growth chart used). The maternal BP was 150/98, 3+ of protein was present in the urine.

Learning outcomes

- You should be able to recognise connective tissue, gastrointestinal and dermatological conditions that occur during pregnancy.

- You should be able to recommend when invasive diagnostic testing is required and decide which type of test should be used.

- You should be able to describe how to detect psychiatric disorders during antenatal care.

- You should be able to recognise the effects of medications for psychiatric disorders on the mother and fetus during the pregnancy and on the neonate after birth.

Essential Human Development, First Edition. Edited by Samuel Webster, Geraint Morris and Euan Kevelighan

Connective tissue disorders

Connective tissue (CT) disorders can be more easily understood by thinking about the basic science behind the clinical picture. Connective tissue is widespread in the body, providing extensive structural support. It exists in many diverse forms giving it many unique properties. In its simplest form it is made up of cells and an extracellular matrix (ECM). The ECM is composed of glycosaminoglycans (GAGs) and proteoglycans (PGs), which are large, negatively charged, hydrophilic molecules that attract water and give the ECM a high water content (over 90%). Within the ECM exist cells that produce and maintain the ECM, and it is the specialisation of these cells that gives rise to the unique features of each connective tissue type (Table 13.1).

Connective tissue disorders may be inherited. The known heritable conditions include:

- Marfan syndrome;
- Ehlers–Danlos syndrome;
- osteogenesis imperfecta;
- Alport syndrome;
- epidermolysis bullosa.

Each of these disorders has a genetic basis resulting in defective synthesis and incorporation of a critical connective tissue component. In contrast, some connective tissue disorders have an autoimmune basis, with antibody-directed destruction of target proteins. The result is the dysfunction of structurally normal tissue following autoimmune breakdown. These conditions include:

- systemic lupus erythematosus;
- scleroderma;
- Sjögren syndrome;
- rheumatoid arthritis.

During pregnancy a range of immunological changes take place that can affect connective tissue disease progression.

Systemic lupus erythematosus

Systemic lupus erythematosus (SLE) is an autoimmune disease that can present as a varied spectrum of disease manifestations and in pregnancy may follow a benign, asymptomatic course, or may be complicated by severe maternal and fetal compromise. Diagnosis of SLE can be difficult as its symptoms are similar to other, more common conditions. The American

Table 13.1 Types of connective tissue cells.

Cell type	Specialist function
• Fibroblasts	• Produce collagen and elastin
• Adipocytes	• Lipid production and storage
• Osteocytes/osteoblasts	• Bone synthesis
• Chondrocytes/chondroblasts	• Cartilage matrix production
• Endothelial cells/pericytes	• Line blood vessels

Table 13.2 Diagnosis of systemic lupus erythematosus is made if at least four of the symptoms described here are present in the patient.

Organ affected	Clinical manifestation
Central nervous system	Psychiatric: psychosis, mood/anxiety disorder; Seizures
Skin/mucosa	Photosensitivity, discoid rash, facial (malar) rash, oral ulcers
Kidneys	Cellular casts; Persistent proteinuria >0.5 g/day
Blood	Thrombocytopenia; Leucopenia/lymphopenia; Haemolytic anaemia
Connective tissue	Non-erosive arthritis, pleurisy, pericarditis
Immunological disorder (presence of autoantibodies)	Anti-DNA, anti-Smith, antiphospholipid antibodies

College of Rheumatology has set out diagnostic criteria for the diagnosis of SLE, which include at least four (but not all) of the symptoms described in Table 13.2.

Fetal considerations

Transfer of antibodies (anti-Ro and anti-La) across the placenta can have fetal manifestations that persist into the neonatal period. The spontaneously resolving neonatal lupus rash (seen in 5% of anti-Ro or anti-La positive patients) persists for up to 6 months. The rash is similar in distribution and appearance to the maternal rash and is photosensitive. It requires no treatment and has no long-term effects.

The other neonatal condition resulting from maternal SLE is far more serious, and permanent, but can be identified, investigated and treated during the antenatal period. Autoimmune destruction of the conducting systems of the heart causes a progressive dysfunction of the atrioventricular node by fibrosis and the subsequent progression through first- and second-degree heart blocks to complete heart block (seen in 2% of anti-Ro or anti-La positive patients). This is permanent and requires pacing of the heart in early neonatal life. There is a 30% mortality rate associated with this dysfunction. Higher mortality rates are associated with a coexistent myocarditis and effusion. Investigation in the neonatal period includes electrocardiography (ECG) and echocardiography (ECHO) following review by the neonatology team.

Treatment of SLE in pregnancy

Immunosuppressive agents and anti-inflammatory analgesics are the mainstay of treatment in SLE, and women may be very well controlled on them. However, special consideration should be given to the potential side effects of certain drug classes.

- NSAID (non-steroidal anti-inflammatory drug) analgesia should be stopped. Alternatives (paracetamol, codeine) should be used if pain relief is required.
- Oral steroids (prednisolone) are safe in pregnancy but long-term use will require intravenous steroids in labour. Maintenance doses may be increased to treat flares.
- Hydroxychloroquine is commonly used in SLE management. It is safe to continue.
- Azathioprine is safe in pregnancy.
- Cytotoxic drugs with an immunosuppressive effect (methotrexate, cyclophosphamide) are contraindicated.
- Mycophenolate mofetil is contraindicated in pregnancy.

Antiphospholipid syndrome and SLE

Antiphospholipid syndrome (APLS) and SLE must not be confused but are closely related. SLE may be associated with the presence of antiphospholipid antibodies (anti-cardiolipin and lupus anticoagulants). To diagnose antiphospholipid syndrome these antibodies (with or without a pre-existing diagnosis of SLE) must be associated with an adverse clinical outcome, as defined by the 2006 International Consensus Statement for the classification of antiphospholipid syndrome (Table 13.3).

Marfan syndrome

In pregnancy, Marfan syndrome is associated with a high risk of cardiac complications but it is a multisystem disease and complications may be varied. An autosomal dominant

Table 13.4 The effects of Marfan syndrome on different systems. The risks for pregnancy are discussed in the text.

System	Association/complication
Central nervous system	Dural ectasia Degenerative disc disease Dysautonomia
Cardiovascular	Mitral valve prolapse Aortic root dilatation Aortic aneurysm Mitral regurgitation Bicuspid aortic valve
Respiratory	Pneumothorax Fibrosis Emphysema Obstructive lung disease Middle lobe hypoplasia
Skeletal	Arachnodactyly Scoliosis Pectus excavatum/carinatum High arch oral palate Hypermobility Osteoarthritis
Ophthalmic	Glaucoma Retinal detachment Lens subluxation Visual deterioration (myopia)

condition, Marfan syndrome, is caused by dysfunction of the *FBN1* gene, which codes for the production of fibrillin-1, and is found on chromosome 15. Fibrillin-1 is essential for elastin production, an important component in the ECM of the aorta, ligaments and eyes (Table 13.4).

Special considerations in pregnancy:

1. Because of defective elastin exacerbated by the physiological changes in pregnancy, the risk of aortic rupture and dissection is increased. Clinicians should be aware of the signs and symptoms, and a low threshold for investigation is vital.
2. The risk of rupture and dissection is increased if the aortic root diameter exceeds 4 cm. For women whose aortic root diameter is greater than 4.5 cm, delaying pregnancy until after aortic root repair is advisable after discussion with cardiothoracic surgeons/cardiologists. Regular echocardiography scans (ECHO) should form part of the antenatal care (every 3 months).
3. Patients with an aortic root graft or prosthetic valves need anticoagulation. Ideally a plan should be made pre-conceptually as warfarin is teratogenic.
4. Hypertensive patients may be taking potentially teratogenic medications. Angiotensin converting enzyme inhibitor (ACE) or receptor blocker (ARB) medications need alteration either pre-conceptually or early in pregnancy (<6 weeks).

Table 13.3 Diagnostic factors for antiphospholipid syndrome.

Diagnostic class	Outcome	Examples
Clinical outcome	Thrombosis	Arterial, venous, small vessel
Clinical outcome	Pregnancy	Three miscarriages <10 weeks
		One fetal loss >10 weeks Premature delivery <35 weeks with known pre-eclampsia or intra-uterine growth restriction
Immunological	Raised titre of anti-cardiolipin antibody	Two samples >12 weeks apart
Immunological	Raised titre of lupus anticoagulant	Two samples >12 weeks apart

Table 13.5 Classification of Ehlers–Danlos syndrome.

Clinical type	ED syndrome class type
Classical	1 and 2
Hypermobility	3
Vascular	4
Kyphoscoliosis	6
Dermatosparaxis	7

Ehlers–Danlos syndrome

This is a heterogeneous group of disorders that have defective collagen production in common (Table 13.5). Vascular Ehlers–Danlos syndrome (type 4) carries the highest risk in pregnancy, and the mortality risk to the mother in these cases may be as much as 1 in 4. It is caused by a mutation in the *COL3A1* gene located on chromosome 2, which encodes the collagen alpha-1(III) protein of type III collagen. It is an extensible protein that is a major component of vascular tissues and skin. Vascular Ehlers–Danlos syndrome presents with thin, translucent skin, easy bruising and fragility of arteries, gastrointestinal structures, and the uterus.

Special considerations in pregnancy should be given to the following complications when planning antenatal care and counselling patients:

1. Increased pain and joint dysfunction (increased incidence of pubic symphysis dysfunction and sacroiliac joint instability).
2. Pre-term labour and cervical weakness (may be painless).
3. Pre-term pre-labour rupture of membranes.
4. Uterine rupture.
5. Precipitous labour, cervical weakness and poor pelvic floor support.
6. Risk of bleeding as antepartum haemorrhage (APH) and postpartum haemorrhage (PPH), vessel rupture and aneurysm.
7. Vaginal trauma and poor healing.
8. Fetal intrauterine growth retardation (IUGR).

Symphysis pubis dysfunction

Symphysis pubis dysfunction is caused by the laxity of the pubic symphysis joint due to hormonal changes that occur in pregnancy affecting connective tissues. Symphysis pubis dysfunction occurs in around one-quarter of all pregnancies.

The mother may experience excruciating, persistent lower abdominal and lower back pain. The discomfort is worsened while walking, climbing stairs, standing and getting out of bed. On examination, the tenderness is present over the symphysis pubis region and the sacroiliac joint. The signs sometimes extend to the gluteal area, and the patient may have limited hip movement. Her gait might be affected by pain. The neurology findings are normal.

Differential diagnosis should include:

- Obstetric causes such as preterm labour, placental abruption and chorioamnionitis.
- Urinary tract infection.
- Constipation or other gastrointestinal problems.
- Lower back pain syndromes such as arthritis, lumbar disc lesions or sciatica.
- Bone and soft tissue infections such as tuberculosis.
- Femoral vein thrombosis.
- Tumours.

No curative treatment exists for symphysis pubis dysfunction. Physiotherapy and regular analgesia are advisable.

Backache

Backache is very common in pregnancy. It is associated with increased lordosis of the lumbar spine, increased body weight and increased laxity of the back muscles.

Differential diagnosis should include sciatica, cauda equina syndrome, a slipped or herniated disc, or other neurological disorders.

An appropriate exercise programme and minimisation of strain to the back are advisable for managing backache during pregnancy. Analgesia is prescribed after exclusion of other neurological disorders.

Carpal tunnel syndrome

Carpal tunnel syndrome is caused by the entrapment of the median nerve in the carpal tunnel of the wrist. It usually starts in the second half of pregnancy and affects about 20% of pregnant women. A patient typically complains of wrist pain, weakness and/or numbness over the first three digits, which sometimes interferes with her sleep.

The main risk factor associated with carpal tunnel syndrome in pregnancy is fluid retention, which may increase pressure within the carpal tunnel and irritate the median nerve. Wrist splinting and analgesia are the first choices for treatment. Surgical management is curative but rarely required because the problem almost always resolves after pregnancy.

Hyperemesis gravidarum

Hyperemesis gravidarum is a condition that causes severe nausea and vomiting in pregnancy, usually between 4 and 10 weeks gestation, with weight loss of more than 5% of body weight, dehydration, ketonuria and electrolyte disturbance (mainly hypokalaemia). It should be differentiated from physiologically normal nausea and vomiting in pregnancy, which although debilitating does not meet the above criteria and responds well to simple medical interventions.

The pathology behind hyperemesis gravidarum is unclear. Studies have found links with contributing factors including a rising beta-human chorionic gonadotrophin (BHCG) level, upper gastrointestinal dysmobility (i.e. decreased gastric mobility, relaxed intestinal muscles), hepatic abnormalities, thyroid function abnormalities, lack of dietary vitamin B_6, *Helicobacter pylori* infection or an immunological response to the 'foreign' fetus.

Differential diagnosis includes:

- Multiple pregnancy.
- Molar pregnancy.
- Endocrinology, e.g. hyperthyroidism or diabetic ketoacidosis (DKA).
- Gastrointestinal tract pathology, e.g. liver pathology, pancreatitis, gastroenteritis or peptic ulcer disease.
- Urinary tract pathology, e.g. pyelonephritis or urinary tract infection (UTI).
- Neurology, e.g. brain tumour or migraine.

Diagnostics tests useful in suspected hyperemesis gravidarum include:

- Urine dipstick test to confirm ketosis and exclude UTI.
- Blood tests including a full blood count (FBC), urea and electrolytes (U&E), liver function tests (LFTs), thyroid function test (TFT), amylase, BHCG, and vitamin B_6 level.
- Ultrasound scan in early pregnancy.
- Ultrasound abdomen scan, including kidneys, ureters and bladder.

Treatment of hyperemesis gravidarum requires aggressive management in a hospital setting. These patients are in need of intensive hydration and symptomatic treatment with antiemetic drugs and vitamins. Diet in the early stage of the condition is limited to a light diet only.

Gastroesophageal reflux disease (GORD)

The main symptom of gastroesophageal reflux disease (GORD), or acid reflux, is a burning sensation behind the sternum (also known as heartburn). It occurs in about 50% of pregnant patients. The discomfort usually improves after pregnancy. GORD does not affect pregnancy outcomes.

There are two major contributing factors causing GORD. Firstly, an increased level of progesterone decreases smooth muscle mobility. Secondly, the growing uterus obstructs the gastrointestinal system. As a result mobility of the oesophagus decreases, lower oesophageal sphincter tone decreases, gastric tone and contractions decrease, intestinal mobility decreases (mainly of the small intestine) and biliary contractility decreases.

Differential diagnosis of heartburn symptoms include the epigastric pain of pre-eclampsia and mid-chest pain of myocardial infarction, other cardiac conditions, or peptic ulcer disease. The diagnosis of GORD is based mainly upon the history taken from the patient in combination with the patient's symptoms. In less obvious cases an electrocardiogram (ECG), troponin T test or gastroscopy should be performed urgently.

The patient suffering from GORD should be advised about changes to diet including eating small, frequent meals, and avoiding caffeine, carbonated drinks and spicy food. Treatment in GORD is symptomatic. Gaviscon is usually the first-choice medication.

Constipation

Constipation is a very common symptom in pregnancy. It is the consequence of adaptations to pregnancy and sometimes the side effect of iron medications often prescribed for pregnant women. Increased progesterone levels are responsible for decreased smooth muscle motility, and the growing uterus often obstructs the gastrointestinal tract.

A light diet with increased amounts of fibre and water can help. Long-term treatment with laxatives is not normally required.

Haemorrhoids

Haemorrhoids are also a very common problem in pregnancy. Haemorrhoids become swollen in the anal canal as physiological changes in pregnancy cause decreased smooth muscle tone (progesterone effect) and veins become enlarged. Constipation can also have a role in haemorrhoid development.

Diet modification and symptomatic treatment with laxatives and topical haemorrhoid cream are recommended.

Varicose veins, varicosities

Varicose veins present with symptoms of painful legs with swollen, blue, rope-like veins. For the same reasons as other effects of progesterone levels during pregnancy, varicosities are classified as physiological skin changes caused by the enlarging uterus putting additional pressure on major blood vessels (such as the inferior vena cava), weight gain, and loss of venous elasticity and smooth muscle tone. There are often associated hereditary factors, with the first episode occurring during pregnancy.

Patients developing varicose veins during pregnancy should wear compression stockings. The treatment is usually symptomatic, and rarely surgical.

Dermatological conditions in pregnancy

Clinical history and examination can often differentiate easily between conditions that pre-dated the pregnancy and those that have arisen during the antenatal period (Table 13.6). Of those that arise in pregnancy, a further differentiation should be made between the normal physiological changes seen in pregnancy and those that reflect an underlying pathology. Correct identification of dermatological conditions arising in pregnancy is important as they may have fetal implications

Table 13.6 Dermatological conditions seen during pregnancy.

Pre-existing	Normal physiological changes	Pregnancy related
Eczema	Hyperpigmentation	Obstetric cholestasis
Psoriasis	Spider naevi	Viral rashes
Hidradenitis suppurativa	Palmar erythema	Polymorphic eruption
Acne	Haemangiomas	Pemphigoid gestationis
Human papillomavirus (HPV) condylomata acuminata	Striae gravidarum	Prurigo of pregnancy
	Postpartum alopecia	Drug reactions
	Oedema	

requiring additional monitoring, and may be a cause of fetal mortality.

When taking a patient's medical history you should include:

- the presenting complaint;
- history of the presenting complaint;
- past obstetric history;
- past medical history;
- drug history;
- allergies;
- family history.

Specific pregnancy-related conditions

Polymorphic eruption of pregnancy

Although specific to pregnancy, this condition has a benign clinical course with no known fetal implications. Usually starting in the third trimester the characteristic appearance is of a red urticarial rash over the abdomen. Umbilical sparing is classically described, and the rash may spread to the thighs, rarely the legs. Treatment is with symptomatic relief for itching and topical creams. Resolution is spontaneous following delivery.

Obstetric cholestasis

Obstetric cholestasis is characterised by a severe itch, in the absence of a rash and with abnormal liver enzymes (characteristically raised bile acids and alanine aminotransferase). This is a diagnosis made after exclusion of other causes. The itching may be severe enough to cause significant sleep deprivation. Treatment is with symptomatic relief and chelating agents to reduce the concentration of bile salts. Both itching and abnormal liver function usually resolve after delivery, but postnatal resolution should be confirmed. Further maternal morbidity may be caused by the increased incidence of postpartum haemorrhage and the iatrogenic intervention to deliver. Fetal risks include prematurity (from early delivery) and sudden intrauterine death for which no accurate predictive test is available.

Pemphigoid gestationis

Pemphigoid gestationis also presents most commonly in the third trimester, and this dermatological condition characteristically starts in the periumbilical area and radiates to the trunk and extremities. The rash is vesicular with associated bullae. Clinical suspicion is supported by the histological confirmation of subepidermal blistering. The underlying pathogenesis is an autoimmune process, and a number of autoimmune conditions may be identified from the woman's history. Treatment may require intravenous steroids in addition to the standard symptomatic treatments.

Dermatological manifestations of viral disease

Rashes associated with a viral prodrome or following significant exposure to another infected person all warrant further clinical review in pregnancy. Viral exposure may be teratogenic to the fetus and associated with serious malformations. Maternal immunosuppression caused by pregnancy leads to increased susceptibility to viruses and a more severe clinical course. Early diagnosis and treatment reduces mortality and morbidity for both the mother and the fetus.

If vesicular rashes are present suspect a varicella zoster virus infection. In cases with non-vesicular rashes consider parvovirus B19, rubella or measles.

Immunoglobulin testing (for IgM and IgG antibodies) can confirm both acute exposure and previous immunity and should be requested. For measles and varicella zoster infections immunoglobulin treatments are available (human normal immunoglobulin and varicella zoster immune globulin respectively).

Psychiatric disease in pregnancy

Mental health may have wide-ranging effects on the mother, newborn, partner and family. Psychiatric disorders may be part of a normal grief reaction (in response to the death of a fetus or neonate) and as such may be transient. Persistent grief reactions leading to depression and withdrawal, or pre-existing conditions such as schizophrenia, depression or bipolar disorder, may become chronic and as such, need specialist management antenatally, intrapartum and postnatally.

Pre-conception care should include careful counselling and advice on the following topics:

- Ensuring reliable contraception to prevent unplanned pregnancies or pregnancies conceived while taking teratogenic medications.
- Risks of stopping, reducing or changing medications.
- Risks of relapse and deterioration in the antenatal and postpartum periods.
- Implications for antenatal management.
- Risks and benefits of breastfeeding and the implications of medications.

Screening

Ideally, when the patient is referred from the primary care provider for booking, a referral letter should indicate previous illness. When screening patients, various questionnaires and assessment tools are available. A detailed history at booking will identify women at risk or in need of specialist input, and focused directed questioning should elicit:

- Current mental health issues and treatments (especially medication history).
- Previous metal health issues and treatments (e.g. depression, bipolar disorder, schizophrenia).
- Previous postnatal complications (e.g. postnatal depression or psychosis).
- Family history with regards to mental health issues.
- Previous pregnancy outcomes and complications, both maternal and fetal.

The UK National Institute for Health and Care Excellence (NICE) guidance specifically advises asking three directed questions:

1. *During the past month, have you often been bothered by feeling down, depressed or hopeless?*
2. *During the past month, have you often been bothered by having little interest or pleasure in doing things?*
3. *Do you feel this is something you want help with?* [if an answer is Yes to questions 1 or 2]

Medication in pregnancy

Lithium

Maternal complications

Toxicity is evidenced clinically by tremor, arrhythmias (cardiac), confusion, renal failure, ataxia and dysarthria. Lithium level tests should be performed monthly in pregnancy and then weekly from 36 weeks. During labour and the postnatal period therapeutic levels should be checked. Care should be taken with fluid balance and in monitoring any conditions that may alter renal function (PPH, dehydration) and hence lithium toxicity.

Fetal complications

First-trimester teratogenic effects include Ebstein anomaly (rare at 1/20 000 incidence), other cardiac defects (more common at 8–60/1000 incidence) and fetal hydantoin syndrome.

Breastfeeding

High levels of lithium pass into breast milk. Monitor baby for toxicity.

Special considerations

These include regular monitoring of serum concentrations in the mother to ensure that the therapeutic range is maintained.

Selective serotonin reuptake inhibitors (SSRIs)

Maternal complications

SSRIs are safer than tricyclic antidepressants (TCADs) in overdose but withdrawal may precipitate depression and suicide. SSRIs include citalopram, fluoxetine and sertraline.

Fetal complications

- All infants exposed to SSRIs should be monitored for withdrawal (irritable and jittery baby) and problems with feeding.
- Specifically, paroxetine in the first trimester is teratogenic (linked to heart defects) and all SSRI medications are associated with an increased incidence of persistent pulmonary hypertension in the neonate.
- Fluoxetine is the safest in pregnancy.

Breastfeeding

Trace amounts of SSRIs are found in the milk but breastfeeding is not contraindicated.

Benzodiazepines

Maternal complications

Toxic in overdose and risk of dependency.

Fetal complications

Associated with cleft palate and neonatal 'floppy baby' syndrome.

Special considerations

Consider stopping or reducing benzodiazepine medications in pregnancy, and include a neonatal review.

Breastfeeding

Drugs with a long half-life should be avoided and caution employed if used when breastfeeding a premature infant.

Antipsychotics

Maternal complications

Antipsychotic medications typically reflect their mode of action. Dopamine antagonists cause extrapyramidal side effects (worse with depot preparations) and hyperprolactinaemia. As a result, subfertility can be a problem. Olanzapine is associated with significant weight gain and the risk of gestational diabetes.

Fetal complications

Clozapine (a second-generation atypical antipsychotic) is associated with a risk of fetal agranulocytosis.

Breastfeeding

Drugs with a long half-life should be avoided and caution employed if used when breastfeeding a premature infant.

Antiepileptic drugs (valproate, carbamazepine, lamotrigine)

The risk of complications during pregnancy is increased in women with epilepsy because of the effects of a seizure on the fetus and the side effects of some antiepileptic drugs.

Valproate and carbamazepine are associated with a small increase in the risk of congenital abnormalities including neural tube defects, cardiac defects, facial defects and hypospadias. Lamotrigine may have an association with increased risk of cleft lip and cleft palate. Epileptic patients taking more than one antiepileptic drug have a higher risk of having a baby with congenital defects than a patient on monotherapy.

Pre-conceptual counselling in conjunction with an epilepsy specialist should include a review of medication. Options include switching to single agent therapy, changing the agent to a less teratogenic class, and using the smallest possible dose to achieve a seizure free state.

Maternal complications

A higher than normal dose of folic acid is recommended for women of childbearing age with epilepsy or those expecting to become pregnant. High-dose folic acid (5 mg orally, once daily) is prescribed to women taking antiepileptic medication and should be commenced in the pre-conceptual period.

With the physiological changes of pregnancy antiepileptic drugs are often metabolised more quickly than usual, leading to an increased risk of seizure in 20–35% of pregnant women with epilepsy. Lamotrigine plasma levels drop significantly in pregnant women so regular monitoring of serum levels is advised along with modifications to dosing. After birth patients can resume pre-pregnancy doses of antiepileptics. A neurologist should optimise a patient's antiepileptic drugs pre-pregnancy and review her during pregnancy to adjust doses accordingly. Close postnatal follow-up is essential.

Fetal complications

In addition to the increased risk of congenital abnormalities with some antiepileptic drugs, some babies are born predisposed to blood clotting problems. Vitamin K_1 administered at birth protects against this and other causes of haemorrhagic disease of the newborn.

Breastfeeding

Lamotrigine passes into breast milk but its effects on the baby are unknown. The advantages of breastfeeding outweigh the disadvantages of exposing the baby to lamotrigine.

Clinical case

Case features

Pre-eclampsia was suspected and admission arranged for investigation. An admission cardiotocograph (CTG) showed a fetal bradycardia, which did not improve and subsequently Jane's baby was born by emergency caesarean section.

The immediate impression is of severe fetal distress on the maternal background of pre-eclampsia and a fetal background of IUGR. At this gestation and in this scenario, a category 1 caesarean section was the correct decision.

Case investigations

There are several parallel lines of investigation in this case:

1. Fetal investigation identified a growth-restricted fetus and the admission CTG highlighted acute fetal compromise. With no other CTG traces to review it must be treated as a terminal bradycardia and every effort made to deliver the fetus immediately

2. Maternal investigation acutely will be aimed at establishing the severity of the pre-eclampsia (LFT, U+E, FBC, quantification of urinary protein) and preparing the mother for emergency surgery (coagulation screen, group and save). Continuous BP, pulse and oxygen saturations is essential.

3. Differentiating superimposed pre-eclampsia from a renal lupus flare is complex as many of the biochemical features are common to both (increased protein loss, low platelets, renal dysfunction and hypertension). Differentiating the two conditions requires multidisciplinary input and further investigation (rising antibody titres, urinary renal casts, falling complement fractions/raised complement split products Ba and Bb).

4. Antibody measurement long term for making the formal diagnoiss of SLE.

Case conclusions

Future pregnancies in this woman will be consultant managed, jointly with medical input. Her SLE and history of

SUMMARY

pre-eclampsia will mean that the following investigations and interventions will be warranted:

- Aspirin to reduce the risk of recurrent pre-eclamptic toxaemia (PET) (heparin is not indicated without a formal diagnosis of APLS) and uterine artery Doppler assessment.
- Avoid conception within 6 months of an SLE flare to reduce complication risks.
- Increased BP and urine monitoring.

- Serial ultrasound for fetal biometry, liquor and umbilical artery Doppler assessment in order to identify IUGR early if it recurs.
- Anti-Ro and anti-La antibody measurement in order to quantify the risk of fetal heartblock/neonatal cutaneous lupus.
- Medication review should be done ideally pre-conceptually.

Key learning points

- Connective tissue disorders have a diverse spectrum of multisystem symptoms but the obstetric complications carry significant morbidity and mortality risks to both the mother and fetus.
- Psychiatric disease is common in pregnancy and an important consideration for postnatal management and follow-up.

- Nausea and vomiting, constipation, heartburn, haemorrhoids, varicose veins, backache and carpal tunnel syndrome are common symptoms in pregnancy. They are associated with the hormonal changes of pregnancy.

 Now visit **www.wileyessential.com/humandevelopment** to test yourself on this chapter.

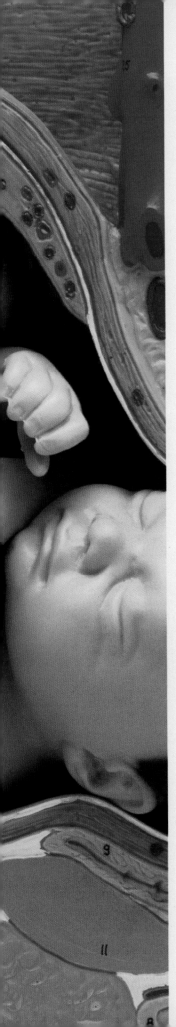

CHAPTER 14
Multiple pregnancy and other antenatal complications

Marion Beard

Case

A 27-year-old woman presents at antenatal clinic following assessment by her midwife. She is 34 weeks gestation in her first pregnancy with dichorionic diamniotic twins. She has a raised body mass index (32 kg/m² at booking). Over the past 2 days she has felt increasingly unwell, with a worsening headache, nausea, and pain to the epigastrium and right upper quadrant. In the past 2 hours she has experienced blurring of vision and reports feeling anxious.

The midwife records a blood pressure of 175/112 mmHg using a manual sphygmomanometer, and on dipstick testing of the urine there is prominent proteinuria (+++).

The obstetrician notes bilateral pitting pedal oedema, extending to the knees. The patient's partner is concerned that her face has become noticeably puffy. On examination the peripheral reflexes are brisk with three beats of ankle clonus bilaterally. The woman appears agitated, restless and distracted. Cardiotocographic monitoring of the twins shows reduced variability of both fetal heart rates.

Learning outcomes

This chapter should help you to:

- Understand the importance and mechanism of chorionicity.
- Appreciate the additional risks of multiple pregnancy to mother and fetuses.
- Understand the main means of monitoring multiple pregnancy.
- Appreciate the effects of the common medical conditions arising in pregnancy and how multiple pregnancy might exacerbate these.
- Understand delivery options and management for multiple pregnancy.

Essential Human Development, First Edition. Edited by Samuel Webster, Geraint Morris and Euan Kevelighan

Incidence of twins and chorionicity

Around 2–3% of births are of twin babies. The incidence has doubled with the advent of assisted reproductive technologies since 1980. As twin pregnancies carry more risks for both mother and babies, the guidance around assisted reproduction has changed to reduce the risk of multiple pregnancy, particularly of higher order multiples. The IVF default in the UK is therefore transfer of a single embryo. While this inevitably reduces the chances of conceiving, it is effective in reducing the morbidity of multiple gestation.

Whether conception is spontaneous or assisted, if two ova are fertilised these dizygotic fetuses will have different genotypes, separate placentas and membranes. They may therefore be different genders. Dizygotic twins may be notable in some families with an element of heritability, and are more common in some ethnic groups and geographical regions. The reasons for this superfertility, where ova may be produced by both ovaries simultaneously, are likely to be multifactorial. An example is the potential fertility boost from regular consumption of phytoestrogens (yam) coupled with genetic predisposition in the Yoruba people of southern Nigeria.

Monozygotic conceptions are sporadic events so rates are equivalent around the world. In this case, one fertilised egg splits to form two embryos. The timing of this division will determine the extent to which they share a placenta or gestational sac, known as chorionicity (Figure 14.1). They will be genetically identical, the same sex, and with early division (< day 4 post-fertilisation – the morula stage) each will have their own placenta and sac. Approximately 10% of dichorionic, diamniotic (DCDA) twins will therefore be identical.

If the division occurs between days 4 and 8 as the blastocyst forms, the embryos will share a placental mass to varying extents but each will have its own amniotic sac (see Figure 14.1). Vascular anastomoses between their circulations are likely. These monochorionic, diamniotic (MCDA) twins are at risk of twin-to-twin transfusion syndrome (TTTS) where changing flow through the anastomoses can lead to hypovolaemia in the donor twin and hypervolaemia with cardiac failure in the recipient twin. The early changes can be insidious and later can be more rapid, with the mother reporting sudden changes in abdominal shape. Fortnightly scans from 16 weeks to 24 weeks are offered to women with monochorionic twin pregnancies to monitor for intertwin differentials in amniotic fluid volume and growth velocity. Changes in these can be indicative of decompensation of vascular equilibration making both fetuses vulnerable to demise.

With later division in the blastocyst stage (days 9–12) when implantation has occurred, the placenta and sac are shared. These are monochorionic, monoamniotic (MCMA) twins. These comprise only 1% of monozygotic pregnancies (1/5000 total pregnancies). Although the risks of TTTS are slightly

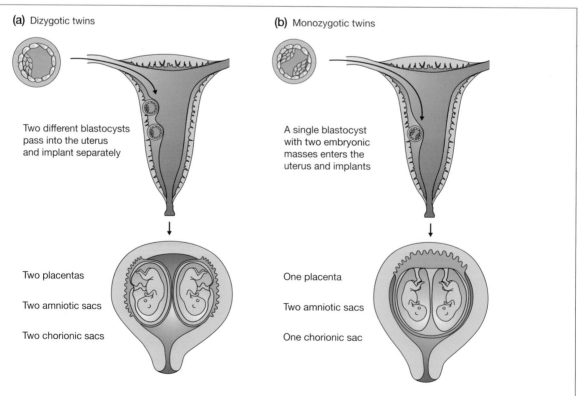

(a) Dizygotic twins

Two different blastocysts pass into the uterus and implant separately

Two placentas

Two amniotic sacs

Two chorionic sacs

(b) Monozygotic twins

A single blastocyst with two embryonic masses enters the uterus and implants

One placenta

Two amniotic sacs

One chorionic sac

Figure 14.1 Diagram of monozygotic (identical) twins and dizygotic (fraternal) twins in utero. (Source: S. Webster and R. de Wreede (2012) *Embryology at a Glance. Reproduced with permission of John Wiley & Sons, Ltd.*)

lower due to a more balanced pressure system in the placental circulation, the free movement of the fetuses around one another increases the risk of cord entanglement with potential for asphyxia rising with advancing gestation.

With division at an even later stage when the embryonic disc is forming (beyond day 13), varying degrees of conjoined twins may arise. These rarely reach viability and if successfully delivered may require extensive surgery with a high rate of mortality. Spontaneous higher-order multiple pregnancy is very rare. Less than 1/8000 spontaneous pregnancies are triplets where all three fetuses survive beyond 24 weeks, and can be a combination of mono- and dizygotic conception. Only twins will be considered for the remainder of the chapter.

Identification of twin conception

The monozygotic multiple pregnancy is a sporadic event but the risk of dizygotic conceptions is increased in the following situations:

- Previous multiple gestation or strong family history thereof.
- Extremes of reproductive age, particularly when the mother is over 40 years old at conception.
- Multiparity.

The woman pregnant with twins may produce more human chorionic gonadotrophin (hCG) to sustain the establishment of a greater total placental mass, and so may experience exaggerated early pregnancy symptoms. These include extreme fatigue, severe nausea and vomiting, and hyperemesis gravidarum. If a quantitative serum βhCG is measured this may be unexpectedly high, although this is not consistently found. Pregnancy symptoms are notoriously difficult to correlate to hormone levels, and high beta-hCG is not predictive of multiple conception. Hyperemesis should always be a trigger for an early pregnancy scan to exclude multiple pregnancy or gestational trophoblastic disease such as hydatidiform mole.

In most cases, twin pregnancy is identified at the dating scan at 10–13 weeks gestation (Figure 14.2). The first scan is a

time of great excitement in any pregnancy, and the unexpected finding of twin fetuses can be overwhelming for a family.

At this point referral to an obstetrician is made and a plan for antenatal care and delivery is arrived at jointly with the mother. This initial meeting is important from a counselling point of view as the couple's pleasure at the thought of the 'instant family' may be tempered by the revelation that the pregnancy has suddenly become high risk.

Risks to the fetus

In the discussion of chorionicity and its potential effects above, it can be seen that the extent to which the intrauterine space, the amniotic sac and the placental vasculature are shared has considerable impact on the risks to the wellbeing of the fetuses.

Around 20% of twin pregnancies will **miscarry** one fetus. This may be revealed by bleeding and passage of the fetus or there may be a silent demise. In many cases the pregnancy can continue as a singleton but the mother should be advised that there is a five-fold risk of progression to loss of the second fetus. Early demise of one twin may be an incidental finding on ultrasound scan or at delivery.

Intrauterine growth restriction with fetal weight less than 10th centile for gestation is seen in around one-fifth of dichorionic twin pregnancies and in one-third of monochorionic twin pregnancies. The metabolic and synthetic demands on the placenta increase substantially as the second trimester progresses. Monitoring the growth of the fetuses by ultrasound is a key element of surveillance. Scanning from 24 weeks onwards with biometry of head and abdominal circumference at fortnightly or monthly intervals will reassure that growth is maintained on centile curves for gestation. Other ultrasound markers of good placental function are the adequacy of amniotic fluid volume and forward flow through the umbilical cord (umbilical artery Doppler).

The rate of fetal **anomaly** is higher in dizygotic pregnancies as each fetus carries its own risk. This includes the risks of trisomy such as Down syndrome. Structural anomaly and neuromotor conditions not predictable antenatally, such as cerebral palsy, are increased approximately threefold in monozygotic pregnancies.

Biochemical screening for aneuploidy is less helpful than the identification of ultrasound markers in multiple gestation. The detailed scan offered to all women at 18–20 weeks looks for structural skeletal, abdominal wall, central nervous system, urogenital, craniofacial and cardiac anomaly in each fetus. In the event of a discordant severe anomaly, where one fetus is affected and the other is apparently healthy, selective termination may be offered. In DCDA twins the risks of this mid-trimester procedure include infection as the termination is via amniocentesis with intracardiac potassium chloride injection, and of premature labour. This is potentially before or around the limit of viability (23–24 weeks gestation) so can threaten the healthy twin. If the procedure is successful, the demised twin will remain in utero until delivery.

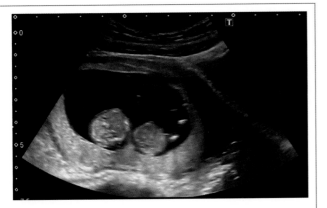

Figure 14.2 Ultrasonograph of twin gestation.

If selective feticide is opted for in the case of monochorionic twins, injected potassium chloride would be transported to the healthy twin. For this reason ablation of the appropriate umbilical cord is done using laser or occlusion. In fetuses sharing a placenta the effect of iatrogenic or spontaneous co-twin death after 24 weeks can be acute, with significant haemodynamic shift causing death, neurological damage or cardiac failure in the survivor. **Intrauterine death** of a single fetus can also precipitate preterm delivery.

The risk of **preterm delivery** is high in multiple pregnancies. In many cases this will be iatrogenic. There may be a need for 'in hours' delivery with suitably senior staff to be present if there are known obstetric complications or where caesarean section delivery is needed, and to deliver at a suitable gestation. Spontaneous preterm delivery may be due to the increased fetal mass in utero causing uterine stretch, painless cervical dilatation, or the combined effects of pro-labour hormones from the twins.

The aim is for the babies to arrive at a sufficiently mature gestation but prior to significant deterioration in placental function. Stillbirth and perinatal death is a risk, most likely due to the increasing demands on a maturing high-output placenta with consequent reduction in its function. For this reason current guidance recommends delivery of dichorionic twins at 37–38 weeks, and at 36–37 weeks for monochorionic diamniotic twins. The specific risks of cord entanglement for monoamniotic twins mean that their delivery should be by caesarean section at around 32 weeks. These may all be brought forward if there is clinical indication – for example, if there is a suggestion that one or both fetuses is becoming compromised and would be best cared for ex utero *with neonatologist support*.

Caesarean section itself is much more common in multiple pregnancies with twin gestations, having an approximately 60% risk of one or both babies being delivered abdominally. This itself is a risk to the babies as there are higher rates of respiratory difficulties in those delivered by caesarean section compared with a vaginal delivery.

Delivery itself is a risk for the twin, particularly the aftercoming twin. Ultrasound scans at later gestations include description of the order of presentation (i.e. Twin 1, Twin 2) with these descriptors being used consistently so as to allow for meaningful serial measurement of the fetuses. If the first twin is cephalic there is no contraindication to normal vaginal delivery unless there are other reasons for caesarean section. The second twin may change position after the first is delivered, and although the ideal is for another cephalic presentation, breech delivery is possible. In the case of an awkward transverse lie then manoeuvre of the second fetus can help achieve vaginal delivery. This can be by external manipulation through the maternal abdomen or by internal podalic version, where the fetal foot is grasped and moved through the cervix so as to deliver by the breech. If there is a delay before delivery of the second twin of more than 30 minutes, the risk of morbidity to that twin increases rapidly. Use of ventouse can be helpful for a cephalic presentation to stabilise the head and to expedite delivery. Recourse to caesarean section for the second twin may be required if signs of distress develop and vaginal delivery is not imminent.

Risks to the mother

In addition to the shared risks of many conditions with negative impact on the fetus (TTTS, intrauterine infection and the consequences of fetal anomaly), the twin pregnancy places unique stresses on the mother. Pre-existing medical conditions may be exaggerated or unmasked and pregnancy-specific conditions are significantly more likely to occur.

The unpleasant **symptoms of normal pregnancy** mediated by the effects of hormonal and mechanical shifts, such as ligament softening leading to musculoskeletal pain and gastro-oesophageal reflux, are more pronounced and have earlier onset. These can be particularly difficult to manage as they may reduce the enjoyment of the pregnancy with limitations on normal mobility and food consumption.

Iron-deficiency **anaemia** is common in pregnancy and is generally effectively treated by supplementing iron orally or parentally. There is a higher iron requirement in a twin pregnancy therefore healthcare staff need to be alert to the clinical features of anaemia and an additional full blood count is useful in the second trimester. An insidious anaemia is then less likely to be encountered at the routine 28-week review, at which time there is less opportunity to increase circulating iron and depleted iron stores in time for a safe delivery.

Pregnancy increases the background risk of **thrombosis** 5- to 10-fold, and multiple gestation will increase this further due to the mass effect of the large uterus causing venous stasis, particularly in the pelvis. Mode of delivery will also affect this as caesarean section will multiply this again by 10 (i.e. non-pregnancy venous thromboembolism risk × 100). At any hospital admission the use of thromboprophylaxis with low molecular weight heparin should be considered following assessment.

The woman who enters a twin pregnancy with **diabetes** considerably multiplies her risks of stillbirth and fetal loss, caesarean section and pregnancy-induced hypertension or pre-eclampsia. In women embarking on pregnancy with normal glucose homeostasis there is an increased likelihood of developing gestational diabetes, and they are more likely to require insulin should this occur. Diabetic multiple pregnancies are frequently complex with a need for high levels of contact between the mother and the team caring for her.

Mental health in these high-risk pregnancies is beginning to be a focus of research interest. Increased levels of postnatal depression have long been acknowledged in multiple pregnancies, and community services need to be alert to this possibility. The emotional effects of the intense antenatal care inherent to a twin pregnancy are less well understood. Our assumption is of reassurance through surveillance, but a significant proportion of women may become anxious and low in mood as their gestation advances. During this time their awareness of the risks of a twin pregnancy increases and there is a danger of reassuring the healthcare team while causing stress to the mother. The balance aiming for effective monitoring of the pregnancy without causing alarm and anxiety is likely only to be achieved on an individual basis, and all personnel involved need to consider the psychological impact of what we do. The involvement of the woman, her partner and family in planning care is fundamental to meeting her needs.

Hypertensive disorders of pregnancy are more common and are likely to be earlier in onset in the twin pregnancy. The two most impactful conditions are pregnancy-induced hypertension (gestational hypertension) and pre-eclampsia. The former may precede the latter. If there are other risk factors for hypertension, current recommendation is that low-dose aspirin is offered from 12 weeks until delivery. This is thought to reduce aggregation in the microcirculation of the placenta, improving perfusion and hence nutrient transfer at the placental interface.

Risk factors for hypertensive disorders include primiparity, obesity, previous hypertension in pregnancy or first-degree family history of this, advanced maternal age, and interdelivery interval of more than 10 years. Stroke and fetal compromise can be a direct consequence of sustained hypertension, and antihypertensives may be considered if the trend is upwards.

Pre-eclampsia is a pregnancy-specific condition with a classic triad of hypertension, proteinuria and oedema. The latter is not required for diagnosis. The basic blood pressure and urine dip monitoring that takes place at each antenatal visit is to exclude this condition, which affects up to 10% of all pregnancies. There is a considerable spectrum from the very mild, progressing to eclampsia with maternal seizures and acute organ failure in 0.25% of all UK pregnancies. This has halved in the past 30 years due to implementation of treatment protocols including antihypertensives and neurostabilisation to reduce the risk of seizure and stroke. The morbidity of pre-eclampsia arises from its multisystemic effects. As a disorder of endothelial dysfunction, end organs (CNS, renal, liver, eyes, placenta) are affected, and in its fulminant form a rapid cascade into multiple organ dysfunction then failure can be seen. The more insidious onset pre-eclampsia can sufficiently impair the placental function to compromise fetal growth and vitality, increasing the risk of intrauterine fetal death.

Clinical case

Review of case

The case presented as an introduction is suggestive of pre-eclampsia in a twin pregnancy. The woman has three risk factors for hypertensive disorders (obesity, primiparity and multiple gestation). As these would have been evident from booking, low-dose aspirin could be recommended to reduce risk. Of concern is the recent deterioration – she now feels unwell, and there is a need for urgent attention to attenuate the potential for harm to her as priority, and secondarily to her babies.

Admission is indicated. If seizure occurs, resuscitation should be undertaken. Baseline urea and electrolytes, liver function including urate, full blood count and coagulation screen should be requested. A group and save serum should be taken with intravenous access via a cannula. A urine sample should be obtained for urine protein estimation via spot protein:creatinine ratio, and in view of the woman's malaise an indwelling urinary catheter would be helpful, allowing rest and accurate urine output measurement as part of fluid haemostasis monitoring. Pulmonary oedema is a potential complication so restriction of fluids to avoid overload can help retain body water in the intravascular space. Due to reduced mobility, borderline dehydration and her pregnancy she should be prescribed low molecular weight heparin to avoid thromboembolism. She needs frequent observations recorded on a HDU chart, and senior clinicians should be informed and involved in her management.

There are four elements of the woman's presentation of particular concern:
1. Her blood pressure is very elevated. This may have been creeping upwards with potential to affect the placenta causing fetal growth restriction, but the level of hypertension is now at a level where there is immediate risk of haemorrhagic stroke to the mother. Antihypertensive medication is indicated. Labetalol, an alpha- and beta-adrenergic antagonist felt to be safe in pregnancy on the basis of extensive and long term use, can be useful in lowering blood pressure. The goal should not be to achieve dramatic reduction as there is the possibility of a relative hypotension leading to placental hypoperfusion and fetal compromise. A modest reduction to achieve BP of around 140/90 is achievable with least harm. If the BP remains difficult to control or is labile, consideration of intravenous antihypertensives such as labetalol or hydralazine infusion is appropriate.

2. The recent onset of feeling unwell, shaky and 'jittery' in the context of the woman's hyperresponsive peripheral tendon reflexes may indicate neuroelectrical instability. Eclamptic seizure is rare but can be life-threatening for both mother and fetuses. An infusion of magnesium sulphate causes neurological depression to effectively reduce the risk of seizure, and has a small antihypertensive effect. Monitoring of magnesium levels is unhelpful as levels will always be too high with an infusion ongoing; the balance of therapeutic effect against toxicity

is measured on a clinical basis, by monitoring of deep tendon reflexes, pulse and respiration rate.

3. Cardiotocograph (CTG) monitoring of the fetuses has shown reduced variability of the fetal heart rate. This indicates a loss of physiological reserve, potentially from hypoxaemia from placental failure. These babies are likely to do better with a preterm delivery rather than watchful waiting as they are showing signs of compromise.

4. There has been a recent onset of general malaise, restlessness, nausea and subcostal/epigastric pain. In the context of pre-eclampsia, hepatic subcapsular haemorrhage needs to be excluded. Biochemistry to assess liver function will show elevated transaminases and urate, coagulation will be deranged with thrombocytopenia, and there will be tenderness at the liver edge. HELLP syndrome (Haemolysis, Elevated Liver enzymes, Low Platelets) is a severe and life-threatening complication of pre-eclampsia where deposition of fibrin in small vessels coupled with disordered hepatic synthetic function can lead to disseminated intravascular coagulation. Resuscitation if needed and prompt delivery can be lifesaving for mother and fetuses.

It is likely that this mother will require delivery without delay. Whether there is sufficient time to give antenatal corticosteroids to improve the respiratory surfactant production in the fetuses will depend on her initial responses to therapy and the overall clinical picture.

Following delivery she will still be at risk, as up to *50% of seizures occur* postpartum. Monitoring of her blood pressure and general condition should be continued in the community until 6 weeks postpartum. She is at increased risk of pre-eclampsia in any future pregnancy, and long term she is more likely to experience cardiovascular pathology such as hypertension and ischaemic heart disease.

Key learning points

- Multiple gestation carries significant morbidity for the mother and her fetuses.
- Monitoring during the antenatal period aims to identify conditions such as impaired or discordant fetal growth, anomaly or TTTS at an early stage.
- Ultrasound scanning is a key tool in effective antenatal monitoring of twins.
- The traditional 'two patients' framework of obstetric practice is complicated by a third patient in twins, and these challenging pregnancies can reveal, precipitate or worsen maternal medical conditions. These include the pregnancy-specific conditions such as pre-eclampsia.
- The clinical case presented demonstrates a severe and deteriorating acute presentation and gives examples of management to protect the mother and to optimise the wellbeing of her babies.

 Now visit **www.wileyessential.com/humandevelopment** to test yourself on this chapter

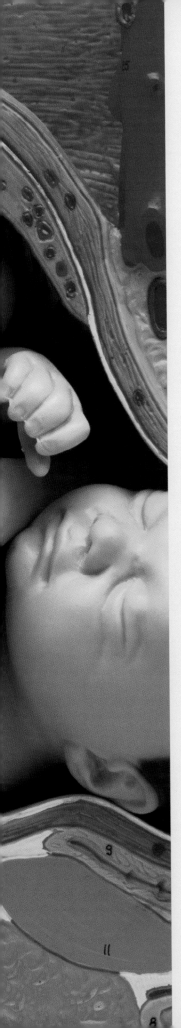

CHAPTER 15

Problems in late pregnancy

Deepa Balachandran Nair

Case

A 37-year-old primigravida at 33 weeks gestation presents to the A&E with abdominal pain and bleeding *per vaginum*. She reports the pain to be constant and severe. She estimates that she has lost about half a cupful of fresh blood. Her antenatal course had been uneventful except for a high blood pressure noted on the last antenatal check-up at 32 weeks, but this did not require medication.

On presentation, she was conscious and oriented, her pulse rate was 100 beats per minute (bpm) and her blood pressure was 140/80 mmHg. Abdominal examination showed the uterus to be corresponding to 34 weeks gestation, tense and tender. The fetal heart was heard at 150 bpm.

Learning outcomes

- You should be able to suspect the causes of bleeding during pregnancy from presenting symptoms and recommend appropriate management.

- You should understand the potential importance of reduced fetal movements, and the management of women presenting with reduced fetal movements.

- You should be able to define prolonged pregnancy and understand the risks associated with it.

Essential Human Development, First Edition. Edited by Samuel Webster, Geraint Morris and Euan Kevelighan
© 2018 John Wiley & Sons, Ltd. Published 2018 by John Wiley & Sons, Ltd.

Antepartum haemorrhage

Antepartum haemorrhage is defined as vaginal bleeding occurring after 24 weeks gestation and before the birth of the baby.

Antepartum haemorrhage complicates 3–5% of pregnancies. There are a variety of causes such as placenta praevia (low-lying placenta), placental abruption (premature separation of the placenta), cervical ectropion and cervical polyp. It is of unknown origin in approximately 50% of cases (Figure 15.1). In general, placental causes are of more serious consequence to the mother and fetus.

Placenta praevia

Normally, the placenta is implanted into the upper segment of the uterus. When the placenta is implanted into the lower uterine segment it is referred to as placenta praevia. The risks associated with this condition are primarily due to the fact that the lower uterine segment undergoes changes in late pregnancy in preparation for the onset of labour, predisposing to bleeding and prematurity of the baby. In addition, it lacks contractile capacity compared with the upper segment, making it more difficult to control bleeding following placental separation.

Placenta praevia can be broadly classified into:
1. Major praevia, when the placenta covers the internal os either partially or completely.
2. Minor praevia, when the placenta is in the lower uterine segment but not reaching the internal os.

Browne's classification divides placenta praevia into four groups (Figure 15.2):

    Grade 1 – placenta in the lower uterine segment, not reaching the internal os.

    Grade 2 – placenta in the lower uterine segment, just reaching the internal os.

    Grade 3 – placenta partially covering the internal os.

    Grade 4 – placenta completely covering the internal os.

Incidence and risk factors

Placenta praevia complicates about 1 in 300 pregnancies and is associated with a number of risk factors (Table 15.1).

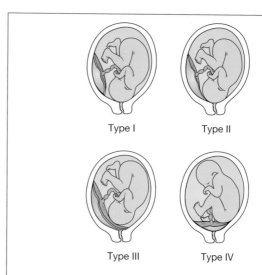

Figure 15.2 Types of placenta praevia.

Presentation and diagnosis

Placenta praevia usually presents as painless vaginal bleeding commonly occurring towards the end of the second trimester or thereafter. Classically there are a series of minor bleeding episodes referred to as "warning" haemorrhages before a major bleed. On examination tachycardia and hypotension are usually proportionate to the amount of blood loss. The size of the uterus corresponds to the gestational age and the uterus is soft, non-tense and non-tender. Malpresentations are more common with placenta praevia. Even in the case of cephalic presentation, the presenting part is usually high as the low-lying placenta prevents engagement of the fetal head. There may be palpable contractions indicating that the woman is in labour, which has led to shearing away of the placenta from its bed causing the bleed.

In clinical practice, a low-lying placenta is first diagnosed on the 20-week scan performed primarily to assess for fetal anomalies. If a major placenta praevia (a placenta covering the os either partially or completely) is seen on this scan a repeat scan is performed at 32 weeks to ascertain if the placenta is no longer low-lying. If a minor placenta praevia is diagnosed a repeat ultrasound scan is performed at 36 weeks gestation. In either case, earlier scans may be warranted if the patient presents with vaginal bleeding. Most cases of minor placenta praevia diagnosed at 20 weeks do not remain as placenta praevia in

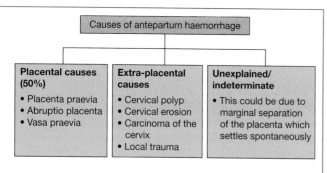

Figure 15.1 Causes of antepartum haemorrhage.

Table 15.1 Risk factors associated with placenta praevia.
• Advancing maternal age
• Multiparity
• Multiple pregnancy
• Prior caesarean delivery
• Cigarette smoking
• Unexplained elevation of maternal serum alpha-fetoprotein (AFP)

later gestations due to the differential growth of the upper and lower uterine segments as pregnancy progresses. This is referred to as apparent placental migration. Transabdominal ultrasound is typically used, but a transvaginal ultrasound is equally safe in cases of placenta praevia and is more sensitive. In cases where there is a doubt in the diagnosis after a transabdominal scan, a transvaginal ultrasound is recommended for confirmation. Colour Doppler is useful in the diagnosis of adherent placenta especially in a previously scarred uterus where there is an increased risk of this.

Prior to the wide availability of ultrasound, vaginal examination was performed in theatre in cases of clinically suspected placenta praevia with all preparations in place to proceed with a caesarean section (this was referred to as examination in a 'double set-up'). During vaginal examination the fornices are palpated first to check for the boggy feel of the placenta. Examination is abandoned in the presence of a boggy mass felt either through the fornices or through the os or if examination provokes bleeding. Clinical examination to diagnose placenta praevia, however, is rarely required in present-day clinical practice.

Management

Basic resuscitative measures are instituted in a patient presenting with major haemorrhage. A multidisciplinary approach involving a senior obstetrician, anaesthetist, midwife, neonatologist and haematologist is employed. Alongside stabilisation of the patient in terms of airway, breathing and circulation, the extent of ongoing haemorrhage is assessed. If she continues to bleed or is in labour, an emergency caesarean section is performed. If the bleeding has stopped, she can be managed expectantly.

The expectant management for placenta praevia was first described by Macafee. The aim is to limit the morbidity and mortality resulting from iatrogenic prematurity to the baby and only deliver the baby if absolutely necessary. Antenatal corticosteroids are administered to all women with placenta praevia at about 28 weeks gestation or earlier if they have had 'warning' haemorrhages prior to that. Anti-D should be administered after an episode of bleeding to non-sensitised rhesus D-negative women (see Chapter 12).

Admission to hospital is recommended by 32–34 weeks gestation in women with major praevia with significant 'warning' haemorrhages. Blood should be cross-matched and available for use should the need arise.

Women with an ultrasound diagnosis of major placenta praevia and no antepartum haemorrhage should be offered elective caesarean section at 38–39 weeks gestation. These patients need not be admitted to hospital unless bleeding occurs. They should, however, be advised about the risks of major bleeding should they go into labour and the need to come to the maternity unit urgently in that case. They should avoid sexual intercourse, always have a companion to help in case haemorrhage arises, and be within a short distance of the hospital.

Caesarean section in cases of placenta praevia can be challenging. There is an increased risk of bleeding during entry into the uterus due to engorged vessels in the lower uterine segment, and through possible separation of the placenta to facilitate delivery of the baby. The risk of postpartum haemorrhage is increased due to reduced contractility of the lower uterine segment and failure of the vessels of the placental bed to constrict. Typically, uterine incision should be followed by careful separation of the placenta to identify the bag of membranes and subsequent rupture of the membranes to deliver the baby. Sometimes, however, it becomes necessary to cut through the placenta to deliver the baby. Maternal and fetal outcomes are rarely compromised by cutting through the placenta. In centres with access to interventional radiology bilateral uterine artery catheterisation can be performed prior to caesarean section. This allows for embolisation to be carried out without delay if there is severe haemorrhage.

In minor placenta praevia, if the lowest edge of the placenta is more than 2 cm from the cervical os vaginal delivery is possible. If it is less than 2 cm from the os, bleeding with cervical dilatation is very likely and hence caesarean section is recommended.

Type 2 posterior placenta praevia is otherwise known as 'dangerous' placenta praevia. On trying to dip the head into the maternal pelvis there is typically slowing of the fetal heart owing to compression of the placental cord and prompt recovery on release of pressure. This is known as the Stallworthy sign. Caesarean section is always recommended for this type of placenta praevia.

Adherent placenta

The incidence of adherent placenta has increased in recent years in parallel with rising caesarean section rates. Adherent placenta is believed to occur due to injury to the decidua basalis of the endometrium during surgery. This layer normally acts as a barrier to penetration of trophoblastic tissue into the myometrium. Adherent placenta can be divided into the following three types (Figure 15.3):

1. Placenta accreta – when there is loss of the normal plane of cleavage between the placental tissue and the myometrium; the placenta is adherent to uterine wall.

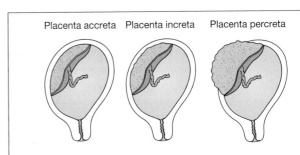

Figure 15.3 Types of adherent placenta.

2. Placenta increta – when the placenta penetrates through the myometrium.
3. Placenta percreta – when the placenta penetrates through the myometrium and onto the serosa. When penetration occurs beyond the serosa there may be further invasion of the placental tissue into the bladder, parametrium or rarely impingement onto the ureters.

Diagnosis

A high index of suspicion for adherent placenta is required in those with a previous caesarean section and a low-lying anterior placenta on ultrasound. These women should have a colour Doppler ultrasound scan to diagnose adherent placenta. Magnetic resonance imaging (MRI) is of limited diagnostic value.

Management

Morbidly adherent placenta is an important cause of maternal morbidity and mortality. Multidisciplinary involvement with input from a senior obstetrician, anaesthetist, haematologist, neonatologist, and interventional radiologist, and planning of delivery is required. A placenta praevia with evidence of adherence of placenta to uterine wall is one of the few present-day indications for a classical caesarean section. The baby is delivered through a vertical midline incision on the upper segment of the uterus and the placenta is left untouched with the cord ligated. The placental tissue usually becomes necrosed over a period of time postnatally. These women are followed up with serial beta-human chorionic gonadotrophin (BHCG) measurements and ultrasound scans to confirm resolution. However, the patient needs to be compliant with follow-up as this approach can have complications of sepsis and secondary postpartum haemorrhage.

Abruptio placentae

Placental abruption refers to the premature separation of a normally situated placenta. It has also been referred to as accidental haemorrhage.

Abruption may be revealed when blood insinuates between the membranes and the uterine wall causing vaginal bleeding, or concealed when the blood is retained between the detached placenta and the uterus, or a combination of the two. Concealed haemorrhage is less common, but usually carries greater risks to the mother and baby as the extent of hemorrhage may not be readily appreciated, diagnosis is delayed and the risks of consumptive coagulopathy are higher.

Sher and Statland classification of abruption

Grade 1 – diagnosis following delivery by recognition of a retroplacental clot.
Grade 2 – clinical signs and symptoms of abruption, fetus alive.

Grade 3 – abruption leading to intrauterine fetal demise:
3a – with no evidence of maternal coagulopathy;
3b – associated with maternal coagulopathy.

Incidence and risk factors

Abruptio placentae complicates about 1 in 200 deliveries. The most common condition associated with abruption is hypertension of some form. Other risk factors are enumerated in Table 15.2.

Presentation and diagnosis

Abruptio placentae usually presents as vaginal bleeding associated with abdominal pain. Pain is typically described as severe and constant as opposed to the intermittent contraction pain. However, it should be borne in mind that labour is the most common cause promoting separation of the placenta. Hence about 50% of those with abruption are in labour and may describe intermittent worsening of pain with contractions. Tachycardia may indicate the level of hypovolaemia. The blood pressure may be misleading as a significant proportion of these women may have been hypertensive and the normal blood pressure following the bleed may still be indicative of intravascular volume depletion. Abdominal examination classically shows a tense and tender uterus. In milder cases of abruption the uterus may be irritable. Classical features of a tense and tender uterus with height of the uterine fundus more than the period of gestation are more evident in a concealed abruption. Also the uterus may not be tender when the placenta is located posteriorly. Speculum examination will give an idea of ongoing blood loss and vaginal examination will help establish whether the patient is in labour. Cardiotocography (CTG) monitoring is recommended for women with antepartum haemorrhage and will show abnormalities in cases of significant abruption. In severe cases of abruption (grade 3) intrauterine fetal demise occurs. Maternal coagulopathy

Table 15.2 Risk factors for abruptio placentae.

- Previous abruption
- Low birthweight
- Preterm pre-labour rupture of membranes
- Pre-eclampsia
- Thrombophilias
- Multifetal gestation
- Hydramnios
- Increasing age
- Increasing parity
- Cigarette smoking
- Cocaine use
- Abdominal trauma
- External cephalic version
- Uterine leiomyoma

ensues in about 30% of severe cases. In general, severity of the abruption depends on the interval between onset of symptoms and presentation.

History and clinical examination is of paramount importance in the diagnosis of abruption. Ultrasound is not sensitive (sensitivity <30%) for the diagnosis of abruption, especially acutely, since clots and the placenta have the same sonographic appearance. The main role of ultrasound is to rule out a low-lying placenta as the cause of the bleed. In term or near-term women, when there is a high index of clinical suspicion, an amniotomy may be done. This usually shows blood-stained liquor, which further supports the diagnosis.

A low-lying placenta should be excluded by ultrasound prior to undertaking a digital vaginal examination in any woman presenting with vaginal bleeding.

Management

Intensive resuscitation and multidisciplinary involvement is the cornerstone in the management of abruption. Further management would depend upon the severity of abruption, maternal condition and fetal status.

If there is reasonable certainty about the diagnosis, the fetus is viable and vaginal delivery is not imminent an emergency caesarean section may be the best option. If there is uncertainty about the diagnosis and no evidence of fetal compromise, continuous monitoring of the mother and fetal heart can be done with the aim of intervening in case of abnormality in the fetal heart rate or maternal deterioration. Delay in delivery of the baby in case of abruption can result in poor neonatal outcome.

In cases where intrauterine fetal demise has occurred, the goal is to achieve an atraumatic vaginal delivery as quickly as possible. An amniotomy can often accelerate labour in such situations, and augmentation with oxytocin may be required (Table 15.3). Oxytocin should, however, be used with caution since the uterus may have a tendency towards hypertonicity in this situation. If delivery does not occur within a reasonable time period and there is further deterioration of the maternal status, it may sometimes be necessary to perform a caesarean section even with a dead fetus in order to limit maternal morbidity.

Table 15.3 Benefits of amniotomy in abruptio placentae.

- May provide supportive evidence towards the diagnosis if blood-stained liquor is evident on amniotomy
- Decrease in the amniotic fluid volume may cause better compression of the spiral arteries, decreasing bleeding from the placental site
- Decreased intrauterine pressure may have a role in minimising entry of thromboplastin into the maternal circulation hence reducing chances of maternal coagulopathy

Complications of abruptio placentaa

Maternal

1. **Shock.** It may not be apparent because the blood loss may not all be revealed, and the patient may have been hypertensive prior to the event.
2. **Disseminated intravascular coagulopathy (DIC).** Placental abruption is one of the most common causes of clinically significant DIC in obstetrics. This occurs due to the release of tissue thromboplastin from separation of the placenta into the maternal circulation. It is more common with concealed abruption because intrauterine pressure is higher forcing more thromboplastin into the maternal venous system triggering activation of intravascular coagulation.
3. **Renal failure.** Acute renal failure may occur with severe placental abruption especially if the treatment of hypovolaemia is delayed or incomplete.
4. **Couvelaire uterus.** Also known as uteroplacental apoplexy, this pathological entity was first described by Couvelaire. It is more common in concealed abruption and occurs due to widespread extravasation of blood into the uterine musculature and beneath the uterine serosa. The uterine surface shows multiple areas of ecchymoses, which may be patchy or diffuse. Bleeding into the uterine musculature per se seldom interferes with uterine contractility, and this appearance on its own is not an indication for hysterectomy.
5. **Postpartum haemorrhage.** There is an increased risk of postpartum haemorrhage in abruption due to atony, which may further contribute to maternal coagulopathy.
6. **Sheehan syndrome.** This is characterised by failure of lactation, amenorrhoea, breast atrophy, loss of pubic and axillary hair, hypothyroidism and adrenal cortical insufficiency. It can occur rarely as a complication of severe intrapartum or postpartum haemorrhage.

Fetal

1. Prematurity.
2. Intrauterine hypoxia and fetal demise.

Vasa praevia

This is a unique cause of antepartum haemorrhage in that the blood lost is of fetal rather than maternal origin. Loss of a seemingly minimal amount of blood can be detrimental to the fetus. It is uncommon, with a reported incidence of 1 in 2000 to 1 in 6000 pregnancies. Vasa praevia is usually associated with velamentous insertion of the umbilical cord. It can rarely be suspected on the antenatal ultrasound. The typical presentation is fetal bradycardia or evidence of worsening of the CTG following rupture of membranes associated with vaginal bleeding A high index of clinical suspicion is necessary since urgent delivery by caesarean section is required once the diagnosis is made to minimise neonatal morbidity and mortality. It can result in fetal demise especially following spontaneous rupture of membranes when the diagnosis is unknown. The fetal mortality for this condition can be as high as 60%. Bedside tests like the Apt test or Singer alkali denaturation test can sometimes be performed to confirm the blood to be of fetal origin. These tests, however, seldom influence management.

Other causes of antepartum haemorrhage

The blood loss due to cervical causes of antepartum haemorrhage like ectropion, polyp, local trauma and cervical cancer is usually less in quantity. It may present as a postcoital bleed. It is important to take a cervical smear history in cases of antepartum haemorrhage as sometimes cervical cancer may be first diagnosed in pregnancy. This occurs most often in patients who have not had cervical smears in the past. A speculum examination will demonstrate any cervical pathology.

Often the cause of bleeding cannot be identified even after a thorough history and examination. The bleed in such situations may be due to a marginal separation of the placenta. These pregnancies should be treated as high risk since fetal outcome has been shown to be worse in such pregnancies compared to those not complicated by antepartum haemorrhage.

Reduced fetal movements

Maternal perception of fetal movement first occurs at 18–20 weeks in the first pregnancy and at 16–18 weeks in subsequent pregnancies. Usually perception of movement increases progressively until about 32 weeks, after which time movements plateau but do not decrease. This pattern reflects the maturation of the fetal nervous and musculoskeletal systems. The pattern will also depend on the fetal sleep cycles, which usually last for about 20–40 minutes and seldom last for more than 90 minutes. Several factors affect maternal perception of fetal movement (Table 15.4).

Table 15.4 Factors affecting maternal perception of fetal movement.

Factors increasing perceived fetal movement	Factors decreasing perceived fetal movement
High blood glucose Lying down position Fetal anencephaly	• Drugs: opioids, benzodiazepines, methadone, corticosteroids • Anterior placenta • Maternal cigarette smoking • Fetal spine lying anteriorly • Standing position • Congenital fetal anomalies • Fetal abnormalities affecting the nervous or musculoskeletal systems

Maternal perception of a decrease or alteration in the fetal movement should be regarded as important since approximately 55% of stillbirths are noted to be preceded by decreased fetal movement felt by the mother.

Management

Various methods of assessing fetal movements, like the 'count to 10', 'movement count in 1 hour', and so forth, have been described. However, none of these have been shown to have any benefit. Routine monitoring of fetal movements has also been shown to increase maternal stress and anxiety.

In general, women should be advised to be aware of the baby's movements. If they feel the movements are decreased or absent after 28 weeks gestation, they should be advised to contact their maternity unit. If they are unsure regarding a decrease or alteration in the pattern of fetal movements after 28 weeks, they should be advised to lie down in the left lateral position and count movements for 2 hours. If they feel fewer than 10 movements in these 2 hours of observation they should contact their maternity unit immediately.

When a woman presents with a history of decreased fetal movements, management will depend on the gestational age. In all gestations the initial step is to confirm the presence of the fetal heartbeat. A complete history should be taken to look for factors increasing the risk of adverse pregnancy outcome. This includes factors that predispose to a higher risk of stillbirth, like extremes of maternal age, primiparity, previous bad obstetric history, any form of hypertension in pregnancy, diabetes, obesity, fetal growth restriction, congenital malformations and other genetic or medical factors.

After 28 weeks gestation, if the fetal heart is heard and there are no risk factors noted after a detailed history and examination, the woman can be reassured. However, if there is a significant history of reduced movements and one or more risk factors, she needs to be referred to a maternity unit. In the maternity unit, the first step would be to perform a CTG for a period of at least 20 minutes. If the perception of reduced fetal movements persists despite a normal CTG, or if there are one or more risk factors identified, she should have an ultrasound scan to assess fetal wellbeing.

At a gestation of less than 24 weeks, the presence of the fetal heartbeat should be confirmed. If the woman has not perceived fetal movements by 24 weeks, she should be referred to a fetal medicine specialist to rule out disorders of the fetal neuromuscular system.

Between 24 and 28 weeks gestation, again the fetal heartbeat should be confirmed. There is no evidence to recommend a CTG at this gestation. If there are risk factors for fetal growth restriction an ultrasound assessment should be undertaken.

Prolonged pregnancy

The International Federation of Obstetrics and Gynaecology (FIGO) defines prolonged pregnancy as pregnancy more than

294 days or 42 completed weeks from the last menstrual period (LMP).

This, however, assumes that ovulation occurs 14 days after the LMP. Hence there may be an overdiagnosis of prolonged pregnancy if there is an error in estimation of LMP or delayed ovulation. Dating of pregnancy from the 11–14-week ultrasound, which is routinely performed in the UK, reduces the incidence of prolonged pregnancy.

Prolonged pregnancy, post-term pregnancy, post-dates and postmaturity have variously been used to describe the same entity. Whilst prolonged and post-term pregnancy may be synonymous, post-dates is a questionable term, and postmaturity refers to a specific clinical syndrome features of which are enumerated in Table 15.5.

Features of postmaturity syndrome can be seen even in neonates born earlier than 42 weeks gestation. It occurs in about 10% of prolonged pregnancies and indicates a pathologically prolonged pregnancy.

Incidence and risk factors

The incidence of prolonged pregnancy would depend on the reliability of estimation of gestational age and induction practices. In general the incidence is about 10%. The most common cause of prolonged pregnancy is an error in the estimation of gestational age. Risk factors associated are as enumerated in Table 15.6.

The main concern with prolonged pregnancy is the increase in perinatal mortality. Compared to that at 40 weeks the perinatal mortality as is two-fold higher at 42 weeks and four-fold higher at 43 weeks. The pathology of prolonged pregnancy is poorly understood. In some women there is uteroplacental insufficiency beyond a particular gestational age hence increasing risks like oligohydramnios, meconium aspiration and birth asphyxia, whereas in some the risks associated are due to continuing placental function like macrosomia and shoulder dystocia. These lead to increased maternal morbidity due to perineal trauma, increased operative vaginal delivery, caesarean section and postpartum haemorrhage.

Table 15.5 Features of postmaturity syndrome.

- Wrinkled appearance of baby
- Peeling of skin
- Meconium-stained skin and nails
- Long nails
- Calcified skull
- Thin body with loss of subcutaneous fat
- Little or no vernix
- No lanugo
- Alert look

Table 15.6 Risk factors for prolonged pregnancy.

- Previous prolonged pregnancy (risk of recurrence 20%)
- Primigravidity
- Family history of prolonged pregnancy
- Male fetal gender
- Maternal obesity
- Fetal factors like anencephaly, adrenal insufficiency, X-linked sulfatase deficiency

Prolonged pregnancy is also associated with increased maternal anxiety.

Management

The options for management of prolonged pregnancy are two-fold: expectant management or induction of labour. NICE recommends that all women should be advised about the risks of prolonged pregnancy and given the option of induction of labour between 41 and 42 weeks. Membrane sweep can be offered prior to this as it has been shown to increase the chances of spontaneous onset of labour. In case the woman declines induction of labour, antepartum fetal surveillance in the form of twice-weekly CTG and ultrasound estimation of amniotic fluid volume is recommended, although evidence on the ideal form of fetal surveillance in prolonged pregnancy is limited.

Continuous intrapartum CTG monitoring is recommended because of the increased risk of intrapartum stillbirth.

Clinical case

Case discussion

From the history and examination findings, the diagnosis is likely to be placental abruption. The risk factors of note in this case are advanced maternal age, primiparity and possible gestational hypertension. APH associated with abdominal pain is typical of abruption. The amount of blood lost may, however, exceed estimates as there may be a concealed component, explaining the abdominal pain. Again, the blood pressure may be misleading since the woman may have been previously hypertensive and an apparently normal blood pressure may still mean that she

could rapidly decompensate with continuing intravascular volume depletion. As the fetal heartbeat is present, it is probably a grade 2 abruption.

Prompt resuscitative measures are required. This includes establishment of adequate venous access in the form of two large-bore (14–16G) venous cannulas. Bloods are taken for a full blood count, group and cross match (4–6 units), baseline renal and liver biochemistry and coagulation profile. Multidisciplinary and senior involvement is essential. In particular the anaesthetist and neonatal team need to be informed immediately to facilitate further

Summary

resuscitation and stabilisation of mother and baby. Fetal status should be assessed by cardiotocography. Review of the maternity notes is helpful to identify any risk factors as is review of the previous ultrasound reports to rule out placenta praevia. Once a low-lying placenta is excluded, vaginal examination can be performed to see if the woman is in labour. If the diagnosis of abruption is certain and delivery is not imminent, the safest option is emergency caesarean section. If, however, bleeding has stopped, the woman is stable and the CTG shows the fetus to be un-compromised, further fetal monitoring with CTG will indicate any detrimental change in the in utero environment. A plan for prompt intervention in case of any change should be in place. Following delivery, postpartum haemorrhage should be anticipated and managed appropriately.

Key learning points

- Placenta praevia and abruption are the two important causes of antepartum haemorrhage causing adverse maternal and neonatal outcomes that need to be con-sidered in a woman presenting with antepartum haem-orrhage. These, however, contribute to only 50% of cases of antepartum haemorrhage.
- Prompt resuscitation of the mother through multidisci-plinary and senior involvement is the priority in signifi-cant antepartum haemorrhage.
- Maternal perception of reduced fetal movements is as-sociated with subsequent stillbirth.
- The first step when a woman presents with reduced fetal movements at any gestation is to establish the presence of the fetal heartbeat. This can be done with a hand-held Doppler.
- Cardiotocography is done to establish fetal wellbeing when over 28 weeks gestation.
- Prolonged pregnancy is defined as pregnancy beyond 42 completed weeks of gestation. It is associated with adverse fetal and maternal outcomes.
- NICE recommends offering induction of labour to all women between 41 and 42 weeks to avoid risks associ-ated with prolonged pregnancy.
- If the woman declines induction of labour, twice-weekly CTG and measurement of amniotic fluid volume is rec-ommended beyond 42 weeks.

Now visit **www.wileyessential.com/humandevelopment** to test yourself on this chapter.

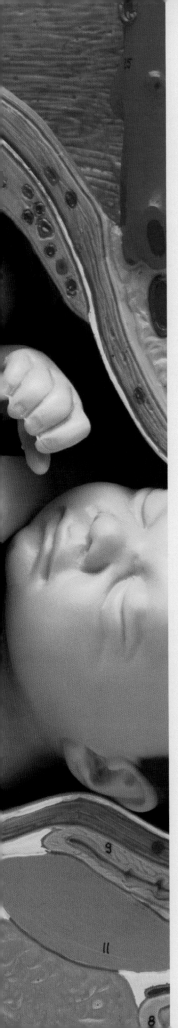

CHAPTER 16
Fetal growth and tests of fetal wellbeing

Maitreyee Deshpande

Case

You are visiting Chloe who is 18 years old and in her first pregnancy. Chloe is an enthusiastic dancer and was training for a dance competition. Although this is an unplanned pregnancy, she is delighted with the news and is well supported by her mother.

She has a BMI of 19 kg/m^2. She smokes 20 cigarettes a day. Her only regular medication is oral iron tablets as prescribed by her general practitioner. Her blood pressure is 100/60 mmHg, her pulse is 86 beats per minute and regular.

A dating scan today has confirmed her gestation as 12 weeks and 3 days. Her midwife has requested review to arrange further antenatal follow-up.

Learning outcomes

This chapter should help you to be able to:

- Define fetal growth restriction (FGR) and small for gestational age fetus (SGA).
- Recognise risk factors for fetal growth restriction.
- Explain screening and diagnosis of SGA.
- Understand tests of fetal wellbeing including cardiotocography (CTG).
- Understand the basic principles of management of pregnancies complicated by fetal growth restriction.

Essential Human Development, First Edition. Edited by Samuel Webster, Geraint Morris and Euan Kevelighan
© 2018 John Wiley & Sons, Ltd. Published 2018 by John Wiley & Sons, Ltd.

Definition and types of fetal growth restriction

Routine antenatal care aims to identify fetal growth restriction (FGR) in the general obstetric population. Fetal growth restriction refers to failure of the fetus to achieve its genetic growth potential. Small for gestational age (SGA) is defined as an estimated fetal weight (EFW) or abdominal circumference (AC) less than the 10th centile, and severe SGA as an EFW or AC less than the third centile.

FGR is not synonymous with SGA. SGA fetuses can be constitutionally small, thus not all SGA fetuses will have FGR. However, FGR is highly likely in a severe SGA fetus. It is important to differentiate between the two entities as FGR implies pathological causation.

There are two types of FGR. In symmetric fetal growth restriction the head size and trunk are reduced in parallel. Early-onset symmetrical FGR can be a constitutionally small SGA fetus or can be caused by chromosomal problems, congenital anomaly and congenital infections. Asymmetric FGR is usually associated with pathological conditions such as pre-eclampsia or placental insufficiency. Due to inadequate supply of blood flow to the fetus redistribution of the blood flow occurs with more blood flowing to the important organs such as brain, heart and adrenal glands. This is known as the 'brain-sparing' effect. Consequently less blood flows to the liver and kidney causing discrepancy in abdominal circumference (lower) and head circumference (same/spared) of the fetus.

Diagnosis of fetal growth restriction

Ultrasound scan for fetal growth includes measurement of fetal abdominal circumference (AC), head circumference (HC) and femur length (FL). Estimated fetal weight can be calculated using these parameters. These measurements are plotted on a centile chart. The use of a customised growth chart can significantly improve the detection rate of FGR. For accurate assessment of growth velocity scans should be performed at least 3 weeks apart.

SGA is diagnosed when AC, or EFW, is below the 10th centile. Comparison of fetal HC and AC will indicate if a fetus is asymmetrically small. If the HC and AC are both below the 10th centile the fetus is symmetrically small. If either the HC or the AC are small while the other is normal, the fetus is asymmetrically small. Typically the HC is spared and the AC is reduced.

Screening for fetal growth restriction

Accurate prediction of pregnancies at risk of FGR would enable increased monitoring. Currently prediction is done by identifying risk factors based on the history, maternal serum screening and serial measurement of symphysis fundal height (SFH).

Determination of fetal size is a complex process with multiple variants such as maternal body mass index (BMI), ethnicity and socioeconomic status. Though there are recognised risk factors for SGA it is difficult to predict how the risk factors interact with each other in an individual woman. The guidance from the Royal College of Obstetricians and Gynaecologists (RCOG) has divided the risk factors into major and minor, as illustrated in Table 16.1.

Several biochemical substances released from the placenta, including pregnancy-associated plasma protein A (PAPP-A), have been studied for prediction of FGR. PAPP-A is a large glycoprotein produced by the placenta and decidua. It has several functions, including prevention of recognition of the fetus by the maternal immune system, matrix mineralisation and angiogenesis. A low level of PAPP-A is descriptive of poor early placentation and may result in adverse pregnancy outcomes. A first-trimester low level of PAPP-A (<0.415 MoM) is a major risk factor for FGR.

Women with one major risk factor for FGR will need serial assessment of fetal growth and umbilical artery Doppler from 26–28 weeks. Women with three or more minor risk factors can be further screened with uterine artery Doppler at the 20-week scan. If maternal uterine artery Doppler shows high resistance the patient should be referred for serial ultrasound scans.

Fetal surveillance

Once FGR is diagnosed, additional assessments of fetal wellbeing are indicated. Some of the common tests of fetal wellbeing are outlined below.

Umbilical Doppler

Doppler assessment of blood flow in the umbilical artery is the primary surveillance tool. It is shown to reduce perinatal mortality and morbidity in FGR cases. As the pregnancy

Table 16.1 Risk factors for fetal growth restriction (FGR): minor and major risk factors.

Minor risk factors	Major risk factors
• Maternal age >35 years	• Maternal age >40 years
• IVF singleton pregnancy	• Smoker >11 cigarettes per day
• Nulliparity	• Paternal SGA
• BMI <20	• Cocaine use
• BMI 24–34.9 kg/m²	• Daily vigorous exercise
• Smoker 1–10 cigarettes per day	• Previous SGA baby
• Low fruit intake pre-pregnancy	• Previous stillbirth
• Previous pre-eclampsia	• Maternal SGA
• Pregnancy interval <6 months	• Chronic hypertension
• Pregnancy interval >60 months	• Renal impairment
	• Diabetes with vascular disease
	• Antiphospholipid syndrome
	• Heavy bleeding in pregnancy
	• PAPP-A <0.4 MoM

BMI, body mass index; MoM, multiples of median; PAPP-A, pregnancy-associated plasma protein A; SGA, small for gestational age.

progresses diastolic flow in the umbilical artery increases and placental resistance falls. A pulsatility index/resistance index (PI or RI) is used to measure resistance in the umbilical artery. If the PI is greater than +2 standard deviations above the mean for the gestational age, it indicates reduced perfusion of the placenta and a risk of fetal hypoxia. Absent or reversed end-diastolic flow in the umbilical artery is strongly correlated with fetal distress and intrauterine fetal death (Figure 16.1).

Amniotic fluid volume

Ultrasound evaluation of the amniotic fluid that surrounds the baby in utero is a routine part of a fetal wellbeing scan. It can predict deficient fluid (oligohydramnios) and excess fluid (polyhydramnios) as both are linked with increased perinatal morbidity.

Two methods that are routinely used in practice to measure amniotic fluid are single deepest vertical pool (SDVP) or amniotic fluid index (AFI). SDVP refers to the vertical dimension of the largest pocket of amniotic fluid, which must not contain umbilical cord or fetal extremities.

Using SDVP measurements the following definitions apply:

- Oligohydramnios: depth of 0 to 2 cm
- Normal fluid: depth of 2.1 to 8 cm
- Polyhydramnios: depth of more than 8 cm

AFI is the sum of maximum vertical pool measurements from the four quadrants of the uterus.

Using AFI measurements the following definitions apply:

- Oligohydramnios: depth of 0 to <5 cm
- Normal fluid: depth of 5 to 25 cm
- Polyhydramnios: greater than 25 cm

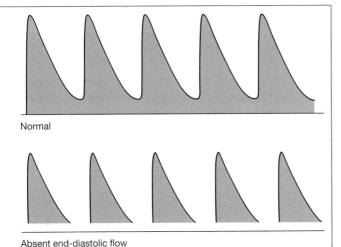

Normal

Absent end-diastolic flow

Figure 16.1 Normal and absent end-diastolic flow in the umbilical artery measured by Doppler ultrasound scanning. The absent end-diastolic flow indicates increased resistance to flow within the umbilical arteries.

Redistribution of blood flow in FGR cases results in blood flowing away from the kidneys to vital structures such as brain and heart. This causes reduced urine output and reduced amniotic fluid. Precise measurement of amniotic fluid via ultrasound is difficult and hence has limited value as a fetal surveillance tool. Amniotic fluid is a dynamic complex and can gather in irregular pockets around the fetus. Both SDVP and AFI correlate poorly with actual amniotic fluid volume.

Cardiotocography (CTG)

Fetal cardiac behaviour is regulated through sympathetic and parasympathetic signals and by vasomotor, chemoreceptor and baroreceptor mechanisms. Pathological events such as fetal hypoxia modify these signals and also the fetal cardiac response. These effects can be visualised on the CTG.

During CTG an external ultrasound transducer monitors the fetal heart and a tocodynanometer records frequency of the uterine activity. There are three features of the fetal heart rate recorded on the CTG – the baseline, beat-to-beat variability and the presence of accelerations or decelerations.

- **Baseline fetal heart rate:** The static fetal heart rate in between periodic changes is a baseline fetal heart rate. It falls with advancing gestational age as a result of maturing fetal parasympathetic tone.
- **Fetal heart rate variability:** This is the difference between the upper and lower limits of the baseline heart rate over a short period of time. Normal baseline variability reflects a normal fetal autonomic nervous system.
- **Fetal heart accelerations:** These are increases in the baseline fetal heart rate of at least 15 bpm lasting for at least 15 seconds. The presence of accelerations on the CTG is a good sign and indicates a reactive fetus.
- **Fetal heart decelerations:** These are transient reductions in fetal heart rate of 15 bpm or more, lasting for more than 15 seconds. Fetal decelerations may indicate fetal hypoxia. Late decelerations are decelerations that start after a contraction and often have a slow return to baseline.

Early decelerations (occurring with uterine contraction) are uncommon, benign and usually associated with head compression (Figure 16.2).

Variable decelerations are intermittent periodic slowings of the fetal heart rate with rapid onset and recovery (Figure 16.3). Time relationships with the contraction cycle are variable and they may occur in isolation. They may be associated with cord compression.

It is 'non-reassuring' if variable decelerations occur with more than half of the mother's contractions and the fetal heart rate drops from the baseline by 60 bpm or less and takes 60 seconds or less to recover for more than 90 minutes, or if the drop is greater than 60 bpm and takes more than 60 seconds to recover, lasting for up to 30 minutes. It would also be non-reassuring if late decelerations occur for up to 30 minutes or if the baseline fetal heart rate is between 161 and 180 bpm.

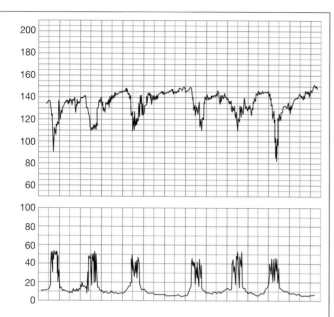

Figure 16.2 A cardiotocograph (CTG) showing early decelerations.

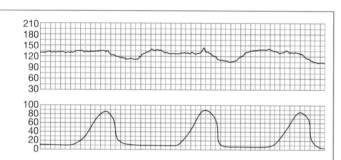

Figure 16.3 An abnormal cardiotocograph (CTG) showing reduced variability and late decelerations.

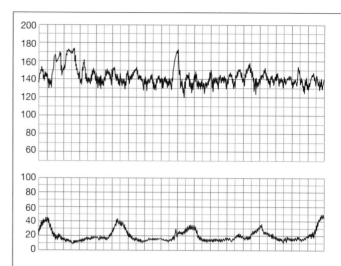

Figure 16.4 A normal cardiotocograph (CTG) in labour.

Table 16.2 Fetal blood sampling (FBS) result and interpretation.	
FBS result (pH)	Interpretation
≥7.25	Normal FBS result. Repeat after 1 hour if CTG remains the same
7.21–7.24	Borderline FBS result. Repeat after 30 minutes
≤7.20	Abnormal FBS result. Consider delivery

CTG, cardiotocography.

The CTG is abnormal if a non-reassuring variable deceleration situation still occurs 30 minutes after beginning conservative methods (below) or if they occur with more than half of the contractions. Similarly, the CTG is abnormal if late decelerations do not improve with conservative measures, are present for more than 30 minutes and occur in more than 50% of contractions. A CTG is abnormal if the baseline fetal heart rate falls below 100 bpm or rises above 180 bpm, or if a single deceleration lasts 3 minutes or more.

A normal CTG in labour is reassuring and unlikely to be associated with fetal hypoxia (Figure 16.4).

If the CTG is non-reassuring or abnormal, conservative methods such as changing maternal position or intravenous fluid should be tried. The patient should be offered fetal blood sampling (FBS) to measure lactate or pH if fetal hypoxia is suspected. Urgent delivery should be carried out if the FBS result is abnormal (Table 16.2).

A normal antenatal CTG is reassuring and confirms fetal wellbeing at the time of the test. However, it is not useful in predicting long-term fetal wellbeing. The presence of unprovoked decelerations (decelerations without uterine activity) is an abnormal feature for the antenatal CTG.

Management of fetal growth restriction

If FGR is diagnosed early in the pregnancy (less than 32 weeks of gestation) further investigations should be performed. These include a detailed anomaly scan to diagnose structural anomalies, karyotyping for chromosomal abnormality and testing for congenital infections such as cytomegalovirus (CMV) and toxoplasmosis. A maternal infection screen should be arranged if risk factors are present, for example syphilis or malaria screening.

In late-onset FGR (after 32 weeks gestation), antenatal management will involve increased fetal surveillance and delivery if there is evidence of either acute or chronic fetal compromise. A balance is required between timely delivery and risks of prematurity. Women with a SGA fetus between 24^{+0} and 35^{+6} weeks of gestation should receive a single course of antenatal corticosteroids (two injections 24 hours apart) to accelerate lung maturity. If umbilical artery flow velocity waveform and fetal monitoring tests are normal, the pregnancy can be continued with regular monitoring. Delivery is usually offered at or after 37 weeks gestation. If the umbilical artery flow velocity waveform is abnormal, delivery is indicated earlier than 37 weeks gestation. Difficult decisions regarding the timing of delivery may be required when Doppler studies show absent end-diastolic velocities in the umbilical artery at extreme prematurity. A senior obstetrician should be involved in deciding timing and mode of delivery. The mode of delivery will depend upon the gestation of the pregnancy, fetal and maternal condition, cervical Bishop score and the presentation of the fetus. Overall in the presence of FGR labour can be poorly tolerated and there is a higher likelihood of delivery by caesarean section.

Clinical case

Case follow-up

In Chloe's case, multiple risk factors for FGR were identified including her smoking habit, low BMI, possibly vigorous exercise, being a dancer, and poor nutrition. Chloe was therefore scheduled for serial assessment of fetal growth and umbilical artery Doppler from 28 weeks.

Case conclusion

Chloe's ultrasound scan at 32 weeks showed tailing off of fetal growth with abdominal circumference falling below the 50th centile. Chloe had two 12 mg intramuscular injections of dexamethasone 24 hours apart to accelerate fetal lung maturity. She was scheduled for weekly fetal umbilical Doppler studies and growth scans fortnightly. At 36 weeks she presented with reduced fetal movements and her scan showed reduced end-diastolic flow on umbilical artery Doppler. She was offered an urgent induction of labour. She required an emergency caesarean section in labour for presumed fetal distress and her baby boy weighed 2.2 **kg**.

Key learning points

- A small for gestational age fetus (SGA) is defined by an estimated fetal weight (EFW) or abdominal circumference (AC) less than the 10th centile and severe SGA as an EFW or AC less than the 3rd centile.
- The presence of risk factors for FGR will warrant consultant-led antenatal care with serial growth scans.

- CTG is used in pregnancy to monitor fetal heart rate and uterine contraction frequency.
- Umbilical artery Doppler is a primary surveillance tool in monitoring fetuses with growth restriction.
- An abnormal umbilical artery Doppler is an indication for early delivery. A fine balance is needed between timely delivery and risks of prematurity.

 Now visit **www.wileyessential.com/humandevelopment** to test yourself on this chapter.

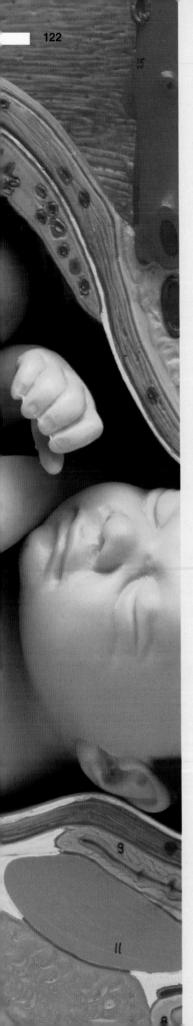

CHAPTER 17
The eye in pregnancy and the newborn

Part 1: The white pupil (leucocoria)

Colm McAlinden

Case

An 18-month-old child is brought to the local general practitioner by her parents. They are concerned as they have noticed her left pupil appears white in colour (leucocoria), particularly in dim lighting conditions and in some recent photographs (see Figure 17.10). The right pupil is normal. They are also concerned as the left eye is turned inwards slightly (strabismus). She has had no previous eye problems and there is no family history of eye disease. Her past medical history is unremarkable with no current or past medication and no known drug allergies. She has met all the normal developmental milestones.

Learning outcome

- You should be able to recognise the signs and symptoms of conditions of the eye that can occur during pregnancy and in the newborn and describe their causes.

Essential Human Development, First Edition. Edited by Samuel Webster, Geraint Morris and Euan Kevelighan
© 2018 John Wiley & Sons, Ltd. Published 2018 by John Wiley & Sons, Ltd.

Differential diagnosis of paediatric leucocoria

Retinoblastoma

Retinoblastoma is a malignant tumour arising from the primitive retinoblasts of the developing retina. It is the most common primary intraocular malignancy of childhood, accounting for 3% of all childhood cancers. It results from a mutation in the *RB1* gene (chromosome 13q14) with a worldwide incidence of 1 in 15–20 000, with no racial or gender predilection. Presentation is at approximately 2 years of age in somatic cases but younger at 12 months in genetic cases. Leucocoria occurs because the white tumour reflects light and blocks the normal red reflex of the retina. The tumour is intraocular and usually curable for 3–6 months after the initial sign of leucocoria.[1] Late diagnosis delays treatment and increases the risk of systematic metastasis and decreased survival rates.[2]

Retinoblastoma may be either genetic (germline/heritable) or somatic (sporadic/non-heritable). Approximately 90% of cases are somatic with no family history and are unilateral. Approximately one-third of these somatic cases may arise from new germline mutations, which may be passed on to offspring. Overall, 60% of cases are unilateral, which may be either genetic or somatic, and 40% are bilateral, which are genetic.[3]

Leucocoria is the most common initial sign but other clinical features may include strabismus, reduced vision, epiphora (watery eye), orbital inflammation and an acute red eye. Fundoscopy reveals a white retinal mass (Figure 17.1) with either growth into the vitreous (endophytic) or into the subretinal space (exophytic) with or without calcification. Complications include optic nerve invasion, anterior segment involvement (glaucoma, iris heterochromia, phthisis bulbi), extraocular spread and metastasis to the bone marrow, liver and lungs. The two key investigations are ultrasound and mutation testing, which may be performed via peripheral blood or from a tissue sample (following enucleation). Mutation testing helps distinguish genetic and somatic cases, which has important implications for the risk to relatives and future siblings and offspring. Treatment requires multidisciplinary input and is usually managed via a specialised centre. Treatment options are guided by the staging and include laser, cryotherapy, radiotherapy, chemotherapy and enucleation.

Congenital cataract

Cataract is defined as an opacification of the crystalline lens of the eye. Congenital and infantile cataract affects approximately 1 in 4000 live births (Figure 17.2).[4] Two-thirds of cases are bilateral and the cause can be identified in half of these cases. The most common cause is genetic (usually autosomal dominant) but other causes include metabolic disorders and intrauterine infections. In unilateral cases, a cause is only identified in 10% of cases, and is usually sporadic without systemic disease or family history. Unilateral cases usually occur in healthy full-term infants,[5] and the cataract morphology is important as this may indicate the likely aetiology. Other signs may include leucocoria, nystagmus or strabismus. As amblyopia is likely to occur, prompt expert opinion is required with a view to cataract surgery. Cataract surgery in children is highly specialised and is associated with a higher incidence of complications than in adults. Paediatric input may also be required to investigate possible causes (Table 17.1) and treatment of underlying disorders. Following cataract surgery, refractive error and amblyopia needs to be treated, and options include spectacles (including multifocal/bifocal lenses), contact lenses, occlusion therapy (patching) and cycloplegic eye drops.

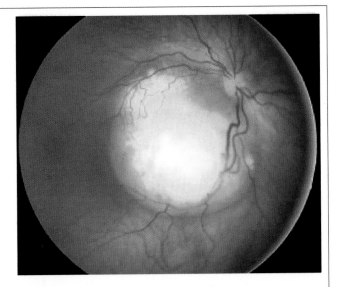

Figure 17.1 Endophytic retinoblastoma. (Source: © Aerts et al. (2006) http://ojrd.biomedcentral.com/ articles/10.1186/1750-1172-1-31. Used under http:// creativecommons.org/licenses/by/2.0.)

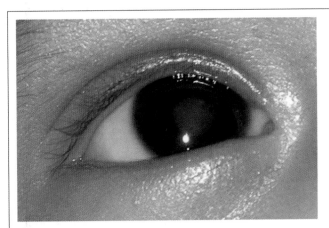

Figure 17.2 Congenital cataract. (Source: Courtesy of Denice Barsness, CRA/CPMC Department of Ophthalmology, San Francisco.)

Table 17.1 Main causes of congenital cataract.

Chromosomal	Trisomies – Down, Patau, Edward syndromes Monosomies – Turner syndrome Deletions – 5p (cri-du-chat syndrome), 18p, 18q Microdeletion – 16p13 (Rubinstein–Taybi syndrome) Duplications – 3q, 10q, 20p
Syndromic	Craniosynostosis – Apert and Crouzon syndromes Craniofacial – Smith–Lemli–Opitz and Hallermann–Streiff–François syndromes Dermatological – Cockayne syndrome, incontinentia pigmenti, hypohidrotic ectodermal dysplasia, ichthyosis, naevoid basal cell carcinoma syndrome, Rothmund–Thomson syndrome, eczema Neuromuscular – Alström syndrome, myotonic dystrophy, Marinesco-Sjögren syndrome Connective tissue – Marfan, Alport and Conradi–Hünermann–Happle syndromes, spondyloepiphyseal dysplasia Anterior segment dysgenesis – Peters' anomaly, Axenfeld–Rieger syndrome
Metabolic	Carbohydrate – galactosaemia, galactokinase deficiency, hypoglycaemia, mannosidosis Lipids – abetalipoproteinaemia Amino acid – Lowe syndrome, homocystinuria Sphingolipidoses – Niemann–Pick disease, Fabry disease Minerals – Wilson's disease, hypocalcaemia Phytanic acid – Refsum's disease
Endocrine	Diabetes mellitus, hypoparathyroidism
Infective	Toxoplasma, rubella, herpes, measles, influenza, poliomyelitis, syphilis
Others	Drugs (steroids), trauma, radiation

Retinopathy of prematurity (ROP)

ROP is a proliferative retinopathy that affects premature (<32 weeks) neonates of low birthweight (≤1.5 kg). ROP was first reported in 1942 and became the leading cause of childhood blindness. The cause was due to the use of supplementary oxygen, which improved preterm survival but caused blindness. Controlled oxygen therapy was introduced, which saw a decrease in ROP but a rise in neonatal death.[6] Oxygen delivery is now a balancing act between ROP and survival.

During normal development the retina remains avascular until 4 months gestation. After the fourth month, vascular complexes extend from the optic disc towards the peripheral retina. These vascular complexes reach the nasal retina by 8 months gestation, but do not reach the temporal peripheral retina until 1 month after birth. In prematurity, growth factor suppression due to hyperoxia and loss of maternal-fetal interaction results in the inhibition of retinal vascularisation. This leads to retinal hypoxia, which stimulates growth factor-induced vasoproliferation, which can cause a retinal detachment. In prematurity, controlled oxygen administration decreases ROP but does not eliminate it.[7]

Premature (<32 weeks) or low-birthweight (≤1.5 kg) infants should be screened and the main treatment option is laser photocoagulation (transpupillary diode laser). Vitreoretinal surgery is considered in cases of ROP-associated retinal detachment.

Coats disease

Coats disease is a rare idiopathic retinal telangiectasia resulting in small multifocal outpouchings of retinal vessels with intraretinal and subretinal exudates (Figure 17.3), and

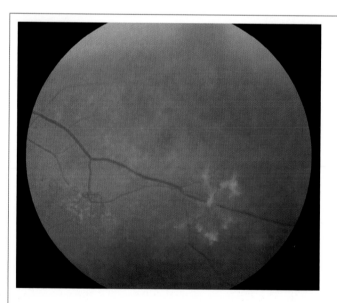

Figure 17.3 Coats disease. (Source: Courtesy of Denice Barsness, CRA/CPMC Department of Ophthalmology, San Francisco.)

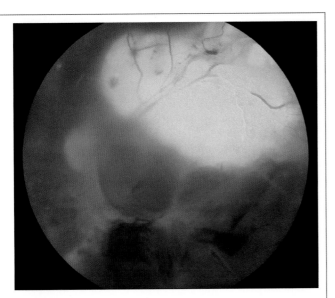

Figure 17.4 Exudative retinal detachment associated with Coats disease. (Source: Courtesy of Denice Barsness, CRA/CPMC Department of Ophthalmology, San Francisco.)

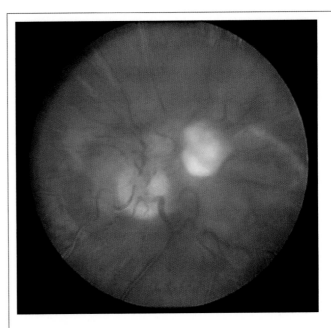

Figure 17.5 Toxocariasis. (Source: Courtesy of Denice Barsness, CRA/CPMC Department of Ophthalmology, San Francisco.)

frequently an exudative retinal detachment (Figure 17.4). It is usually unilateral, and 75% of cases occur in boys. Presentation is usually in the first decade of life with symptoms of visual loss, strabismus or leucocoria. Complications include glaucoma, uveitis, cataract and phthisis bulbi. Treatment aims to control exudation, and options include laser photocoagulation, anti-vascular endothelial growth factor (VEGF) agents, or cryotherapy. In cases of exudative retinal detachment, vitreoretinal surgery may be required.

Toxocariasis

The nematodes *Toxocara canis* and *Toxocara cati* are parasitic roundworms that infect dogs, other canids and cats. Ova excreted in the faeces are inadvertently ingested by humans, typically children. The larvae penetrate through the gut and spread to the liver, lung, skin, heart and brain (visceral larva migrans) or to the eye (ocular toxocariasis: Figure 17.5). The death of larvae induces a severe inflammatory reaction followed by granulation. The presenting symptoms and signs depend on the severity, as it may appear as a localised white elevated retinal granuloma, localised inflammation of ocular structures or as a diffuse endophthalmitis. In addition, vitreous traction bands associated with macular dragging may occur as well as a tractional retinal detachment, and chronic inflammation may lead to the development of a cataract. The diagnosis is based on history – for example, contact with puppies or eating dirt (pica) – lesion morphology and supportive laboratory data such as serum enzyme-linked immunosorbent assay (ELISA) titres, aqueous humour ELISA Toxocara titers and other diagnostic imaging such as optical coherence tomography, fluorescein angiography and ultrasound. Management

is primarily aimed at treating complications arising from intraocular inflammation and vitreous membrane traction.[8]

Persistent fetal vasculature (PFV)

The hyaloid vascular system is present within the vitreous cavity during embryogenesis and normally this vasculature regresses during the second trimester. PFV refers to a group of disorders associated with the persistence of various components of the hyaloid system. It usually presents with unilateral leucocoria and can be classified as anterior, posterior or mixed, depending on the affected ocular structures. A varied degree of fibrogial and vascular proliferation may be observed within the vitreous cavity, and the affected eye may be slightly smaller. Other ocular findings may include cataract, a fibrovascular membrane behind the crystalline lens that places traction on the ciliary processes, glaucoma and retinal detachment. PFV is present from birth and early detection is imperative as vitreoretinal surgery may be successful in selected cases.[9]

Retinal astrocytoma

Retinal astrocytoma is a benign and rare tumour, which may present in childhood with leucocoria. Isolated retinal astrocytomas are usually not associated with systemic disease whereas multiple or bilateral astrocytomas are usually associated with tuberous sclerosis. Approximately 50% of patients with tuberous sclerosis will have retinal astrocytomas. Rarely, there are also associations with neurofibromatosis and retinitis

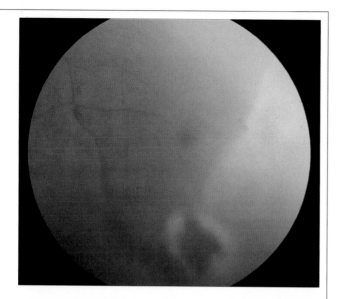

Figure 17.6 Familial exudative vitreoretinopathy (FEVR). (Source: Courtesy of Denice Barsness, CRA/CPMC Department of Ophthalmology, San Francisco.)

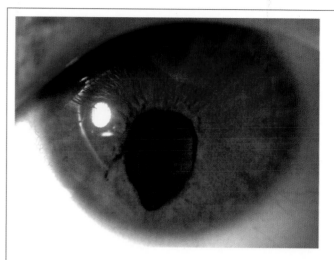

Figure 17.7 Iris coloboma. (Source: Courtesy of Denice Barsness, CRA/CPMC Department of Ophthalmology, San Francisco.)

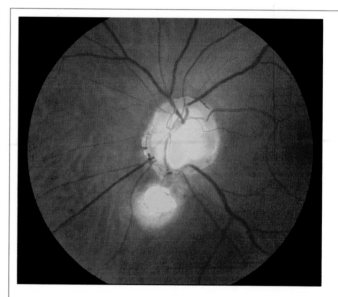

Figure 17.8 Posterior coloboma. (Source: Courtesy of Denice Barsness, CRA/CPMC Department of Ophthalmology, San Francisco.)

pigmentosa. The tumour appears as a flat or elevated yellow-white retinal mass, which may be translucent or calcified. Treatment is not usually required.

Familial exudative vitreoretinopathy (FEVR)

FEVR is a progressive condition similar to ROP characterised by failure of vascularisation of the peripheral temporal retina, but it is not associated with prematurity or low birthweight (Figure 17.6). Inheritance is usually autosomal dominant, or rarely X-linked or autosomal recessive, with high penetrance and variable expressivity. Clinical signs include an abrupt cessation of peripheral vasculature at the equator, peripheral vitreous bands, vascular tortuosity, telangiectasia and neo-vascularisation. There may also be vascular straightening and temporal dragging of the disc and macula. Complications include tractional retinal detachment, subretinal exudation (akin to Coats disease), cataract, vitreous haemorrhage and glaucoma. Treatment in the form of laser photocoagulation and cryotherapy may be beneficial, and vitreoretinal surgery may be performed in selected cases of retinal detachment.

Coloboma

A coloboma is a defect or absence of part of an ocular structure resulting from incomplete closure of the embryonic fissure (Figures 17.7 and 17.8). The embryonic fissure usually extends from the optic disc to the pupil margin, and hence a coloboma may affect the complete length of the embryonic fissure (complete coloboma) or partially (coloboma of the optic disc, choroid, retina, ciliary body or iris; see Figure 17.7). A large choroidal coloboma may present as leucocoria.

Myelinated nerve fibres

In normal eyes, the myelination of the optic nerve ends at the cribriform plate, but in eyes with myelinated nerve fibres, the ganglion cells retain oligodendroglia (the cells responsible for myelination). They are whiter, larger and denser than cotton wool spots or retinal infiltrates (Figure 17.9). They are almost always connected to the optic disc, run within the retinal nerve fibre layer, and in the vast majority only affect one eye.

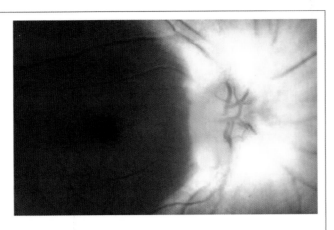

Figure 17.9 Myelinated nerve fibres.

Systemic associations include neurofibromatosis (type 1) and Gorlin syndrome. Most cases remain unchanged and stable, without progression or development in the alternate eye. No treatment is required, although they may cause visual field defects and can be associated with other ocular features such as high myopia, anisometropia and amblyopia.[10,11]

Vitreoretinal dysplasia

Vitreoretinal dysplasia is a non-attachment of the retina due to an arrest in development of the vitreous and retina. It results in a retrolental mass with leucocoria. It may occur in isolation or in association with systemic abnormalities including Norrie disease, Patau syndrome, incontinentia pigmenti and Walker–Warburg syndrome.[12]

Clinical case

Case discussion

Leucocoria is not an uncommon presentation to general practitioners and other healthcare professionals (Figure 17.10 and Table 17.2). It may also be an incidental finding by any doctor during a consult or medical examination. It may indicate a life-threatening, vision-threatening or benign condition. Hence it is imperative, following history taking, that all children presenting with leucocoria undergo dilated fundoscopy as part of the clinical examination.

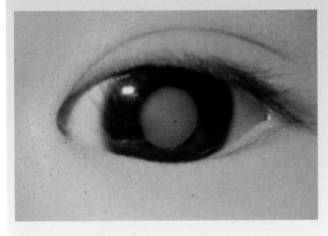

Figure 17.10 White pupil (leucocoria). (Source: Courtesy of Denice Barsness, CRA/CPMC Department of Ophthalmology, San Francisco.)

Table 17.2 Summary of the main causes of leucocoria.

Lens	Cataract
Vitreous	Persistent fetal vasculature (PFV)
Retina	Retinoblastoma
	Coats disease
	Retinopathy of prematurity (ROP)
	Familial exudative vitreoretinopathy (FEVR)
	Coloboma
	Astrocytoma
	Myelinated nerve fibres
	Vitreoretinal dysplasia
Infection	*Toxocara*

SUMMARY

Key learning points

- Retinoblastoma is a malignant tumour involving the retina with a worldwide incidence of 1 in 15–20 000. This must be considered in the differential with any child presenting with leucocoria.

- Children with suspected leucocoria must undergo a dilated fundal examination as part of the clinical examination.

REFERENCES

1. Dimaras H, Kimani K, Dimba EA, et al. Retinoblastoma. *Lancet* 2012;379:1436–1446.

2. Leal-Leal C, Flores-Rojo M, Medina-Sanson A, et al. A multicentre report from the Mexican Retinoblastoma Group. *Br J Ophthalmol* 2004;88:1074–1077.

3. Denniston AKO, Murray. PI. *Oxford Handbook of Ophthalmology*, 2nd edn. Oxford University Press; 2009.

4. Rahi JS, Dezateux C. Measuring and interpreting the incidence of congenital ocular anomalies: lessons from a national study of congenital cataract in the UK. *Invest Ophthalmol Vis Sci* 2001;42:1444–1448.

5. Rahi JS, Dezateux C. Congenital and infantile cataract in the United Kingdom: underlying or associated factors. British Congenital Cataract Interest Group. *Invest Ophthalmol Vis Sci* 2000;41:2108–2114.

6. Campbell K. Intensive oxygen therapy as a possible cause of retrolental fibroplasia; a clinical approach. *Med J Aust* 1951;2:48–50.

7. Hellstrom A, Smith LE, Dammann O. Retinopathy of prematurity. *Lancet* 2013;382:1445–1457.

8. Arevalo JF, Espinoza JV, Arevalo FA. Ocular toxocariasis. *J Pediatr Ophthalmol Strabismus* 2013;50:76–86.

9. Goldberg MF. Persistent fetal vasculature (PFV): an integrated interpretation of signs and symptoms associated with persistent hyperplastic primary vitreous (PHPV). LIV Edward Jackson Memorial Lecture. *Am J Ophthalmol* 1997;124:587–626.

10. Straatsma BR, Foos RY, Heckenlively JR, Taylor GN. Myelinated retinal nerve fibers. *Am J Ophthalmol* 1981;91:25–38.

11. Tarabishy AB, Alexandrou TJ, Traboulsi EI. Syndrome of myelinated retinal nerve fibers, myopia, and amblyopia: a review. *Surv Ophthalmol* 2007;52:588–596.

12. Kanski J, Bowling B. *Clinical Ophthalmology: A Systematic Approach*, 7th edn. Elsevier Saunders; 2011.

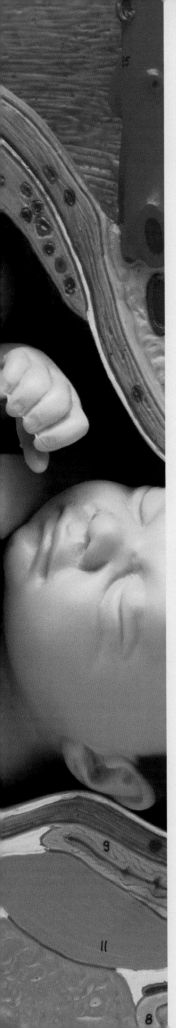

CHAPTER 17

The eye in pregnancy and the newborn

Part 2: The eye during pregnancy

Colm McAlinden

Case

A 24-year-old primigravida at 35 weeks gestation presents with a 1-week history of blurred vision, photopsia and headaches. Best corrected visual acuity is 6/12 in each eye (no improvement with pinhole) and fundoscopy reveals widespread retinal haemorrhages, cotton wool spots, hard exudates at the macula and swollen optic discs. Physical examination reveals a blood pressure of 210/130 mmHg and peripheral oedema. Pre-pregnancy blood pressure was 120/80 mmHg. A 24-hour urine sample reveals 6.8 g of protein.

Learning outcome

- You should be able to recognise the signs and symptoms of conditions of the eye that can occur during pregnancy and describe their causes.

Essential Human Development, First Edition. Edited by Samuel Webster, Geraint Morris and Euan Kevelighan
© 2018 John Wiley & Sons, Ltd. Published 2018 by John Wiley & Sons, Ltd.

Introduction

Pregnancy has many effects on the physiology of the human body, which assist in fetal survival and development as well as maternal preparation for parturition.[1] In addition to physiological changes, pathological changes may occur de novo or from existing clinical or subclinical conditions. We will consider the main physiological and pathological ocular changes to the eye.

Physiological changes

Cornea and crystalline lens

One of the most common problems in pregnancy is dry eye syndrome due to the disruption of the lacrimal acinar cells.[2] Generally, there is a poor correlation between clinical signs of dry eye syndrome, such as fluorescein tear break-up time, and symptoms, such as gritty or burning eyes.[3] Contact lens wearers may have more symptoms and may have to cease lens wear until after pregnancy. Lack of sleep, excessive computer use and long hours in warm, dry or air-conditioned environments can worsen dry eye symptoms. Artificial tear drops can be used regularly for symptomatic relief during pregnancy and treatment of any associated lid abnormalities such as blepharitis and meibomian gland dysfunction.

The cornea can change in curvature, thickness and sensitivity during pregnancy, principally in the later stages of pregnancy.[4] The curvature and corneal thickness increase and the sensitivity decreases. These changes are thought to occur due to oedema in the cornea.[5,6] Similar transient changes may occur to the crystalline lens including a reduction in the amplitude of accommodation.[7] Therefore patients may present in pregnancy with difficulty reading, particularly if they have pre-existing uncorrected hyperopia (**long-sighted**). Krukenberg spindles (pigment deposition on the corneal endothelium) have been reported to appear early in pregnancy in some women without other signs of pigment dispersion syndrome and these usually decrease in late pregnancy and postpartum.[8]

Intraocular pressure

Intraocular pressure (IOP) decreases throughout pregnancy in all three trimesters; this may be due to increased aqueous outflow, decreased scleral rigidity and episcleral venous pressure, and generalised acidosis during pregnancy.[9] This effect may be even greater in patients with ocular hypertension.[10] IOP typically returns to normal levels postpartum.

Ocular adnexa

During pregnancy, the ocular adnexa may be affected by melasma (chloasma, or mask of pregnancy), which is an increase in skin pigmentation.[11] Melasma may also occur with oral contraceptive use. Spider angiomas may also appear around the eyes and face.[12] Both of these usually resolve postpartum. Bilateral but more often unilateral ptosis may occur during pregnancy or postpartum.[13]

Pregnancy-specific ocular disease

Pre-eclampsia and eclampsia

Both pre-eclampsia and eclampsia can result in a number of ocular complications. Visual symptoms affect approximately 25% of patients with severe pre-eclampsia, and 50% with eclampsia, with blurred vision being the most common symptom.[14] Other symptoms include headache, photopsia, diplopia and visual field defects. Although retinal haemorrhages (blot or flame), Elschnig spots, cotton wool spots and oedema secondary to arteriolar damage can occur, the most common ocular feature is severe arteriolar spasm, which is observed as vasoconstriction of the retinal arterioles.[15] The above signs are commonly seen in hypertensive retinopathy. The suggested mechanisms of these changes include endothelial damage, ischaemia and hormonal changes.[16]

Serous retinal detachment can also occur; it affects less than 1% of pre-eclamptic patients. However, it occurs in approximately 10% of eclamptic patients.[17] Women with HELLP syndrome (Haemolysis, Elevated Liver enzymes and Low Platelet count) are seven times more likely to develop a serous retinal detachment.[18] Temporary blindness due to cortical cerebral oedema has also been reported in up to 15% of women with pre-eclampsia and eclampsia.[19] Presenting symptoms usually include visual disturbances, headache, hyperreflexia and clonus.

Central serous retinopathy (CSR)

CSR is a condition resulting from subretinal fluid accumulation (at the level of the retinal pigment epithelium) that leads to a shallow detachment of the sensory retina. Patients usually present with a sudden reduction in vision but may have other symptoms such as a central scotoma or metamorphopsia (distortion). Due to the elevation of the retina, patients usually have a hyperopic shift in their refractive error. Basic ophthalmic examinations such as visual acuity, refraction and fundoscopy are likely to reveal the diagnosis. The Amsler grid is a very sensitive test and is useful to demonstrate symptoms such as metamorphopsia and central scotomas (Figure 17.11).[20] This grid is also useful in other macular conditions.

Whilst the aetiology of CSR is unknown, pregnancy (particularly third trimester) is a significant risk factor. Other associations include adult men (20–50 years), type A personality, stress, Cushing's disease and drug-induced (e.g. corticosteroids). Optical coherence tomography (OCT) may be used to help establish a diagnosis and in the monitoring of the condition. Fluorescein angiography is a useful investigation in many retinal diseases, and although there is no evidence that fluorescein is teratogenic, it is avoided in pregnancy as it can cross the placenta

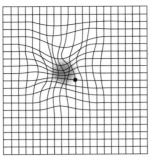

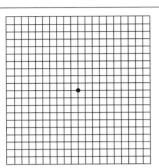

Figure 17.11 Amsler grid; left – normal appearance; right – the appearance to a patient with metamorphopsia.

and there is greater permeability of the blood–brain barrier in the fetus.[21] The vast majority of cases resolve spontaneously 1–2 months postpartum and do not require treatment. Persistent cases may respond to argon laser treatment or photodynamic therapy. Although choroidal neovascularisation is rare, it is important to monitor and advise of the risk.[22]

Occlusive vasculopathies

In most cases of ophthalmologic features associated with pre-eclampsia, there is a good visual recovery except in cases of Purtscher-like retinopathy, which is a rare condition resulting from retinal arteriolar embolism from amniotic fluid. It presents postpartum with sudden-onset marked visual loss with fundoscopic features including haemorrhages and cotton wool spots. Purtscher-like retinopathy is also associated with hypercoagulability and pancreatitis.[23] Other occlusive vasculopathies, including central and branch occlusions of retinal arteries or veins, have been reported in pregnancy (Figures 17.12 and 17.13).[17]

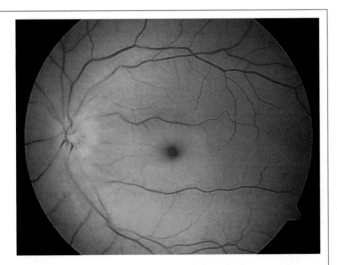

Figure 17.12 Old central retinal artery occlusion with ischaemic oedema of the macula. (Source: Courtesy of Carl Zeiss Meditec.)

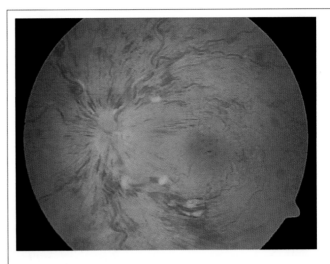

Figure 17.13 Central retinal vein occlusion with papillary oedema, flame-shaped hemorrhages in the nerve fiber layer, and cotton wool spots. (Source: Courtesy of Carl Zeiss Meditec.)

Disseminated intravascular coagulopathy (DIC) can occur in cases of obstetric complications such as placental abruption, complicated abortion, intrauterine fetal death or eclampsia. Widespread clotting can result in occlusion of choroidal vessels leading to secondary serous retinal detachments.[24]

Pre-existing ocular disease during pregnancy

Diabetic retinopathy

Diabetic retinopathy (DR) is the most common ocular condition affected by pregnancy (Figure 17.14). This refers to patients with pre-existing diabetes and DR, not patients who develop gestational diabetes, which does not appear to increase the risk of developing DR. The standard treatment for proliferative DR is panretinal photocoagulation, but at present it is not possible to adequately predict who will progress and regress without treatment. However, risk factors for the progression of DR in pregnancy include hypertension and inadequate glycaemic control prior to pregnancy. Proliferative retinopathy can be asymptomatic and it is therefore important for diabetic women with DR to be closely monitored during pregnancy and postpartum. Diabetic maculopathy is part of DR and is the main cause of visual loss rather than proliferative retinopathy. Focal laser photocoagulation was previously the main option for diabetic maculopathy, but recently new treatment options in the form of anti-vascular endothelial growth factor (anti-VEGF) therapies have become available. However, unfortunately, there are no safety data about the use of these agents during pregnancy.

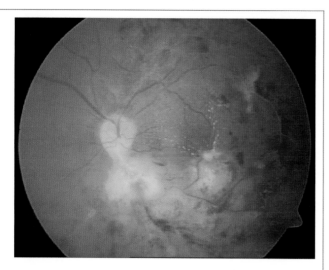

Figure 17.14 Proliferative diabetic retinopathy with extensive lipid exudation, large cotton wool spots, flame-shaped and dot-blot hemorrhages and clinically significant macular oedema. (Source: Courtesy of Carl Zeiss Meditec.)

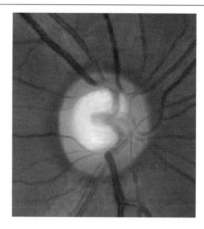

Figure 17.15 An optic disc suspicious of glaucoma: vertical cup to disc ratio 0.6, vessel bayoneting and visible lamina cribrosa pores.

Uveitis

Uveitis refers to inflammation of the uvea, commonly classified in terms of the anatomical structures affected or by aetiology. For cases of chronic non-infectious uveitis, during pregnancy women experience fewer flare-ups perhaps due to immune and hormonal changes. However, after delivery, women are at a higher risk of rebound flare-ups and should be counselled to seek urgent medical attention due to the risk of secondary complications of uveitis such as cataract and glaucoma.[25,26]

Glaucoma

Although glaucoma is primarily a condition affecting the older population, it can affect any age group (Figure 17.15). As previously mentioned, IOP tends to decrease during pregnancy, which is beneficial for glaucoma as the only treatment option at present for this neuropathy is IOP reduction. However, during pregnancy not all women will have a reduction in IOP and hence control may become problematic. The majority of patients with glaucoma manage the condition with medical therapy (IOP-lowering eye drops) but one must consider systemic absorption and potentially harmful effects to the fetus.[27] Although many factors govern the most appropriate management option, alternatives such as surgery and laser therapy should be considered in pregnancy. One such laser therapy is selective laser trabeculoplasty, which following a recent systematic review was found to be as effective as medical therapy in terms of IOP reduction.[28]

Sheehan's syndrome

Sheehan's syndrome (SS) is characterised by anterior pituitary infarction and necrosis secondary to postpartum haemorrhage and obstetric shock. The pituitary gland is physiologically enlarged during pregnancy due to the effects of lactotrophs, and is thus susceptible to the effects of rapid depletion of blood volume and systemic hypotension leading to infarction. It is a rare cause of hypopituitarism in developed countries due to advances in obstetric care but remains common in underdeveloped countries. Patients with SS have varying degrees of anterior pituitary hormone deficiency, from single pituitary hormone insufficiency to total hypopituitarism. The presentation may be acute (acute pituitary failure) or slowly progressive, which is more common. Due to the varying degrees of deficiency, symptoms can be markedly different from patient to patient, but the more common symptoms tend to be failure to lactate, fatigue and amenorrhoea. From an ophthalmological point of view, this is a vision-threatening condition. Compression of nearby structures such as the optic chiasm can result in visual field defects, and compression of the cavernous sinus can injure cranial nerves III, IV and VI resulting in ophthalmoplegia. Cranial nerve III is most commonly involved, which in addition to ophthalmoplegia can result in a dilated pupil and lid ptosis.[29]

Hyperthyroidism

Hyperthyroidism may present as a new diagnosis in pregnancy, affecting up to 0.1–0.4% of pregnancies, but the more common presentation is relapse of previously controlled hyperthyroidism.[30] The most common cause of hyperthyroidism is Graves' disease – due to thyrotropin receptor-stimulating antibodies (TRAb).[31] Graves' disease typically exacerbates in the first trimester, and some of the common symptoms overlap with symptoms of early pregnancy such as increased appetite, nausea and vomiting, heat intolerance, and irritability or anxiousness. It may also exacerbate postpartum.[31]

Ophthalmological signs include lid retraction, lid lag on downgaze, lagophthalmos, proptosis and extraocular muscle restriction. Optic nerve compression due to extraocular muscle thickening at the orbital apex can cause visual loss, reduced colour vision, visual field defects and an afferent pupillary defect. Additional signs that may be present include reduced blink rate, blood vessel injection, chemosis and dry eye.[32] Management is required using a multidisciplinary approach with input from the obstetrician, endocrinologist and ophthalmologist.

Idiopathic intracranial hypertension

This is an idiopathic syndrome with raised intracranial pressure; it was previously termed pseudotumour cerebri or benign intracranial hypertension. Symptoms can include headache, transient visual obscurations (usually lasting for seconds and typically precipitated by postural changes), diplopia, photopsia, pulsatile tinnitus, and nausea and vomiting. The headache may waken the patient from their sleep but improves on rising and then becomes worse during the day. Clinical signs include papilloedema (Figure 17.16) with normal brain magnetic resonance imaging. There will be an increased opening pressure on lumbar puncture with normal cerebrospinal fluid (CSF) composition, and visual fields may be severely constricted. A bilateral or unilateral sixth nerve palsy may be present (a false localising sign) causing diplopia but no other neurological signs.[33]

This condition is classically associated with obesity, significant recent weight gain and pregnancy. In pregnancy, the probable reason is due to increased weight gain. Other associations include various medications (e.g. oral contraceptive pill, nalidixic acid, hypervitaminosis A, tetracyclines, ciclosporin, lithium and steroids, including withdrawal).

Non-pregnant management options include lumbar puncture, weight loss, ceasing associated drugs, and acetazolamide. CSF diversion procedures (lumboperitoneal or ventriculoperitoneal shunt) may be considered if vision deteriorates or headaches persist. Optic nerve sheath fenestration is indicated for visual loss without headache. In the context of pregnancy, there is no increased risk of fetal loss, and acetazolamide may be used after 20 weeks gestation. An intense weight loss programme is contraindicated in pregnancy. In cases without visual compromise, close observation with visual field testing is recommended but in cases with visual compromise, optic nerve sheath fenestration, shunting and repeat lumbar punctures should be considered. The use of steroids is controversial.[34]

Toxoplasmosis

Primary infection in pregnancy with the protozoan parasite *Toxoplasma gondii* is rare, especially in the UK. Spread is via cat faeces and eating undercooked meat. Primary infection in immunocompromised women is associated with a higher risk of disseminated illness with chorioretinitis and encephalitis. Latent ocular toxoplasmosis may also reactivate during pregnancy with negligible risk of congenital toxoplasmosis to the fetus. Maternal infection (high IgM and IgG antibodies) may warrant starting spiramycin to decrease the risk of fetal infection, and if vertical transmission occurs, anti-toxoplasmosis therapy should be considered. Fetal infection may be diagnosed with high IgM antibodies in the fetal blood or amniotic fluid, and cerebral ventriculomegaly may be seen on ultrasound scanning, but in most cases the ultrasound scan is normal.[35]

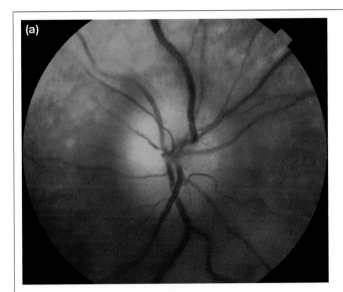
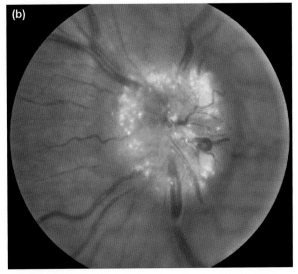

Figure 17.16 (a) **Early papilloedema with indistinct disc margins, elevation and hyperaemia**. (Source: Courtesy of Tim Cole, Topcon GB.) (b) **Established papilloedema with the addition of cotton wool spots**. (Source: Courtesy of Denice Barsness, CRA/CPMC Department of Ophthalmology, San Francisco.)

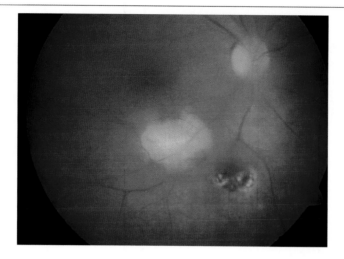

Figure 17.17 Acute toxoplasmosis recurrence with an older atrophic scar. (Source: Courtesy of Carl Zeiss Meditec.)

Clinical case

Case discussion

Visual problems are very common during pregnancy and doctors should have a firm understanding of the various ocular conditions that may occur for the first time in pregnancy or pre-existing conditions that are modified by pregnancy. The diagnosis of the case presentation is pre-eclampsia with hypertensive retinopathy. Pre-eclampsia is common but can become a life-threatening condition for the mother and fetus. The patient should be referred immediately to an obstetric department with a view to delivery of the baby. No specific ophthalmological intervention is required as the hypertensive retinopathy is likely to resolve either partially or fully following delivery.

Key learning points

- A range of physiological changes occur to the eye during pregnancy including changes to the tears, cornea, lens, refractive error and intraocular pressure.
- Pathological problems in pregnancy can be grouped into new ocular disease developing during pregnancy, such as pre-eclampsia-related hypertensive retinopathy, or the modification of pre-existing ocular disease by pregnancy, such as diabetic retinopathy.

 Now visit **www.wileyessential.com/humandevelopment** to test yourself on this chapter.

FURTHER READING

Dimaras, H., Kimani, K., Dimba, E.A., *et al.* (2012) Retinoblastoma. *Lancet* 379, 1436–1446.

Errera, M.H., Kohly, R.P. and da Cruz, L. (2013) Pregnancy-associated retinal diseases and their management. *Survey of Ophthalmology* 58, 127–142.

Hellstrom, A., Smith, L.E. and Dammann, O. (2013) Retinopathy of prematurity. *Lancet* 382, 1445–1457.

Kesler, A. and Kupferminc, M. (2013) Idiopathic intracranial hypertension and pregnancy. *Clinical Obstetrics and Gynecology* 56, 389–396.

Schultz, K.L., Birnbaum, A.D. and Goldstein, D.A. (2005) Ocular disease in pregnancy. *Current Opinion in Ophthalmology* 16, 308–314.

SUMMARY

REFERENCES

1. Chesnutt AN. Physiology of normal pregnancy. *Crit Care Clin* 2004;20:609–615.

2. Schechter JE, Pidgeon M, Chang D, et al. Potential role of disrupted lacrimal acinar cells in dry eye during pregnancy. *Adv Exp Med Biol* 2002;506:153–157.

3. Nichols KK, Nichols JJ, Mitchell GL. The lack of association between signs and symptoms in patients with dry eye disease. *Cornea* 2004;23:762–770.

4. Park SB, Lindahl KJ, Temnycky GO, et al. The effect of pregnancy on corneal curvature. *CLAO J* 1992;18:256–259.

5. Weinreb RN, Lu A, Beeson C. Maternal corneal thickness during pregnancy. *Am J Ophthalmol* 1988;105:258–260.

6. Riss B, Riss P. Corneal sensitivity in pregnancy. *Ophthalmologica* 1981;183:57–62.

7. Milazzo S, Mikou R, Berthout A, et al. Understanding refraction disorders and oculomotor problems during pregnancy. *J Fr Ophtalmol* 2010;33:368–371.

8. Duncan TE. Krukenberg spindles in pregnancy. *Arch Ophthalmol* 1974;91:355–358.

9. Efe YK, Ugurbas SC, Alpay A, et al. The course of corneal and intraocular pressure changes during pregnancy. *Can J Ophthalmol* 2012;47:150–154.

10. Qureshi IA. Intraocular pressure and pregnancy: a comparison between normal and ocular hypertensive subjects. *Arch Med Res* 1997;28:397–400.

11. Moin A, Jabery Z, Fallah N. Prevalence and awareness of melasma during pregnancy. *Int J Dermatol* 2006;45:285–288.

12. Beard MP, Millington GW. Recent developments in the specific dermatoses of pregnancy. *Clin Exp Dermatol* 2012;37:1–4; quiz 5.

13. Sanke RF. Blepharoptosis as a complication of pregnancy. *Ann Ophthalmol* 1984;16:720–722.

14. Schultz KL, Birnbaum AD, Goldstein DA. Ocular disease in pregnancy. *Curr Opin Ophthalmol* 2005;16:308–314.

15. Wagner HP. Arterioles of the retina in toxaemia of pregnancy. *JAMA* 1933;101:1380–1384.

16. Dinn RB, Harris A, Marcus PS. Ocular changes in pregnancy. *Obstet Gynecol Surv* 2003;58:137–144.

17. Errera MH, Kohly RP, da Cruz L. Pregnancy-associated retinal diseases and their management. *Surv Ophthalmol* 2013;58:127–142.

18. Vigil-De Gracia P, Ortega-Paz L. Retinal detachment in association with pre-eclampsia, eclampsia, and HELLP syndrome. *Int J Gynaecol Obstet* 2011;114:223–225.

19. Borromeo CJ, Blike GT, Wiley CW, et al. Cortical blindness in a preeclamptic patient after a cesarean delivery complicated by hypotension. *Anesth Analg* 2000;91:609–611.

20. Amsler M. L'Examen qualitatif de la fonction maculaire. *Ophthalmologica* 1947;114.

21. Halperin LS, Olk RJ, Soubrane G, et al. Safety of fluorescein angiography during pregnancy. *Am J Ophthalmol* 1990;109:563–566.

22. Liew G, Quin G, Gillies M, et al. Central serous chorioretinopathy: a review of epidemiology and pathophysiology. *Clin Experiment Ophthalmol* 2013;41:201–214.

23. Miguel AI, Henriques F, Azevedo LF, et al. Systematic review of Purtscher's and Purtscher-like retinopathies. *Eye (Lond)* 2013;27:1–13.

24. Cogan DG. Ocular involvement in disseminated intravascular coagulopathy. *Arch Ophthalmol* 1975;93:1–8.

25. Wakefield D, Abu El-Asrar A, McCluskey P. Treatment of severe inflammatory eye disease in patients of reproductive age and during pregnancy. *Ocul Immunol Inflamm* 2012;20:277–287.

26. Kump LI, Cervantes-Castaneda RA, Androudi SN, et al. Patterns of exacerbations of chronic non-infectious uveitis in pregnancy and puerperium. *Ocul Immunol Inflamm* 2006;14:99–104.

27. Razeghinejad MR, Tania Tai TY, Fudemberg SJ, et al. Pregnancy and glaucoma. *Surv Ophthalmol* 2011;56:324–335.

28. McAlinden C. Selective laser trabeculoplasty (SLT) vs other treatment modalities for glaucoma: systematic review. *Eye (Lond)* 2014;28:249–258.

29. Kilicli F, Dokmetas HS, Acibuc F. Sheehan's syndrome. *Gynecol Endocrinol* 2013;29:292–295.

30. Patil-Sisodia K, Mestman JH. Graves hyperthyroidism and pregnancy: a clinical update. *Endocr Pract* 2010;16:118–129.

31. Lazarus JH. Thyroid function in pregnancy. *Br Med Bull* 2011;97:137–148.

32. Ehler JP, Shah CP, Fenton GL, et al. *The Wills eye manual: office and emergency room diagnosis and treatment of eye disease.* Philadelphia: Lippincott Williams & Wilkins; 2008.

33. Biousse V, Bruce BB, Newman NJ. Update on the pathophysiology and management of idiopathic intracranial hypertension. *J Neurol Neurosurg Psychiatry* 2012;83:488–494.

34. Kesler A, Kuperminc M. Idiopathic intracranial hypertension and pregnancy. *Clin Obstet Gynecol* 2013;56:389–396.

35. Collins S, Arulkumaran S, Hayes K, et al. *Oxford Handbook of Obstetrics and Gynaecology,* 3rd edn. Oxford: Oxford University Press; 2013.

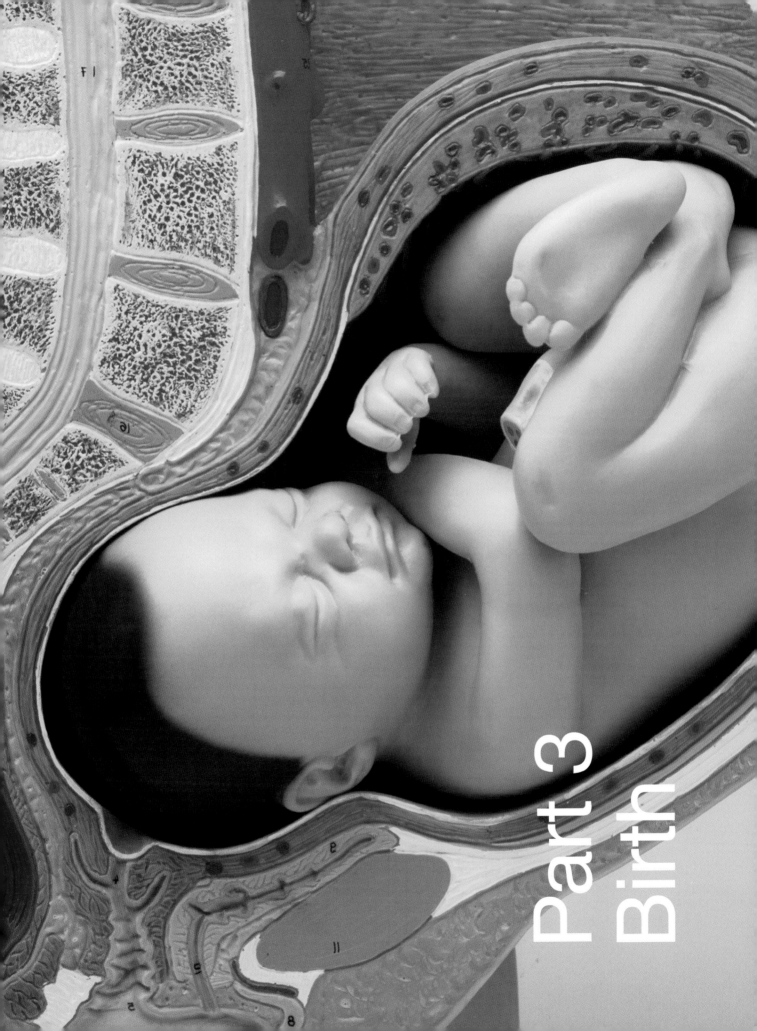

Part 3
Birth

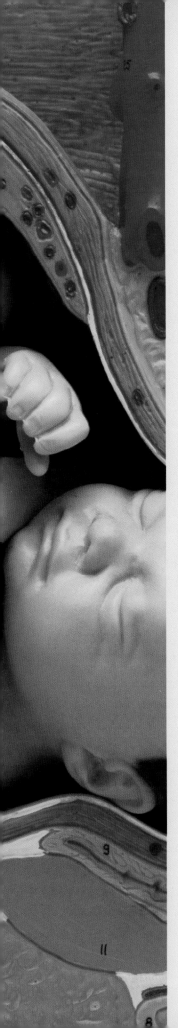

CHAPTER 18
Normal labour

Euan Kevelighan

Case

A 28-year-old G2P1 at 41^{+3} days (Term + 10) presents to the labour ward triage centre contracting 3 in every 10 minutes. Her antenatal course has been uncomplicated. Her previous pregnancy resulted in the vaginal delivery of a healthy 2-year-old girl weighing 3.5 kg.

On abdominal examination the lie is longitudinal, with cephalic presentation and 2/5ths palpable per abdomen. Pelvic examination reveals a fully effaced cervix that admits two fingers equating to 4 cm of dilatation. The membranes are intact. She is uncomfortable and requesting analgesia.

Learning outcomes

By the conclusion of this chapter you will be able to:

- define and describe the three stages of labour;
- describe a normal vaginal delivery;
- understand difference between first and subsequent labours;
- understand the importance of a partogram;
- describe benefits and side effects of the different types of analgesia used in labour;
- define important notations in obstetrics;
- describe useful drugs and doses administered in labour.

Essential Human Development, First Edition. Edited by Samuel Webster, Geraint Morris and Euan Kevelighan

Labour

Labour is the process of birth, resulting in the expulsion of fetus, placenta and membranes from the uterus. It is divided into three stages of unequal length:

1. **First stage:** the onset of labour until the cervix is fully dilated. It is further subdivided into:
   (a) Latent phase – onset of contractions until the cervix is fully effaced and dilated up to 3 cm.
   (b) Active phase – from 3 cm until full cervical dilatation.
2. **Second stage:** from full dilatation until delivery of baby. It also is subdivided into two phases:
   (a) Propulsive – from full dilatation until head reaches the pelvic floor.
   (b) Expulsive – when woman has irresistible desire to bear down/push until baby is delivered.
3. **Third stage:** from delivery of the baby until expulsion of the placenta and membranes.

Labour is diagnosed when a woman has painful, regular uterine contractions with cervical effacement and dilatation. Other factors associated with the onset of labour include a mucous "show" (operculum) and spontaneous rupture of fetal membranes "the waters breaking".

The cause of onset of labour is unknown. Part is mechanical as preterm labour is more common in women with an overstretched uterus, for example polyhydramnios and multiple pregnancy. Prostaglandins have a role as a cervical membrane sweep (releasing prostaglandins) increases the chances of a woman going into labour when performed in late pregnancy.

Definitions

Effacement: incorporation of the cervical canal into the lower uterine segment from the internal os downwards, reducing the distance between the internal os and the external os, until the internal os effectively disappears.

Dilatation of the cervix: refers to changes in the external os. The nulliparous cervix is tubular, with the internal os the same diameter as the external os. After vaginal delivery the cervix is changed, and the multiparous cervix has an external os with a larger diameter than its internal os. The primiparous cervix has to efface before it can dilate. The multiparous cervix undergoes effacement and dilatation simultaneously. Therefore second and subsequent labours tend to be more rapid than primigravida labours.

Caput: oedema of the scalp due to pressure of the head against the rim of the cervix.

Moulding: overlapping of the vault bones – the shape of the skull alters so the engaging diameters become shorter (Figure 18.1).

Engagement: descent of the biparietal diameter through the pelvic brim. If the head is at the level of the ischial spines it must be engaged unless there is caput. When the head is engaged not more than 2/5ths can be felt abdominally. Engagement usually occurs before labour is established in primigravidae and after in multigravidae women.

Lie: the relation of the long axis of the fetus to the mother. It may be longitudinal, oblique or transverse. Only a longitudinal lie is normal.

Presentation: the part of the fetus in the lower pole of the uterus, for example cephalic, vertex or breech.

Attitude: the posture of the fetus, for example flexion, deflexion or extension. The normal attitude is full flexion when normal presentation is a vertex.

Position: the relationship of the presenting part to the mother's pelvis. The denominator is used to describe the position of baby with respect to the mother's pelvis, for example LOL or LOA.

- Denominator – arbitrary part of presentation:
- occiput in vertex presentation;
- sacrum in breech presentation;
- mentum in face presentation.

The denominator denotes the position of the presenting part with reference to the pelvis (Figure 18.2).
The eight possible positions of the fetal head are: DOA, LOA, LOT (LOL), LOP, DOP, ROP, ROT (ROL) and ROA (see below).

Station of the fetal head: the relationship of the head to ischial spines. By notation the ischial spines (see Chapter 2) are designated station *zero*. When the head is above the spines, it is said to be at −1, −2, −3 or −4 cm. If the head is below the spines the notation is +1, +2, +3 or +4 cm. The station can only be determined by vaginal examination.

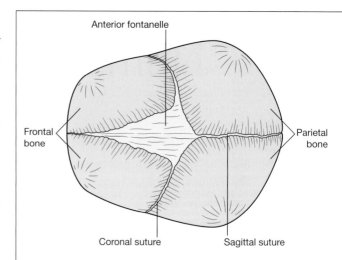

Figure 18.1 The fetal skull. When moulding occurs the sagittal suture becomes obliterated as the parietal bones overlap.

Mechanism of normal labour

This involves a sequence of passive movements of the head of the baby as it descends through the birth canal. The head usually presents in transverse position, the commonest position being left occipito-lateral (LOL). As the head descends it flexes and when the neck is fully flexed the presenting diameter is the suboccipito-bregmatic diameter (9.5 cm). The leading part of the head is known as the vertex. Further descent of the vertex occurs and the head is fully engaged when 0/5ths of it are palpable per abdomen. Rotation of the fetal head occurs, to the left occipito-anterior (LOA) position. Descent continues and the occiput rotates anteriorly at the level of the pelvic floor (ischial spines). The head is now direct occipito-anterior (DOA) – short rotation. This is known as internal rotation.

The part of the fetal head that first reaches the pelvic floor rotates anteriorly. In a well-flexed fetal head this is the vertex, so the occiput rotates anteriorly (Figure 18.2). In cases where the fetal head is deflexed or extended, occipital rotation is likely to be posteriorly resulting in an occipito-posterior fetal diameter (11.5 cm), which is much less likely to deliver vaginally – long rotation.

The occiput is below the pubic symphysis. Further maternal pushing with contractions results in descent and delivery of the fetal head by extension. The shoulders are now in the pelvic cavity but are in the left oblique diameter. The shoulder diameter is known as the bisacromial diameter (distance between the acromion processes) and measures 11 cm. The head rotates naturally to come into line with the shoulders (the occiput is in line with the fetal spine). This is known as restitution. Further descent results in the shoulders rotating to bring the bisacromial diameter into the anteroposterior plane of the pelvic outlet. The head rotates so that the occiput comes into line with the left maternal thigh. This is known as external rotation.

The anterior shoulder is delivered by lateral flexion of the fetal trunk posteriorly. The posterior shoulder is delivered by lateral flexion of the trunk anteriorly and the rest of the baby follows easily (Figure 18.3).

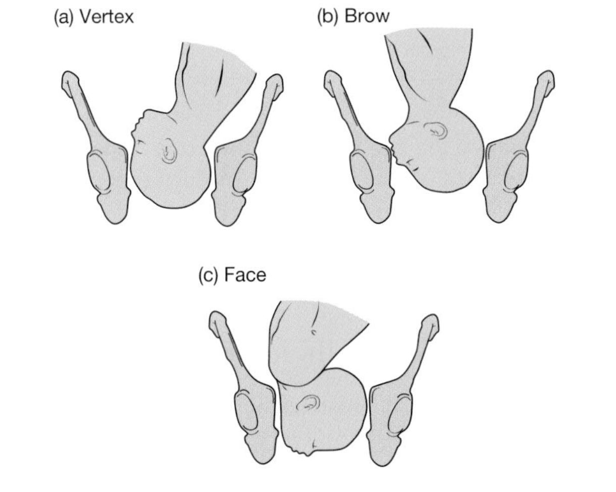

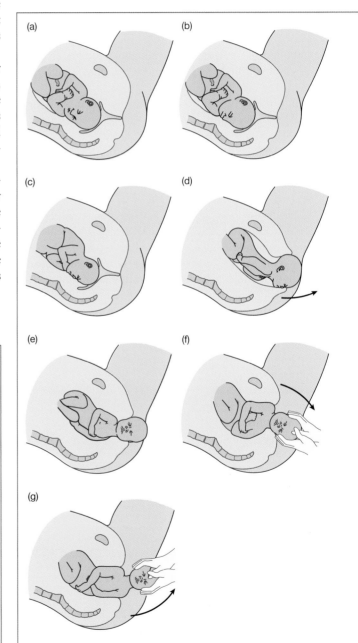

Figure 18.3 Diagram of normal labour mechanism.

Figure 18.2 Flexion of the fetal neck with descent into the pelvis. (a) A vertex presentation with a flexed neck. (b) A brow presentation with neck deflexion. (c) A face presentation with extension of the neck.

The normal rate of cervical dilatation is 0.5–1 cm/hour in nulliparous woman, and usually 1–2 cm/hour in a multiparous woman. During labour it is usual for the uterus to contract three or four times every 10 minutes, with contractions lasting 45 to 60 seconds. The duration of labour can vary widely and depends on when active labour commences. Generally a first labour may be 10–12 hours in length while a subsequent labour is usually shorter at approximately 6 hours (Table 18.1).

Management of labour

When in the first stage of labour the woman and fetus are regularly assessed:

- Pulse, blood pressure, temperature and respiratory rate.
- Urinalysis.
- Abdominal palpation: lie, presentation and engagement of the fetal head.
- Contractions: strength (by palpation), duration (timed) and frequency (timed).
- Analgesia requirements: include Entonox (gas and air), pethidine, remifentanil and/or epidural.
- Vaginal examinations: for degree of effacement, dilatation of cervix, length and position of cervix (in latent phase labour), station of presenting part (in relation to ischial spines), position of presenting part (if head presenting common positions are DOA, LOA, ROA or OP), presence of caput or moulding.

The fetal heart rate pattern is assessed via intermittent auscultation or electronically via cardiotocography (CTG). In low-risk patients intermittent auscultation using a Pinard stethoscope or sonicaid (using Doppler) is acceptable. If the patient has risk factors, for example small for gestational age, epidural, meconium-stained liquor or is on an oxytocin drip, then continuous CTG monitoring is recommended.

In low-risk women, auscultation should be performed every 15 minutes during and after a contraction for 60 seconds in the first stage of labour, and every 5 minutes in the second stage.

Table 18.1 The differences between primigravida and multigravida labour.

Primigravida	Multigravida
Inefficient uterine action Prolonged labour common if untreated	Uterine action efficient – dystocia (abnormally slow labour) rare
Rupture of uterus virtually unknown	Risk of uterine rupture
Risk of cephalopelvic disproportion and fetal trauma. In general, the size of the fetus is related to the mother's size	Disproportion and trauma rare if mother has had a previous vaginal delivery

Once the cervix is fully dilated and the fetal head is on the pelvic floor the woman is encouraged to push with contractions. She will often get an irresistible urge to push. As the head descends the perineum distends and the anus dilates. The midwife supports the perineum during delivery to prevent precipitous delivery and reduce the risk of vaginal tearing. If the patient has an epidural in situ this abolishes the urge to push, so often an hour is allowed before pushing is commenced. The head is born by extension and the accoucheur feels the fetal neck to exclude the presence of the umbilical cord. The head restitutes and undergoes external rotation, and with lateral flexion the anterior shoulder slips under the pubic symphysis. The baby is delivered onto the mother's abdomen by the shoulders. The umbilical cord is clamped and cut. It is common practice to delay cord clamping by 1 minute in uncomplicated deliveries as this reduces the risk of anaemia in infants.

Active management of the third stage of labour reduces postpartum haemorrhage (PPH). Active management includes:

- Administering an oxytocic drug (often Syntometrine® – see 'Useful drugs in obstetrics and their actions' later).
- Clamping and cutting the umbilical cord (delaying cord clamping does not increase the risk of PPH).
- Delivering the placenta by controlled cord traction.

The oxytocic is given with the delivery of the anterior shoulder of the baby. Active management of third-stage labour therefore begins during the second stage. Signs of placental separation are: the cord lengthens, the uterine fundus rises and there is a gush of blood. The manoeuvre of controlled cord traction is known as the Brandt–Andrews method and involves pulling on the cord while applying countertraction on the uterus to prevent uterine inversion. The placenta and membranes are thoroughly inspected to ensure they are complete. Retained placental tissue is associated with both PPH and infection. Some patients request a physiological third stage. They are not given an oxytocic and delivery of the placenta occurs passively. This increases the risk of PPH.

The labia, vagina and cervix are inspected for lacerations and sutured if necessary. The fundus of the uterus should be well contracted close to the level of the umbilicus. The estimated blood loss is documented. This is usually less than 500 mL.

The partogram and its importance

A partogram is a graphic representation of the woman's progress in labour (Figure 18.4). Once a patient is admitted in labour a partogram is commenced. This illustrates cervical dilatation, descent of the fetal head, and uterine contractions with frequency, and records all routine observations of mother and baby including fetal heart rate, colour of liquor, mother's pulse, blood pressure and drug therapy.

The example shown in Figure 18.4 is for a patient who is a Gravida 4 Para 3 at Term +1 (one day over her due date),

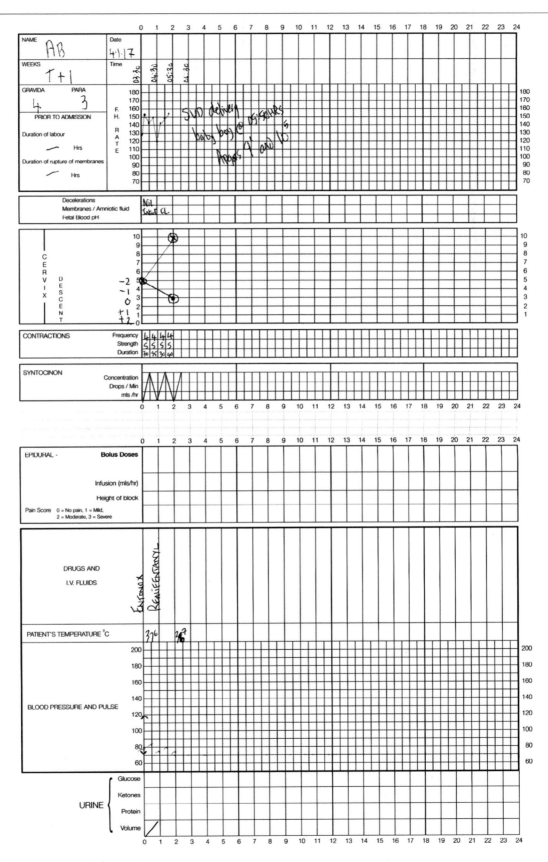

Figure 18.4 An example of a partogram.

admitted in established labour and whose cervix is 5 cm dilated.

Her labour progressed rapidly and her cervix was fully dilated 2 hours later at 05.30. The fetal head had also descended from station –2 to the ischial spines (station zero). The woman had four contractions every 10 minutes and the strength of contractions was strong (S). The duration of the contractions varied between 30 and 40 seconds. The membranes around the baby were initially intact but later ruptured and clear (Cl) liquor noted *per vaginum*. The fetal heart rate was recorded every 15 minutes.

Other useful information on this partogram include that the woman used Entonox® ('gas and air') initially for analgesia before having remifentanil patient-controlled analgesia sited. No oxytocin (Syntocinon®) was required as labour progressed rapidly, which is in keeping with having had three vaginal deliveries in the past. Other parameters included in this partogram include the patient's pulse, blood pressure, temperature and urine output. In this case the patient's vital signs were normal and she did not void urine during her short labour.

The partogram is very useful as it highlights slow progress in labour, for example delay in cervical dilatation or failure of the head to descend. For more information on using partograms to diagnose failure to progress in labour see Chapter 19.

Analgesia in labour

Pain relief in labour depends on the mother's preference, how painful the contractions are and the anticipated length of labour (Table 18.2).

Table 18.2 Pharmacological methods of pain relief.

Drug	Method	Indication for use	Effectiveness	Side effects	Duration
Oxygen/nitrous oxide	Inhalation 50/50 mixture of oxygen and nitrous oxide	First and second stage of labour	Mild	Faint, nausea and vomiting	Short-acting during inhalation
Pethidine	Intramuscular 50–150 mg	First stage	Mild – takes 'edge' off pain	Nausea and vomiting. Respiratory depression in newborn – naloxone used to reverse this effect	3–4 hours
Pudendal nerve block	Infiltration of right and left pudendal nerves (S2–S4) just below ischial spines	For operative vaginal delivery (in second-stage labour)	Moderate/good analgesia		45–90 minutes
Perineal infiltration	0.5% lidocaine at posterior fourchette	To facilitate episiotomy and/or before suturing tears/episiotomies	Effective local analgesia within 5 minutes		45–90 minutes
Remifentanil PCA (patient-controlled analgesia)	Intravenous (powerful opiate that does not cross the placenta)	For patients in whom epidural is contraindicated or who wish a less complete analgesic block	Good		
Epidural anaesthesia	Injection of 0.25–0.5% bupivacaine via catheter into extradural space (L3–L4)	First and second stage Caesarean section (CS)	Complete pain relief in >95% within 20 minutes	Transient hypotension (preload with i.v. fluids) Decreased mobility Dural puncture <1/100 Increased length of second-stage labour	Continuous infusion with top-ups every 3–4 hours
Spinal anaesthesia	0.5% bupivacaine into subarachnoid space	Operative delivery, e.g. forceps or CS Manual removal of placenta	Complete pain relief within few minutes	Respiratory depression	Single injection – wears off after 3–4 hours

Non-pharmacological methods include acupuncture, homeopathy and hypnosis. Educating women what to expect with labour pain can help reduce anxiety and the sense of loss of control. There is strong evidence that a trusted companion present throughout the labour and delivery reduces pain relief requirements.

Useful drugs in obstetrics and their actions

Syntocinon = synthetic oxytocin – an octapeptide that causes rhythmical uterine contractions, can be administered IV or IM. Acts in 2 minutes when given i.m. It is used to ensure efficient uterine action in dystocia and also as a uterotonic in postpartum haemorrhage.

Ergometrine – 500 µg (0.5 mg) injected i.v. acts within 40 seconds and persists for 30 minutes. Takes 6 minutes to act when given i.m. It causes tetanic contractions (prolonged spasm). It is used for postpartum haemorrhage and the main side effects are nausea, vomiting and hypertension. It is contraindicated in hypertension and cardiac disease.

Syntometrine = a combination of 10 IU of oxytocin and 0.5 mg of ergometrine. This is used for the active management of the third stage of labour. It is given as an intramuscular injection into maternal thigh as the anterior shoulder appears under the pubic symphysis. It is also useful in treatment of postpartum haemorrhage.

Clinical case

Case conclusion

The fetal heart is 145 bpm and regular. The mother's vital signs are normal. Due to increasing pain she requests epidural anaesthesia. Since she is in established labour this is sited and within 20 minutes she is completely pain free. Continuous CTG is commenced and the fetal heart pattern remains reassuring. Her membranes rupture spontaneously 2 hours later, and on vaginal examination she is 7 cm dilated and no cord is palpable. The position of the fetal head is LOA, and the leading part of the fetal head is at the level of the ischial spines (station zero). The epidural is topped up an hour later as the patient complains of painful contractions. Three hours later the midwife notices that the perineum has distended somewhat. Vaginal examination confirms that the cervix is fully dilated and the fetal head is at introitus. The patient has no urge to push as the epidural is providing complete pain relief. With encouragement the woman delivers a live baby boy weighing 2.4 kg. As the anterior shoulder is delivered the midwife gives an i.m. injection of Syntometrine into the maternal thigh to accelerate the third stage of labour. The baby cries at birth and cord clamping is delayed for 1 minute.

The placenta delivers 3 minutes later and the perineum is checked and intact. Blood loss is estimated at 250 mL. The uterus is well contracted.

Key learning points

- Labour is divided into three stages of unequal length.
- The diagnosis of labour is only made when a woman has painful, regular uterine contractions with evidence of cervical effacement and dilatation.
- There are significant differences between a first-time labour and subsequent labours. A partogram is a graphic representation of labour. It provides essential information about the progress of the labour.

- There are many methods of pain relief in labour. These range from Entonox providing partial relief, to epidural and spinal analgesia, which result in complete pain relief.
- It is important to know obstetric definitions, including positions of the head, station, lie, presentation and attitude of the fetus.
- Three common drugs used in labour are oxytocin, ergometrine and Syntometrine.

 Now visit **www.wileyessential.com/humandevelopment** to test yourself on this chapter.

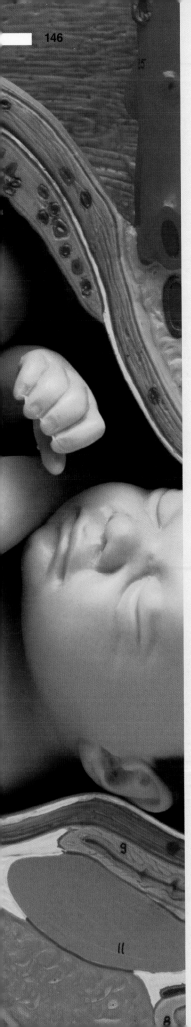

CHAPTER 19
Abnormal labour

Franz Majoko

Case

DE was a 23-year-old woman in her first pregnancy who was admitted with a 3-hour history of spontaneous onset of contractions at 40 weeks gestation. Palpation confirmed a term pregnancy with cephalic presentation and the head was 3/5 palpable. Contractions were 2–3 in 10 minutes of moderate strength with duration of 45 seconds. The fetal heart rate was normal. Cervical dilatation was 4 cm and membranes ruptured spontaneously during examination, draining clear amniotic fluid. Maternal observations were normal.

When she was reassessed after 4 hours, cervical dilatation was still 4 cm and the head was 3/5 palpable. An infusion of Syntocinon® 10 IU in 500 mL of normal saline was commenced and the rate was increased at half-hourly intervals to achieve four contractions in 10 minutes with duration between 45–60 seconds. She was re-examined after 2 hours and cervical dilatation was 7 cm and the head was 2/5 palpable. When the infusion rate was 24 mL/h and contractions were five in 10 minutes fetal heart decelerations were noted. The Syntocinon infusion rate was reduced. Fetal blood sampling (FBS) was performed and the result was normal. The Syntocinon infusion was continued at the reduced rate. An hour after the FBS decelerations in the fetal heart rate were persisting and a further FBS was considered but on examination the cervix was fully dilated with the head at spines.

Learning outcomes

- You should be able to define abnormal progress in labour.
- You should be able to use a partograph to identify poor progress in labour.
- You should be able to identify factors associated with abnormal labour.
- You should be able to describe options for the management of abnormal labour.
- You should be able to define preterm labour.
- You should be able to describe the factors associated with spontaneous preterm delivery.
- You should be able to describe the management of spontaneous preterm labour.
- You should be able to describe methods used for prediction and prevention of preterm labour.
- You should be able to describe methods of induction of labour.
- You should be able to describe indications for induction of labour.
- You should be able to describe complications of induction of labour.

Essential Human Development, First Edition. Edited by Samuel Webster, Geraint Morris and Euan Kevelighan
© 2018 John Wiley & Sons, Ltd. Published 2018 by John Wiley & Sons, Ltd.

Definitions

Labour that is described as **normal** has spontaneous onset of uterine contractions with a cephalic presentation at term (37–42 weeks), with no use of oxytocic drugs to augment contractions or use of an epidural, resulting in a vaginal birth of a baby in good condition.

Abnormal labour occurs when anatomical and/or functional abnormalities of the fetus, pelvis, uterus and cervix interfere with the normal course of labour and delivery.

Several terms are used interchangeably to describe abnormal labour and these include **dystocia**, **dysfunctional labour**, **prolonged labour** or **failure to progress**. The term 'abnormal labour' will be used in this chapter.

Although the term 'abnormal labour' also includes preterm labour, induction of labour and precipitate labour, these will only be considered briefly in this chapter. Very rapid labour (precipitate labour) can cause injuries to the birth canal as well as lead to injury to the baby due to its rapid passage through the birth canal.

The incidence of abnormal labour is difficult to determine but it is estimated that it may complicate 17–37% of labours.

Diagnosis

The correct diagnosis of labour is important in the management of a labouring woman as misdiagnosis may lead to unnecessary intervention. The active phase of labour is diagnosed when there is regular, painful uterine activity and progressive cervical dilatation of 4 cm or more. It has recently been suggested that in multiparous women, the active phase of labour may start at cervical dilatation of 5–6 cm.

Our knowledge of progress in labour was gained through the work of Friedman, and later Philpott and Castle, who studied thousands of labours resulting in uncomplicated vaginal births enabling the setting of time limits and progress milestones that define normal labor. In the 1950s Friedman studied labour systematically, and in 1954 introduced the concept of a partogram by graphically depicting the dilatation of the cervix during labour. In 1972, Philpott and Castle developed Friedman's concept into a tool for monitoring labour by adding the 'alert' and 'action' lines to the graph. The World Health Organization (WHO) later modified the partograph. The WHO partograph was designed to monitor not only the progress of labour, but also the condition of the mother and the baby. The advantage of the partograph over written clinical notes is the visual impact that enables early recognition of abnormal labour and thereby early interventions to correct the abnormality (see Figure 18.4). The UK's National Institute for Health and Care Excellence (NICE) and WHO advocate use of the partograph in monitoring progress for all women in the active phase of labour.

When using the partograph the diagnosis of abnormal progress is made if cervical dilatation is more than 2 hours to the right of the alert line.

Causes of abnormal labour

The causes of abnormal labour are traditionally considered under the 3 Ps:

- Passages – pelvis, soft tissues.
- Passenger – size, flexion, moulding, position.
- Powers – uterine contractions.

An additional 2 Ps are sometimes considered:

- Practitioner – interference, failure to respond/correct dysfunctional labour.
- Patient – parity, pain relief.

The causes and their appropriate interventions will be considered in turn, but in clinical practice there are large areas of overlap.

Passages

Feto-pelvic disproportion occurs when the disparity in the size or shape of the maternal pelvis (Figure 19.1) and fetal head prevents safe vaginal delivery. This diagnosis is not made by assessing the size of the baby or pelvic capacity radiologically prior to labour. It may be suspected in maternal short stature (<150 cm), high head at term or previous difficult vaginal delivery. Feto-pelvic disproportion is a functional diagnosis made when regular, strong uterine contractions fail to cause descent of the presenting part. Use of the partograph is helpful for early diagnosis.

Cervix

Occasionally, despite strong regular contractions, the cervix does not dilate. In most cases, the cause of this is unknown but sometimes the cervical resistance may be due to scarring resulting from previous surgery such as cone biopsy. When labour needs to be induced, cervical preparation with

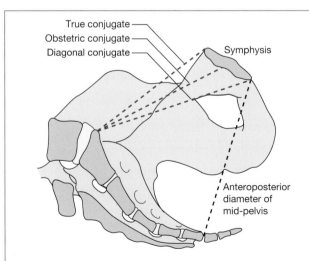

Figure 19.1 The bones of the pelvis and pelvic dimensions.

prostaglandins before stimulating contractions is advisable. Stimulating uterine contractions with an unfavourable cervix may result in failure of cervical dilatation leading to an avoidable caesarean section.

Delivery by caesarean section is the most effective solution to problems of the passage.

Passenger

The size of the fetus, and/or the presenting diameter of the head may result in abnormal progress in labour.

Size

Fetal macrosomia and anomalies such as hydrocephalus are associated with abnormal labour. Macrosomia is often defined as birthweight above 4000 or 4500 g, and its incidence ranges from 1 to 10% depending on the definition used.

Malposition

In most labours the vertex (Figure 19.2) is the presenting part with a diameter of 9.5 cm, with a fully flexed head in an occipito-anterior position. When the head is deflexed, a brow presentation with a diameter of 13 cm is encountered and vaginal birth is not feasible despite normal pelvic dimensions. Further deflection of the head results in a face presentation, which has a diameter of 9.5 cm. In an occipito-transverse position, the presenting diameter is 11.5 cm (occipito-frontal) and a rotational assisted delivery is usually required to achieve a vaginal birth. In 5% of labours, the fetal head rotates to the occipito-posterior position during descent through the pelvis.

Malpresentation

This includes breech, face, brow and shoulder presentations (Figure 19.3). Breech presentation is the most common

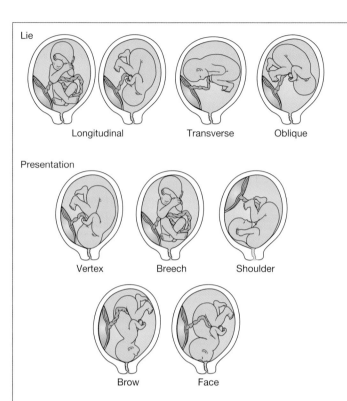

Figure 19.3 The lie and presentation of the fetus.
(Source: S. Webster and R. de Wreede (2012) *Embryology at a Glance*. Reproduced with permission of John Wiley & Sons, Ltd.)

malpresentation, occurring in 3–4% of pregnancies at term. It is preferable to make a diagnosis prior to the onset of labour, when external cephalic version may be offered. Since publication of the results of a term breech trial few planned vaginal breech deliveries are conducted. The majority of babies presenting by the breech are delivered by caesarean section, but sometimes the diagnosis is made late in the second stage when vaginal breech delivery is the most appropriate delivery option.

Shoulder, brow and some face presentations are delivered by caesarean section.

Powers

The strength of uterine contractions is assessed clinically by palpation, which is subjective and liable to wide inter-observer variation. Contractions are considered adequate if the frequency is 3–4 in 10 minutes, with duration of more than 40 seconds and strong on palpation. In research studies the uterine contractile force can be quantified by the use of an intrauterine pressure catheter, which allows for direct measurement and calculation of uterine contractility reported in Montevideo units (MVUs). For contractions to be considered adequate, the force produced must exceed 200 MVUs during a 10-minute period. Intrauterine pressure catheters are used only for research purposes because they are invasive procedures.

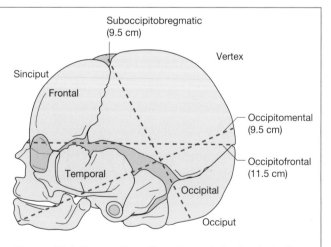

Figure 19.2 Presenting diameters of the fetal skull.

Problems of uterine contractions can be of frequency, intensity, coordination or a combination of these. When there is uncoordinated uterine action the contraction pattern fails to result in cervical effacement and dilatation.

Inadequate uterine action is corrected by use of intravenous oxytocin (Syntocinon). A dilute solution of oxytocin, such as 10 IU in 500 mL normal saline, is administered through an infusion pump and is titrated against uterine contractions. The infusion is started at a dose of 1 mU/min and increased at 30-minute intervals until regular strong contractions with a frequency of 3–4 in 10 minutes are achieved. The dosage may be reduced or stopped if the frequency of contractions is more than five in 10 minutes. Electronic monitoring of the fetal heart rate is advisable when oxytocin is used to augment uterine contractions. A reassessment of progress should be made within 4 hours of starting augmentation to confirm response to the intervention and avoid obstructed labour. Oxytocin can cause uterine overactivity where the contractions may be excessively long or excessively frequent, affecting placental blood flow and causing fetal distress.

Oxytocin cannot be used to overcome mechanical obstruction to delivery and its misuse can result in uterine rupture especially in multiparous women.

Patient

Parity has an effect on duration of labour, and nulliparous women have longer duration compared to multiparous women (Figure 19.4). The cervical dilatation at which the active phase commences is different in multiparous women, at 5–6 cm.

Epidural analgesia is associated with a longer duration of labour through a motor block and may contribute to a prolonged second stage. These cases have also been associated with an increase in oxytocin use and operative vaginal delivery. However, use of epidural for analgesia during labour does not result in a statistically significant increase in caesarean delivery.

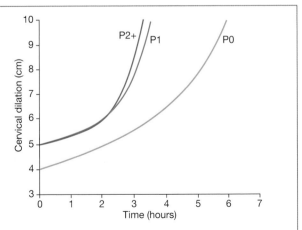

Figure 19.4 Cervical dilatation with time in nulliparous versus multiparous women.

Pre-labour rupture of membranes precedes onset of contractions in 6–12% of women, and labour whose onset is preceded by spontaneous rupture of membranes tends to be longer.

Practitioner

Some actions by the practitioner, such as misdiagnosis in the latent phase of labour, may increase the risk of prolonged labour.

Types of abnormal labour

Abnormal labour falls into two broad groups, either **prolonged** or **arrest** of labour progress.

Prolongation problems

The major problem with prolonged labour is a lack of agreement on the normal time for the length of labour. In the active management of labour pioneered by O'Driscoll, 1 cm/h was considered as the slowest rate of dilatation, and augmentation of contractions was started when the rate of cervical dilatation was below this. Some 10–12% of nulliparous women in spontaneous labour dilate at a rate of 0.5–0.6 cm/h. The mean duration for the active phase of labour is 10 h in primigravid and 6 h in multiparous women. If cervical dilatation extends more than 2 h to the right of the alert line on the partograph, labour is considered to be prolonged.

The most common cause of prolonged labour is inefficient uterine contractions. This problem is most often overcome by use of an oxytocin infusion.

Disproportion is usually diagnosed retrospectively after a prolonged labour culminating in a caesarean section. Prolonged labour is the leading indication for primary caesarean deliveries.

Primary dysfunctional labour

This is the commonest abnormal labour pattern in which the rate of cervical dilatation is less than 1 cm/h in the active phase. It is estimated to occur in 26% of spontaneous primigravid labours and 8% of multiparous women. The first intervention is augmentation of uterine contractions with Syntocinon. This is successful in improving cervical dilatation in 80% of women. However, if labour is greater than 4 hours to the right of the alert line, the caesarean section rate increases to 34%. Oxytocin should be used with caution in multiparous women because of the risk of uterine rupture in non-responders.

Secondary arrest

This is arrest of cervical dilatation or of descent of the presenting part. The active phase of labour commences normally but cervical dilatation stops or slows prior to full dilatation. This is usually due to relative feto-pelvic disproportion associated with malposition such as occipito-posterior or transverse positions. Secondary arrest is rare in multiparous women, at 2% incidence. In nulliparous women, 70% respond to oxytocin. The caesarean section rate in non-responders is 83% compared to 5.6% in responders. Secondary arrest is associated with a high instrumental delivery rate. Strong contractions are needed for flexion, and time should be allowed for rotation to occur.

Arrest problems

Arrest disorders cannot be properly diagnosed until the patient is in the active phase and has had no cervical change for two or more hours with the contraction pattern exceeding 3–4 in 10 minutes lasting more than 40 seconds. Uterine contractions must be considered adequate to correctly diagnose arrest of dilation. Arrest of descent indicates feto-pelvic disproportion (CPD). CPD may be absolute or relative. Absolute CPD is rare and occurs because the pelvis has smaller than normal dimensions. Relative CPD occurs more frequently with a normal size pelvis but a larger presenting diameter due to malposition of the baby's head, such as occipito-posterior where the presenting diameter is 11.5 cm.

A caesarean section is required in dealing with absolute CPD. In relative CPD associated with malposition, spontaneous rotation of the fetal head may occur with stronger contractions, or an assisted vaginal birth such as rotational forceps or ventouse may be conducted.

Effects of prolonged labour

Prolonged labour has both immediate and long-term effects:
- Maternal exhaustion and ketosis resulting from dehydration and anaerobic metabolism are frequent problems that need to be treated.
- Increased likelihood of operative delivery (forceps, vacuum and caesarean section) and associated trauma to the genital tract.
- Increased risk of postpartum haemorrhage especially from uterine atony.
- Fetal hypoxia and risk of hypoxic injury.
- Increased risk of puerperal sepsis (endo/myometritis) as a result of prolonged rupture of membranes.
- Maternal psychological effects such as dissatisfaction with birthing experience and anxiety regarding future births.
  Failure to identify prolonged labour and intervene early leads to obstructed labour.

Obstructed labour

Obstructed labour means that the fetus cannot descend through the pelvis despite adequate uterine activity because there is an insurmountable barrier preventing its descent.

Obstruction usually occurs at the pelvic brim so that a significant proportion of the head remains palpable per abdomen. Complications arising from obstructed labour can be avoided if the diagnosis is made early and appropriate action is taken. In multiparous women uterine rupture is likely to occur if operative intervention is not performed in a timely manner. Some women develop vesico-vaginal fistulae as a result of prolonged compression of the anterior vaginal wall and bladder by the presenting part.

Preterm labour

Introduction

Preterm labour is defined as regular uterine contractions associated with cervical change after 24 weeks and before 37 completed weeks of pregnancy. Preterm labour complicates 6–10% of pregnancies. Approximately 75% of preterm births occur as a result of spontaneous preterm labour, while in 20–25% it results from intervention for a maternal or fetal condition. Preterm labour is associated with a high level of morbidity due to respiratory distress syndrome (RDS), bronchopulmonary dysplasia or intraventricular haemorrhage and is responsible for 50% of childhood neurological disabilities. It accounts for 50–75% of perinatal mortality.

The diagnosis is made when palpable painful contractions lasting longer than 30 seconds with frequency of at least two in 10 minutes accompany cervical changes such as in position, consistency, length and dilatation and occurring before 37 weeks. There is a high false positive rate: 80% of women with presumptive diagnosis of preterm labour will not have preterm delivery.

Risk factors/aetiology

Preterm labour has multiple aetiologies. It may represent an early activation of the normal labour process or a pathological mechanism. There are some risk factors/markers associated with preterm labour (Table 19.1). The strength of association of the risk markers has wide variation but women with

Table 19.1 Risk factors for preterm labour.

Maternal
- Severe maternal disease (diabetes, hypertension)
- Urinary tract infection
- Febrile illness (pneumonia, malaria)
- Low socio-economic status
- Maternal age <18 or >40
- Uterine abnormalities (fibroids, bicornuate)
- Previous preterm birth/late miscarriages

Fetal/placental
- Congenital anomaly
- Multiple pregnancy
- Intrauterine infection

a history of preterm birth have a 20–40% risk of recurrence. Preterm pre-labour rupture of membranes (PPROM) precedes 30–40% of cases of preterm labour.

Management of preterm labour

The interventions in a woman presenting in preterm labour are directed at inhibiting/reducing contractions to delay delivery and optimising fetal status prior to preterm birth.

Tocolysis

Tocolytic drugs inhibit myometrial contractions and may prolong pregnancy by 2–7 days. The delay in delivery can allow time for the administration of a complete course of corticosteroids for fetal lung maturation or to facilitate in utero transfer to a tertiary neonatal facility. A number of agents have been used to suppress uterine contractions including ethanol, beta-agonists, calcium channel blockers, prostaglandin synthetase inhibitors, nitric oxide donors and oxytocin receptor antagonists. Most tocolytic drugs have potential for maternal complications (Table 19.2).

Contraindications to tocolysis include antepartum haemorrhage, chorioamnionitis, cervical dilatation more than 3 cm, fetal compromise such as IUGR with fetal heart rate abnormality, severe pre-eclampsia or eclampsia as well as unstable maternal haemodynamic condition.

Corticosteroids

Corticosteroids reduce the incidence and severity of neonatal RDS, intraventricular haemorrhage and necrotising enterocolitis and thus decrease neonatal morbidity and mortality. Dexamethasone and betamethasone are the most frequently used drugs for fetal lung maturation. There is a risk of maternal pulmonary oedema when antenatal corticosteroids are used in combination with tocolytic agents, especially in women with infections, fluid overload and multiple pregnancy. The dose of betamethasone is two doses of 12 mg administered intramuscularly 24 hours apart, whereas dexamethasone is four doses of 6 mg intramuscularly every 12 hours. Pulmonary oedema does not appear to occur when corticosteroid is used alone.

Delivery

Preterm babies are more susceptible to trauma during delivery compared to term babies. The birth should be in a facility that provides neonatal intensive care and attended by a team experienced in neonatal resuscitation. Non-vertex presentation occurs frequently in preterm labour hence the importance of confirming presentation by ultrasound upon admission if necessary. The preterm fetus with breech presentation is at risk of cord prolapse and head entrapment. Given the higher morbidity and mortality of preterm vaginal breech delivery, especially at a gestational age less than 34 weeks, caesarean section is recommended. However, a preterm fetus with a cephalic presentation can have a vaginal birth.

Prevention and prediction of preterm labour

Prevention of preterm labour may involve reducing the risk/factors shown in Table 19.1. These approaches include improvement in quality of life but have not been shown to reduce the incidence of preterm labour. Some focus has also been directed towards detection of preterm contractions or cervical change prior to the onset of labour. The risk markers/factors for preterm labour have low predictive value. There continues

Table 19.2 Tocolytic drugs including their frequently encountered side effects.

Drug	Mechanism of action	Dosage	Side effects
Terbutaline	β_2-agonist Decrease free intracellular calcium ions	0.25 mg subcutaneous 20 minutes to 3 hourly 0.05–0.35 mg per minute intravenously	Hypotension Tachycardia Pulmonary oedema
Magnesium sulphate	Intracellular calcium antagonism	4–6 g bolus in 20 minutes and then 2–3 g/h	Flushing Headaches Muscle weakness
Nifedipine	Calcium channel blocker	10 mg every 15 minutes (four doses) then 20 mg orally 4–6 h	Hypotension Headache Flushing
Indometacin	Prostaglandin inhibitor	50–100 mg PR 50 mg orally 6 h	Ductus arteriosus constriction Oligohydramnios
Atosiban	Oxytocin antagonist	6.75 mg intravenous bolus then 18 mg/h for 3 h followed by 6 mg/h for 45 h	Tachycardia Hypotension Flushing

to be interest in tests that have higher predictive value for pre-term birth and these include cervical length measurement and fetal fibronectin.

Transvaginal ultrasound scanning (TVS) cervical assessment

Cervical effacement and lower uterine segment changes pre-date cervical dilatation. A TVS to detect cervical changes, shortening and funnelling, may be useful in prediction of subsequent preterm birth, especially in women with risk markers. Patients with cervical length less than 2.5 cm are believed to be at higher risk of preterm labour.

Fetal fibronectin

The presence of fetal fibronectin in cervical/vaginal secretions after 24 weeks gestation suggests the detachment of fetal membranes from the decidua and therefore increased likelihood of preterm birth. The usefulness of the fibronectin test lies in the predictive value of a negative test, which is 99%. If the test is negative, less than 1% of women will give birth within the next 14 days. However, the predictive value of a positive test is low. Twenty percent of women with a positive test are likely to deliver in the next week or two.

Induction of labour

Induction of labour (IOL) is a process of initiating labour artificially when it is felt that the risk to the mother or fetus is greater than the benefit of allowing the pregnancy to run its natural course. About 20% of the labours in England and Wales are induced.

Indications for induction may be maternal or fetal. Some of the common indications for IOL are post-maturity, ruptured membranes, suspected intrauterine growth restriction (IUGR) and maternal medical problems such as obstetric cholestasis, hypertensive disorders and diabetic disease in pregnancy.

Prior to commencing the process of induction of labour a cervical assessment is made to decide on the method of induction. A Bishop score is recorded (Table 19.3) and a cardiotocograph (CTG) is performed to confirm fetal wellbeing.

Various cervical ripening methods are available to maximise the success of induction of labour in women with an unfavourable cervix. Mechanical methods of induction are among the oldest methods to initiate labour and were developed to promote cervical ripening and the onset of labour by stretching the cervix. They have largely been replaced by pharmacological agents, especially prostaglandin E2 preparations.

Methods of induction of labour

Mechanical

Mechanical methods include laminaria and balloon catheters. Their advantages, compared with pharmacological methods, include simplicity, lower cost and fewer side effects.

Pharmacological

Prostaglandins have been used for induction of labour since the 1960s. In the UK, vaginal prostaglandins are the most commonly used induction agents. The preparations of vaginal prostaglandin E2 (PGE2) include gels, tablets and pessaries. The induction regimens used vary considerably in the number of applications of each medication used, the dosages used and time intervals between doses. Sustained-release pessaries such as dinoprostone 10 mg have been developed to reduce the number of applications needed during the induction process. Prostaglandins have been shown to be safe and efficacious and PGE2 is the preferred method of induction of labour.

Misoprostol is a synthetic PGE1 analogue that is gaining widespread use for induction of labour. It is associated with a higher risk of hyperstimulation. It is not currently used in the UK for induction of labour when the fetus is alive.

Other methods

Amniotomy: When the Bishop score is ≥9, labour may be induced by artificial rupture of membranes and Syntocinon without the need for cervical ripening.

Membrane sweep: This involves performing an internal vaginal examination and digitally sweeping the fetal membranes. It releases endogenous prostaglandins, which increases the chance that the patient will go into spontaneous labour in the next 48 hours. The membranes should not be ruptured by the procedure

Complications of induction of labour

The complications of induction of labour vary with the method used and include hyperstimulation, fetal distress and uterine rupture as well as failed induction.

Hyperstimulation: This can be either tachysystole (more than five contractions in 10 minutes over a period of at least 20 minutes), or hypertonic contraction lasting for more than 2 minutes in association with changes in the fetal heart trace.

Table 19.3 Modified Bishop score.

Characteristic	Score			
	0	1	2	3
Dilatation (in cm)	Closed	1–2	3–4	5
Length (in cm)	>4	3–4	1–2	0
Consistency	Firm	Medium	Soft	–
Position	Posterior	Central	Anterior	–
Head station	–3	–2	–1, 0	+1, +2

This occurs in up to 5% of PGE-induced labour and more frequently with the use of misoprostol.

Hyperstimulation may also occur with the use of oxytocin infusion. Excessive uterine contractility is managed by reducing or stopping the oxytocin infusion or removing PGE from the vagina. Tocolysis may be required and immediate delivery by caesarean section may be required if fetal heart changes persist.

Fetal distress: Abnormal CTG changes are usually associated with increased frequency or strength of uterine contractions. A tocolytic drug such as terbutaline may be administered, and if an oxytocin infusion was in use this should be stopped. A caesarean section may be required if the fetal heart rate does not return to normal.

Failed induction: There is no standard definition for what constitutes a failed induction of labour. Failure to establish labour after one cycle of treatment occurs in 15% of cases. If induction fails, the woman's condition, fetal wellbeing and the pregnancy in general should be fully reassessed. The subsequent management options include a further attempt to induce labour or a caesarean section. If it is decided to continue with induction, the timing should depend on the clinical situation and the woman's wishes.

Induced labours have higher intervention rates and therefore labour should be induced only for medical reasons. There is increased requirement for epidural analgesia and operative delivery.

Clinical case

Case investigations

Progress in labour was monitored by periodic examinations at which the level of the presenting part and cervical dilatation were assessed. When concerns for fetal wellbeing arose due to decelerations in the fetal heart, fetal blood sampling (FBS) was performed. The fetal scalp pH was 7.33. If the CTG remains a concern, an FBS is usually repeated within the hour. A decision had been made to perform another FBS but as she was now in the second stage of labour an assisted delivery was performed.

Case conclusion

This was a case of primary dysfunctional labour due to inadequate uterine contractions. The correct action of augmenting contractions by use of an oxytocin infusion was undertaken and there was good response in that within 2 hours cervical dilatation had increased and descent of the fetal head had occurred. The partograph is useful in the diagnosis of abnormal progress in labour, and timely intervention may prevent obstructed labour (Figure 19.5, on the following page). In the second stage delivery can be expedited by use of either forceps or ventouse extractor. It was decided to expedite the delivery by use of forceps. A baby girl was delivered with Apgar scores of 7 and 10 at 1 and 5 minutes respectively.

Key learning points

- Any patient in labour is at risk of abnormal labour regardless of parity or an anatomically adequate pelvis.
- The progress in labour of all women in the active phase should be plotted on a partogram for the early identification of abnormal labour.
- The initial aims of management of preterm labour are to slow the onset of labour and aid development of the fetus with corticosteroids.

(Continued)

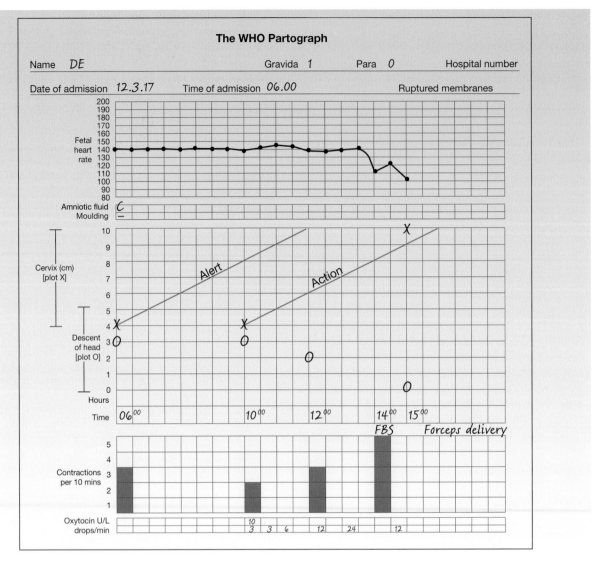

Figure 19.5 The partograph for the clinical case.

 Now visit **www.wileyessential.com/humandevelopment** to test yourself on this chapter.

CHAPTER 20
The puerperium

Fran Hodge

Often neglected, the puerperium is a time of extensive change. This period covers the 6 weeks following delivery during which time the physiological changes of pregnancy are reversed. There is a tendency to regard the puerperium as a period of lower risk compared with pregnancy and delivery, whilst in actual fact the risks of some conditions such as thrombotic events are significantly increased. Therefore it is not a period to be overlooked.

Case study

A 28-year-old mother of three is seen 4 weeks after her emergency caesarean section under general anaesthetic for cord prolapse. She has been married for 6 years and her two other children are aged 4 years and 18 months. She usually works as a receptionist. She had intended to breastfeed her baby; however, she suffered with mastitis and cracked nipples so started formula feeding 1 week ago.

She appears low in mood, is tearful and admits to having some difficulties coping with her three young children. She recalls having been treated for mild depression while she was in college in her late teens.

Learning outcomes

- You should be able to discuss the physiological changes that occur in the 6 weeks following childbirth.
- You should be able to perform a basic postnatal check-up and support new mums with breastfeeding.
- You should be able to identify women at risk of and/or developing postnatal depression.
- You should be aware of diagnosis and management of mastitis, secondary PPH and sepsis.

Essential Human Development, First Edition. Edited by Samuel Webster, Geraint Morris and Euan Kevelighan
© 2018 John Wiley & Sons, Ltd. Published 2018 by John Wiley & Sons, Ltd.

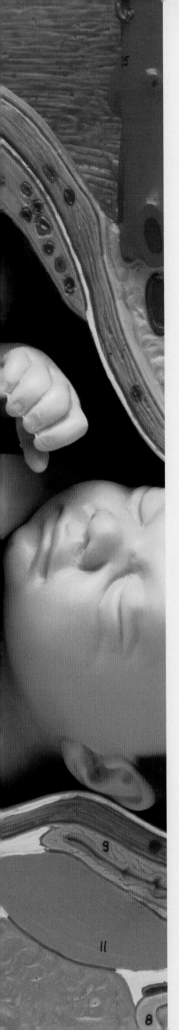

Physiological changes

Week 1

The uterus contracts almost immediately after delivery. Afterpains are common in the first 3–4 days following this. The lochia will initially be fresh red although quickly changes to old blood and eventually to a yellow-white discharge. The large expansion in blood volume should gradually reduce over the first week although the prothrombotic changes persist after this time.

Week 2

The uterus is usually back within the pelvis by around 14 days postnatally. The lochia persists for around 2–3 weeks and should reduce in quantity over that time. Glomerular filtration rate remains raised although significantly lower than initially postpartum.

Week 6

It takes around 6 weeks for the cardiovascular changes to entirely reverse. Therefore that is the time frame required for blood pressure and oedema to return to normal. The thrombotic changes of pregnancy are also reversed by this week.

Week 12

By now the physiological dilatation of the renal tract should have resolved. Alongside this the glomerular filtration rate will also have returned to normal.

Postnatal care

This should include a full examination and full blood count prior to discharge. Debriefing of the event should be performed by the person conducting the delivery. A postnatal appointment should be offered at 6 weeks if indicated. Adequate analgesia should be prescribed and this will vary with mode of delivery although often simple paracetamol and ibuprofen will suffice. The woman's risk of thrombosis should be assessed, and compression stockings and low molecular weight heparin prescribed as necessary.

Urine should be voided every 6 hours of urination during labour, and attempts made to encourage this if not, such as running a tap, while attempting to urinate. If no urine emerges within 6 hours of delivery the bladder volume should be formally assessed and catheterisation performed if necessary. Rhesus-negative women require anti-D within 72 hours of delivery. MMR immunisation should be offered if the woman was found to be seronegative for rubella during her antenatal period. Information should be provided on wound care, hand hygiene, pelvic floor exercises, contraceptive advice, information regarding the local breastfeeding group, and a physiotherapy referral made if indicated.

The woman should also be advised which symptoms warrant medical evaluation following her discharge. These would include increased blood loss, fainting, palpitations, fever, abdominal pain, headache and visual disturbance, shortness of breath, chest pain and unilateral leg symptoms. The risk of domestic abuse should be considered.

The UK's National Institute for Health and Care Excellence (NICE) guidance from 2006 requires each woman to have an individualised postnatal care plan.

Examination

The following aspects should be included in any postnatal examination:

Breasts – engorgement, discharge, erythema, temperature, abscess.
Abdomen – uterine size, tenderness, wound healing/discharge.
Perineum/vagina – uterine size, lochia, wound healing.
Legs – swelling, erythema, tenderness.
Chest/other areas as indicated.

Postnatal exercise

Early mobilisation is always promoted in order to reduce the risk of thrombotic events. Breathing exercises are particularly important in the postoperative patient.

Pelvic floor exercises are paramount. Written information regarding these should be given to all women on discharge and a physiotherapy referral may be indicated. This is particularly relevant if there has been an assisted delivery, prolonged labour, complex or extensive perineal trauma, or concerns regarding urinary or faecal continence.

Approximately one in five women will suffer with some degree of urinary incontinence postnatally. And it is important to exclude both urinary retention and fistula formation. All units should have a bladder care protocol, which should be followed in the postnatal period.

Fewer than 1 in 20 women will encounter faecal incontinence, and again a fistula needs to be excluded. This may be due to damage to either the anal sphincter itself or the pudendal nerve during delivery, most commonly caused by third or fourth degree tear and forceps delivery. Again the mainstay of treatment will be physiotherapy; however, surgical repair may be necessary.

If the mode of delivery was caesarean section then physical exercise should remain gentle for the first 6 weeks. Often as women are otherwise fit and healthy and often looking after a newborn in addition to other small children, they push themselves to do too much too soon. It is important to remind them that this is major abdominal surgery. They may gradually increase their activities towards normal levels by around 12 weeks. Core abdominal exercises should not be performed until any excessive deficit (>2 cm) in the rectus muscle has resolved, which may take several months.

Usual activities such as gentle walking can be resumed immediately as soon as the woman feels able, gradually building back up to her usual exercise levels over the coming weeks as her body allows.

Psychological wellbeing

Many women have an idealistic view of pregnancy and delivery and may find it difficult to cope if this is not the case. The birth of a child, however straightforward, is a life-changing event that has a huge psychological impact on any woman. It also adds a new dimension to the whole family dynamic.

The baby blues occur in around half of women and commonly occur on days 3–5. The woman may be tearful and feel overwhelmed and express symptoms of anxiety and depression. These are usually mild and short lasting and an entirely normal response to this emotional event; however, if they persist then a specialist opinion should be sought as approximately 10% of women will develop postnatal depression. Diagnosis can be difficult as normal emotional changes associated with the puerperium may be mistaken for symptoms of depression, or alternatively a woman displaying depressive symptoms may be dismissed as experiencing normal emotions. Failure to diagnose promptly can have a long-term detrimental effect on the mother-child relationship.

Once diagnosed, postnatal depression can usually be adequately treated with behavioural therapies and medication. If required the woman should ideally be seen for this within 1 month, but always within 3 months. Appropriate medications include selective serotonin reuptake inhibitors (SSRIs) or tricyclic antidepressants although in breastfeeding fluoxetine, citalopram and escitalopram should be avoided if possible in favour of medications such as sertraline and paroxetine. Lithium and clozapine do not have a role during breastfeeding. Alternative therapies such as St John's wort should not be used during pregnancy and breastfeeding. As with treatment of many conditions, the lowest effective dose should be used for the shortest possible time. If the woman exhibits any suicidal ideation, reduced function, symptoms persisting for over 6 weeks, panic attacks or obsessional thoughts, feelings of guilt or worthlessness then an urgent referral may become necessary. Specialist psychiatric input is desirable, and many regions have a perinatal mental health team equipped to deal with such cases.

Around 1 in 500 women will develop puerperal psychosis. This condition does have a familial element and specialist psychiatric input is imperative. Over half of cases will present in the first week and 90% by 12 weeks. The onset is usually sudden with a rapid deterioration. They usually present as a mixed-affective, schizophrenic or manic state with symptoms such as excessive anxiety, delusions, hallucinations and irrational thoughts. There may be an element of confusion, and symptoms are often not constant. A prolonged stay in a mother-and-baby unit may be necessary.

Women at increased risk are those with a previous history of significant psychiatric illness in addition to a lack of social support and poor relationship in addition to recent life events and those suffering with the baby blues. Primiparous women and those with delivery complications are also thought to be at increased risk. The risk of recurrence is around 20%; however, this may be reduced by a long inter-pregnancy interval.

In the last CEMACH (Confidential Enquiries into Maternal and Child Health) report 2006–2008 there were 29 deaths of women with associated psychiatric disorders. There were nine cases of suicide, three of drug misuse, 16 medical (including substance abuse) and one accident. The majority of these women were white, married, aged over 30 and employed. Those involved with substance misuse were more likely to be young, single and unemployed. However, it is important to remember that suicide risk is not always associated with a lower socioeconomic status and more than half of them will have had a previous psychiatric condition.

Rarely women will develop post-traumatic stress disorder. This is not limited to women who have had what healthcare professionals may deem a complex delivery. Women with no complications at all may still suffer this condition, and often something as simple as a delay in obtaining adequate analgesia may have a negative impact on the woman's perception of events. This is particularly common in women experiencing precipitate deliveries. There is no known medication suitable for treating this condition and it should be managed using behavioural therapies.

To reduce the risk of developing these conditions they should be screened for at 4–6 weeks postnatally and again at 3–4 months. The simple screening tool recommended is shown in Box 20.1.

Lactation and breastfeeding

The benefits of exclusive breastfeeding for the first 6 months of a baby's life were noted in 1984, when it was shown to be associated with a lower risk of neonatal death compared with other methods, in addition to a reduction of gastrointestinal and to a lesser degree respiratory infections and atopic conditions. The risk of sudden infant death syndrome is reduced, and there is some protection from chronic conditions such as obesity, diabetes mellitus, Crohn's disease and lymphoma. From

> **Box 20.1 Screening for postnatal depression**
>
> - During the past month have you often been bothered by feeling down, depressed or hopeless?
> - During the past month have you often been bothered by having little interest or pleasure in doing things?
>
> If answer is yes to either of these go on to ask:
> - Is this something you feel you need or want help with?

the maternal point of view it is known to reduce the risk of postpartum haemorrhage if it is immediate, and to reduce the risk of both ovarian and breast cancer in addition to osteoporosis risk reduction. It may delay the return of fertility: whilst the woman remains amenorrhoeic there is a pregnancy risk of only 2% in the first 6 months of exclusive breastfeeding. It may also help to accelerate her weight loss, and of course it promotes bonding with her newborn.

Breast milk is easily digested by the baby and provides an efficient energy source. As long as the mother is herself not deficient, with the exclusion of vitamin D, breast milk alone provides complete nutrition and allows adequate growth for the first 6 months of life. For adequate vitamin D sunlight exposure is required. If this is not likely then the World Health Organization (WHO) recommends that all babies and children under 5 years receive a supplement of vitamin D, although this is not required if a baby is taking over 500 mL of formula a day, or if breastfeeding mums took a vitamin D supplement during their pregnancy.

Physiology of breastfeeding

Lactation is stimulated following delivery by the rapid reduction in oestrogen levels coupled with the increase in prolactin and oxytocin. Prolactin is secreted from the anterior pituitary and results in increased milk production while oxytocin is secreted from the posterior pituitary and leads to milk ejection. Prolactin levels are high throughout the pregnancy, but milk is not produced due to the inhibition of prolactin by the high levels of oestrogen and progesterone. It is the rapid reduction of these following the delivery of the placenta that removes the blockade of the prolactin effect allowing milk production to commence (Figures 20.1 and 20.2).

Allowing the baby to suckle at the breast will further increase the prolactin levels resulting in the alveoli of the breast producing milk. It is said that the baby effectively orders its next meal by taking the current one as the prolactin levels will peak around 30 minutes after suckling commences. Therefore increased suckling leads to increased prolactin levels, in turn resulting in increased milk production, and this effect is critical for the establishment of breastfeeding and the reason

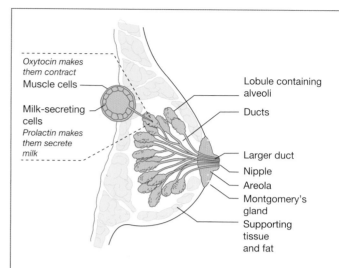

Figure 20.2 Hormonal effects on breast anatomy.

for unrestricted feeding to be recommended. Prolactin levels will remain elevated throughout feeding; however, after a few weeks there is less of a relationship between the quantity of prolactin and the quantity of milk produced. It is known that prolactin levels peak at night making night-time feeds important for maintaining supply and the raised prolactin levels will leave the mum feeling relaxed and sleepy.

Suckling will also stimulate the release of other pituitary hormones include gonadotrophin-releasing hormone (GnRH), follicle-stimulating hormone (FSH) and luteinising hormone (LH), and it is this that will suppress ovulation and therefore menstruation whilst exclusively breastfeeding, although this should not be relied upon for contraception.

The increased levels of oxytocin released will cause the myoepithelial cells surrounding the alveoli to contract causing the milk within the alveoli to flow along the duct resulting in milk ejection (see Figure 20.2). Oxytocin levels are altered more rapidly than those of prolactin. Milk ejection may also be triggered by emotional stimulus, such as the woman touching or simply seeing her baby. She may become aware of an active oxytocin reflex by a tingling sensation prior to or during a feed, by noticing milk flowing when she thinks of her baby

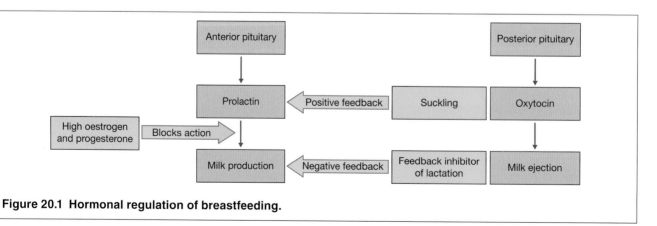

Figure 20.1 Hormonal regulation of breastfeeding.

or hears it cry. She may leak milk from the contralateral breast during feeding and notice continued milk ejection if the feed is interrupted. The baby will be seen to take slow, deep sucks with a pause for swallowing which may be audible and she may become thirsty during a feed. In the early days she may be aware of the uterus contracting and causing increased blood flow at this time. However, the absence of these signs does not mean that the reflex is not active, simply that she is not aware of it. Oxytocin release also allows her to feel a state of calm and reduced stress and assists in the bonding process.

Further control of milk supply is by a polypeptide known as feedback inhibitor of lactation. As the name suggests it prevents the production of more milk to prevent the breasts from becoming over-full. It is this that helps to regulate the rate of milk production according to how much the baby is taking and therefore how much it needs.

On average a woman's milk will 'come in' by approximately 48 hours. This may be later if delivery was by caesarean section, and can be encouraged by skin-to-skin contact between mother and baby and frequent unlimited suckling. This should not be painful, and if it is the positioning should be checked. It is often associated with around 24 hours of engorgement and discomfort. During this time simple analgesia, a non-underwired bra and use of a hot compress will help to relieve these symptoms.

Prior to this the breasts produce only small amounts of colostrum in response to suckling. This is rich in protein, white blood cells and antibodies, in particular IgA, and is more than adequate to sustain the baby over these first few days. Up to 40 mL of colostrum will be produced on day 1. By day 3 there is in the region of 300–400 mL being produced, and this increases to 500–800 mL by day 5. During the second week the milk is known as transitional and this becomes mature milk by the end of the second week.

Good attachment technique is the key to successful breastfeeding. As part of the baby-friendly initiative many units now have lactation advisors to assist women whilst in hospital and also when at home if required. This can be crucial to success particularly in an age where discharge home may be as early as 2 hours post-delivery. During feeding the baby's mouth should be wide open and contain the areola and more breast tissue below than above. Its bottom lip should be pursed outwards and it should be taking deep, long sucks with pauses for audible swallowing. The baby's cheeks should remain rounded, the chin should touch the breast whilst the nose remains free. Initially it may be uncomfortable as the baby latches on successfully although it should not be painful. Where feeding is successful the baby will have plentiful dirty nappies, the woman should be aware of the breasts softening and the nipple should be rounded and not misshapen by the end of the feed.

If feeding becomes painful she should be examined for signs of mastitis, commonly caused either by milk stasis or infection. Milk stasis occurs due to inefficient drainage of the breast, often caused by poor attachment or limiting feed lengths. Signs of mastitis include unilateral pain, erythema, a palpable lump, pyrexia and flu-like symptoms. A blocked duct may also present in a similar manner but without the pyrexia and systemic symptoms. Both are treated with continued feeding/expressing from the affected side and again a hot compress. If pyrexia is present prompt treatment with flucloxacillin or erythromycin should be commenced for 10–14 days. The woman may develop a localised abscess, which may respond to the same antibiotics; however, if this is extensive or there is little improvement with treatment a surgical review may be required.

Mastitis is most common in the second and third weeks postpartum, and over 75% of cases occur in the first 3 months although it could occur at any stage of feeding. If there is no response to treatment within the initial 12–24 hours then the woman should be referred for a medical review. There was one case of a death from mastitis-associated sepsis in the last triennial CEMACH report (2006-2008) and it may rarely be associated with necrotising fasciitis and toxic shock syndrome.

Secondary postpartum haemorrhage (PPH)

This is defined as excessive blood loss more than 24 hours after delivery. It is most commonly due to either retained products and/or infection. Therefore the treatment would be admission, observation, full examination and septic screen. Usually the uterus will be tender to palpate and the cervical os will be slightly open. Intravenous antibiotics should be administered. Imaging may be undertaken, and this may result in an evacuation of retained products of conception, which should ideally be performed during daytime hours (if the bleeding is not too excessive to warrant immediate surgery) and performed by the most senior obstetrician available. Any tissue obtained should be sent for histology in order to exclude choriocarcinoma.

Sepsis

The incidence of postoperative infection is around 8% and may take the form of endometritis, urinary tract infection or wound infection. Sepsis is the presence of infection with systemic signs and is defined as severe once there is associated organ dysfunction.

Signs and symptoms may include a marked pyrexia (above 38°C) or hypothermia, persistent tachycardia (above 90 bpm), tachypnoea (above 20 breaths/min), leucopenia, hypoxia, hypotension, oliguria, diarrhoea and vomiting, abdominal pain and impaired consciousness. However, the absence of these symptoms does not exclude the diagnosis.

Puerperal sepsis requires prompt diagnosis and treatment. Despite this it may rapidly become life threatening and it is not a condition to be overlooked in any postnatal woman presenting with a pyrexia. In fact deaths from sepsis had increased in the last triennial CEMACH report (2006–2008) with 14 of the 29 cases occurring after delivery (three after caesarean, eight after spontaneous vaginal delivery, one following miscarriage and two after terminations). Overall there are in the region of 10 maternal deaths a year as a result of sepsis. Once there is severe organ dysfunction the mortality rate is 20–40%, and this rapidly rises to 60% if septic shock is present. Severe sepsis requires a multidisciplinary approach with the involvement of physicians and microbiologists and may require admission to an intensive care unit. Barrier nursing should be undertaken.

The commonest site is the genital tract, specifically endometritis of the uterus. Other sites could include the breast, urinary tract, lung, skin and soft tissue, the gastrointestinal tract or pharynx.

Sepsis requires admission, observations, full septic screen including full blood count, urea and electrolytes, C-reactive protein (CRP), serum lactate, high and low vaginal swabs, blood culture, wound culture, urine culture, sputum culture and appropriate imaging as indicated. If the woman has a serum lactate above 4 mmol/L or significant hypotension then aggressive fluid replacement is also indicated. Facial oxygen may be given to maintain oxygen saturations, and in severe sepsis steroids may be required. Pain, pyrexia and a tachycardia in a postnatal woman should warrant intravenous antibiotics and a senior review.

The observations should be frequent and extensive – ideally recorded on a MEOWS (Modified Early Obstetric Warning System) chart including the respiratory rate – often omitted but crucial in the full assessment of the unwell patient. She will require broad-spectrum intravenous antibiotics according to local protocol – every hour of delay in administration is linked to increased mortality rates. In addition to this an urgent and regular senior review should be sought.

Overall management is therefore largely supportive with removal of the septic focus if possible and consideration of blood products and thromboprophylaxis as indicated.

Group A streptococcus (*Streptococcus pyogenes*) can easily be spread from the throat to the perineum as it is responsible for around 10% of pharyngitis cases. A careful history of recent illness or exposure to illness such as pharyngitis, impetigo and cellulitis should therefore be taken. If a woman with a sore throat has fever of greater than 38°C, tonsillar exudates (pus on the tonsils) and large cervical lymph nodes then antibiotics should be given.

Analgesia using non-steroidal anti-inflammatory drugs (NSAIDs) should be avoided as NSAIDs will hinder the polymorphs dealing with the group A streptococcus. Thirteen cases of maternal deaths in the CEMACH report of 2006–2008 were associated with this pathogen. Postnatal care in the community does not routinely include observations or examination; however, if a woman displays any symptoms suggestive of sepsis these should be performed as appropriate.

Other common pathogens include *Escherichia coli, Staphylococcus aureus, Streptococcus pneumoniae*, methicillin-resistant *Staphylococcus aureus, Clostridium septicum* and *Morganella morganii*. Pain out of proportion to the signs and symptoms may suggest a deep-seated infection and warrants consideration of necrotising enterocolitis (NEC) and myositis.

Severe sepsis in the postnatal woman remains a rare event, therefore many healthcare workers have a low index of suspicion. The signs can be generalised and non-specific and a woman can deteriorate very rapidly. It is therefore crucial to consider this diagnosis in patients that present.

Thrombotic conditions

The prothrombotic changes of pregnancy persist for several weeks following delivery and although the majority of these events occur antenatally the greatest risk is actually during the puerperium.

The CEMACH report of 2006–2008 contains eight cases of fatal pulmonary emboli. Six cases were after caesarean section and two following spontaneous vaginal delivery (SVD). Many units will have their own local guidance regarding the postnatal prescription of low molecular weight heparins (LMWH), and it is therefore important that these are adhered to. The current guidance from the Royal College of Obstetricians and Gynaecologists (RCOG) suggests that high-risk women require treatment for 7 days with LMWH and compression stockings, and this should be continued for longer if there are ongoing risk factors. Of course this should only be administered in the absence of any contraindications such as active bleeding, bleeding tendency such as haemophilia, thrombocytopenia, acute stroke within the last month, severe renal or liver disease, and uncontrolled hypertension.

High-risk women would include those with two or more persisting risk factors, a body mass index above 40, having undergone an emergency caesarean (class I, II or III) or an elective caesarean with one other risk factor. Also those with an inherited thrombophilia, previous thrombotic event and those receiving antenatal LMWH should be given a 6-week course of LMWH postnatally. After this time the risk of a fatal PE is minimal.

Risk factors for a thrombotic event include previous deep vein thrombosis (DVT), inherited or acquired thrombophilia, medical comorbidities, age over 35, obesity (BMI >30 in pre/early pregnancy), parity of three or above, smoking, paraplegia or significant varicose veins. Obstetric risk factors include multiple pregnancy and assisted reproductive therapies, pre-eclampsia, caesarean section, postpartum haemorrhage of over 1 litre requiring transfusion, and prolonged labour with mid-cavity rotational delivery. New-onset potentially reversible risk factors could include surgery in the puerperium, admission and immobility, long-distance travel over 4 hours and systemic infection requiring admission.

Peripartum cardiomyopathy

Although peripartum cardiomyopathy is very rare, any woman presenting within 6 months of delivery with breathlessness, oedema or orthopnoea and signs of tachypnoea or tachycardia should undergo a chest X-ray and echocardiogram in order to rule out this condition.

Clinical case

Case study

The woman's full blood count and thyroid function tests are normal. She is commenced on a small dose of citalopram. She is reviewed again in 2 weeks and appears stable. She joins a local support group for women with postnatal depression. Her husband is very supportive and her mother arranges to help her with the care of the two older children 2 days a week. She is referred for cognitive therapies and within 1 year is medication free and remains under regular review.

Key learning points

- Complications may arise in the postpartum period – it is important to look for and treat sepsis, postpartum haemorrhage and mastitis promptly.

- Postnatal depression is relatively common and has a high recurrence rate in subsequent pregnancies.

 Now visit **www.wileyessential.com/humandevelopment** to test yourself on this chapter.

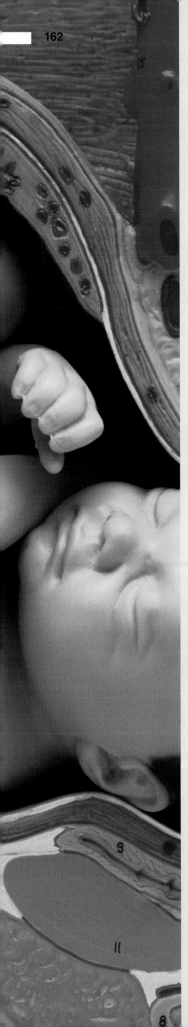

CHAPTER 21
Obstetric emergencies

Benjamin Chisholme and Euan Kevelighan

Case

A 40-year-old woman with two previous vaginal deliveries and three caesarean sections presents to the labour ward at 31 weeks with a massive antepartum haemorrhage. A 20-week booking scan had shown a low-lying placenta. On examination her pulse is 120 bpm and blood pressure 80/40 mmHg. Oxygen saturation is 87% in air. She is tachypnoeic at 26 breaths per minute. There is at least 2500 mL blood on bedsheets.

The ST2 in obstetrics summons help asking for the obstetric registrar and consultant, anaesthetists and senior paediatrician. Resuscitation is commenced following A, B, C – the ST2 provides the patient with oxygen via a facemask at a flow rate of 15 L/min. The patient is conscious and able to communicate but a little agitated.

The ST2 inserts two wide-bore (grey or orange) Venflons® and takes blood for full blood count, urea and electrolytes, clotting screen, group and cross-matching of six units initially, liver function tests and blood glucose. One litre of Hartmann's crystalloid is infused rapidly through each cannula and two units of O-negative blood, which is stored in the labour ward fridge. The abdomen is soft and fetal heart is present at 80 bpm.

The major haemorrhage protocol is instituted involving consultant haematologist, transfusion laboratory and porters to take blood samples and retrieve blood from laboratory. What would you do next?

Learning outcomes

- You should be able to describe how to respond to an obstetric emergency and outline the underlying principles involved.

- You should be able to describe the common causes of obstetric emergencies.

- You should be able to recognise complications of pregnancy and labour, and recommend appropriate investigations and management.

Initial management of obstetric emergencies

Obstetric emergencies may arise with little or no warning and are frightening and stressful for all involved. A well-rehearsed, systematic approach and effective teamwork are essential in what may be a chaotic and emotionally charged situation.

Priority must be given by the obstetric team to the stabilisation of the mother, on whom the fetus is physiologically dependent. This chapter provides an overview of the most common obstetric emergencies other than pre-eclampsia, which is dealt with in Chapter 11.

Approach to obstetric emergencies

As with any medical emergency an ABC approach is used, with some modifications to take pregnancy into account (Box 21.1).

Resuscitation

Cardiopulmonary resuscitation is difficult and less effective in pregnancy. A pregnant woman's oxygen requirement is increased, her airway is compromised by laryngeal oedema and her diaphragm splinted by the uterus. Reduced gastric emptying and relaxation of the lower oesophageal sphincter increase the risk of aspiration pneumonitis. These problems are compounded by obesity and the presence of the gravid uterus. In addition to its high demand on the circulation, the gravid uterus compresses the inferior vena cava and reduces maternal cardiac output from as early as 20 weeks gestation and by up to 70% at term. This can be relieved by tilting the woman 30° to her left using pillows, a wedge or the rescuer's knees. Alternatively, the uterus is displaced manually to the left and towards the woman's head.

If the woman remains collapsed after 4 minutes of CPR, perimortem caesarean section should be performed. This may need to be done in non-sterile conditions with minimal equipment but can be lifesaving for the woman by improving maternal venous return.

Training in the management of obstetric emergencies is available from a number of organisations. ALSO® (Advanced Life Support in Obstetrics – http://www.aafp.org) and PROMPT (PRactical Obstetric Multi-Professional Training – http://www.promptmaternity.org/) provide regular sessions around the UK. Maternity units should also run their own regular 'skills-and-drills' refresher sessions for their multidisciplinary team.

Causes of maternal collapse

Maternal collapse is defined as 'severe respiratory or circulatory distress that may lead to a sudden change in level of consciousness or cardiac arrest if untreated'. It may occur in pregnancy, during labour or in the puerperium and may have non-obstetric causes (Figure 21.1). For example, cardiac disease is the leading indirect cause of maternal death and may only become apparent when the cardiovascular system is subjected to the physiological demands of pregnancy.

Immediate help should be sought if there is evidence of maternal compromise including:

- an obstructed airway;
- respiratory rate <5 or >35 breaths per minute;
- pulse rate <40 or >140 bpm;
- systolic blood pressure <80 mmHg or >180 mmHg;
- sudden reduction of level of consciousness, unresponsiveness or seizure.

Modified Early Obstetric Warning Scores (MEOWS) may help recognise women at risk before they reach the point of collapse. Pulse rate, blood pressure, temperature, respiratory rate, oxygen saturation and level of consciousness are measured and combined to calculate a numerical score and determine the intervention required. Bedside MEOWS charts are helpful only if used correctly. It is insufficient to simply chart deterioration without summoning help when indicated (Figure 21.2).

Box 21.1 The ABC approach to an obstetric emergency

If the woman is unresponsive CALL FOR HELP using the local system for summoning the obstetric emergency team. This team should include a senior midwife, obstetrician, anaesthetist, neonatologist and someone to act as a scribe to record events. Position the woman in a 30° left lateral tilt, or shift the uterus to the left, to reduce aorto-caval compression and increase maternal venous return.
   Assess:
- AIRWAY – Give high-flow oxygen and maintain airway with chin-lift if necessary.
- BREATHING – Look, listen and feel for respiratory effort for 10 seconds.

- CIRCULATION – Assess pulse, skin tone and perfusion by checking capillary refill.
If there is no sign of life, start CPR following the basic life support (BLS) algorithm until help arrives.

   Simultaneously, place two wide-bore cannulas and obtain blood for full blood count, group and save, coagulation screen, liver function, urea and electrolytes, glucose and lactate. If sepsis is suspected, obtain blood for culture. Record all vital signs. If there is bleeding request at least four units of blood to be cross-matched. Give intravenous fluid resuscitation (with caution if the patient is hypertensive or eclamptic).

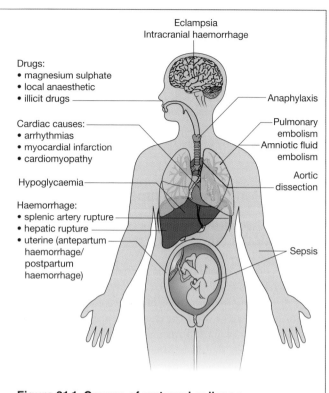

Figure 21.1 Causes of maternal collapse.

Massive obstetric haemorrhage

Massive obstetric haemorrhage may be defined as blood loss of greater than 1500 mL with resulting hypotension and tachycardia, requiring transfusion of four or more units of blood with a fall in haemoglobin greater than 40 g/L. It may occur antepartum (between 24 weeks gestation and labour), intrapartum (between the onset of labour and completion of delivery) or postpartum.

Postpartum haemorrhage (PPH) is the most common presentation and is a leading cause of maternal death worldwide. It is further divided into primary PPH, which is blood loss of more than 500 mL within 24 hours of delivery, and secondary PPH, which is defined as a blood loss of more than 500 mL between 24 hours and 12 weeks after delivery. Secondary PPH is usually caused by infection.

The physiological changes of pregnancy such as increased cardiac output, plasma volume expansion, increased red cell mass and increased production of clotting factors enable healthy women to compensate for blood loss. A significant amount of circulating volume may be lost before the signs of hypovolaemia develop. Large volumes of blood may also be sequestered in the uterus or abdomen, so haemorrhage may not be immediately visible and women may appear clinically well before deteriorating rapidly.

Management

Call for help and follow the ABC approach. Cross-match four units of blood. Follow the local obstetric haemorrhage protocol, which should involve a senior obstetrician, midwife and haematologist.

Determine which of the four Ts (poor uterine tone, trauma, retained placental tissue or poor clotting) may be responsible for bleeding (Box 21.2). Palpate the uterus for tone and remove clots to enable contraction. Emptying the bladder also helps the uterus contract into the pelvis. Ensure the placenta was delivered complete. Suture any bleeding points in the vagina or cervix.

If there is massive haemorrhage, clotting factors, fibrinogen and platelets may be exhausted or diluted by the administration of intravenous fluids. Disseminated intravascular coagulopathy (DIC) may occur leading to uncontrollable bleeding and death. As blood transfusion replaces only red cells, it may be necessary to give platelets, fibrinogen and

---

Box 21.2 Causes of obstetric haemorrhage may be categorised as the 'Four Ts'

Tone

Poor uterine tone results in failure to contract (atony) and close the spiral arteries in the placental bed. Uterine atony is the most common cause of haemorrhage.

It is associated with prolonged labour, babies weighing over 4 kg, multiple pregnancy, maternal obesity and maternal age greater than 40 years.

Trauma

Caesarean section, episiotomy, operative vaginal delivery using forceps or suction extraction and babies weighing more than 4 kg may all result in trauma to the cervix, vagina and perineum or internal structures such as the uterus and broad ligaments.

Tissue

Bleeding may occur if the placenta is retained (>30 minutes after oxytocin injection). Retained placental fragments remain attached and continue to bleed causing primary or secondary haemorrhage. It is vital to examine the placenta after delivery to ensure it is intact.

Thrombin

Haemorrhage or pre-eclampsia causes consumption of platelets and clotting factors.

Disseminated intravascular coagulopathy (DIC) can develop resulting in uncontrollable, spontaneous bleeding. Blood components are replaced with advice from a haematologist.

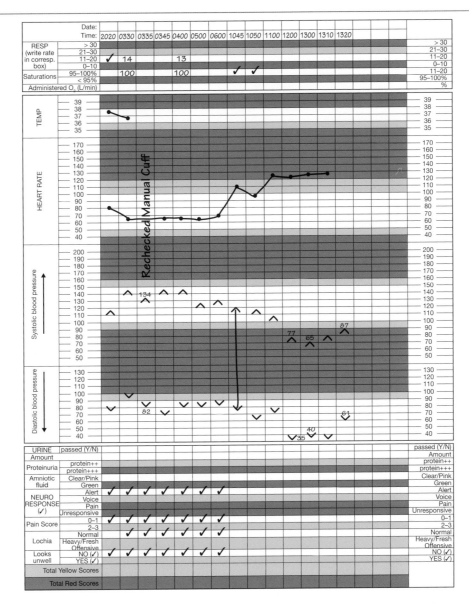

Figure 21.2 A poorly completed Modified Early Obstetric Warning Scores (MEOWS) chart. Few parameters were recorded and the score was not calculated. The patient, who had internal bleeding, had hypotension and tachycardia for more than an hour before help was summoned.

clotting factors as either fresh frozen plasma or cryoprecipitate. In pregnancy, fibrinogen levels are naturally raised; a low fibrinogen level in the presence of bleeding is an ominous sign.

The first and simplest measure to stop bleeding due to atony is to vigorously massage the uterus to encourage contraction. If this fails, use bimanual compression of the uterus (Figure 21.3).

Uterotonic drugs are given following delivery to increase uterine contractions that help to close the spiral arteries in the placental bed and reduce haemorrhage.

Synthetic oxytocin (Syntocinon®) is usually given intramuscularly in the third stage of labour to encourage uterine contraction and prompt delivery of the placenta. If there are risk factors for PPH, it may be followed with a continuous infusion. Its side effects include hypotension and fluid retention.

Ergometrine can be given intravenously or intramuscularly, sometimes in combination with oxytocin (as Syntometrine®). The mechanism of action of ergometrine is unclear, but it causes strong contractions in a relaxed uterus. Its side effects include nausea and vomiting. It is also a vasoconstrictor so should be avoided in women with pre-eclampsia or hypertension.

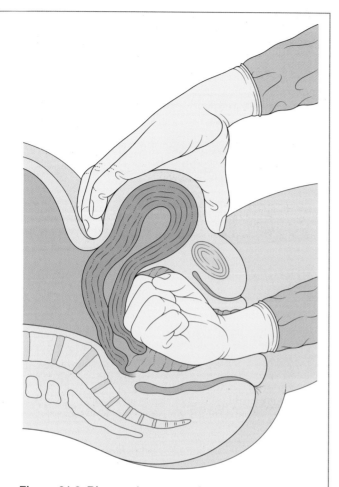

Figure 21.3 Bimanual compression.

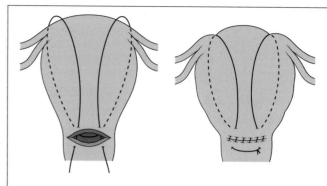

Figure 21.4 B-Lynch suture.

Emergency hysterectomy can be life-saving in a case of very severe haemorrhage but is considered to be a last resort.

Venous thromboembolism

Until relatively recently venous thromboembolism (VTE) was the leading direct cause of maternal death in the UK. It is now third, behind sepsis and eclampsia/pre-eclampsia, and is responsible for 0.79 deaths per 100 000 maternities. This improvement is probably due to greater awareness of VTE, better identification of women at risk and the use of thromboprophylaxis.

Pathophysiology

Pregnancy is a naturally prothrombotic state that probably evolved to prevent haemorrhage during childbirth. Considering Virchow's triad of factors that contribute to thrombosis, there is **hypercoaguability** due to an increased production of clotting factors, and the potential for **stasis** of blood due to reduced mobility and compression by the gravid uterus of the pelvic vessels. Should sepsis, pre-eclampsia or trauma intervene, the third factor, **endothelial dysfunction**, becomes present.

In addition, other interventions and disorders during pregnancy may increase the risk; hyperemesis in early pregnancy causes dehydration, caesarean section reduces mobility and causes endothelial injury, and antiphospholipid syndrome results in hypercoaguability.

Symptoms

While a degree of swelling in the lower limbs is often normal in later pregnancy, deep vein thrombosis (DVT) is suggested by calf pain, swelling, ankle oedema, localised redness, increased temperature of the affected leg or engorged superficial veins. Compression of the pelvic veins may produce thrombi in the iliofemoral veins presenting with low abdominal pain or thigh pain. DVT may present with few symptoms, or remain

If there is no response, the prostaglandin F2α analogue carboprost (Hemabate®) may be used. PGF2α provokes uterine contractions but it is contraindicated in pelvic infection, severe cardiac, renal, hepatic and pulmonary disease, and may cause vomiting, flushing and bronchospasm. It must be used with caution in asthmatics. As a rule of thumb, if a patient is still bleeding and a second dose of carboprost is being considered, she should be prepared for theatre and possible surgical management.

Surgical options include examination of the uterus and cervix under anaesthetic, along with evacuation or repair of any bleeding points. Uterine packing or the placement of a saline-filled tamponade device such as the Bakri balloon may be considered. Opening the abdomen and placing a B-Lynch suture to compress the uterus is an approach that may stop uterine bleeding (Figure 21.4).

Where facilities and expertise exist, the uterine or internal iliac arteries can be occluded by the placement under radiological guidance of intravascular balloons or sponges. This technique is known as uterine artery embolisation.

ⓘ Risk factors 21.1 Venous thromboembolism

Pre-existing
- Previous venous thromboembolism

Heritable thrombophilia:
- Antithrombin deficiency
- Protein C deficiency
- Protein S deficiency
- Factor V Leiden
- Prothrombin gene G20210A

Acquired (antiphospholipid syndrome)
- Persistent lupus anticoagulant
- Persistent moderate/high-titre anticardiolipin antibodies or β2 glycoprotein 1 antibodies
- Medical comorbidities (e.g. heart or lung disease, systemic lupus erythematosus, cancer, inflammatory conditions, nephrotic syndrome, sickle-cell disease, intravenous drug use)
- Age >35 years
- Obesity (BMI >30 kg/m²) either pre-pregnancy or in early pregnancy
- Parity ≥3

- Smoking
- Gross varicose veins
- Paraplegia

Obstetric
- Multiple pregnancy, assisted reproductive therapy
- Pre-eclampsia
- Caesarean section
- Prolonged labour, mid-cavity rotational operative delivery
- PPH (>1 litre) requiring transfusion

New-onset/transient
- Surgical procedure in pregnancy or puerperium

Potentially reversible
- Hyperemesis, dehydration
- Ovarian hyperstimulation syndrome
- Admission or immobility (≥3 days)
- Systemic infection
- Long-distance travel (>4 hours)

---

occult until it embolises to the pulmonary artery resulting in pulmonary embolism (PE).

Pulmonary embolism should be suspected if a woman complains of any sudden-onset shortness of breath. Other symptoms, such as pleuritic chest pain or haemoptysis, may develop later. Rarely, massive pulmonary emboli may occur presenting with severe pain, hypotension, tachycardia, syncope or collapse, and death.

Prevention of VTE

The Royal College of Obstetricians and Gynaecologists in the UK has published comprehensive guidelines for prevention and treatment of venous thromboembolism in pregnancy and the puerperium. It recommends that all pregnant women should be offered a risk assessment to determine the level of intervention required. Those at high risk may be offered prophylactic low molecular weight heparin (LMWH) throughout pregnancy and for 6 weeks following delivery. LMWH may be considered for those at intermediate risk, while for those at lower risk mobilisation and good hydration may be all that is required.

LMWH does not cross the placenta and is considered safe in pregnancy. Warfarin is teratogenic in the first trimester and should be avoided in late pregnancy due to the risk of fetal, neonatal or maternal haemorrhage. Women already taking warfarin may need continued anticoagulation treatment with

heparin instead. All anticoagulants should be stopped and reviewed if there is vaginal bleeding or signs of labour.

Investigation and management of deep vein thrombosis (DVT)

Where there is strong suspicion of DVT anticoagulation with LMWH should be offered until the diagnosis is excluded, preferably by using Doppler ultrasound. Magnetic resonance imaging or conventional contrast venography may be required to exclude iliac vein thrombosis.

If no thrombus is found treatment should be stopped. If the symptoms and clinical suspicion of DVT persist anticoagulation should be continued and investigations repeated a week later. Measurement of D-dimer, a product of fibrin degradation that may rise in DVT, is not a recommended diagnostic factor in this case as it may rise naturally in pregnancy.

If DVT is confirmed anticoagulation with LMWH should be offered and may be converted to warfarin postnatally. Mothers may breastfeed while taking heparin or warfarin.

Investigation and management of suspected pulmonary embolism (PE)

Pulmonary embolism must be considered as a possible cause of any sudden-onset shortness of breath or maternal collapse. The ABC approach to resuscitation should be followed.

The patient may also be tachycardic and have a raised jugular venous pressure. An electrocardiogram may reveal the $S_1Q_3T_3$ pattern of right heart strain sometimes seen in PE, but this is non-specific and may be seen in normal pregnancy. Echocardiography may reveal pulmonary hypertension.

Arterial blood gas sampling may reveal hypoxia (reduced P_aO_2) due to reduced perfusion of the lung supplied by the occluded artery, and reduced P_aCO_2 as a result of acidosis and hyperventilation.

A chest X-ray can be helpful to exclude other causes of the patient's symptoms such as pneumothorax or pneumonia. The patient can be reassured that chest X-rays are not thought to be harmful to the fetus at any stage of pregnancy. X-ray features of pulmonary emboli include effusion, atelectasis and wedge-shaped infarcts but films may also appear normal.

Doppler scanning of the legs is performed if a DVT is suspected. If DVT is diagnosed, the patient is offered anticoagulation with LMWH, which is the same treatment regimen for pulmonary embolus and may avoid the radiation exposure associated with further investigations such as ventilation/perfusion lung (*V/Q*) scanning and computed tomography pulmonary angiography (CTPA). If *V/Q* scanning or CTPA are required, women should be counselled of the slightly increased risks that these tests pose for childhood cancer in the fetus and breast cancer in the mother, respectively.

Massive, life-threatening pulmonary embolism is treated with intravenous unfractionated heparin, medical thrombolysis or surgical embolectomy.

Shoulder dystocia

Shoulder dystocia describes an inability of the fetus's shoulders to pass through the birth canal after the head has emerged (Figure 21.5). It is an obstetric emergency. It is diagnosed when vaginal cephalic delivery requires additional manoeuvres to deliver the baby when gentle traction has failed; it is a rare but serious complication affecting less than 0.7% of deliveries. Usually the anterior shoulder is impacted against the pubic symphysis. Rarely the posterior shoulder impacts against the sacral promontory.

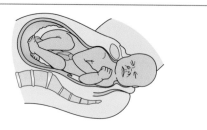

Figure 21.5 Shoulder dystocia.

Pathophysiology

Shoulder dystocia results from impaction of the fetal shoulder against the maternal symphysis pubis. The risk factors for shoulder dystocia are associated with large babies, or those with shoulders wider than the diameter of the maternal pelvis that they are attempting to pass through. Previous shoulder dystocia is associated with recurrence rates of between 3.7 and 12% although the true risk may in fact be higher as women may be offered caesarean section in subsequent pregnancies. Other risk factors include fetal macrosomia, maternal diabetes, maternal obesity, prolonged or augmented labour, and instrumental delivery

Most cases occur with no identifiable risk factors so birth attendants should be vigilant for shoulder dystocia during any delivery.

Complications

Traction on the baby's head should be gentle and axial. If excessive traction, particularly downward, is applied during shoulder dystocia the brachial plexus may be injured resulting in Erb's palsy (see Chapter 22). While 65–90% of Erb's palsies resolve, some are permanent. During a traumatic delivery the baby may also suffer fractures to the clavicle or humerus, hypoxic brain injury, acidosis or intrapartum death. Mothers may suffer perineal injury, haemorrhage and psychological trauma.

Management

Shoulder dystocia is an emergency; the multidisciplinary obstetric emergency team, including a neonatologist, should be called immediately. The mother should stop pushing to prevent further impaction of the shoulders in the maternal pelvis. Never apply pressure to the uterine fundus.

External manoeuvres are attempted first. The simplest is to place the mother in McRoberts' position, lying prone with hips flexed onto the chest by two assistants. This increases the relative anterior-posterior diameter of the maternal pelvis to help the fetal shoulders pass. Normal axial traction is applied to attempt to deliver the fetal head. Downward, lateral pressure on the mother's suprapubic area, from the direction of the fetal back (Rubin 1 manoeuvre), augments the effect of McRoberts' position by reducing the distance between the fetal shoulders.

If external manoeuvres fail, internal manoeuvres are attempted. These include:
- Exerting pressure on the posterior aspect of the anterior shoulder to rotate shoulders into the wider oblique or transverse diameters (Rubin 2).
- If unsuccessful Rubin 2 may be combined with wood screw – pressure on the anterior surface of the posterior shoulder: the aim is to rotate the shoulders through 180 degrees.

Box 21.3 To remember shoulder dystocia management think 'HELPERR'

Do not spend more than 30 seconds on each manoeuvre:
- H = call for help – midwives, senior obstetrician, neonatologist and anaesthetist.
- E = (evaluate for) episiotomy – may need this for internal manoeuvres.
- L = legs into McRoberts' position – hyperflexion of hips and abduction of thighs.
- P = suprapubic pressure to posterior aspect of anterior shoulder. Can be continuous pressure or rocking movements (like CPR).
- E = enter pelvis – perform internal manoeuvres.
- R = Roll over onto 'all fours' (Gaskin manoeuvre). This increases the anteroposterior diameter of pelvis and facilitates other manoeuvres.
- R = Repeat manoeuvres

- If this fails try a reverse Woods' screw – rotate in the opposite direction to the Woods' screw. If successful the shoulders will rotate up to 180 degrees and deliver.
- Remove the posterior arm and shoulder. The obstetrician inserts a hand and sweeps the posterior fetal arm across the fetal chest and face releasing the posterior shoulder.

Attempting to replace the fetal head in the birth canal (Zavanelli's manoeuvre) and performing a caesarean section, or surgically dividing the mother's pubic symphysis to open the pelvis, are both measures of last resort.

Cord prolapse

Cord prolapse is rare, with an incidence of 0.1–0.6%. It occurs when the umbilical cord emerges from the cervix alongside or beneath the presenting part of the fetus. The cord may be compressed or occluded by spasm due to handling or contact with air. The fetal blood supply is then compromised leading to fetal distress, disability or stillbirth if the baby is not delivered immediately. By identifying umbilical cord presentation before the membranes are ruptured and avoiding vaginal delivery, cord prolapse may be prevented. However, many cases of cord prolapse occur following spontaneous rupture of fetal membranes before the head has engaged in pelvis. Routine vaginal examinations during labour should include palpation for the cord.

There are many risk factors for cord prolapse that make it more likely that the cord is delivered before the fetus. For example, a cord suspended freely in excess fluid around a small baby whose head is not engaged is likely to be expelled with the fluid when the membranes are ruptured. Cord or placental abnormalities also increase the risk.

Management

Call for help. Elevate the presenting part of the fetus and keep it there to relieve cord compression. Placing the mother in the Trendelenburg position (head down), or on all fours, and filling the maternal bladder with warm saline may also be helpful. If at home, the mother must be transferred to hospital immediately and supportive measures continued on the way. The fetal heart rate must be monitored. No attempt should be made to replace the cord above the presenting part, and handling should be minimised to prevent vasospasm.

The mode of delivery depends on an assessment of the cervix and the position and station of the fetal head. An operative vaginal delivery may be performed if the situation is favourable and it is likely to be achieved rapidly. At anything less than full cervical dilatation an emergency caesarean section is performed.

Amniotic fluid embolism

Amniotic fluid embolism (AFE) can evolve with remarkable speed. It shares many of the features of anaphylaxis, pulmonary embolism, severe sepsis and acute cardiac events. It is the fourth leading direct cause of maternal death, with an incidence of 1.9 per 100 000 maternities in the UK. Previously regarded as almost always fatal, more recent fatality rates of

---

⊘ Risk factors 21.2 Cord prolapse

General
- Multiparity
- Birth weight <2.5 kg
- Prematurity (<37 weeks)
- Fetal anomaly
- Breech presentation
- Transverse, oblique or unstable lie
- Second twin
- Polyhydramnios
- Unengaged presenting part
- Low-lying/abnormal placenta

Procedure-related
- Artificial rupture of membranes
- Manipulation of fetus after rupture of membranes
- During external cephalic version of a breech baby

> **⚠ Risk factors 21.3 Amniotic fluid embolism**
>
> - Maternal age >35
> - Placenta praevia
> - Placental abruption
> - Caesarean section
> - Instrumental delivery
> - Pre-eclampsia

15–30% have been reported, perhaps due to improved recognition and management.

Pathophysiology

The entry of amniotic fluid into the maternal circulation can occur at any time between the onset of labour to a few hours postpartum, although deaths have been attributed to AFE during surgical termination of pregnancy, caesarean section and following abdominal trauma. Typically, the patient becomes clammy, hypotensive, dyspnoeic and cyanosed. Seizures, cardiac arrest and disseminated intravascular coagulopathy (DIC) may follow. Pulmonary vasospasm in response to amniotic fluid may cause acute right-sided heart failure followed by left ventricular failure and pulmonary oedema.

Traditionally, it was assumed that fluid containing fetal squames such as vernix or hair embolised to the maternal pulmonary circulation in a manner similar to a blood clot in a pulmonary embolism. Subsequently, an immune-mediated mechanism has been proposed given that AFE shares some features of sepsis and anaphylaxis. This suggests AFE causes an anaphylactoid response to substances present in amniotic fluid including platelet-activating factor, cytokines, bradykinin and arachidonic acid. The precise mechanism remains unknown.

Management

There is no diagnostic test for AFE and it is difficult to differentiate from other causes of sudden maternal collapse. Treatment is supportive and involves maintaining maternal circulation and oxygenation, and addressing any coagulopathy by replacing depleted blood components. This requires expert advice from a haematologist. While no specific therapies improve survival, immediate resuscitation and supportive care, including the management of DIC, are essential. If the fetus remains in utero, immediate caesarean section is usually required to optimise maternal resuscitation.

Uterine inversion

Uterine inversion occurs when the uterus turns inside out during or after delivery The inversion can be minor or complete. It is rare, occurring in approximately 1 in 3500 vaginal deliveries

and even less frequently during caesarean section. It is more common in developing countries, possibly because deliveries are more likely to be managed by untrained birth attendants. Uterine inversion usually presents with haemorrhage, with or without shock. There may be abdominal pain or a vaginal mass, and the uterus may not be palpable abdominally. Hypotension may be disproportionate to blood loss due to neurogenic bradycardia, which may lead to cardiac arrest.

Pathophysiology

A number of risk factors are associated with uterine inversion, including an atonic uterus, a morbidly adherent placenta, manual removal of the placenta, precipitate labour, a short umbilical cord, placenta praevia and some connective tissue disorders.

The severity of a uterine inversion can be identified. In the first degree the inverted fundus reaches the cervical ring, in the second degree it passes through the cervical ring but remains in the vagina, in the third degree the fundus extends to the introitus, and in the fourth degree both the uterus and vagina are inverted.

Management

The collapsed patient will require resuscitation while the uterus is replaced, either manually or by using hydrostatic pressure and insufflating the vagina with warm saline (O'Sullivan's technique). Replacement should be performed promptly to prevent the uterus becoming oedematous. To avoid further haemorrhage, the placenta should not be removed until the uterus is replaced.

Fetal distress in the second twin

Approximately 16 women per 1000 had a multiple birth in the UK in 2011, and the rate has risen sharply since 1980 with the more widespread use of assisted reproduction.

Although many clinicians offer caesarean section for monochorionic twins, monochorionic and diamniotic twins may be delivered vaginally unless there are clinical reasons for caesarean section, such as a breech presentation or a previous uterine scar. Elective caesarean section poses risks to the mother, and does not reduce the risk of fetal/neonatal death or morbidity compared to planned vaginal delivery.

Risks to the second twin

Obstetric complications including malpresentation, cord prolapse and postpartum haemorrhage are more common in twin pregnancies. The risks are greater for the second twin, whose cord blood gases deteriorate more rapidly probably due to impaired placental function after delivery of the first twin. Typically, the second twin is delivered within 30 minutes of the first.

Second twins delivered vaginally at term have an increased risk of death, particularly due to intrapartum anoxia. Elective birth at 36–37 weeks is therefore recommended as it reduces the risk of serious adverse outcomes for the infant.

Pathophysiology

The most common causes of distress during delivery of the second twin are placental abruption, umbilical cord prolapse or tetanic contraction of the uterus. The second twin must be delivered by the quickest possible route.

Management

The obstetric emergency team should be called and the patient prepared for emergency delivery by obtaining good intravenous access, blood for grouping and saving, and following the ABC approach.

If the second twin has a cephalic presentation instrumental vaginal delivery may be attempted, although vacuum extraction (e.g. ventouse, or Kiwi devices) should not be used before 34 weeks gestation.

A breech presentation may be delivered vaginally by reaching into the uterus and grasping the feet. A second twin in a transverse lie may be turned by external manipulation (external cephalic version) or by reaching in for one or both feet and converting it to a breech presentation (internal podalic version).

If sufficient expertise to perform these manoeuvres is not available, or attempts fail, the second twin should be delivered immediately by caesarean section.

Clinical case

Case management

The patient is transferred urgently to theatre and delivered by emergency caesarean section. A live baby boy weighing 1.5 kg and in poor condition is resuscitated by paediatricians and transferred to the neonatal intensive care unit.

The patient continues to bleed due to uterine atony. Uterotonics are given including 10 IU oxytocin i.v., ergometrine 500 µg i.v. and carboprost 250 µg i.m. repeated every 15 minutes (maximum of eight doses). An oxytocin infusion of 40 IU in 500 mL of saline is also commenced. Despite these measures the bleeding persists and a B-Lynch suture is considered. Despite compression of the uterus the post-partum haemorrhage persists and the patient is haemodynamically unstable. The consultant haematologist provides advice via telephone including transfusion with packed red cells, fresh frozen plasma and cryoprecipitate. Due to the extent of the blood loss the patient develops disseminated intravascular coagulation (DIC) with deranged clotting. The consultant obstetrician performs a hysterectomy in order to save the woman's life. Fortunately this stops the bleeding and further transfusion of blood, fresh frozen plasma (containing clotting factors) and platelets correct the DIC. The patient is transferred to the intensive treatment unit and extubated later the same day.

Case conclusions

The following day the patient is transferred back to a high-dependency unit on labour ward. She makes an excellent recovery. Her baby boy progresses well on the neonatal unit and is discharged home at 35 weeks, that is, 4 weeks post-delivery.

This patient had a life-threatening haemorrhage – her risk factors were low-lying placenta (placenta praevia) and multiple previous births (this was her sixth baby), both of which predispose to PPH and uterine atony. It is sometimes said in obstetrics that 'it is the APH that weakens and the PPH that kills'. It is important to perform hysterectomy before the patient becomes moribund.

Key learning points

- Obstetric emergencies often occur without prior warning.
- A structured approach following A, B and C of resuscitation (airway, breathing and circulation) is strongly recommended.
- Regular simulation practice via skills and drills in a multidisciplinary setting (midwives, anaesthetists and obstetricians) allows practising rare obstetric emergencies in a safe learning environment, e.g. shoulder dystocia, massive obstetric haemorrhage, maternal collapse and cord prolapse.

 Now visit **www.wileyessential.com/humandevelopment** to test yourself on this chapter.

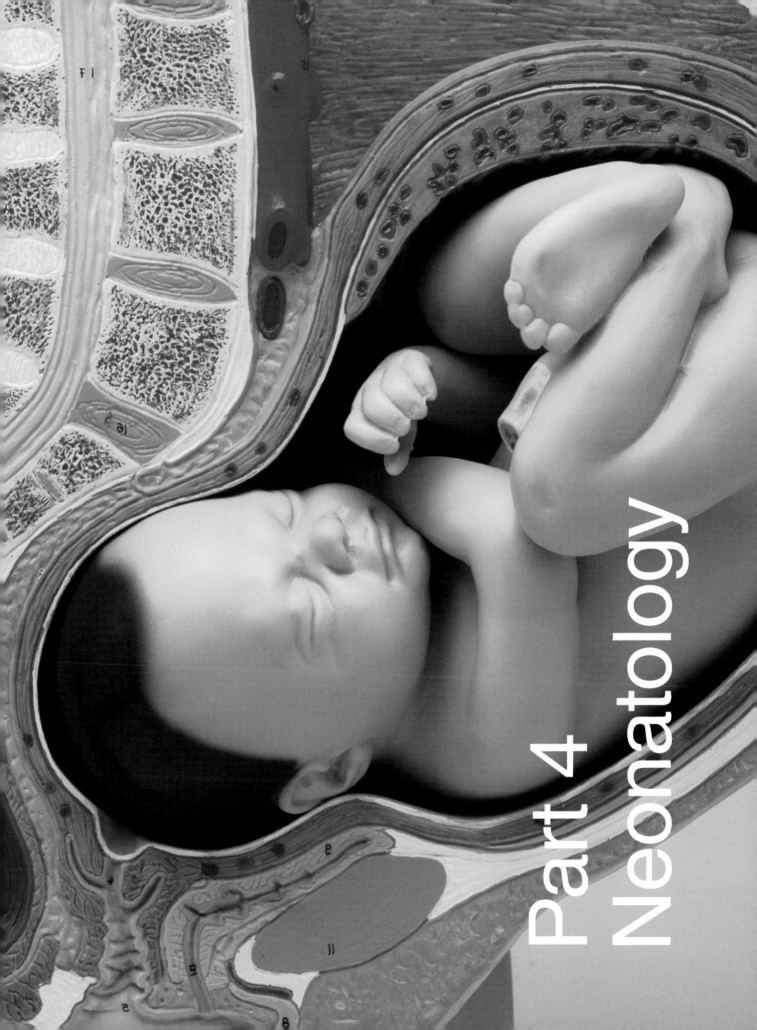

Part 4
Neonatology

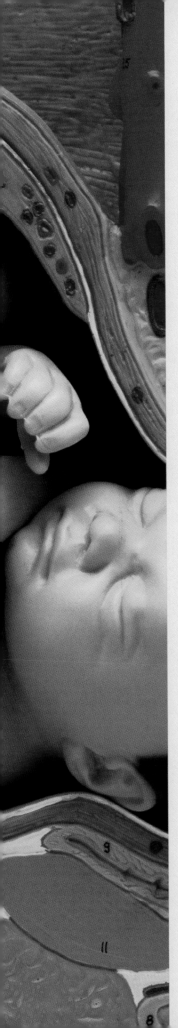

CHAPTER 22

Newborn resuscitation and newborn examination

Nitin Goel and Jamie Evans

Case

The paediatrician has been asked to attend an emergency caesarean section delivery of a 41-week gestation baby. Mother is 28 years old and this is her first pregnancy. She had complete antenatal care and the pregnancy has been uncomplicated. The baby is expected to be of good size. She was admitted a few hours ago and during the monitoring it was noted that there is presence of meconium in the amniotic fluid. Over the last half hour or so, the fetal heart rate trace has been of concern.

At delivery the baby is noted to be quite large and there was some difficulty in extraction of baby, requiring use of forceps. The paediatrician receives the baby, who is floppy, pale and not breathing, with a slow heart rate. There is also bruising and swelling of the scalp.

Learning outcomes

- You should be able to recognise when a newborn baby needs resuscitation.
- You should be able to describe the physiology of perinatal hypoxia.
- You should be able to describe the methods of newborn resuscitation and choose the most appropriate methods for each situation.
- You should be able to describe how to examine a newborn baby.

Newborn resuscitation

Birth is a relatively hypoxic experience, as babies undergo a transition from the placenta as the organ of gas exchange to the baby's lungs. Should there be any delay or problem with this process, babies may require help to establish breathing, and occasionally to re-establish the heart's pumping action. Most babies require either minimal or no resuscitation at birth, but it is essential to be well prepared in case the need arises. Being aware of the history of the pregnancy and labour will help in identifying babies at risk of requiring resuscitation at birth. Despite this, some babies with no antenatal risk factors may need support at birth (Box 22.1). It is estimated that only 1 in 2000 deliveries will actually need both ventilation and chest compressions. Everybody involved in the care of newborns should be trained in basic newborn resuscitation, and a trained resuscitator should be present at high-risk deliveries. In the UK, the Resuscitation Council runs regular Newborn Life Support (NLS) courses in various hospitals across the country. It is mandatory for the professionals involved in newborn resuscitation to be trained in NLS and recertified every 4 years. The International Liaison Committee on Resuscitation (ILCOR) reviews the current evidence every 5 years and updates the NLS guidelines accordingly.

Differences from adult resuscitation

There are fundamental differences in newborn resuscitation compared with all other ages. These are:

- babies are small, wet and cold;
- lungs are full of fluid;
- lung inflation is new;
- chest compressions are more effective due to cartilaginous rib cage.

Myocardial depression in newborn babies is secondary to the lack of adequate aeration and gas exchange in lungs, unlike adults where the arrest is mainly cardiac in origin and cardiac compression and defibrillation play a major role.

During labour babies pushed through the birth canal experience some hypoxia (lack of oxygen) and hypoperfusion, as placental supply is interrupted momentarily during every uterine contraction. A normal fetus responds to this by redirecting blood to vital organs (brain, heart and adrenals) and away from the skin, bowel and muscles. The heart rate drops and blood pressure rises as part of the 'diving reflex'. This is also accompanied by episodes of anaerobic metabolism resulting in some acidosis. Normal babies are prepared for this stress and their brains can withstand hypoxia much longer than adults. If the stress is overwhelming and prolonged, or the fetus is not well enough to adapt to physiological responses, then babies are unwell at birth and need support in the form of aeration and ventilation of lungs. Chest compression is used in a few cases and only to assist the heart in delivering oxygenated blood to the coronary arteries and the heart muscle.

Physiology of perinatal hypoxia

At the onset of acute hypoxia, the fetal breathing movements, driven by the respiratory centre, become deeper and more rapid. The P_aO_2 falls and the fetus soon loses consciousness; the respiratory centre stops functioning and regular breathing ceases, with the fetus entering a period of **primary apnoea**. The heart is still beating, albeit at a lower rate, using anaerobic metabolism from glycogen in the fetal heart. The blood pressure is unchanged due to vasoconstriction and restriction of blood flow to vital organs. The circulation is thus maintained but at a cost of increasing lactic acid as a by-product of anaerobic metabolism (Figure 22.1).

Box 22.1 Babies at risk of needing resuscitation

- Prematurity (<37 weeks gestation), especially <30 weeks gestation
- Antepartum haemorrhage
- Signs of fetal compromise on maternal monitoring
- Meconium staining of liquor – signifies fetal distress in utero
- Small/large for gestational age
- Maternal medications/general anaesthesia at delivery
- Maternal infection/chorioamnionitis/pre-eclampsia
- Congenital abnormalities
- Events at delivery – cord prolapse, difficult extraction, birth trauma, prolonged labour
- Breech delivery
- Instrumental delivery – use of ventouse or forceps

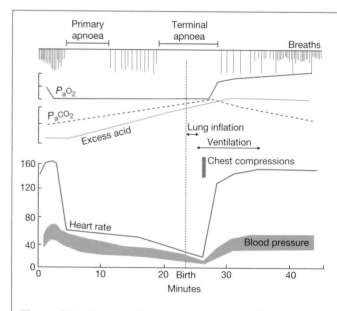

Figure 22.1 The physiological stages of primary and terminal (or secondary) apnoea in perinatal hypoxia, with resuscitation commenced at 23 minutes.

If the insult continues and the fetus is not delivered, primitive spinal centres are released from suppression by higher breathing centres. This results in a series of gasping breaths, and if these gasps fail to aerate the lungs, they fade away because of increasing lactic acidosis. The fetus then enters **secondary** or **terminal apnoea**. If this continues, the heart muscle ceases to function, blood pressure falls and without intervention the fetus can die. The whole process can take about 20 minutes.

A baby who is not breathing at delivery can be in either primary or secondary apnoea. In primary apnoea with a clear airway the baby will make gasping movements, aerate the lungs and recover spontaneously; this can be assisted by physical stimulation in the form of drying and wrapping the baby. This is usually done on a specific piece of equipment that has an overhead heater, a surface to lay the baby on, and equipment to allow full resuscitation (Resuscitaire®). In contrast, a baby in secondary apnoea has passed the gasping stage and will not recover without vigorous resuscitation ranging from active aeration of the lungs to chest compressions and, rarely, the use of medications.

Unfortunately in the delivery room one cannot differentiate whether the baby is in primary or secondary apnoea. Thus all the babies are assumed to be in secondary apnoea and resuscitation is followed in step-wise fashion starting from physical stimulation to more advanced steps depending on the requirement.

Assessment and care at birth

After the cord is clamped and cut, most babies will breathe or cry actively within a minute of birth and do not need any support. **Thermoregulation** is an essential part of newborn care. Babies arrive from a warm in utero environment to a cold external atmosphere. They are wet with amniotic fluid, are small in size with a relatively large surface area, so they lose heat rapidly and can become hypothermic. If this is prolonged it can lead to hypoxia and acidosis. This can be prevented by drying and wrapping in pre-warmed towels, placing the baby on a warm Resuscitaire or in direct contact with the mother's skin, and ensuring the delivery room is warm and draught free.

The next step is the initial assessment, which involves the following in order:
- COLOUR of trunk, lips and tongue, visible as soon as the baby is delivered. Extremities are usually slightly dusky in newborns (acrocyanosis).
- TONE – felt as soon as the baby is handled.
- BREATHING – noted simultaneously, can take a couple of minutes to regularise.
- HEART RATE – listened straight afterwards with a stethoscope.

The above are reassessed at regular intervals during the resuscitation and the responses guide subsequent steps.

Traditionally **Apgar scores** (Table 22.1) have been used to assess the baby's condition at birth and regular intervals (1, 5

and 10 minutes). This score has limited significance and is often recorded retrospectively and subjectively. It does not aid in the active resuscitation process. A persisting poor Apgar score at 10 minutes is a poor prognostic sign.

A centrally pink baby, with well-flexed posture and good tone, crying and breathing regularly with a heart rate exceeding 100 bpm needs no further support and should be handed over to the midwifery team/parents.

A baby who is dusky-pale in colour, floppy, not breathing adequately with a slow heart rate needs further intervention as detailed below.

Resuscitation at birth

The earlier resuscitation is instituted, the better the outcome. In the past methods like rocking the baby, tapping on hips, respiratory stimulants, intragastric oxygen and so forth were used with apparent success; all of these were potentially harmful, have now been discredited and are not used. Despite these methods, the babies recovered, indicating that the majority of babies are in primary apnoea and do not require any intervention.

The usual order of approaching newborn resuscitation is:
- dry and cover the baby;
- assess colour, tone, breathing and heart rate;
- airway;
- breathing;
- chest compressions;
- drugs.

Airway

The first step is to **open the airway**. For that the **head should be in a neutral position** (Figure 22.2), neither too extended nor too flexed, to avoid obstruction of the airway. Most of the time this is all that is needed for floppy babies and some babies will start making respiratory efforts. Mechanical obstruction is rarely the cause, but can occur with blood, thick mucus, vernix or meconium. Active suction is not recommended as it may cause more harm by vagal stimulation. In cases of

Sign	Score 0	Score 1	Score 2
Colour	Pale/blue	Blue extremities	Completely pink
Heart rate	Absent	<100/min	>100/min
Reflex response	No response	Grimace	Cough/sneeze
Muscle tone	Flaccid	Some flexion	Well flexed
Respiration	Absent	Weak	Good cry

Table 22.1 Apgar scoring. Scores from each row are combined to give an Apgar score.

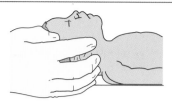

Figure 22.2 The neonatal head in a neutral position.

meconium staining of liquor, suctioning under direct vision is recommended if the baby is floppy and unresponsive. A crying baby has an open airway, which does not need intervention.

Airway manoeuvres

If the above methods do not elicit a response the baby requires **inflation breaths**, which are five sustained 2–3-second positive-pressure breaths delivered via a soft, suitably sized mask (snugly covering the mouth and nose) at pressures of about 30 cmH$_2$O. The baby is again reassessed. If there is an increase in heart rate this denotes the strategy for lung aeration is working, so some more positive-pressure breaths are required. These are given as **ventilation breaths** at 30 per minute, shorter than the inflation breaths at about 1 second each, at pressures of about 20 cmH$_2$O. After 30 seconds reassess the situation and continue if the heart rate is maintained but respiration is still not regularised. It is recommended now that the resuscitation should be **commenced in air**, with oxygen only considered for babies who have persistently low oxygen saturations despite resuscitation.

To improve the airway opening in a floppy baby the following manoeuvres can be applied:
- **Head neutral and chin support** – keeping finger on bony part of chin near the tip.
- **Jaw thrust** – moving the jaw forwards using fingers under each side of lower jaw (Figure 22.3). This can be done using a single hand or both the hands.
- Use of **oropharyngeal (Guedel) airway** – can be used in place of jaw thrust if an extra pair of hands is not immediately available.

Most babies will respond to the above airway manoeuvres. Occasionally a more secure airway is needed, in cases where there are copious secretions or meconium obstructing the airways, or if prolonged resuscitation is contemplated. This can be done by **endotracheal intubation** by a skilled paediatrician. It also allows the operator to concentrate on other tasks. In preterm babies, surfactant can be administered through this.

If the heart rate does not improve after inflation/ventilation breaths, then check whether the head position is still neutral and that the seal of the mask covering the mouth and nose is good. With effective inflation breaths the chest will rise and fall. Seeing the chest movements is the only way to ensure that lungs are getting aerated. If, despite good chest movements and effective ventilation breaths, there is no improvement in heart rate, chest compressions should be started.

Chest compressions

If despite lung aeration there is persisting bradycardia, chest compressions are required. A second pair of hands is needed for providing compressions, so it is essential to call for help early. This stage is reached because there is persisting hypoxia and acidosis due to which the heart muscle has ceased to pump. The main aim of chest compressions is to pump oxygenated blood into the coronary arteries to re-establish effective heart pumping. During the compression phase blood is squeezed from the chest by the increased pressure in the thoracic cavity, whereas during the relaxation phase the chest refills with blood.

The way to perform chest compression is to press the sternum over its lower third, which can be identified by placing both thumbs just below an imaginary line joining the nipples (Figure 22.4). The whole chest is gripped with both hands, placing the thumbs together at the front and fingers on the back at the spine. The lower third of the sternum is compressed downwards regularly by about one-third of the anteroposterior depth of the chest. Care is taken to press the sternum only and not to compress the ribs, which may be injured. An alternative method is to use two fingers perpendicular to the chest while the back is supported. This is less effective and fingers tend to slip and may cause bruising over the chest.

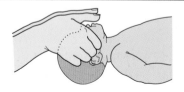

Figure 22.3 Jaw thrust manoeuvre.

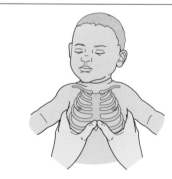

Figure 22.4 The locations of the hands, fingers and thumbs during neonatal chest compression.

As mentioned previously, both the compression and recoil are important and the aim is not to produce effective blood flow for the whole body, but to shift some oxygenated blood into the coronary arteries. The current guidelines state a ratio of 3:1 chest compressions to breaths, aiming at a rate of 90 compressions and 30 breaths in a minute. This ensures adequate aeration of the lungs in between compressions.

Drugs

If despite effective ventilation and chest compressions there is persistent bradycardia or no response, drugs should be considered. This is a rare event and the general outcome is not favourable. This stage is reached when persisting hypoxia leads to severe metabolic acidosis, myocardial dysfunction and exhaustion of energy stores. Before commencing drugs ensure that lung aeration has been achieved and effective cardiopulmonary resuscitation has been performed.

The aim is to deliver drugs rapidly and as close as possible to the heart. This is best achieved by placing an umbilical venous catheter (UVC). This is preferred over peripheral venous cannulation, as in circulatory failure peripheral access is difficult to obtain and the drug is unlikely to reach the heart. UVC is easy to obtain and all the necessary drugs can be given through it (Figure 22.5).

Table 22.2 lists drugs used in neonatal resuscitation. During the administration of drugs ventilation breaths and cardiac compressions are continued with assessments at regular intervals to monitor response and guide further action. If despite effective resuscitation the heart rate remains undetectable for 10 minutes, then it would be reasonable to stop further resuscitation as any further survival is likely to be associated with severe neurological disability in the long term.

Table 22.2 Drugs used in neonatal resuscitation.

Drug	Preparation	Dosage	Action
Sodium bicarbonate	4.2% or 8.4%	1–2 mmol/kg	Improving cardiac function by correcting acidosis
Adrenaline	1:10000	10 µg/kg	Increase cardiac output
Dextrose	10%	2.5 mL/kg	Provide energy to the heart
Saline	0.9%	10 mL/kg	As fluid volume
Adrenaline	1:10000	30 µg/kg	Further dose in case of non-response

Other scenarios

- **Meconium-stained liquor.** If the baby is active and crying, no further support or active suction is required. In the case of a floppy baby covered in thick meconium with no respiration, the airway should be inspected under direct vision of a laryngoscope and any particulate matter in the oropharynx should be cleared out with gentle suction.
- **Baby has acceptable heart rate but remains blue.** Check for any airway obstruction. If airway and breathing are satisfactory check for oxygen saturations using a pulse oximeter to rule out causes of cyanosis.
- **Baby is pale, shocked and breathless.** This could be due to acute blood loss during delivery, which can occur with placental abruption. These babies will need urgent volume replacement in the forms of crystalloids or group O Rh-negative blood.

Post-resuscitation care

Once the baby has been stabilised the parents need to be updated and further care should be planned depending upon the extent of resuscitation and the clinical status of the baby. Written communication is vital, and comprehensive, factual and accurate notes detailing the resuscitation have to be completed as soon as possible.

Therapeutic hypothermia

Therapeutic cooling has been shown in multicentre trials to improve outcomes of death and disability following a perinatal hypoxic event. Following an insult, some cells will immediately die, but over the subsequent few days as the body attempts to heal, inflammatory mediators flood to the damaged area and this inflammatory cascade triggers late-onset apoptotic cell death.

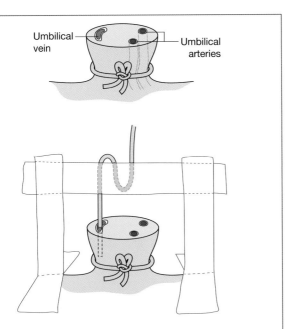

Umbilical vein

Umbilical arteries

Figure 22.5 Umbilical venous catheterisation.

If during the first 6 hours of life the baby can be cooled to a temperature of 33–34°C this process can be slowed and to some extent halted. Cooling is normally performed for 72 hours before the baby is slowly rewarmed over a 12-hour period. Cerebral function monitoring is continued during this time, and reversion of the trace to normal during the cooling period is a positive prognostic factor.

Adverse effects of cooling include coagulation defects, impaired cardiac function, fat necrosis, thrombocytopenia, hypokalaemia, and worsening of persistent pulmonary hypertension of the newborn (PPHN). Following the period of cooling, the baby will need neurological assessment including reflexes, tone, power and feeding. Babies will require a MRI scan, which is usually done at 10–14 days of life, and full follow-up with a developmental check at 6 months and 2 years of age.

Examination of the newborn

After a baby is born an initial check is performed by either the midwife or a paediatrician attending the delivery. This check is usually confined to ensuring that the infant looks well and that there are no major abnormalities. The parents themselves look at the baby and not uncommonly may pick up some anomalies or birthmarks. The initial check is then followed up by a full detailed examination, also called the 'postnatal baby check'. Newborn physical examination is one of the most valuable health screening tests, as early detection and management of anomalies may affect the long-term outcomes. This forms a part of the National Health Service screening programme in the UK, called the Newborn and Infant Physical Examination (NIPE) programme. NIPE clearly defines the goals, target conditions and competency standards.

Timing of examination

Many babies are currently discharged home before 8 hours of age. The advice from the NIPE programme is that there is no optimal time to detect all abnormalities, and it is considered that the overall risk associated with babies going unscreened is greater than if babies are examined early. Hence, all babies should be offered the examination before discharge even if this is at or before 6 hours. It is essential to make sure that all babies are examined before 72 hours. A second examination is performed at 6–8 weeks, usually by the general practitioner in the community.

Who should examine the baby?

Babies should be examined by a trained practitioner who has the time to talk and listen to the mother. This could be a trained midwife, a trained nurse practitioner, or paediatrician. There is an increasing preference for midwives to perform this examination.

Aims of newborn examination

Before the actual examination it is essential to check maternal, family, pregnancy and perinatal history in detail. Ensure the baby stays warm, that appropriate hand washing is done and that a parent is present during the examination. The aims are:

- To detect **whether baby is well** or requires some observation or treatment.
- To diagnose **any obvious congenital abnormalities** with a detailed head-to-toe examination.
- To **measure birthweight and head (maximum occipito-frontal) circumference**.
  To **perform a specific screening** examination targeting the following:
  (a) **Heart:** to listen to the heart sounds and feel femoral pulses to rule out any congenital heart disease. The problems may range from minor self-resolving defects to more complex ones. This examination may be supplemented with checking the baby's oxygen saturation by a pulse oximeter, depending on local unit protocol.
  (b) **Hips:** to ensure bilateral hip stability, ruling out any developmental dysplasia of the hip (DDH). DDH is due to the malformation of the ball-and-socket joint of the hip, and may not be always present at birth. The examination is done by performing Ortolani's and Barlow's manoeuvres (as described below). If any dislocatable/dislocated hips are noted, then they are referred to the orthopaedic team. Early diagnosis and treatment is essential to prevent any future problems with mobility. About 1–2 in 1000 babies will have hip problems that need operative treatment. In some cases ultrasound may be used as a screening tool to identify babies at risk, for example in babies born by breech delivery or if there is a history of a first-degree relative with DDH.
  (c) **Eyes:** to examine eye movements and check red reflexes (Figure 22.6) in both eyes via ophthalmoscope. This is not done to check the vision. It is common to see small subconjunctival haemorrhages; they resolve spontaneously. Absence of a red reflex can point towards eye problems including congenital cataracts and retinoblastoma. Urgent ophthalmic review is needed.

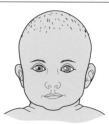

Figure 22.6 Red reflex eye test. In this case the right eye has a normal reflex, the left eye does not.

A cataract is a clouding of the normally clear and transparent eye lens. Retinoblastoma is a fast-growing cancer of eye, with one of the best cure rates among paediatric cancers. About 2–3/10000 babies will have eye problems needing treatment.

(d) **Testes:** in male babies, to feel whether both testes have descended into the scrotum. Undescended testes need to be followed up but they do sometimes descend spontaneously over the next few months. No descent up to 1 year after birth may require surgery, as it can lead to subfertility, or in rare cases malignancy. In the case of bilateral undescended testes, these babies need to be assessed carefully, especially if there is hypospadias (the urethral meatus is abnormally placed anywhere underneath the line of glans or along the penile shaft, see Figure 43.5). In these cases there is a chance that the baby could actually be a virilised baby girl due to congenital adrenal hyperplasia.

- To review any **problems suspected from antenatal screening**, family history or the events of labour, for example any anomalies observed during fetal ultrasound scanning, risk of any inherited disorders, maternal risk factors for sepsis, difficult labour, meconium stained liquor and so forth.
- To initiate appropriate treatment and arrange for **advice and follow-up where indicated**, for example hepatitis vaccination, phototherapy for jaundice, cleft lip or palate feeding support, scans for antenatal dilated renal pelvis and so forth.
- To address any **parental concerns**.
- To check that the baby has passed **urine and meconium**.
- To identify any **social issues** like parental substance abuse, mental health problems, learning difficulties or poor housing, and to alert the appropriate professional groups.
- To provide **health education advice** with regards to breastfeeding, cot death prevention and safe transport in cars.

Apart from the specific screening mentioned above, the following basic steps can act as an aid for top-to-toe examination.

Face – Check for any obvious dysmorphic features. Look for any recognisable chromosomal or genetic syndromes. Observe the tongue, and look for micrognathia.

Skin – Check colour in terms of pink, pale or cyanosed, and check for a rash, birthmarks, or jaundice (best to assess in bright light). Erythema toxicum neonatorum is a common newborn rash present in the first few days of life, and resolves spontaneously. Mongolian blue spots are benign self-resolving pigmented skin areas commonly seen in Afro-Caribbean, Asian and Latino babies.

Head – Check for moulding or swelling, caput succedaneum (subcutaneous oedema), abrasions, forceps marks or cephalohaematoma (subperiosteal haematoma). Look at the head shape. Feel the anterior and posterior fontanelles. Rule out premature fusion of skull bones (craniosynostosis).

Ears – Check the sizes, positions and shapes of the ears. Look for any preauricular tags or pits.

Mouth – Feel the gums for cysts or teeth, the hard and soft palate for clefts, and check the rooting reflex. Epstein's pearls are small inclusion cysts in the midline of the hard palate that resolve spontaneously.

Chest – Check for signs of respiratory distress, the shape of the chest, nipples and breath sounds.

Abdomen – Check the umbilicus, the two arteries and one vein. Look for any umbilical hernia or granuloma, and check the surrounding area for redness, pus or a foul smell. A single umbilical artery may be associated with other anomalies. Palpate for the spleen, liver and kidneys.

Genitalia – (male described previously); female: examine the labia. A small amount of mucus or blood at the vagina is normal.

Legs and feet – Check for any deformities like club foot (talipes equinovarus). The majority are positional and resolve with gentle massage and physiotherapy (see also Chapter 42).

Arms and hands – Check for extra digits, fused digits, the shape of the hands, and look for single palmar creases.

Neurology – Check tone and posture. A full-term healthy baby will have a flexed posture with arms adducted and hips abducted. Do the 'pull to sit' examination and check the Moro reflex (arms adduct widely and then abduct in response to a loss of support). Look for symmetry.

Spine – In ventral suspension feel along the spinous processes and examine the spine and sacral dimple carefully. Any midline anomalies, skin, hair or blind-ending cleft anomalies warrant further review.

Hips – Perform an **Ortolani test** to rule out dislocated hips (Figure 22.7). Examine to determine if there is any asymmetry of the legs or groin creases by straightening out the legs. This should return a dislocated head to the acetabulum. Place a middle finger over the greater

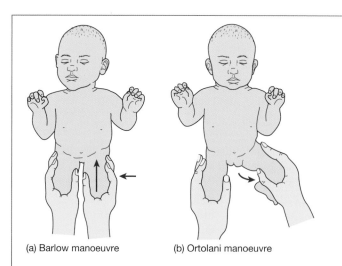

(a) Barlow manoeuvre   (b) Ortolani manoeuvre

Figure 22.7 The Barlow and Ortolani tests for hip anatomy.

trochanter, a thumb over the medial thigh and the palm over the knee. Have the knees fully flexed at a 90° angle to the hip. Then pull each leg in turn away from the pelvis, abduct and externally rotate the hip, pressing forwards with the middle finger. If the hip is dislocated a clunk will be felt as the femoral head slips forwards into the acetabulum. If there is resistance to full hip abduction this may be due to a dislocated hip that is unable to be relocated to the acetabulum.

Perform the **Barlow test**, which should dislocate a dislocatable hip. Hold the legs as above and abduct to 70°. Test each in turn by pressing forwards and medially with the fingers. A clunk may be felt if the hip relocates into the acetabulum. Then press backwards and laterally with the thumb (reversed procedure). Again a clunk will be felt if the hip dislocates from the joint. Dislocatable hips may settle in the first few days; however, follow-up should still be arranged. In addition, the hips may feel loose (unstable or clicky) on the Barlow test but not be dislocatable, and again this should settle shortly after birth.

The outcome of the newborn check is recorded in the maternity notes and the baby's personal child health records ('Red book'), which is held by the parents and reviewed by health professionals at each visit over the early years of life. Early diagnosis of a significant issue or abnormality may make all the difference to a baby's subsequent health. For minor deviations from normal (birthmarks, fusion of the toes, extra digits), parental anxiety can be minimised with reassurance.

Up to one-fifth of healthy newborns may be found to have a minor anomaly; most of these are of no importance (Box 22.2). These babies are at approximately a 3% risk of having a major anomaly. However, if there are multiple minor anomalies, then the risk of an accompanying major malformation rises. Fortunately very few babies fall in such a category.

Box 22.2 Examples of common minor neonatal abnormalities

- Folded-over ears
- Hyperextensibility of thumbs
- Syndactyly of the second and third toes
- Single palmar crease
- Polydactyly, especially if familial
- Umbilical hernia, especially in Afro-Caribbean babies
- Single umbilical artery
- Hydrocele
- Fifth-finger clinodactyly
- Simple dimple just above the natal cleft
- Undescended testes
- Single café-au-lait spot
- Single ash-leaf macule
- Capillary or strawberry haemangioma
- Accessory nipples

Birth injuries

Whilst babies are generally well equipped for the process of birth, there are many injuries that can occur during this process due to the baby's size or position, or due to manoeuvres or equipment used to help deliver the baby.

Caput succedaneum

Caput succedaneum is the most common injury, as mentioned above. It is superficial oedema or bruising at the presenting part of the head. This can be extensive, extending past suture lines but should not be boggy. It resolves quickly.

Cephalohaematoma

This is bleeding present in the periosteum of the bone and therefore should be limited by the suture lines. It is also very common and most often occurs in the parietal area. This usually heals within weeks and needs no further treatment.

Generalised bruising

Babies can be very bruised following delivery depending upon their presentation during birth. Breech presentations tend to have buttock or genitalia bruising. A baby with face presentation tends to have facial bruising, and quick deliveries can leave babies with a facial petechial rash.

Preterm babies are often bruised, and this is important to remember as these babies may have higher levels of jaundice. Any birth injuries or birthmarks must be documented to avoid unnecessary child protection issues when seen in the community.

Cuts and lacerations

The most common cuts and lacerations seen following birth are in instrumental deliveries. Forceps blades can cause facial bruising and even laceration of the skin, and the ventouse cap causes chignon and can sometimes be associated with skin loss and bleeding.

Rarely, lacerations from scalpels occur during emergency caesarean section deliveries and can usually be treated with steristrips. Injuries may also occur from fetal scalp electrodes.

Fractures and palsies

Erb's palsy: This is caused by stretching of the cervical nerve roots (namely C5–6) of the brachial plexus. It most commonly occurs where there is shoulder dystocia or during breech delivery. It causes a limp arm, flexed fingers and pronated wrist and this position is typically called the 'waiter's tip' position.

Clavicle fracture: Another reason for a limp arm following shoulder dystocia or difficult delivery is fracture of the clavicle. This is usually picked up due to high suspicion at delivery or reduced use of the arm. However, as part of the routine baby examination the clavicles must be checked. Babies with this condition may require some pain relief.

Klumpke's palsy: This occurs less commonly but is also an injury to the cervical roots (C7–8) of the brachial plexus. It causes weakness of the hand muscles and difficulty in wrist extension.

Facial nerve palsy: This most commonly occurs following forceps delivery and is most easily seen when the baby is crying.

All of these injuries tend to resolve spontaneously with little intervention, but rarely nerve injuries may cause a permanent paralysis.

Clinical case

Case investigations

The baby is brought to the pre-warmed Resuscitaire and assessed. The colour is pale/dusky, tone is decreased and baby is not breathing. The heart rate is slow and the baby is covered in some light-green meconium. The airway is therefore inspected under direct vision by laryngoscope and no meconium is seen in the oropharynx. The baby is then dried, stimulated and wrapped. By now the baby is about 1 minute of age. Head is positioned in neutral, but no respiratory effort results. The baby is then given five sustained 2–3-second positive-pressure breaths via a suitable mask covering mouth and nose, at 30 cmH$_2$O. This results in increased heart rate, but no respiratory effort. Ventilation breaths are then continued at 30 per minute at a lower pressure of 20 cmH$_2$O. After about a minute, the baby takes its first gasps of breaths and then starts crying. The colour rapidly improves from pale/dusky to pink. The heart rate is regular and normal and baby is breathing regularly by 3–4 minutes of age. The tone gradually improves and the baby becomes quite active. The baby is then assessed for any gross abnormalities and handed over to the midwife and parents. The paediatrician documents the resuscitation and gives an Apgar score of 1 at 1 minute, 9 at 5 minutes and 10 at 10 minutes.

The baby then stays with mother and breastfeeds in the postnatal ward. During the routine postnatal check the next day, the paediatrician notes the large swelling on the scalp, which is limited by the suture margins. The paediatrician reassures the parents that this is possibly a cephalohaematoma and will spontaneously resolve with time. Rest of the examination is normal including a thorough check for other birth injuries. The baby has symmetrical Moro's reflex, thus ruling out any brachial plexus injury and clavicle fracture.

Case conclusion

This was an example of a term newborn that needed brief support in the transition from fetal to newborn life. The baby was assessed and resuscitated in an organised manner resulting in good outcome. Thorough postnatal examination revealed a minor birth injury, consistent with the events around delivery.

Key learning points

- The majority of babies at birth require either minimal or no resuscitation. Some babies, in particular those at risk, need help with the transition from the fetal to the newborn period.
- Professionals involved in newborn care should be trained in newborn resuscitation. Newborn resuscitation is different to that of adults as it is mainly respiratory in origin. Adequate aeration of lungs is the primary aim.
- Use of drugs in neonatal resuscitation is rare and the outcome is generally not favourable.
- Thorough head-to-toe examination of a newborn baby between 6 and 72 hours of age is essential to ensure the baby is well and to rule out any anomalies.
- Particular emphasis is placed upon heart, hips, eyes and testes examinations.
- The examination is an ideal time for health promotion advice, including breastfeeding and cot sleeping care.

 Now visit **www.wileyessential.com/humandevelopment** to test yourself on this chapter.

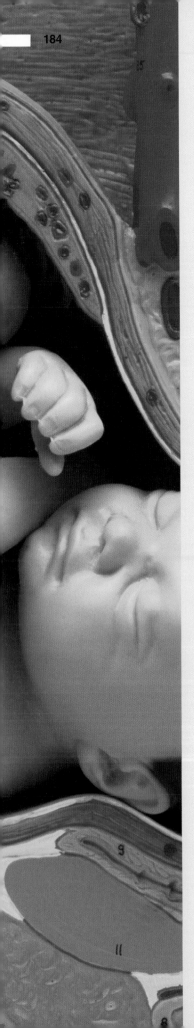

CHAPTER 23

Newborn feeding, jaundice and maternal diabetes

Geraint Morris

Case

Anna was born at 39 weeks, weighing 3.8 kg with a 1-minute Apgar score of 8, and a 5-minute score of 9. Anna is the first child for her mother, Jane, who is recovering well from labour. Jane is 26 years old and was diagnosed with polycystic ovary syndrome (PCOS) 2 years ago. Her consultant prescribed clomifene citrate to increase her chances of conceiving. Jane begins breastfeeding Anna, but after 2 weeks is suffering from sore nipples and is struggling to feed Anna on demand, which occurs approximately every 4 hours. Jane understands the benefits of breastfeeding and is keen to continue but unsure if she should, or if she will be able to. She is considering using formula feed to supplement or replace breastfeeding.

Learning outcomes

- You should be able to describe the benefits of breastfeeding to a new mother.
- You should be able to describe the effects of maternal diabetes on the fetus and predict potential complications at birth and for the neonate.

Introduction

The majority of babies will not need any intervention following birth and will feed almost immediately. Babies have all the innate reflexes that will allow them to do this. Even though feeding involves an immensely complex set of neuromuscular activities requiring the newborn to breathe, suck and swallow in a coordinated way, most infants seem to get this right with little effort.

Poor feeding may indicate a problem such as cleft lip and/or palate, hypoxic ischaemic encephalopathy, infection or a neuromuscular abnormality.

The birth of a baby, especially the first baby, is clearly an anxious time for many parents, and new parents will appreciate the support and guidance of a skilled midwife to help with handling, feeding and changing their new baby, as well as looking out for any signs of ill-health.

Breastfeeding

The UK has seen a steady rise in the number of new mothers choosing to breastfeed at birth over the last 10 years or so. This may have been due to a concerted effort on behalf of health professionals and other organisations to promote breastfeeding (Table 23.1). However, at the time of writing, whilst a majority of women choose to commence breastfeeding, most will choose to change to formula feeding within the first 6 weeks. There may be a number of reasons for this including the cultural perception of breastfeeding (e.g. ethnic minority groups tend to have higher breastfeeding rates; there may still be a negative attitude about breastfeeding in public areas), practical difficulties (e.g. with technique), convenience (e.g. fathers cannot feed their babies, issues related to women returning to work), failure and fear of failure (a small minority of breastfed babies do not get enough milk and become dehydrated) and health reasons (e.g. HIV infection or certain maternal medications that may be harmful to the breastfed infant) (see also Chapter 20).

Formula feeding

Many infant milk formulas are available commercially; the goal of the manufacturers has been to make their product as similar to breast milk as possible. However, most formula milks have been adapted from cows' milk, and contain little or no bioactive compounds as compared with breast milk, but will be nutritionally adequate as an infant feed until about 6 months old. Term infants will need approximately 40–60 mL per kilogram body weight per day on the first day, rising by 30 mL/kg/day for each subsequent day to approximately 150 mL/kg/day for the first 6 months of life.

Different types of formula milk have been produced in recent years for specific purposes.

Vitamin K

Breast milk and commercial formula milks are nutritionally adequate for most term infants but levels of vitamin K are low in babies at birth. Haemorrhagic disease of the newborn is a coagulopathy resulting from vitamin K deficiency that manifests in the newborn period. Infants may present with bleeding from the umbilicus, mucous membranes and the gut ,or with intracerebral bleeding. Infants of mothers who have been on anticonvulsant medication or antituberculous medication during pregnancy are at higher risk. This condition may be effectively prevented by giving a vitamin K supplement to all babies shortly after birth.

Vitamin D

Vitamin D deficiency in newborn infants may be getting commoner, and may often be unrecognised. It may be secondary to maternal vitamin D deficiency in the first instance, and if untreated in the newborn baby, may lead to rickets (see Chapter 37). Infants at highest risk are those from dark-skinned groups, particularly families living a mainly indoor lifestyle, and especially in winter months. Sunlight exposure is effective in boosting vitamin D Levels, and foods rich in vitamin D should be recommended (e.g. oily fish, eggs, mushrooms). However, many recommend that newborn infants, particularly those at risk, should receive vitamin D supplementation for the first year of life.

Weaning and milk feeding in older infants

Whilst the best age at which to commence babies on solid food remains controversial, weaning is generally started in Western countries at around 6 months old when babies can tolerate the

Table 23.1 The benefits of breastfeeding.	
Benefits to baby	**Benefits to mother**
• Lower incidence of gastroenteritis • Lower incidence of ear and respiratory infections • Lower incidence of obesity and diabetes • Lower incidence of urinary infections • Lower incidence of constipation • Lower incidence of eczema and allergic disease • Lower risk of necrotising enterocolitis • Possible improved neurodevelopment • Possible lower incidence of sudden infant death	• Readily available, no preparation needed • Low cost • Lower risk of breast cancer • Lower risk of ovarian cancer • Possible greater sense of achievement • Possible improved bonding • Uses up calories • Delayed return of ovulation and menstruation

higher solute load that solid foods possess. Weaning too early runs the risk of sodium overload on immature kidneys, whilst late weaning means that some nutrients, notably iron, may become deficient.

Breastfeeding can be safely continued for as long as mothers are prepared to do so, but mothers seldom breastfeed for more than a year or two. Provided infants are given a varied range of solid foods from the time of weaning, nutritional problems will be rare. However, an over-reliance on milk, which is relatively poor in iron, may cause iron deficiency, which may result in anaemia, and may be linked with poorer neurological development. Formula feeding beyond 6 months is also safe, and can be substituted by cows' milk at around 1 year; however, many 'follow-on' milks are now available, which provide extra nutrients, particularly iron, for infants at these ages.

Neonatal jaundice

In the days and weeks following birth, there is a rapid fall in the quantity of circulating haemoglobin and rapid destruction of red blood cells. The haem groups released in this process are converted to biliverdin and then to bilirubin by macrophages. The bilirubin is bound to albumin and carried to the liver, where the hepatocytes conjugate the bilirubin by the action of glucuronyl transferase. This conjugated bulirubin, which is now water soluble, is excreted mainly into the bile ducts and from there into the intestine, where it is further converted into urobilinogen and stercobilin. Stercobilin is excreted in the stool whereas the urobilinogen re-enters the circulation (Figure 23.1). Most of the circulating urobilinogen is taken up by the liver and re-secreted ('entero-hepatic circulation'), but a small proportion is excreted by the kidneys.

Because of the relative immaturity of the newborn liver and the unusually high quantity of bilirubin that is produced at this time of life, it is very common for babies to become visibly jaundiced in the first 2 weeks of life.

In the majority of these babies, provided the jaundice is only due to the normal breakdown of haemoglobin ('physiological jaundice'), no treatment is required. However, the difficulty is in gauging the severity of jaundice simply from looking at the baby. Some babies, particularly if there is pathological haemolysis, will become severely jaundiced, and the level of conjugated bilirubin in the bloodstream becomes toxic to the central nervous system. This may result in a condition called 'kernicterus', in which there may (or may not) be an initial bilirubin encephalopathy with poor feeding, hypo- or hypertonia, lethargy, seizures and even death, and later a more chronic neurological abnormality including athetoid cerebral palsy, dystonia, deafness, visual impairment and abnormal eye movements.

It is therefore important to identify those babies with severe jaundice, as this can be treated easily with good hydration and phototherapy, which involves placing the baby on or under a light source that emits light at the blue end of the visual spectrum. This helps to convert bilirubin to water-soluble isomers that can then be excreted by the kidneys and liver without having to undergo conjugation.

Haemolytic disease of the newborn (HDN)

This is a condition caused by a mismatch between the blood groups of the unborn baby and the mother. Red cells carrying rhesus or other (e.g. ABO, Kell, Kidd, Duffy) blood group antigens from a fetus may enter the maternal circulation during a feto-maternal haemorrhage, usually at or around the time of a placental abruption, birth, miscarriage or abortion. If the mother does not have these antigens (i.e. if she is negative for these blood groups), her immune system may generate IgM antibodies to them. IgM does not tend to cross the placental barrier so the fetus is not affected. However, in later pregnancies, when the mother will have produced more IgG antibodies, the IgG antibodies pass into the fetus and these attach to

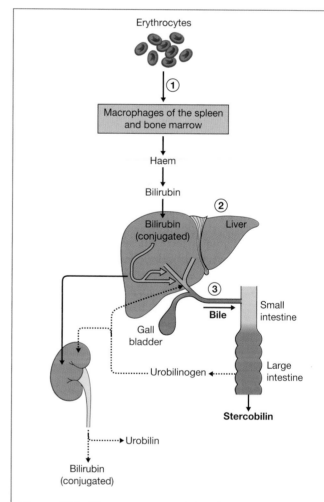

Figure 23.1. The processes of the destruction of red blood cells and excretion or recycling of their components.

the fetal red cells inducing haemolysis (see also Chapter 12). The degree to which the haemolysis occurs depends on the quantity of antibodies that passes through the placental barrier, which depends on the extent of the immune response. Rhesus antigens are particularly likely to induce HDN.

HDN may cause severe fetal anaemia and jaundice in the newborn infant within 24 hours of birth. Severe anaemia may lead to cardiac failure and severe oedema of the fetus (hydrops fetalis). Kernicterus may result from the postnatal accumulation of high bilirubin levels.

Prevention

Rhesus-related HDN may be prevented by administering a specific antibody to rhesus antigens ('anti-D immunoglobulin') to rhesus-negative women following an event that may trigger a feto-maternal haemorrhage (e.g. miscarriage, therapeutic abortion, ectopic pregnancy, invasive prenatal diagnostic tests, caesarean section and normal birth). Antenatal prophylaxis with anti-D is now also recommended for rhesus-negative women.

Treatment

In pregnancies with a high risk of HDN, fetal blood sampling may help gauge the severity of haemolysis, and fetal transfusion can be undertaken to prevent the complications of anaemia.

Phototherapy and good hydration will help to avoid the accumulation of bilirubin, but if the levels rise at a high rate, or to potentially toxic levels, then an exchange transfusion may be needed. This means transfusing maternal blood group-compatible blood into the baby whilst withdrawing the baby's blood at the same rate. This decreases the maternal antibody level in the baby, decreases the rate of haemolysis and decreases the bilirubin concentration in the circulating blood.

Normal growth and maturity

Most newborn babies born in the UK weigh between 2.5 and 4.5 kg. Babies with intrauterine growth restriction (IUGR) or who are small for gestational age (Box 23.1) are at risk of hypoglycaemia and hypothermia and should be monitored for these in the first few days of life. Polycythaemia may also result from chronic intrauterine hypoxia. The commonest cause of IUGR is placental dysfunction, which may be due to maternal smoking or illness such as pre-eclampsia, but further causes include congenital infection, fetal alcohol syndrome, maternal malnutrition or genetic disorders. Babies with IUGR secondary to placental dysfunction tend to feed avidly and may catch up with their genetically determined growth potential in the first few months of life. In severe IUGR, this may not happen and the child may remain small.

See Chapter 24 for the problems associated with prematurity.

Infants of mothers with diabetes

A minority of babies born to mothers with diabetes, because of the maternal vascular complications of diabetes, will have intrauterine growth restriction; however, infants born to mothers with diabetes tend to be bigger than they would be otherwise, especially if the diabetes is poorly controlled. Up to half of these babies will have a birthweight above the 90th centile. During pregnancy if there are high levels of circulating glucose in the mother's circulation, the glucose, being a small molecule, will freely cross the placenta into the fetus's circulation. The fetal pancreatic cells will, in response to the high level of glucose, become hyperplastic and secrete insulin in greater quantities. This hyperinsulinism tends to cause the fetal tissues to grow disproportionately large ('macrosomia'), and this may cause difficulties with the delivery. Following birth, the hypersecretion of insulin may continue for several days, causing hypoglycaemia. This needs to be treated promptly with glucose supplementation, if necessary via the intravenous route, as insulin stops the production of alternative metabolites that normal babies would use to fuel the developing brain, such as ketones and lactate.

Box 23.1 Birthweight terminology

- *Low birthweight* = 1.5 to 2.5 kg
- *Very low birthweight* = 1 to 1.5 kg
- *Extremely low birthweight* = less than 1 kg
- *Premature birth* = birth at less than 37 completed weeks gestation
- *Extreme prematurity* = birth at less than 28 weeks gestation
- *Small for gestational age* = babies who have a birthweight lower than the 10th centile for that gestation (these may not be pathologically small)
- *Intrauterine growth restriction* = babies with evidence of having suboptimal growth for a pathological reason (these babies may not necessarily be small, but have not achieved their growth potential)

Box 23.2 Fetal complications of maternal diabetes

- Birth injury
- Hypoxic ischaemic encephalopathy
- Respiratory distress syndrome
- Congenital heart disease
- Hypoglycaemia
- Hypocalcaemia
- Polycythaemia

SUMMARY

Clinical case

Case investigations

At 2 weeks old Anna weighs 3.7 kg, and it is typical for babies to regain their birthweight by this stage. Jane has soreness in one breast, but there is no sign of mastitis. The nipple and areola of the sore breast have some small cracks.

Jane is referred to a breastfeeding counsellor, and they discuss the benefits of different methods of feeding Anna. The counsellor gives Jane some methods for caring for her nipples after feeding, and advice on feeding from the sore breast first to ensure it is emptied. Jane will also try expressing and storing milk, which may relieve some of the soreness and will enable her husband to bottle-feed Anna expressed breast milk. The counsellor also checks that Anna is latching on to the breast well.

Case conclusions

Jane comments that the support of discussing breastfeeding with someone with experience is helpful in itself, and she feels better about continuing breastfeeding. She will return and speak with the breastfeeding counsellor again if she feels the need. She feels that she is giving Anna the best start in life by breastfeeding and is motivated to continue.

Key learning points

- Breastfeeding has advantages for both the neonate and the mother but many mothers find it difficult to breast-feed, and some who start breastfeeding struggle to continue beyond 6 weeks.

- It is common for newborns to develop neonatal jaundice in the first 2 weeks of life, but it is important to be able to distinguish between this often expected physiological jaundice and more dangerous pathological haemolysis.

 Now visit **www.wileyessential.com/humandevelopment** to test yourself on this chapter.

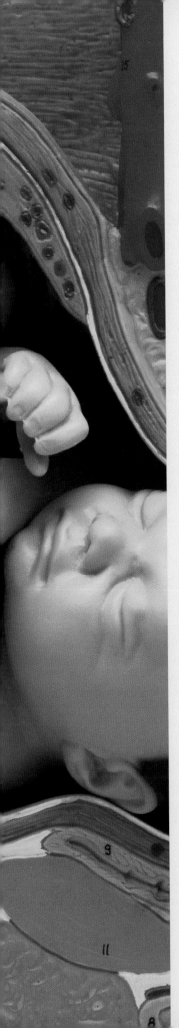

CHAPTER 24
The preterm infant

Nitin Goel

Case

A 24-year-old woman, in her first pregnancy, presents at 25 weeks gestation with a history of rupture of membranes a few hours ago and now has abdominal pain. She is admitted and assessed. She is found to be in active labour. She is given a first dose of steroids and antibiotics. The neonatal team is informed of the possible delivery of an extreme preterm baby. The neonatologist speaks to the mother and provides counselling and information regarding preterm birth at 25 weeks gestation.

Learning outcomes

- You should be able to define preterm birth.
- You should be able to predict the potential needs of preterm neonates born at different gestations periods.
- You should be able to diagnose neonatal conditions associated with preterm birth.

Essential Human Development, First Edition. Edited by Samuel Webster, Geraint Morris and Euan Kevelighan
© 2018 John Wiley & Sons, Ltd. Published 2018 by John Wiley & Sons, Ltd.

Introduction

Preterm birth is defined as birth at less than 37 completed weeks of gestation. The clinical course, management and associated problems depend on the gestation. With decreasing gestation, the intensity of care will increase. Babies born between 35 and 37 weeks gestation are termed 'late preterm' and may not appear preterm, but are still at risk of more problems than full-term babies. Preterm babies at less then 34 weeks will need admission to the neonatal unit. Babies born at less than 30 weeks, and in particular at less than 28 weeks gestation (extreme preterm), will need intensive care support and can have multiple problems in relation to immaturity of various organ systems (Table 24.1). They will need to stay in the neonatal unit for a few weeks to months depending on the clinical problems and support required.

Preterm labour

There can be many reasons why a pregnancy does not complete a full term of more than 37 weeks gestation. Most often the onset of preterm labour is spontaneous with no identifiable cause. Premature rupture of membranes (PROM), chorioamnionitis

(placental inflammation and infection), and antepartum haemorrhage (APH) with placenta praevia or placental abruption are among the most common identifiable reasons. It is difficult to diagnose and predict the onset of preterm labour. A bedside procedure called the **fibronectin test** is performed, which can help to rule out preterm labour. Beyond 22 weeks gestation, the presence of fibronectin suggests the separation of the chorion from the decidua and thus threatened preterm labour. Its presence can predict preterm labour with 37% accuracy, but its absence rules out preterm labour with 99% accuracy.

If there is no impending risk to the mother or the baby, then preterm birth can be delayed by tocolytic medications. This buys some time for the administration of antenatal corticosteroids to the mother.

Antenatal steroid therapy

Various studies have now established that administration of corticosteroids to the mother activates surfactant production and significantly reduces the complications in the preterm baby, such as the severity of respiratory distress syndrome, intraventricular haemorrhage, necrotising enterocolitis, and overall neonatal morbidity and mortality.

They are now routinely prescribed for threatened labour of less than 34 weeks gestation. The effect is optimal only if baby is delivered more than 24 hours but within a week of the treatment.

Care at birth

Keeping the baby warm after birth is of utmost importance in cases of premature birth. Hypothermia is associated with increased morbidity and mortality in preterm babies. It causes increased energy consumption. It can worsen the respiratory distress, leading to hypoxia and acidosis. To prevent this, all care should be taken to keep the baby warm. The delivery room environment should be around 25°C. After birth baby should be placed under a radiant warmer and wrapped in warm towels. It has been proved that babies less than 30 weeks maintain their temperature better if placed in a clear plastic bag immediately after birth, without drying, with face uncovered and head covered with a hat. Then these babies are placed directly under the radiant warmer.

Preterm babies born between 34 and 37 weeks often will not require any more support at birth than a term baby. Most babies born between 30 and 33 weeks gestation are in reasonable condition at birth and often need 'assisted transition' rather than actual resuscitation. They may require some breathing support in the form of continuous positive airway pressure (CPAP)/positive end-expiratory pressure (PEEP) to prevent their premature lung alveoli from becoming collapsed. Babies less than 30 weeks will need the presence of the neonatal team and a senior paediatrician at delivery. If a preterm baby needs inflation breaths, the initial pressures are 20–25 cmH$_2$O, lower than for term gestation.

Table 24.1 Common medical problems associated with prematurity.

Thermoregulation	Hypothermia
Respiratory	Respiratory distress syndrome (RDS) due to surfactant deficiency Apnoea of prematurity Broncho-pulmonary dysplasia (chronic lung disease)
Cardiovascular	Hypotension Patent ductus arteriosus (PDA)
Nutritional	Slow to establish oral feeds Need for parenteral nutrition
Infections	Prone to systemic sepsis Central line infection
Gastrointestinal	At risk of necrotising enterocolitis (NEC)
Neurological	Intraventricular haemorrhage (IVH) Periventricular leucomalacia (PVL)
Metabolic	Hypo/hyperglycaemia Electrolyte imbalances – Na, K, Ca Metabolic acidosis Osteopenia of prematurity (metabolic bone disease)
Haematological	Jaundice Anaemia of prematurity
Ophthalmological	Thrombocytopenia Retinopathy of prematurity

Babies less than 28 week gestation will often require more breathing support in the form of endotracheal intubation and positive pressure ventilation (IPPV) at birth. This also allows the administration of surfactant. Preterm lungs are deficient of surfactant and tend to collapse leading to respiratory distress syndrome. With administration of surfactant, these stiff lungs become more compliant and ventilation becomes easier.

After the initial stabilisation, such babies are then transferred to the neonatal unit for further care. In the neonatal unit, they are kept in a **thermoneutral and humid environment** to minimise heat loss and energy expenditure. This is made possible by keeping these babies in incubators with temperature and humidity control.

Respiratory distress syndrome

Respiratory distress syndrome is also called hyaline membrane disease, or surfactant-deficient lung disease. Surfactant is a mixture of phospholipids and proteins excreted by the type II pneumocytes of the alveolar epithelium in lungs. It acts by reducing surface tension and keeps the alveoli distended. In preterm babies, lungs are still in the early stages of development. Pneumocytes are formed around 22 weeks gestation, and surfactant production starts around 25 weeks onwards (see Chapter 7 and Figure 7.6). Gas exchange is only possible towards the end of the canalicular stage (24–25 weeks).

Babies less than 28 weeks are more prone to this syndrome and often need surfactant administration at birth. Surfactant is available in a natural preparation sourced from pig lung or calf and is directly instilled into lungs via an endotracheal tube, within the first 24 hours after birth. Administration of surfactant significantly reduces the morbidity and mortality.

Apnoea of prematurity

Apnoeas, bradycardia and oxygen desaturations are quite commonly seen in preterm babies. Apnoea is defined as a pause in breathing of more than 20 seconds associated with a decrease in heart rate. Oxygen desaturations without an accompanying lowering of heart rate are often seen, the majority of which are brief and spontaneously resolving. If prolonged they can lead to significant hypoxia and clinical worsening, hence the importance of continuous monitoring of these babies. The lower the gestation, the higher is the frequency of these events. About 80% of babies under 30 weeks gestation will experience them as compared to just 7% of babies between 34 and 35 weeks gestation.

These apnoeas can be central in origin due to immaturity of the brainstem respiratory centre, or due to obstruction in air flow. At times these can be an initial marker of some systemic problem like evolving sepsis, necrotising enterocolitis, intraventricular haemorrhage, significant patent ductus arteriosus, anaemia of prematurity, gastro-oesophageal reflux, seizures, electrolyte imbalances, and so forth.

Management

Management depends on the overall clinical picture, and the frequency and severity of these events. The majority are self-limiting, some need gentle stimulus to the baby, while others may require brief positive-pressure support and occasionally mechanical ventilation. Medications like methylxanthines (caffeine) form the mainstay of treatment for central apnoeas with no underlying cause. These act as central respiratory stimulants, increase minute ventilation and improve diaphragmatic contractility. The most common side effect is tachycardia. It has been shown that in the long term, caffeine helps in improving the neurodevelopmental outcome.

ⓘ Key facts 24.1 Respiratory distress syndrome in the newborn

Clinical signs

- Fast breathing (tachypnoea) with respiratory rate >60/min.
- Subcostal and intercostal recessions.
- Use of accessory muscles, nasal flaring.
- Expiratory grunting – in attempt to keep the alveoli open.

Monitoring

- Oxygen saturations via pulse oximetry.
- Monitoring of heart rate, respiration, blood pressure.
- Blood gas – evidence of respiratory acidosis.

- Chest X-ray – diffuse ground-glass appearance, low volume lungs, air bronchograms (radiolucent bronchial tree surrounded by radio-opaque collapsed/fluid-filled alveoli).

Management

- Temperature maintenance.
- Respiratory support – oxygen/CPAP/mechanical ventilation.
- Intravenous fluids.
- Antibiotics.
- Minimal handling.

Fluid management and nutrition

Adequate nutrition is essential for optimal growth and neurodevelopment of the preterm baby. As the in utero placental nutrition is discontinued prematurely in these babies at a crucial period of neuronal development, it is essential that after birth the same is provided adequately. In utero a fetus more than trebles its weight in the last trimester. Due to rapid growth, their nutritional requirements are quite different from full-term babies.

Babies of more than 34 weeks are mature enough to suck and swallow milk. An appropriately sized baby of this gestation can be fed the same as a term baby. Babies of 30–34 weeks gestation require feeding support via the oro/nasogastric tube, until they are able to suck and swallow efficiently. Breast milk can be expressed and supplemented with protein and calories, in the form of milk fortifiers, and given to these babies to ensure optimum nutrition. In case of non-availability of breast milk, special preterm formula milks can be used.

Very preterm babies of under 30 weeks gestation will need parenteral nutrition as their gut is too immature to handle full enteral feeds. This is provided intravenously via a peripheral or central venous catheter, under strict aseptic conditions. These lines are a potential source of infection and can lead to septicaemia unless strict asepsis is observed during insertion and fluid changes. The daily fluid requirements vary with gestation and age of baby. The starting day 1 volume can be 60–80 mL/kg/day, then increased daily by 10–30 mL/kg up to a maximum of 160–180 mL/kg/day. The constitution of the parenteral nutrition can be adjusted according to the individual baby's requirement in terms of calorie, protein, lipid, electrolyte and mineral content. Regular monitoring of weight, blood glucose and electrolytes is undertaken, and the parenteral nutrition is modified accordingly. Enteral feeds are started simultaneously in very small amounts initially and then gradually built up depending on gestation and feed tolerance. Once full enteral feeds are established, the parenteral nutrition is discontinued, and feeds are supplemented with calories, phosphate, iron and vitamins depending on the gestation and age.

Patent ductus arteriosus

In preterm babies the ductus arteriosus may remain patent after birth. See Chapter 36.

Bronchopulmonary dysplasia (BPD)

Various definitions have been given to BPD. The most common is oxygen dependency beyond 28 days of age. Another definition is oxygen dependency beyond 36 weeks corrected gestational age. 'Chronic lung disease' is often used interchangeably with BPD.

BPD results from multiple factors, most commonly premature surfactant-deficient lungs, pressure and volume injury to lungs from prolonged mechanical ventilation, oxygen toxicity and infection.

The chest X-ray is abnormal with widespread radio-opacity, cystic areas, hyperexpansion and streaky changes. These babies often require prolonged mechanical ventilation and are then weaned onto non-invasive support like CPAP, bilevel positive airway pressure (BiPAP) and high-flow treatment. Some babies are discharged home on low-flow nasal oxygen.

Management

This involves optimisation of ventilation, avoiding high inspiratory pressures and keeping oxygen saturations greater than 92%. Once the baby is stable, active weaning off should be attempted, tolerating higher PCO_2 levels. A course of corticosteroids can be used to facilitate weaning off ventilation, but their short-term benefits have to be weighed against possible long-term adverse neurodevelopmental outcomes. Following extubation, non-invasive methods are used like CPAP, BiPAP and high-flow oxygen. The aim is to keep oxygen saturations between 92 and 95%. Some babies may develop pulmonary hypertension, which can be diagnosed by ECG and echocardiography. These babies need oxygen saturations greater than 95% and their outcome can be poor.

Management also involves adequate nutrition, as these babies require higher calorie intake. Excessive fluids should be avoided and some babies may need a short course of diuretics to ease lung compliance. Haemoglobin should be regularly monitored, and if the packed cell volume (PCV) falls below 40%, a red cell transfusion can be considered.

Necrotising enterocolitis (NEC)

NEC is a potentially fatal illness that mainly affects preterm babies in the neonatal unit. The earlier the gestation and lower the birthweight, the greater the likelihood and higher the morbidity and mortality. Mortality varies from 10 to 30%, particularly in babies of less than 1000 g birthweight. The main predisposing factors are prematurity itself, intrauterine growth retardation, hypoxia and ischaemia due to any cause, significant patent ductus arteriosus (PDA), poor mucosal integrity, abnormal bacterial flora and the presence of substrate (especially hyperosmolar formula milk) in the intestinal lumen.

NEC is associated with inflammation, infection and coagulative necrosis of the bowel wall and may affect any part of the bowel, most commonly the distal small bowel. The bowel wall becomes inflamed and oedematous. In severe cases gas is present in the layers of bowel wall, called pneumatosis, which can be visible on the plain X-ray. This can lead to intestinal perforation with high mortality.

Clinical presentation

The presentation can be insidious, with subtle signs like poor tolerance of milk feeds, mild abdominal fullness, episodes of desaturations and apnoeas, temperature instability, tachycardia and evolving base deficit on blood gas. It can then rapidly progress with marked abdominal distension, tenderness, bilious vomiting, blood in stools, severe acidosis, coagulopathy, shock, perforation and death.

Abdominal X-ray pictures vary from a gasless abdomen to dilated thick-walled bowel loops, intramural pneumatosis (air in the bowel wall) and gas in the portal venous system, and in severe cases free air in the peritoneum.

Staging

Based on the clinical and radiological findings, modified Bell's staging is often used to assess the severity of NEC:

Stage I – suspected NEC, with subtle clinical features.
Stage IIA – mild abdominal signs, dilated bowel loops, blood in stools.
Stage IIB – pneumatosis or gas in the portal venous system.
Stage IIIA – severe symptoms and signs, coagulopathy and shock.
Stage IIIB – perforated bowel, free air in peritoneum.

Management

The baby needs to be nil by mouth, with intensive care and monitoring, ventilation, pain relief, circulatory support and antibiotics. In severe cases, bowel surgery may be needed, but this is associated with high mortality and morbidity.

Many prevention strategies have been suggested and have been proven to work in relation to other factors. Antenatal steroids, avoidance of hypoxic events, use of breast milk, early introduction of trophic minimal feeds (non-nutritive) to improve gut flora, slow advancement of feeds and use of standardised guidelines in the unit all help in reducing the incidence of NEC in the neonatal unit. Several trials recently have shown that probiotics are of significant benefit if given regularly to these preterm babies.

Preterm brain injury/cerebral haemorrhage

Intraventricular haemorrhage (IVH) and white matter changes leading to periventricular leucomalacia (PVL) are the two most common types of cerebral lesions affecting the preterm brain with potential adverse effects on long-term neurodevelopment. Uncommonly cerebellar haemorrhage may be seen. Regular cranial ultrasound screening is undertaken in the neonatal unit to detect these lesions early and for follow-up of progress. MRI of the brain can be used for greater accuracy.

The commonly used classification for IVH is:

Grade I – subependymal/germinal matrix haemorrhage (GMH).
Grade II – intraventricular bleeding with no dilatation.
Grade III – intraventricular bleeding with dilatation.
Grade IV – parenchymal involvement in the form of haemorrhagic parenchymal infarction (due to compression of venous drainage in surrounding parenchyma and resulting infarction).

IVH occurs in about one-quarter of babies less than 1500 g weight (very low birthweight babies). The majority happen within the first 72 hours of birth. The origin is usually from the germinal matrix above the caudate nucleus, which contains a fragile network of blood vessels. The incidence and severity are related to the extent of prematurity, severity of respiratory distress syndrome (RDS), pneumothorax, perinatal asphyxia, fluctuations in blood pressure and coagulopathy, among other factors. Small grade I IVH usually resolves spontaneously without long-term effects.

Large intraventricular haemorrhages can either resolve or progress. The drainage and reabsorption of cerebrospinal fluid (CSF) is impaired due to obstruction to its flow by particulate matter/clots and damage to the arachnoid villi. Over time this leads to a build-up of CSF under pressure leading to post-haemorrhagic ventricular dilatation (PHVD) and hydrocephalus in one-third of cases. Clinically it presents with a significant increase of the head circumference, sutural separation, fullness of the anterior fontanelle, frequent desaturations and apnoea. These babies may need frequent drainage of CSF to relieve pressure by performing lumbar puncture or ventricular taps. In severe cases, a temporary reservoir may be inserted to ease the external drainage of CSF. Ultimately they will require a ventriculo-peritoneal shunt for more permanent drainage of CSF. In cases with severe PHVD requiring shunt, about three-quarters will have some impaired neurodevelopmental outcome, in particular motor delay and cerebral palsy.

White matter injury

White matter changes, particularly in periventricular areas, are commonly seen on preterm cranial ultrasound scans. They are commonly termed periventricular leucomalacia (PVL) and are classified as:

Grade I PVL – periventricular echogenicities or 'flares' lasting ≥7 days.
Grade II PVL – transient echodensities evolving into small localised cysts.
Grade III PVL – evolving into extensive periventricular cystic lesions.
Grade IV PVL – deep white matter involvement with extensive cystic changes.

Often in preterm cranial scans, a peritrigonal 'blush' or 'flare' is seen, which resolves spontaneously. If it persists it is termed PVL. Grade I PVL can be seen in about one-quarter of babies under 32 weeks, while grade II and above is uncommon, seen in 1–2% of babies.

PVL can occur due to antenatal or postnatal events like maternal antepartum haemorrhage, perinatal hypoxia, chorioamnionitis, severe RDS, hypotension, hypocarbia, sepsis and NEC. The pathological hallmark is coagulative necrosis of brain parenchyma with liquefaction and cyst formation.

The whole process can evolve over 2–3 weeks, and this is the usual time when such abnormalities are first detected on cranial ultrasound scan, hence the importance of serial scans in preterm babies.

Clinically the babies will be asymptomatic and it can be an incidental finding on scan. In severe cases there is progressive neurological deterioration with hypertonicity and irritability. Grade I PVL cases have generally a good prognosis. Advanced cystic PVL is associated with adverse neurological outcome in the majority, with spastic diplegia, cerebral palsy and cognitive abnormalities, especially with occipito-parietal lesions.

Retinopathy of prematurity (ROP)

ROP is the abnormal vascular proliferation of the retinal blood vessels in premature babies. If untreated, it can progress to retinal detachment, scarring and blindness. Babies born very prematurely are often subjected to hypoxic and high oxygen states, both of which may lead to development of ROP. Normally retinal vascularisation begins around 16 weeks gestation, with the nasal part of the retina vascularised by 36 weeks gestation and the temporal part by 40 weeks. High levels of oxygen cause retinal vasoconstriction and relative hypoxia, which stimulates the formation of vascular endothelial growth factor (VEGF), which leads to abnormal angiogenesis and vascular proliferation in the retina. Based on the spread of these vessels, ROP can be classified into zones and stages (Figure 24.1).

Zone 1 – centre of retina in the optic disc region, including macula – most aggressive and serious.

Zone 2 – anterior to Zone 1, up to the nasal ora serrata.

Zone 3 – anterior to Zone 2, on temporal side – good prognosis.

Stage 1 – demarcation between avascular and vascular retina, with a thin line in between.

Stage 2 – broad thick ridge between the two.

Stage 3 – extensive neovascularisation – poor prognosis unless treated.

Stage 4 – retinal detachment.

Involvement of the posterior retinal vessels and iris vessels leads to more severe ROP, also called 'Plus' disease.

Regular weekly/biweekly ophthalmic screening is undertaken from 30–32 weeks corrected gestation, in the neonatal unit in all preterm babies born under 32 weeks gestation or less than 1500 g birthweight. Treatment includes laser ablation of the abnormal vessels, and results are usually good if treated early. More recent treatment under trial involves injection of anti-VEGF monoclonal antibodies into the vitreous, in the hope to stop the neovascularisation.

Outcomes following extreme preterm birth

Current bioethics guidelines state that any baby born above 24 weeks gestation will be offered full invasive intensive care from birth and admitted to a neonatal unit, unless it has been agreed that in view of the baby's condition it is not in the baby's best interests. At 23 weeks gestation and below, the outcome is generally poor and active resuscitation is not pursued if baby does not show adequate signs of life at birth. At 23 weeks only one in five babies survive and 85% of survivors will have some disability, whereas at 24 weeks survival is about 40% with a 70% chance of some disability in survivors. The mortality and morbidity improve with increasing gestation, with 80% survival at 26 weeks and only 40% of survivors with some disability.

Discharge of the preterm baby from hospital

Any preterm baby going home after a prolonged stay in the neonatal unit requires careful discharge planning. They require supplementation of feeds in the form of breast milk fortifiers, multivitamins and iron. Nasogastric-fed babies will require parental training about feeding. Routine immunisations are advised from 2 months of age after birth and not the corrected age. Babies at risk of respiratory syncytial virus (RSV) bronchiolitis will require additional protection, with monthly prophylaxis in the form of the monoclonal antibody palivizumab in the appropriate season; 'fast access cards' or letters can be provided to the parents for alerting the paediatric team in hospital on readmissions.

Post-discharge from the hospital, the ex-preterm babies are followed up in a multidisciplinary follow-up neonatal clinic, until 2 years corrected for prematurity. A formal neurodevelopmental assessment is carried out at 2 years.

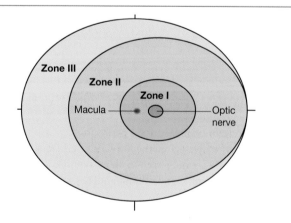

Figure 24.1 Zones of the retina associated with retinopathy of prematurity.

Clinical case

Case investigations

The woman stayed in the labour ward for another day before the baby was delivered. She was able to receive a full course of antenatal steroids before the baby's birth. At birth, the neonatal team were present, prepared for the delivery of an extreme preterm baby, with a birthweight of 650 g. The baby was placed in a plastic bag on a prewarmed Resuscitaire® and the head was covered with a suitable hat. Baby had a good heart rate, was active, with a weak cry, but had inadequate respiratory effort. The team then intubated the baby with an appropriately sized endotracheal tube, gave a dose of porcine surfactant and commenced mechanical ventilation. The baby was admitted to the neonatal unit and transferred into an incubator to maintain warmth and humidity. The initial chest X-ray showed a pattern consistent with respiratory distress syndrome. The baby remained on ventilator support for a week, then was tried briefly on non-invasive support and then back on mechanical ventilation. It was also noted to have a significant patent ductus arteriosus, which was treated with a course of ibuprofen. Finally the baby was off ventilator support by 4 weeks of age, but continued on non-invasive support for another 3 weeks. Chest X-ray showed images consistent with chronic lung disease.

Initially after birth, the baby was on parenteral nutrition consisting of protein, carbohydrate, lipids, electrolytes and trace minerals. Gradually mother's expressed breast milk was introduced via a nasogastric tube and feeding was established. By 3 weeks of age, baby was fully enterally fed. There was a brief period where feeds were withheld due to concerns regarding possible stage I NEC, but that resolved with conservative management and antibiotics. Serial cranial ultrasound scans did not reveal any intraventricular haemorrhage. There was some periventricular flare noted on the day 7 scan, which was not seen in later scans. Retinopathy screen was performed from 32 weeks gestation onwards and was normal. The baby was discharged home fully breastfed at a corrected age of 36 weeks, with a weight of 2.3 kg, with community support and follow-up plans in place.

Case conclusion

The case demonstrates the journey of a baby born 15 weeks earlier than expected. The baby stayed in the neonatal unit for about 3 months and needed management for various issues related to prematurity. This baby had a relatively uncomplicated course and the long-term neurodevelopmental outcome appeared favourable.

Key learning points

- Much of development occurs during the first 30 weeks of pregnancy, and babies born preterm between 35 and 37 weeks typically have good function in most systems but are at greater risk of developing problems than full-term neonates.
- The earlier a baby is born, the more support it will need, with babies born at less than 30 weeks highly likely to need intensive care.

- All body systems of a premature neonate will be underdeveloped, but the respiratory and gastrointestinal systems, and thermoregulation, typically need some form of support in almost all cases.

 Now visit **www.wileyessential.com/humandevelopment** to test yourself on this chapter.

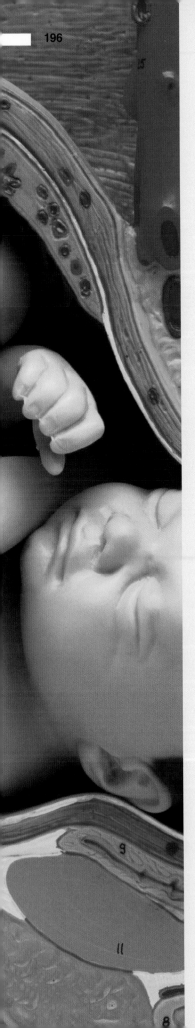

CHAPTER 25
Congenital and perinatal infection

Ian Morris

Case

Harry was born at 33 weeks gestation to Elizabeth, with an Apgar score of 6 at 1 minute and 7 at 5 minutes. He weighs 2.9 kg and on examination his liver and spleen are enlarged. Elizabeth is 34 years old and Harry is her first child. Elizabeth has not noted any illness or infection during her pregnancy. Harry and Elizabeth remain on the neonatal unit and Harry develops some jaundice in his first week, and feeds reasonably well by breast but with some vomiting, diarrhoea and lethargy. His body temperature measured by rectal thermometer is 37.9°C 7 days after birth, and he weighs 2.4 kg at that time. The paediatrician is concerned and considers some further investigations.

Learning outcomes

- Understand the susceptibility of the neonate, especially the pre-term, to infection.
- Be able to describe the routes of transmission of congenital and perinatal infection.
- Know the common causes of congenital infection and their presentation.
- Know the differences between early- and late-onset neonatal infection, and the common organisms involved.
- Be aware of the general and specific management strategies involved in treating infection in the neonate.

Introduction

Infection in the perinatal period is a common and potentially serious problem. Organisms that are harmless at all other stages of life can be devastating when encountered by the fetus. After birth, newborn babies are more vulnerable to bacterial, viral and fungal infections than any other age group as a result of immature immune systems. This is particularly the case in premature infants, and those who are of very low birthweight (VLBW, <1500 g). A low index of suspicion for infection is therefore essential in any sick newborn, and prompt clinical assessment with appropriate investigation and intervention is required. In this chapter we will look at how and when infections are transmitted (see Table 25.1), and understand the clinical presentation and subsequent management of congenitally and perinatally acquired disease.

Congenital infection

Congenital infection refers to an infection transmitted and acquired in utero. Common organisms are listed in Table 25.1, and most are as a result of primary infection of the mother during pregnancy. Some organisms, such as cytomegalovirus (CMV) and herpes simplex virus (HSV), can also occur following reactivation during pregnancy. For some infections, specific measures exist (e.g. the rubella immunisation programme); however, prevention largely consists of general hygiene advice such as good hand-washing, keeping food preparation surfaces clean, and the avoidance of undercooked meats and unpasteurised dairy products.

Diagnosis of a congenital infection antenatally can be challenging, and requires a high index of suspicion. In many of these infections, the mother will be entirely asymptomatic, or experience only mild 'flu-like' symptoms. Potential clues include a maternal rash, miscarriage, premature birth, anomalies on fetal ultrasound, and a history of maternal contact with people known to be infected with a disease. In these instances screening serology to demonstrate seroconversion in the mother may be helpful. Postnatally, a number of clinical features should arouse suspicion of congenital infection (Table 25.2).

Cytomegalovirus (CMV)

CMV may occur following either primary or recurrent maternal infection (1–4% of susceptible women acquire CMV during pregnancy, with reactivation occurring in 10% of seropositive women). The risk of both transmission and clinical sequelae is higher after primary infection, particularly if acquired at earlier gestations. Almost all adults are asymptomatic, as are 90% of infants at birth. However, congenital CMV is the most significant cause of non-genetic sensorineural hearing loss (SNHL) and can cause significant neurological impairment.

Clinical presentation is most typically a triad of jaundice, petechiae and hepatosplenomegaly. Other features include:

Table 25.1 Perinatal infection.

Timing of infection	Acquisition	Route of transmission	Presentation	Common examples
Congenital infection	*In utero*	Transplacental	Anytime from antenatal to years later	CMV Syphilis Toxoplasmosis Rubella Varicella Parvovirus B19
Neonatal infection	Peri-delivery or postnatally	• Transplacental • Ascending via birth canal • Breast feeding • Iatrogenic	• Early onset (<72 hours) • Late onset (>72 hours)	**Bacterial:** Group B streptococcus Gram negative (e.g. *Escherichia coli*) *Listeria monocytogenes* *Neisseria gonorrhoea* *Chlamydia trachomatis* Staphylococcal infections **Viral:** Enteroviruses Herpes simplex virus Varicella zoster virus **Fungal:** *Candida* infections
			• Delayed onset (months to years)	Hepatitis B and C HIV Human papillomavirus

Table 25.2 Common features of congenital infection.

Organ/system	Clinical signs/symptoms
General	Pre-term, intrauterine growth restriction, rash
Brain	Microcephaly, seizures, intracerebral calcifications, developmental delay
Hearing	Sensorineural hearing loss (SNHL)
Eyes	Cataracts, chorioretinitis, microphthalmia, glaucoma
Liver	Hepatomegaly, jaundice, hepatitis
Haematological	Thrombocytopenia/petechiae, anaemia, neutropenia, splenomegaly
Other	Bone abnormalities, pneumonitis, cardiac abnormalities

■ **Antenatal:** Oligo/polyhydramnios, intrauterine growth restriction (IUGR), fetal ascites, non-immune hydrops, prematurity and increased risk of congenital malformations such as talipes.

■ **Neonatal:** Hypotonia, poor feeding, lethargy, temperature instability, 'blueberry muffin' spots, microcephaly, chorioretinitis, cerebral ventriculomegaly and periventricular calcifications. Investigations may reveal anaemia, thrombocytopenia, hyperbilirubinaemia, elevated serum transaminases and raised cerebrospinal fluid (CSF) protein.

If CMV is present in the infant, it is important to establish whether the virus is congenital or acquired as the latter is very unlikely to be of any clinical significance. Diagnosis is with virus isolation (culture or PCR) from urine or saliva, *or* CMV-specific IgM in umbilical cord or infant blood *within the first 3 weeks of life*. The presence of CMV-specific IgG alone is not diagnostic as this may occur with passive transfer from a mother without active infection. Antenatal fetal diagnosis is possible if the virus is isolated in amniotic fluid.

⊙ Key facts 25.1 Cytomegalovirus (CMV)

- Incidence: Commonest congenital infection, affecting 3–4 per 1000 live births.
- Features: Most typically a triad of jaundice, petechiae and hepatosplenomegaly.
- Diagnosis: Virus isolation (culture or PCR) from urine or saliva *within the first 3 weeks of life*, or CMV-specific IgM in umbilical cord or infant blood.
- Treatment: i.v. ganciclovir or oral valganciclovir for 6 weeks.
- Outcome: Overall mortality is low (0.5%), but rises to around 15% in symptomatic infants. Risk of sensorineural hearing loss even if asymptomatic.

Current best evidence suggests that treatment should be limited to those with symptomatic neurological disease, or severe focal organ disease (e.g. severe hepatitis or bone marrow suppression). Treatment has been shown to be effective in preventing hearing deterioration and reducing developmental delay in symptomatic infants, but weekly monitoring for neutropenia, thrombocytopenia and anaemia is required.

Long-term morbidity is high, with studies showing that almost half of symptomatic infants will develop SNHL, learning difficulties, microcephaly and, rarely, visual loss. Significantly, around 10% of asymptomatic infants develop SNHL by 6 years of age (compared to less than 0.5% of the general population). Because hearing is often normal at birth, only 50% of cases of SNHL caused by CMV are expected to be detected by neonatal hearing screening programmes. Overall mortality is low (0.5%), but rises to around 15% in symptomatic infants.

Rubella

Congenital rubella infection is now rare in the UK as a result of rubella immunisation programmes in teenagers. However, some women remain susceptible to the condition on routine antenatal screening, as do migrants from countries without immunisation programmes. Fetal and neonatal problems are uncommon where the virus is acquired after 20 weeks gestation, but in the first trimester it is associated with a 90% risk of fetal transmission, with eye (cataracts, retinopathy, microphthalmia), brain (microcephaly, cognitive impairment) and cardiac malformations, along with SNHL, being the major consequences. The risk of miscarriage and stillbirth is also high. Clinical signs in the neonate are non-specific (see Table 25.2), with diagnosis made in the presence of rubella-specific IgM antibodies in the blood (which persists for 6–12 months after birth), or with viral PCR culture from urine, nasal, throat or blood specimens.

There is no effective treatment for rubella, and termination is considered in most cases where maternal infection is suggested by rising rubella antibody tires. After birth, the infant will continue to excrete the active virus for many months and therefore prevents a risk to non-immune pregnant women.

⊙ Key facts 25.2 Rubella

- Incidence: Very rare in immunised populations.
- Features: Eye, brain and cardiac malformations.
- Diagnosis: Rubella-specific IgM antibodies, or viral PCR culture.
- Treatment: None available.
- Outcome: High risk of miscarriage or stillbirth. SNHL very common.

Toxoplasmosis

Toxoplasma gondii is one of the most common parasitic infections in humans, and is acquired by ingestion of cyst-containing tissues in undercooked meat, or of oocysts excreted by cats and contaminating soil or water. The seroprevalence varies widely between countries (5–80%), and is thought to be around 8% in the UK. The incidence of congenital infection in the UK is around 1 per 10 000.

The risk of maternal-fetal transmission increases with advancing gestational age at the time of maternal infection (from around 5% in the first trimester, to 80% just prior to delivery), with overall transmission rates being about 25%. Conversely, the risk of clinical sequelae is highest if transmitted in the early stages of pregnancy (60–80% in first trimester). Some countries with a higher prevalence screen for the condition antenatally, but this is not current practice in the UK. Where antenatal infection is detected, the mother may be treated with spiramycin in an attempt to reduce transmission of infection and/or severity of its impact on the fetus/newborn.

At birth, the signs are often subtle or absent, with only around 5–10% of infants born to infected mothers manifesting neonatal symptoms. Mortality in this group is around 25%. Common signs at birth may include: prematurity, IUGR, jaundice, hepatosplenomegaly, petechiae, cataract and microphthalmia. When actively investigated, retinochoroiditis and/or intracranial lesions (e.g. calcifications, hydrocephalus, epilepsy) are detected in 17% of infected infants in the postnatal period. Further eye lesions can appear at any stage of life as a result of reactivation of latent cysts in the retina and choroid. Progression to severe neurological impairment is rare (less than 5%), but the extent of milder neurodevelopmental problems is uncertain.

Diagnosis can be made antenatally or postnatally by detection of IgM and IgA by enzyme immunoassay. However, false negative results can occur and serial measurements are often needed where toxoplasmosis is strongly suspected.

Treatment of congenitally infected infants consists of a combination of pyrimethamine and a sulphonamide, along with folinic acid for at least 12 months. These treatment regimens can cause bone marrow toxicity so it is important to monitor for neutropenia and thrombocytopenia.

Syphilis

Syphilis is caused by the bacterium *Treponema pallidum*. Congenital syphilis has seen an increased incidence in recent years, but remains very rare in the UK. Vertical transmission from mother to fetus during pregnancy is around 50% for both primary and secondary infection, and can occur at any stage of pregnancy. Transmission rates are highest for mothers with early stage syphilis and high titres, although it can still be transmitted by women in the latent stages. Antenatal screening is routine in the UK, and treatment with a penicillin-based antibiotic at least 4 weeks prior to delivery prevents congenital infection. Where maternal treatment does not take place or is inadequate, there is a high rate of spontaneous abortion or stillbirth (up to 50%). Other antenatal features include polyhydramnios, intrauterine growth restriction, non-immune hydrops fetalis and preterm labour.

In the neonate, congenital syphilis may present early (in the first 2 years of life), or late. Affected infants are usually asymptomatic at birth, but most develop signs within a few weeks:

- Snuffles (4–22% of newborns, highly infectious discharge).
- Rash (classically vesicobullous or maculopapular, affecting palms and soles and associated with desquamation).
- Severe irritability on handling due to bone pain from periostitis.
- Non-tender generalised lymphadenopathy.
- Hepatosplenomegaly.
- Conjugated hyperbilirubinaemia.
- Anaemia/haemolysis, thrombocytopenia.
- Condylomata lata (wart-like lesions) affecting the borders of the mouth, anus and genitalia.

All infants born to seropositive mothers should be considered to be exposed to syphilis unless there is good evidence of complete treatment and response in the mother. Neonatal diagnosis can be by direct demonstration of *T. pallidum* by dark ground microscopy and/or PCR of exudates from suspicious lesions or body fluids (e.g. nasal discharge). Paired maternal and infant serological testing can also be performed, but serial testing may be required as both false negative and false positive results can occur.

If symptomatic or if serology is suggestive of congenital infection, the infant should be treated with 10 days of intravenous or intramuscular penicillin.

ⓘ Key facts 25.3 Toxoplasmosis

- Incidence: 1 per 10 000 live births.
- Features: Hepatosplenomegaly, petechiae and eye defects, intracranial calcification.
- Diagnosis: Detection of specific IgM and IgA.
- Treatment: 1 year pyrimethamine + sulphonamide + folinic acid.
- Outcome: Mortality up to 25% if symptomatic, long-term neurological sequelae may occur.

ⓘ Key facts 25.4 Syphilis

- Incidence: Extremely rare in the UK.
- Features: Rash on palms/soles, purulent rhinitis, hepatosplenomegaly, periostitis.
- Diagnosis: Direct demonstration on microscopy, or with paired infant/maternal serology.
- Treatment: 10 days i.v./i.m. penicillin.
- Outcome: High incidence of miscarriage or stillbirth without treatment in mother.

Other viral infections

Parvovirus B19

Around 40–50% of pregnant women are susceptible to parvovirus B19, better known as **slapped cheek syndrome**, or **fifth disease**. As well as a blotchy red facial rash, other symptoms in adults include headaches and a mild 'flu-like' illness. No specific treatment is available and most women who acquire the infection during pregnancy will experience no adverse effects, but there is an increased risk of miscarriage if acquired within the first 20 weeks (around 9%). There is also a small but potentially serious risk of fetal anaemia, which can lead to heart failure and fetal hydrops, if acquired in the second trimester. However, there is no evidence of any other congenital or developmental anomaly affecting the neonate or appearing later in childhood.

Varicella (chickenpox)

Chickenpox is a highly contagious infection, spread easily from person to person through direct contact or by coughing or sneezing. Primary maternal infection during pregnancy is uncommon, as most people experience the condition in childhood. However, if infection is acquired during early pregnancy, there is around a 1% chance that a **congenital varicella syndrome** may develop. These infants are usually of low birthweight and can have skin scarring, as well as limb, eye and brain malformations.

An infant whose mother develops signs of chickenpox from 5 days before to 2 days after delivery is at risk of developing chickenpox after birth. The disease is likely to be much more severe than when acquired at other ages, and has a high mortality (up to 30%). Consequently, these at-risk infants should receive varicella zoster immune globulin (VZIG), along with intravenous aciclovir.

Herpes simplex virus (HSV)

Neonatal herpes is rare in the UK, with an incidence around 4 per 100 000 live births. The virus is usually transmitted following exposure to infected genital vesicles during delivery, but can also result from ascending intrauterine infection or from contact with an affected individual postnatally. Transmission is significantly higher with primary rather than reactivated infection, although as the mother is often asymptomatic, neonatal infection is usually unexpected. Diagnosis is with PCR analysis of lesions, blood or CSF.

Affected infants may suffer either localised (skin, eye or mouth lesions), or a more generalised disease. The latter form, involving around one-third of infants, can affect a number of organs and give rise to features such as jaundice, hepatosplenomegaly, disseminated intravascular coagulation and encephalitis. Such disseminated forms have a high mortality (around 20%), even with aciclovir treatment, with many survivors having neurological impairment.

Hepatitis B

Hepatitis B carriage or infection is found throughout the world, but there is a particularly high incidence in developing countries in the Far East and sub-Saharan Africa, where rates are over 10%. There is also an association with intravenous drug use. Consequently, prevalence in the UK can vary widely between regions, and screening of all mothers for hepatitis B surface antigen (HBsAg) is routine in the UK. Mothers are usually asymptomatic carriers, transmitting the virus during labour. Infants who are born to hepatitis B carriers are immunised, and those born to mothers deemed to be at 'high risk' (e.g. hepatitis B e-antigen-positive) are also given hepatitis B immunoglobulin as soon as possible after birth. Immunisation reduces the risk of infection in infants to less than 5%. Without this, most infants will become carriers and risk developing chronic liver disease and cirrhosis in later life. Fulminant hepatitis in the neonatal period is a very rare, but often fatal occurrence.

Hepatitis C

The incidence of hepatitis C in adults in the UK is less than 0.1%, and infection is usually asymptomatic. Transmission to infants is low (around 5%), and is confined to mothers with a high viral load in late pregnancy unless there is concomitant HIV infection. If infants acquire the virus, they have an increased risk of chronic liver disease and hepatocellular carcinoma in later life.

Human immunodeficiency virus (HIV)

HIV infection is still relatively uncommon in pregnancy in the UK, but is highly prevalent in some parts of the world, particularly sub-Saharan Africa. Regions with high levels of immigration and refugees from these areas may therefore see more affected mothers. The virus is principally transmitted vertically during labour, but can also be transmitted transplacentally or via breast milk. Transmission rates can be reduced from around 25–30% without intervention, to less than 1% where risks are eliminated (see Risk factors 25.1), the mother is treated with antiretroviral therapy, the infant is delivered by

---

⚠ Risk factors 25.1 HIV transmission

- High maternal viral PCR load
- Chorioamnionitis
- Prolonged rupture of membranes
- Other sexually transmitted infections
- Vitamin A deficiency
- Invasive procedures during pregnancy or delivery
- Vaginal delivery
- Preterm delivery
- Breastfeeding

elective caesarean section (before labour starts) and the infant is given antiretroviral therapy after birth. Diagnosis is with DNA or RNA PCR. Antibody tests cannot be used before 18 months due to detection of maternal antibody in infant blood. There are usually no signs of infection in the neonatal period, with the development of characteristic opportunistic infections such as *Pneumocystis carinii* in subsequent months.

Early-onset sepsis

Early-onset sepsis (EOS) typically refers to infection presenting in the neonate within 72 hours of life, but definitions vary from 24 hours to 7 days. Infection occurs as a result of exposure to a range of pathogens during birth, combined with a relatively poorly developed immune system. A number of factors are associated with a higher risk of EOS (Risk factors 25.2), and presentation is variable and often non-specific to the source of infection (Box 25.1) Investigations will depend upon the individual presentation, but as a minimum should include a full blood count with differential, C-reactive protein, and blood culture. Urine + CSF microscopy and culture, chest X-ray, blood gas analysis, and swabs of any lesions may additionally be required. It should be remembered that infection markers are often normal in the early stages of infection, and that blood cultures have a high false negative rate. Diagnosis is therefore usually clinical, with a high index of suspicion, and low threshold for intervention required; ensuring infection is treated early and aggressively.

Management

The neonate with sepsis can rapidly deteriorate and so primary management involves supportive care, that is, airway, breathing and circulation. Infants with clear features of sepsis will usually require admission to the neonatal unit for observation and support. Broad-spectrum intravenous antibiotics should be commenced without delay, ensuring that Gram-positive and Gram-negative organisms are covered. Specific choices will depend on local microbiology profiles, but a typical combination would be benzylpenicillin and gentamicin, with appropriate modification once any culture results are available.

Group B streptococcal (GBS) infection

GBS is the most common organism causing bacterial sepsis in the neonatal period. The UK incidence is around 0.5 per 1000 live births, and leads to death in 6% of cases (18% in premature infants). Whilst some countries screen all women for GBS carriage in late pregnancy, the efficacy of this practice in preventing neonatal sepsis is debated, and screening is not routine in the UK. It is estimated that between 25 and 30% of pregnant women have rectal or vaginal colonisation with GBS, and without intervention around 1% of infants born vaginally to these mothers will develop infection. The risk can be increased where a previous sibling has had GBS sepsis, or with other maternal factors (see Risk factors 25.2). In the presence of these risk factors, intrapartum antibiotics for the mother are recommended.

In the infant, onset can be early (majority within 24 hours) or late. The early form typically presents with respiratory distress and septicaemia. Meningitis is more likely if the infant presents later. Where symptoms are present, broad-spectrum intravenous antibiotics are given immediately, whilst a risk-based approach to treatment is used in asymptomatic infants.

Listeria monocytogenes infection

Listeriosis is an uncommon but potentially serious infection in the perinatal period, affecting around 5 per 100 000 live births. The organism is acquired through ingesting soft cheeses, undercooked poultry, and unpasteurised milk; hence the recommendations to avoid such substances during pregnancy. Affected women may be asymptomatic, or develop a 'flu-like' illness, and transmit the organism either transplacentally or via the birth canal. Infection may lead to spontaneous abortion, or premature delivery. An additional characteristic feature is meconium staining of the liquor, even in preterm infants, in whom this is otherwise unusual. Early-onset infection typically presents at or within a few hours of birth, with respiratory distress, septicaemia and a widespread rash. The mortality in these cases is as high as 15–45%. Later-onset disease is usually associated with a meningitis picture, and has a more favourable prognosis. Treatment is with broad-based penicillin agents given intravenously for 2 to 3 weeks.

Gram-negative infection

Infection with Gram-negative organisms such as *Escherichia coli* are much less common than GBS as a cause of early-onset sepsis. However, it can also present as late-onset sepsis, especially in preterm infants undergoing invasive procedures or requiring central intravenous access. All forms can cause significant morbidity and mortality, and require aggressive intravenous antibiotic treatment.

Umbilical infection

A 'sticky' umbilicus is common within a few days at birth, and often occurs as the cord separates through a process of aseptic necrosis. This alone does not require any form of treatment. However, the umbilical area does become colonised with organisms such as *Staphylococcus aureus* and *Staph. epidermidis*,

---

> **(!) Risk factors 25.2 Sepsis at birth**
>
> - Prematurity
> - Prolonged rupture of membranes (>18 hours)
> - Chorioamnionitis
> - Maternal fever in labour (>38°C)
> - Raised maternal infection markers

and sometimes the surrounding skin can become inflamed, or have pus present. In these instances, intravenous antibiotic treatment is initially required.

Eye infections

A sticky eye is very common in the first few days of life, and is usually not infected. Cleansing with cooled, boiled water is sufficient in these instances, and the condition resolves spontaneously. Some cases may be as a result of staphylococcal or streptococcal infection, which will need treatment with topical antibiotic preparations. Other more important causes of eye discharge also need to be considered.

Chlamydia trachomatis is a sexually transmitted organism that is often carried asymptomatically in the genital tract and can cause a purulent eye discharge along with swelling of the eyelids in affected infants. Diagnosis is with immunofluorescent staining of the discharge, and treatment is with a topical tetracycline eye ointment plus oral erythromycin in the most severe cases.

Ophthalmia neonatorum is another cause of purulent conjunctivitis and is caused by gonococcal infection. Where the mother is known to carry this sexually transmitted disease, treatment of the infant with penicillin at birth should prevent problems. However, maternal infection is often asymptomatic and unknown. In these cases, significant discharge and eyelid swelling can occur, which can lead to problems such as corneal ulceration and perforation if left untreated. Topical and systemic treatment with antibiotics is required.

Late-onset sepsis

Late-onset sepsis (LOS) typically refers to infection occurring after 72 hours of life. In the UK this affects around 2–3 per 1000 infants, although the incidence in more vulnerable babies such as those born prematurely is significantly higher. Preterm babies are at added risk due to their immature immune systems, fragile skin that can break down allowing colonising organisms to invade, and exposure to invasive procedures and central intravenous lines.

In LOS, the source of infection is usually from the infants' environment, which can include nosocomial or iatrogenic infection obtained on the neonatal or paediatric unit. For this reason, strict infection prevention measures need to be practised in all units caring for newborn infants, with adherence to hand hygiene, avoidance of overcrowding, sterilising of medical equipment, and judicious use of central intravenous lines and antibiotics. A wide range of viral, bacterial and fungal organisms have been implicated in LOS, but Gram-negative bacteria such as *Klebsiella*, *Pseudomonas* and *E. coli* are responsible for between 20 and 40% of all episodes. These organisms have also been implicated in 'outbreaks' within intensive care environments, and pose a serious risk to infants. As with EOS, clinical features are variable and often non-specific (see Box 25.1), and initial treatment consists of broad-spectrum intravenous antibiotic coverage with appropriate modification once culture results and sensitivities are available.

Box 25.1 Features of neonatal sepsis

- General: Temperature instability (fever or hypothermia), poor feeding, lethargy.
- Gastrointestinal: Vomiting, abdominal distension, early jaundice (<24 hours).
- Cardiorespiratory: Respiratory distress, apnoea, bradycardia/tachycardia.
- Neurological: Irritable, seizures, tense or bulging fontanelle.
- Bloods: Raised C-reactive protein, neutropenia/neutrophilia, thrombocytopenia, hypo- or hyperglycaemia.

SUMMARY

Clinical case

Case investigations

Harry has a positive CRP of 59 mg/L, WBC 24 × 10³/mm³, haemoglobin 165 g/L, haematocrit 48.4%, platelets 164 × 10³/mm³ and negative blood cultures. Upon further investigation the paediatrician discovers that Elizabeth has two cats in her home. IgG assay confirms antitoxoplasmic antibodies in both Harry and Elizabeth. No other infectious agents are found.

Ultrasound scan imaging of Harry's brain finds no intracranial calcifications, but ocular examination discovers chorioretinitis in his right eye. Abdominal examination finds the liver is of normal size and no abdominal distension.

Case conclusions

Harry was diagnosed with congenital toxoplasmosis, and treated with pyrimethamine, trimethroprim, and leucovorin (a folinic acid) for 1 year. At 6 months a follow-up examination shows the formation of a chorioretinal scar in Harry's right eye. At 12 months Harry is meeting expected developmental milestones and no neurological abnormalities are found. His length and head circumference both fall in the 50th centile.

Harry is likely to have few future problems related to his toxoplasmosis because he was diagnosed and treated appropriately. He was generally asymptomatic at birth, also reducing his probability of developing further problems if treated. The chorioretinal scarring may affect his vision, but would probably have become worse without treatment.

Key learning points

- Pathogens that are harmless in children and adults can cause serious problems when acquired congenitally.
- Infection can be acquired at any stage during pregnancy, labour or in the neonatal period, and is a major cause of morbidity and mortality.
- Clinical presentation is highly variable and features are often non-specific.

- At-risk infants can be identified from maternal and labour history, allowing opportunity for early clinical assessment and treatment where appropriate.
- Premature infants are particularly susceptible to infection and warrant extra consideration.

 Now visit **www.wileyessential.com/humandevelopment** to test yourself on this chapter.

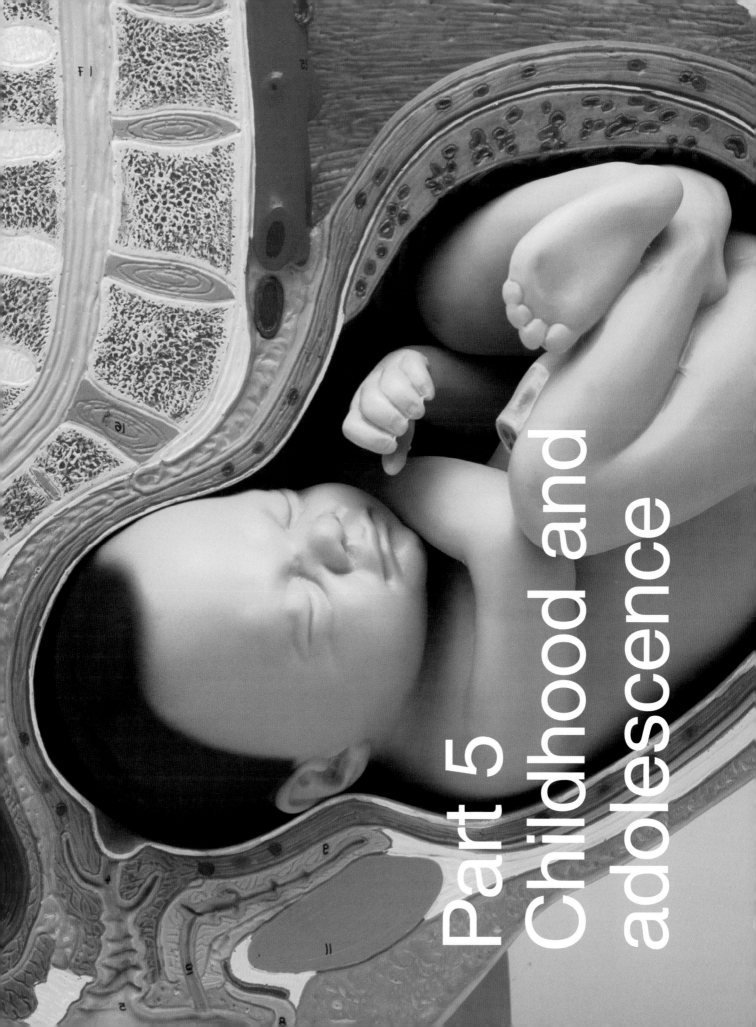

Part 5
Childhood and
adolescence

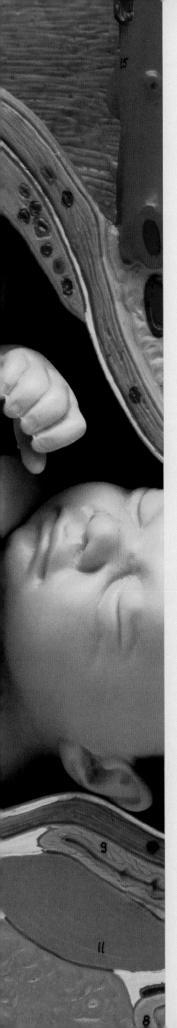

CHAPTER 26
History and examination in childhood

Shabeena Webster and Geraint Morris

Case

Huw is an 18-month-old boy who presented to his family doctor after returning from a holiday abroad. While he and his family were on holiday Huw was taken to the out-of-hours General Practitioner having been unwell for 2 days with a high temperature, poor appetite and a runny nose. The doctor examined him and then commented that even though he did not think Huw had any serious illness, he had heard a heart murmur. He advised the family to take Huw to see their own doctor, Dr Davies, after returning home. By the time Huw saw her, his symptoms were better. Dr Davies took a careful history and examined Huw but could not hear a heart murmur at all. She remembered the family and having seen Huw several times in the past, and noticed that Huw's medical file was quite large but that it contained records of consultations for relatively minor concerns. Dr Davies was able to reassure his parents that the heart murmur had now gone, and that this was a common finding in children who had a fever. Huw's parents were relieved and reassured by the doctor's explanation.

Learning outcomes

- You should be able to describe how the paediatric history and the examination of a child differ from their equivalents in adult practice.
- You should be able to list examples of how abnormalities can be detected by observation rather than by specific tests.

Essential Human Development, First Edition. Edited by Samuel Webster, Geraint Morris and Euan Kevelighan
© 2018 John Wiley & Sons, Ltd. Published 2018 by John Wiley & Sons, Ltd.

Introduction

History taking in paediatrics has many similarities to the way history taking is done in adults, but there are important considerations when dealing with children.

Setting

The examination of a child will be more likely to be successful if the environment in which a child is examined is suitable for a child. A suitable waiting area with friendly and welcoming staff who are at ease with children will go a long way to make children feel relaxed. There should be age-appropriate toys and games to play with.

Background information

Before meeting the child and family, try to collect as much information as possible: What does the referral letter say? Are there any medical issues recorded in the clinical notes/on the hospital databases? Do you need to get any further information before you meet the child? Who is the person accompanying the child – is it their parent/carer/other family member?

Approach to the child

It is important to ensure you know the child's name, age and gender – this will help avoid embarrassment if it is not clear whether a baby is a boy or a girl, and will not only show parents that you have taken the trouble to remember their child's name, but will also reassure them that you have a personal and friendly approach.

It is a matter of practice and experience to know how to speak to a child and to make the conversation appropriate to the child's age and developmental stage. The more practice you have at interacting with children at various ages, the better you will get at this.

In the case of infants and toddlers, it may be perfectly feasible to conduct the whole consultation without moving the child from their parent's knee, but in older children a couch or bed will be necessary. Babies may also be examined on a couch/cot or similar surface.

Who to address – child or parent/carer?

In general, having introduced yourself to the child and carer(s), and established who the accompanying adults are, you should address the child as much as possible to obtain the history. Babies enjoy being talked to and, though you will not gain any factual information from a newborn, you can use your initial interaction to see whether the baby looks well or has any obvious sign of illness. Parents will see that if you speak to their baby, you are showing your skill and professionalism as well as demonstrating that their baby is important to you. As children become older, you will be able to obtain more of the history

directly from them. Even the most reticent adolescent, with the right approach, can give a very coherent history. As with patients of all ages, the aim of the consultation is not just to obtain information but to establish a rapport and a trusting relationship.

The paediatric history

Presenting complaint

This may be a specific symptom such as a cough or a rash; occasionally, however, neither the child nor the carer can pinpoint what is wrong. Children may not understand their symptoms and use terms that may be inaccurate to describe what to them is bewildering. However, given time, the relevant information can be collected.

History of presenting complaint

Once the main symptom(s) has/have been established it is important to explore the main symptom(s) in more depth. If a child is vomiting, check whether the vomiting is projectile, bile-stained, long-standing or frequent. Is there associated abdominal pain, diarrhoea, urinary symptoms or fever?

For presenting symptoms, such as pain check:
- onset/duration;
- frequency, severity, location, radiation, exacerbation and relief;
- effects on lifestyle, anxieties.

Listed in Table 26.1 are common symptoms with which children present under each organ system.

Table 26.1 Common paediatric presenting symptoms and the systems they are linked with.

System	Presenting symptoms
General	Fever, poor feeding, quietness, poor sleep pattern, excessive crying, lethargy
ENT/respiratory	Hearing difficulty, throat pain, stridor, shortness of breath (SOB), cough, wheeze, haemoptysis, chest pain
Cardiovascular	Collapse, murmur, sweating, poor feeding, blueness, shortness of breath
Gastrointestinal	Reduced appetite, difficulty in swallowing, nausea, vomiting, haematemesis, abdominal pain, diarrhoea, constipation, jaundice
Genitourinary	Dysuria, anuria, haematuria, frequency, poor stream, enuresis, haematuria, vaginal discharge
Musculoskeletal	Weakness, pain, deformities, swelling, limp
Neurological	Headache, fainting, dizziness, clumsiness, seizures, abnormal movements, squint, blurred vision
Skin	Rashes, itching, bruising

Past medical history

This is usually shorter than history taking in adults; however, it can be challenging in the case of children with complex medical needs cared for by multiple professionals in various hospitals across the country. Take some time to list relevant factors in the history. Knowing what to leave out is sometimes a matter of experience and practice.

Pregnancy and birth history

This is especially relevant in newborns and infants but may be less relevant in an older child or adolescent. Ask about antenatal scans and tests, problems with delivery, the condition of the child at birth and any neonatal problems.

Feeding and dietary history

Even if the presenting complaint seems unrelated to the gastrointestinal system, taking a history of feeding may help to gauge the severity of an illness. Seriously ill children seldom eat and drink well. If a nutrient deficiency is suspected, for example iron deficiency anaemia, then a detailed dietary assessment is necessary.

Growth and developmental history

Normal growth and development are widely accepted as reliable indicators of good health, and the assessment of a child's health is not complete without measurement of relevant growth parameters and, particularly in the case of a young child, a developmental history. Most parents are encouraged from an early stage to bring their child's health record (the 'red book' in the UK), charting the growth of an infant, to every medical appointment. See Chapter 27 for more detailed information.

Medications

List all medications accurately, including doses and frequency and recent changes. Include drug allergies or sensitivities and highlight these on all medical records and drug charts.

Immunisation

Ask about the child's routine immunisations (Figure 26.1) and any additional vaccinations, for example a BCG (bacille Calmette-Guérin vaccine – protecting against tuberculosis) vaccination received by children at high risk. Enquire about reasons why any were missed.

Family history

Record a genetic family tree including any medical conditions that may be inherited in families. This is particularly important if a genetic condition such as a metabolic disorder

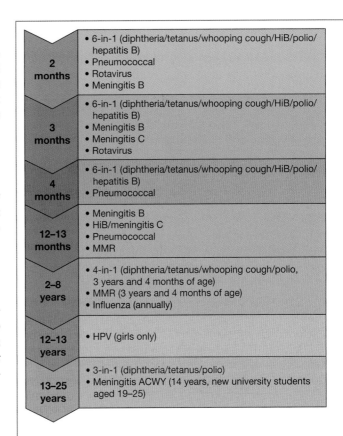

Figure 26.1 The UK immunisation guide.

is suspected. Many paediatric conditions have a genetic basis so this is a vitally important part of the history taking process.

Social history

Ask about who is in the immediate household and any wider support the family has. Ask about the parents' occupations, whether they smoke or own pets, and any other factors in the home environment that may be relevant to the presenting problem. This may be very important if the symptoms might be a result of neglect or abuse. School-related issues and social networks could be discussed if appropriate as well as sexual activity and risk-taking behaviour. It may be advantageous to speak to the child without the parents being present if this kind of discussion is needed – many parents would give their consent to this if adolescents are reluctant to talk in front of them. Remember to ask for another member of staff to act as a chaperone rather than being alone with a child. The more routine this part of the history becomes in your day-to-day work the easier and less embarrassing it will feel to you.

The paediatric examination

Perhaps the most important question one can ask in relation to the examination of a child is: does this child look ill? The answer to that question is difficult to define, and may refer to both acute and chronic illness. Nevertheless it is a question that all doctors who assess children as part of their work must learn to be able to answer. There is no substitute for seeing many well children and many ill children, and learning the difference between them.

Remember to wash your hands, and be alert to all visual clues both on and around the child. Look at the child generally for signs of discomfort or pain, respiratory distress, pallor, dysmorphic features, activity and alertness. Make a note of state of dress, hygiene, dentition, unusual behaviour and the relationship of the child with carers. All these clues can be important if there are concerns about safeguarding. Ask the child and/or carer if you can remove the child's clothes but only enough to enable a satisfactory examination – it is usually possible not to embarrass older children. Start examining areas that are not intimidating or uncomfortable then proceed to further examination once the child is at ease. You may have to abandon a strict examination routine and be opportunistic instead.

If the child is irritable or restless, there may be a few techniques that can be used (e.g. examining the child's soft toy to show what you are intending to do, asking parents/carers to entertain the child, using a toy/mobile phone/game console/television to distract a child) but you may have to ask for help – an experienced paediatric nurse will be able to help calm a child down. If all hope of performing an adequate examination is lost, you may have to just make do with what is possible to achieve, ensure you have addressed any serious concerns and leave the rest until later. It is rarely necessary to restrain a child in order to perform an examination. Firm restraint may become necessary later if a more invasive examination, for example looking in the throat, is needed.

It is beyond the scope of this book to describe detailed examination technique for each system – examination in children is broadly similar to that of adults; however, the range of conditions affecting each system is different in children and hence the examination itself needs to take account of this. To learn about examination of children there is no better way than to watch an experienced paediatrician doing it and then practising many times with children of different ages.

Cardiovascular examination

Bear in mind that the majority of heart problems in childhood are congenital abnormalities. It is therefore especially important to check for femoral pulses, the presence of heart murmurs and oxygen saturations. Note dysmorphic features that may indicate a syndrome associated with congenital heart disease. Common examples would include trisomy 21, Di George and Turner syndromes. You should note the heart rate, respiratory rate, oxygen saturations and blood pressure, all of which normally increase throughout childhood (Table 26.2).

Clubbing may indicate cyanotic heart disease. Skin temperature and capillary refill time – normally this is less than 2

Table 26.2 Paediatric cardiorespiratory values at different ages.

Age (years)	Heart rate (bpm)	Respiratory rate (breaths per minute)	Systolic blood pressure (mmHg)
<1	110–160	30–40	70–90
1–2	100–150	25–35	80–95
2–5	95–140	25–35	80–100
5–12	80–120	20–25	90–110
>12	60–100	15–20	100–120

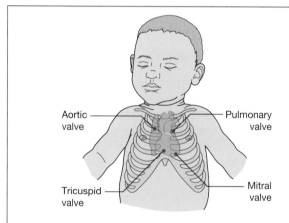

Figure 26.2 Sites of auscultation of the heart.

seconds – will indicate how well perfused the child is. Assessment of the jugular venous pressure is not required in young children.

Auscultation is performed exactly as in adults (Figure 26.2), but remember axillary murmurs (branch pulmonary artery stenosis) and interscapular murmurs (coarctation of the aorta) are commoner in children. The location of a murmur is probably the most useful feature of murmur in childhood in terms of working out its cause.

See Chapter 36 for more details of specific heart abnormalities.

Respiratory examination

Look for clues such as oxygen cylinders and nasal prongs that may indicate chronic lung disease, intravenous access ports and central lines (in patients with cystic fibrosis) and inhalers in asthma.

Clubbing may be a sign of cystic fibrosis in children. Harrison's sulci are two symmetrical horizontal sulci at the lower margin of the anterior thorax, at the attachment of the diaphragm (Figure 26.3). These are a sign of prolonged respiratory distress in children, and most commonly present in children

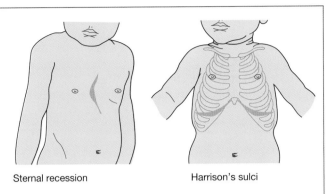

Sternal recession   Harrison's sulci

Figure 26.3 Harrison's sulci, sternal recession.

with asthma with increased respiratory effort over several months. Always check the respiratory rate in childhood – it is a reliable indicator of respiratory difficulty and may be the only obvious abnormality in childhood pneumonia.

Palpating the chest to assess chest movement and percussing for dullness or hyperresonance are not useful in infants and young children, but are informative in older children.

Gastrointestinal examination

Look for clues such as medication, special feeds and supplements. Abdominal examination in children is similar to that in adults.

Neurological examination

The examination technique depends very much on the patient's age. It is not possible to conduct a full examination of the cranial nerves of a young infant as one would in an adult, but much information can be gathered simply by careful inspection. Paediatric neurologists use observation more than any other aspect of examination. Look at posture, gait and movements – are they both normal and symmetrical? Remember to measure head circumference and compare to height/weight centiles on an appropriate chart.

Examine the skin for lesions such as café au lait spots, port wine stains and telangiectasiae, all of which may be important markers of neurological abnormalities in children.

In newborns, infants and younger children, cranial nerves can be assessed by observation of eye, face, tongue, jaw and shoulder movements, testing pupillary reflexes, and testing vision and hearing with age-appropriate methods. In older children, the cranial nerves can be tested similarly to an adult.

In the newborn period, particular emphasis is placed on primitive reflexes (see Chapter 27), head size, fontanelle size and tension, muscle tone, movements and posture. As children grow older, the assessment of muscle bulk and power, tendon reflexes, coordination and sensation becomes easier and more like the adult examination.

Ear and throat examination

This is usually left until last as the young child often needs to be restrained to a certain degree in order for no harm to come to them. It is important to use a good technique and give clear instructions to the parent on how to hold their child.

To examine the ears, ideally the carer holds the child's head to one side against his/her chest with one hand, and the child's arms with the other hand. Turn the child's head to face you to examine the throat. With the aid of a tongue depressor, you should be able to quickly visualise the tonsils, uvula, pharynx and posterior palate. Older children should be able to cooperate independently.

Skin and musculoskeletal system

The skin and musculoskeletal system can be examined much like that of an adult, and again observation is the key skill.

Clinical case

Case discussion

The commonest conclusion to paediatric consultations in general is that the presenting problem is mild, self-limiting or normal. Nevertheless it takes considerable skill to build a rapport with a child and their family such that the family will trust the judgement of the doctor assessing their child. There is an art to showing families that you have taken their concerns seriously without belittling them. Often parents will say that doctors think they are 'over-anxious'. A friendly, age-appropriate approach to the child, a thorough history, a competent examination, and a careful and tactful explanation of the fact that the child does not have anything serious is all that is needed in many paediatric consultations.

Case conclusion

Huw is a normal child, and his heart murmur is an innocent murmur brought on by a self-limiting illness whilst on holiday.

Summary

Key learning points

- Time spent taking a thorough and systematic history will aid the further management of a child.
- There are many similarities to history taking and examination of an adult but a few important additional features that require close attention are necessary in the paediatric medical history.
- Appropriate communication skills when approaching paediatric patients of varying ages comes with practice.

 Now visit www.**wileyessential.com/humandevelopment** to test yourself on this chapter.

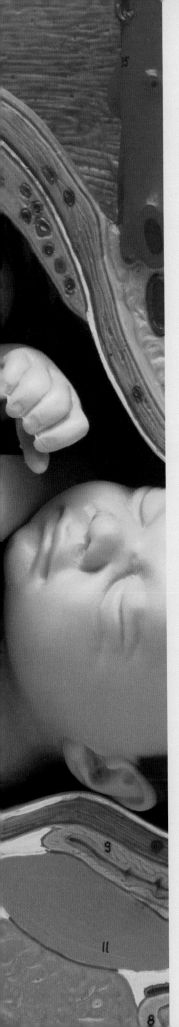

CHAPTER 27
Normal growth and developmental milestones

Bethan Williams

Case

A 9-month-old girl, Mary, presents with concerns regarding her weight gain. She was born at 39 weeks gestation weighing 3.2 kg (75th centile) and currently weighs 6.8 kg (2nd–9th centile). Her length and head circumference both lie on the 50th centile, at 71 cm and 44 cm respectively. She was bottle fed and weaned onto solids at 6 months of age. Her parents have recently separated and her mother is a known substance misuser. Her health visitor has requested a paediatric review to evaluate her health and development.

Learning outcomes

- You should be able to describe the normal physiology of growth, how growth is measured and monitored in children, and be familiar with some of the more common causes for abnormal growth patterns.
- You should be able to describe the normal developmental milestones.

Essential Human Development, First Edition. Edited by Samuel Webster, Geraint Morris and Euan Kevelighan
© 2018 John Wiley & Sons, Ltd. Published 2018 by John Wiley & Sons, Ltd.

Growth

Growth of all body parameters is a fundamental process unique to childhood. Starting from the moment of conception, normal growth occurs as a complex interaction of genetics, hormones, nutritional availability and the environment. Therefore poor growth can result from a number of factors including genetic syndromes, endocrine abnormalities, disease, poor environment or a combination of these.

Factors affecting growth in utero can be different from those affecting postnatal growth. This is illustrated in Table 27.1.

Physiology of growth

Human growth hormone (hGH) is secreted by the anterior part of the pituitary gland. Production is controlled by the hypothalamus via growth hormone-releasing hormone (stimulating production), and growth hormone release inhibitory hormone (GHRIH), also known as somatostatin (inhibiting production). hGH then stimulates hepatic production

of IGF-1 (Figure 27.1). The major functions of this system are:

- increasing collagen and protein synthesis;
- promoting retention of calcium, phosphorus and nitrogen;
- opposing the action of insulin.

hGH is released periodically, usually at night, especially during REM sleep. Acute stress and exercise stimulate hGH release, whereas hyperglycaemia and excess corticosteroids suppress it. It is also under the influence of other pituitary hormones such as thyroid and parathyroid hormones.

Periods of growth

Fetal phase

This is the fastest period of growth, accounting for approximately 30% of eventual height. In the 40-week period of gestation the fetus repeatedly doubles in size, undergoing 42 cycles of cell division before birth, whilst just a further five cycles occur from birth to adulthood. As outlined in Table 27.1, size at birth is determined by the size of the mother and placental

Table 27.1 Comparison of four major growth factors between prenatal and postnatal growth.

Factor	Prenatal	Postnatal
Genetic	Minor effect overall Maternal size important in determining birth size Paternal genetic factors have little effect on birth size Maternal factors tend to override fetal genetic factors in determining prenatal growth	Largely determines final adult height Sex chromosomes have an effect: • XY boys are taller than XX girls • XYY boys are taller than XY boys • XXY boys (Klinefelter syndrome) same height as XY boys • XO girls (Turner syndrome) shorter than XX girls Other genetic conditions that are not X- or Y-linked can also account for short or tall stature
Endocrine	Insulin and insulin-like growth factors (IGFs) are the major prenatal hormones influencing growth: • IGF-2 most important for embryonic growth • IGF-1 most important for later fetal and infant growth Growth hormone has no effect on early growth	Human growth hormone (hGH) is the major hormone controlling growth after birth
Nutrition	Placenta provides all nutrients to growing fetus, therefore essential for growth Placental insufficiency most common cause of intra-uterine growth restriction Placenta also controls hormones necessary for fetal growth Maternal diet influences nutritional availability, particularly important in developing countries	Adequate nutrition is essential for growth Starvation due to lack of substrate availability as a result of poverty, neglect or disease can limit growth potential Obesity occurs mostly as a result of excessive intake of food Poor nutrition may delay the onset of puberty Malabsorption of nutrients may cause reduced growth
Environment	Uterine capacity and placental sufficiency important in providing optimal environment for fetus Multiple pregnancy (e.g. twins) produces smaller babies than singleton pregnancy, but combined weight of multiple babies is greater than that of a singleton implying that placental function is more influential in fetal growth than uterine capacity	The following factors are known to influence growth: • Socioeconomic status • Chronic disease • Emotional status • Altitude (mediated by lower oxygen saturation levels)

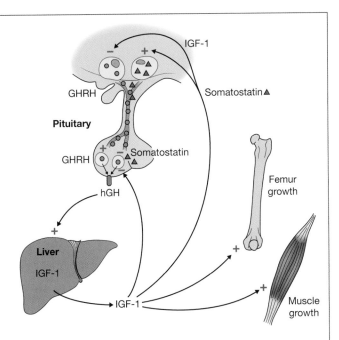

Figure 27.1 The growth axis. GH, growth hormone; GHRH, growth hormone-releasing hormone; IGF-1, insulin-like growth factor 1

nutritional supply, which in turn modulates fetal growth hormones (insulin, IGF-2 and human placental lactogen). In addition to this, maternal smoking and gestational length also influence fetal growth, as do congenital infections. Severe intrauterine growth restriction and extreme prematurity when accompanied by poor postnatal growth can result in permanent short stature. Interestingly, low birthweight can increase the risk of childhood obesity and cardiovascular disease.

Infantile phase

This period encompasses growth between birth and 18 months of age. This is another period of rapid (but decelerating) growth and accounts for 15% of eventual height. A child generally triples their birthweight, increases their length by 50%, and head circumference by one-third during this phase. Here growth is largely dependent on adequate nutrition, but good health and normal thyroid function are also essential. An inadequate rate of weight gain during this growth phase is known as 'faltering growth'.

Childhood phase

This is a slow, steady and prolonged period of growth from 18 months to 12 years of age. It contributes to 40% of final height. The average annual growth during this period is a 5–6 cm increase in height and 3–3.5 kg increase in weight. Whilst growth continues to be influenced by adequate nutrition and good health, the endocrine, genetic and environmental factors have emerging importance here. By the age of

2 years, most children have attained their genetically determined growth centile. Growth hormone and IGF-1 influence on the epiphyses are the main determinants of a child's rate of skeletal growth, and thyroid hormones (particularly thyroxine), vitamin D and steroids also affect cartilage cell division and bone formation. Emotional disturbance in the form of profound, chronic unhappiness can decrease hGH secretion leading to psychosocial short stature.

Pubertal phase

Also referred to as the pubertal growth spurt, this adds 15% to the final height. Rising levels of sex hormones, mainly testosterone and oestradiol, boost hGH secretion leading to rapid growth of long bones. This surge in growth is short-lived as the same sex hormones cause fusion of the epiphyseal growth plates and cessation of growth. By the time a girl has her first menstrual period (menarche) she has completed two-thirds of her pubertal growth spurt and is unlikely to grow more than another 3–5 cm. Boys enter puberty on average 2 years later than girls. This delay in onset lengthens their time in the growth phase, leading to an eventual height greater than that of girls. During the 3–4 years of puberty boys will grow approximately 25 cm, whereas girls will grow 20 cm. Other changes occurring at puberty will be discussed in more detail in Chapter 31.

Measuring growth

The measurement of growth is an extremely important part of the assessment of a child's general health, as reduced growth can indicate underlying pathology. Commonly, three parameters of growth are measured:

- height;
- weight;
- head circumference.

Equipment used to measure height and weight should be regularly calibrated to ensure accuracy of recordings. In children under the age of 2 years height is measured when the child is lying down, whilst in children over the age of 2 years their height is measured when they are standing. It is important when measuring height in the supine position that the legs are held straight; to perform accurately this method needs more than one person. When measuring height with a child standing it is important that shoes are removed, the feet are flat on the floor, the knees are straight, and the head is straight with eyes and ears level. Gentle upward traction bilaterally on the mastoid process is also required. Both these methods are illustrated in Figure 27.2. Measuring height in children with physical disabilities can be more challenging, but is still necessary.

Weight is best measured on electronic scales, with a naked infant, or a child dressed only in underclothes, and no shoes. A wet nappy or heavy jeans or shoes can represent a whole month or even a year's weight gain.

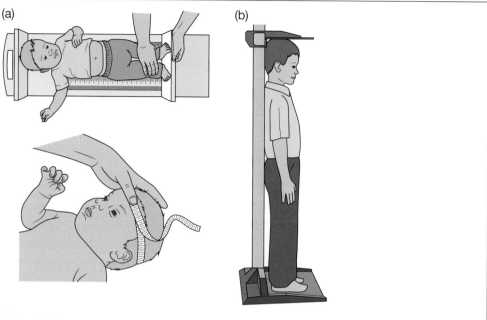

Figure 27.2 Measuring height in children.

The occipito-frontal head circumference is the best measurement for monitoring brain and head growth. A tape is used to measure around the head at the level of the occiput and frontal bone and the greatest of three measurements is recorded. It is also important to review the shape of the head and not just the size.

Once the measurements have been obtained they should be plotted on an appropriate growth chart. Current UK growth charts combine the 1990 UK growth reference data for children at birth and from 4 to 18 years with the World Health Organization (WHO) growth standard for children aged 2–4 years. There are separate charts for boys and girls and these can be found on the websites of the Royal College of Paediatrics and Child Health (RCPCH) (www.rcpch.ac.uk/growthcharts) and the Centers for disease Control and Prevention (CDC) (www.cdc.gov/growthcharts), but there are also separate charts for children with trisomy 21 as their growth profile is different to that of the general population.

The head at birth is disproportionally larger than the body, making up almost one-third of the total body length, compared to the adult ratio of 1:7. The head grows rapidly over the first 2 years, before slowing down, but continues to grow throughout childhood. In the early years, the cranial sutures are open. The posterior fontanelle closes at approximately 8 weeks of age, and the anterior fontanelle closes between 12 and 18 months of age. The sutures are generally fused by the age of 6 years. Measurements indicating a large head, that is greater than the 98th centile (termed macrocephaly) or small head, that is below the 2nd centile (termed microcephaly) are concerning as they could represent underlying brain pathology such as hydrocephalus. However, no one measurement should be taken in isolation (in terms of growth parameter or timing).

In the first 1–2 years of life it is normal for children's growth to cross centiles, but any crossing of centiles at any age should be monitored very closely as it could indicate underlying illness or safeguarding concerns.

The formulae below have been used to estimate growth potential in children:

$$\text{Boy's expected height (mid-parental height centile)} = \frac{\frac{(\text{mother's height} + 12.5\,\text{cm})}{} + \text{father's height}}{2}$$

$$\text{Girl's expected height (mid-parental height centile)} = \frac{\frac{(\text{father's height} - 12.5\,\text{cm})}{} + \text{mother's height}}{2}$$

These formulae have their limitations and should not be used alone especially if parents are at extremes of height. It must also be stressed that single measurements do not predict growth rates; measurements of height and weight (plus head circumference in children under the age of 2 years) should be repeated after a period of at least 4 months for any calculations regarding growth velocity to be interpreted. Usually data will be collected over a period of 12 months for this purpose. These measurements are then plotted on a separate growth velocity chart.

Development

In parallel to growing in size, children will acquire new skills and abilities as their brain develops. This process involves complex interactions of genes and the environment, and Table 27.2 illustrates numerous factors that can also influence these interactions. The genes will determine the potential of the child by providing the basic 'wiring plan' and forming the neuronal connections between different brain regions, whilst the environment influences the extent to which the child achieves that

Table 27.2 Factors influencing development.

Prenatal	Pre- and postnatal	Postnatal
Toxins, infection, drugs, alcohol Ischaemia Nutrition Genetic abnormalities	Parental IQ (IQ may be partially geneti- cally determined, but parental IQ may also influence parenting) Personality	Social environment Cultural factors Nutrition Parenting Physical health Emotional factors; interaction with caregivers

potential, that is experiences 'fine-tune' these connections. It is not always possible to separate out the major contributor in this nature versus nurture phenomenon.

The environment therefore needs to provide for the child's physical and psychological needs in order for optimal development to progress. The needs of a child are very different at different ages; for example, newborns are entirely dependent on their parents for their physical and psychological needs, children of primary school age will be able to meet some of their physical needs and cope with simple social relationships, whereas teenagers can meet their physical needs but are experiencing increasingly complex emotional needs (Figure 27.3).

Previous observational studies have shown that normal development follows a specific sequence in most children and have also provided a range of ages at which children are expected to achieve each skill. Children need to acquire certain skills before they can progress to the next skill; for example, a child must achieve good head control before being able to sit up. These developmental skills are referred to as milestones and can be divided into four separate categories:

1. Gross motor – large movements, e.g. sitting up, walking.
2. Fine motor and vision – small movements, e.g. pencil skills, puzzles.
3. Speech, language and hearing – communication skills, e.g. receptive and expressive language, non-verbal communication.
4. Social behaviour and play – play and self-help skills, e.g. feeding, dressing, toileting, socialising.

These four categories are not mutually exclusive, and some skills may overlap more than one category. Typically, developing children may also show slight variations in their acquisition of skills in the different categories; for example, a child may be slightly more advanced in their gross motor skills than their language skills, or vice versa.

Tables 27.3 to 27.6 demonstrate the normal pattern of development for children, providing the milestone, a description of the milestone and the median age at which that skill is achieved (i.e. the age at which 50% of the standard population achieve that skill).

Tables 27.3 to 27.6 do not provide an exhaustive list of all developmental milestones but are fairly comprehensive. Table 27.7 provides a simple summary of key milestones, which may aid quick revision. (You will note that different authors will quote slightly different median ages.)

Whilst it is important to know what milestones a child should have achieved at specific ages, it is also important to know when to become concerned about a child who is not developing as you would expect them to. This is covered in more detail in Chapter 28.

Primitive reflexes

Persistence of a primitive reflex beyond the age at which it would normally disappear may impair developmental progress and indicate an abnormality of the central nervous system (Table 27.8).

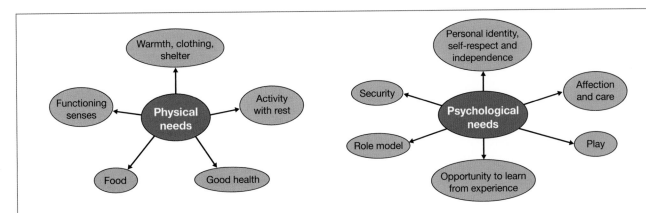

Figure 27.3 A sample of physical and psychological needs of children.

Table 27.3 Gross motor development.

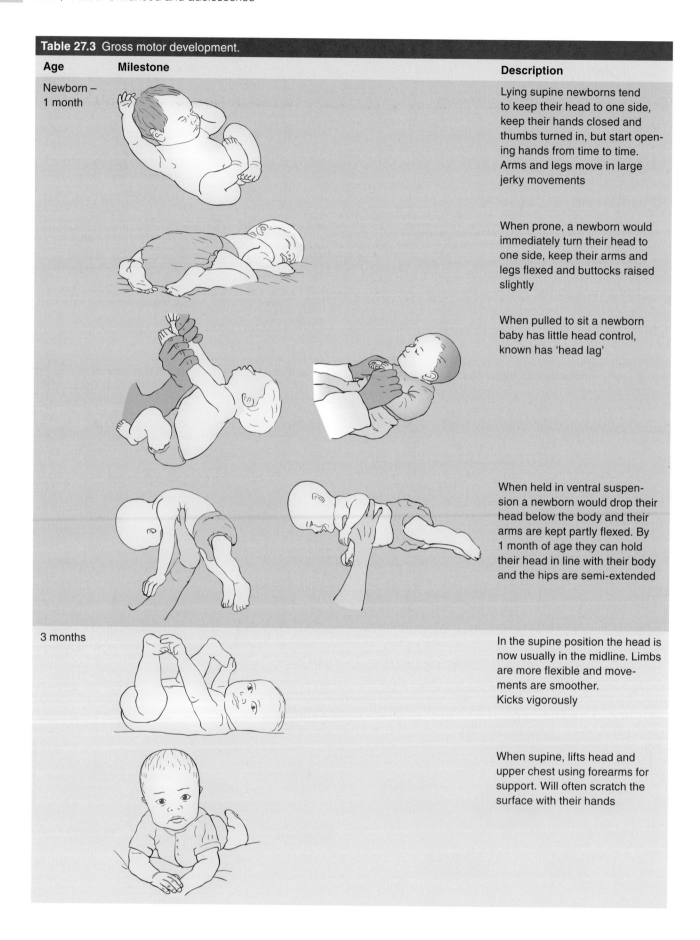

Age	Milestone	Description
Newborn – 1 month		Lying supine newborns tend to keep their head to one side, keep their hands closed and thumbs turned in, but start opening hands from time to time. Arms and legs move in large jerky movements
		When prone, a newborn would immediately turn their head to one side, keep their arms and legs flexed and buttocks raised slightly
		When pulled to sit a newborn baby has little head control, known has 'head lag'
		When held in ventral suspension a newborn would drop their head below the body and their arms are kept partly flexed. By 1 month of age they can hold their head in line with their body and the hips are semi-extended
3 months		In the supine position the head is now usually in the midline. Limbs are more flexible and movements are smoother. Kicks vigorously
		When supine, lifts head and upper chest using forearms for support. Will often scratch the surface with their hands

Age	Milestone	Description

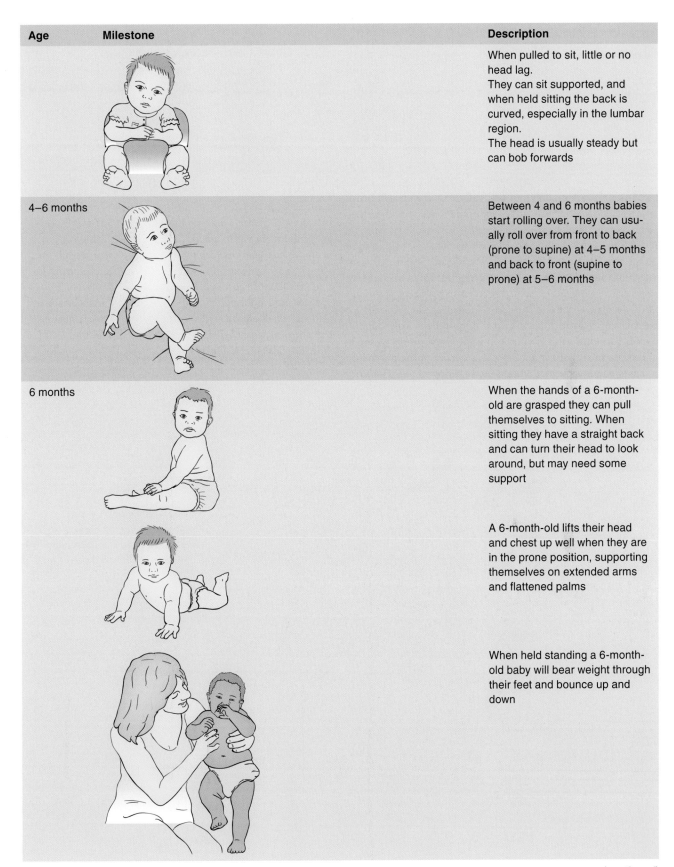

[no age label] — When pulled to sit, little or no head lag.
They can sit supported, and when held sitting the back is curved, especially in the lumbar region.
The head is usually steady but can bob forwards

4–6 months — Between 4 and 6 months babies start rolling over. They can usually roll over from front to back (prone to supine) at 4–5 months and back to front (supine to prone) at 5–6 months

6 months — When the hands of a 6-month-old are grasped they can pull themselves to sitting. When sitting they have a straight back and can turn their head to look around, but may need some support

A 6-month-old lifts their head and chest up well when they are in the prone position, supporting themselves on extended arms and flattened palms

When held standing a 6-month-old baby will bear weight through their feet and bounce up and down

(continued)

Age	Milestone	Description
9 months		Able to pull self into a sitting position. Whilst sitting unsupported can play with a toy without falling over
		When sitting can lean forwards, and turn sideways to pick up toys from the floor
		Able to mobilise around the room either by rolling, or crawling
		Between 9 and 12 months will crawl either on hands and knees, commando crawl or bottom shuffle
		Can pull to stand, holding on for support

Age	Milestone	Description
	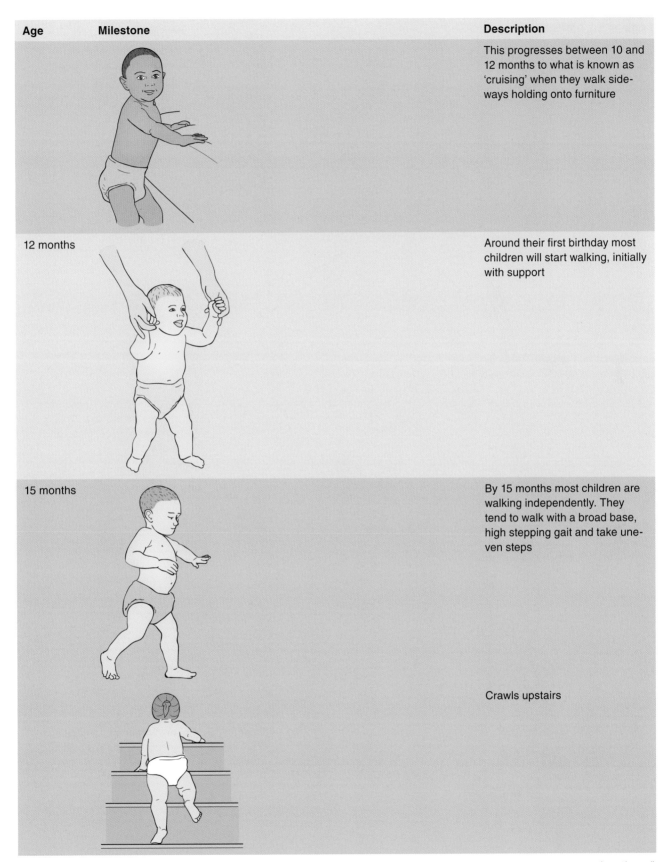	This progresses between 10 and 12 months to what is known as 'cruising' when they walk sideways holding onto furniture
12 months		Around their first birthday most children will start walking, initially with support
15 months		By 15 months most children are walking independently. They tend to walk with a broad base, high stepping gait and take uneven steps
		Crawls upstairs

(*continued*)

Age	Milestone	Description
18 months		Children are usually confident at walking now and are beginning to run with their head held erect. They struggle to negotiate obstacles
		Enjoys pushing large toys
		Able to bend down (or squat) to pick a toy off the floor. This is also referred to as 'stoop and retrieve'
		Walks upstairs with a helping hand or holding on. Would generally descend stairs on their bottoms
		Able to climb onto a chair and then turn around to sit facing forward

Age	Milestone	Description
2 years		Ascends and descends stairs with two feet per step holding onto a rail (or wall)
		Can throw a small ball forwards
		Walks into ball when trying to kick it
		Sits on tricycle but cannot use pedals, will propel by pushing feet along the floor
2.5 years		Can jump with both feet together off a small step

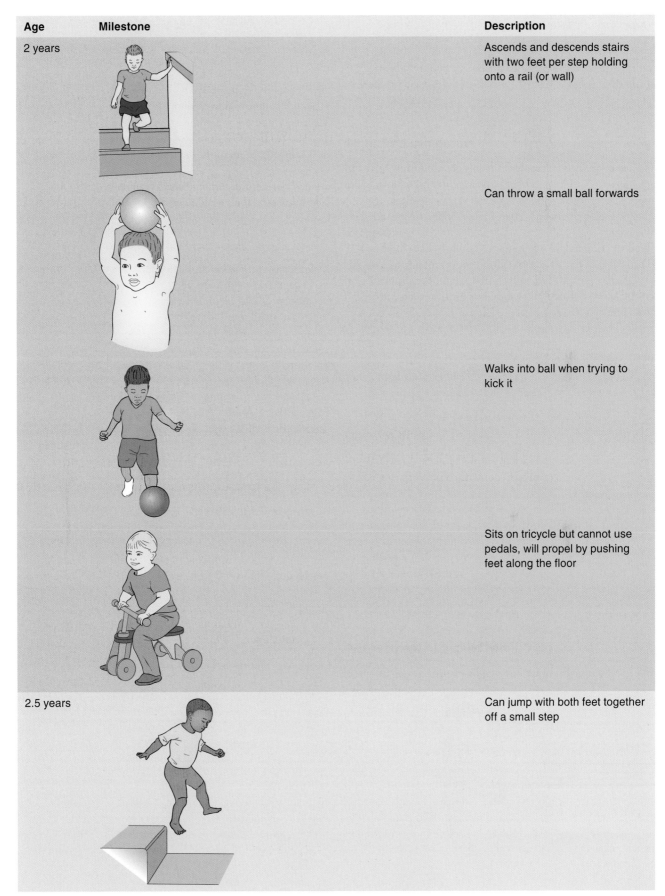

(*continued*)

Age	Milestone	Description

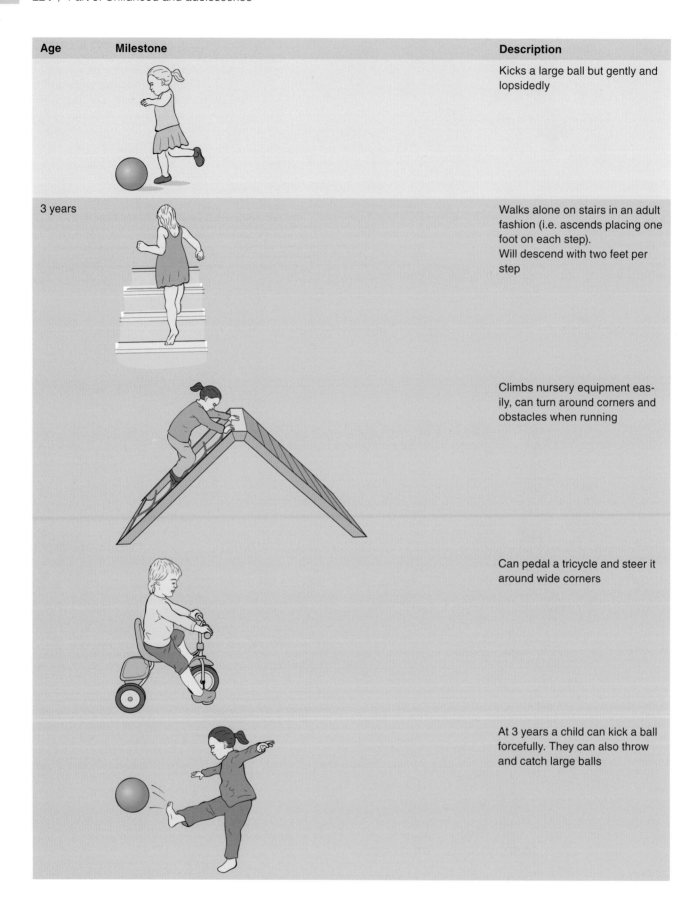

Kicks a large ball but gently and lopsidedly

3 years

Walks alone on stairs in an adult fashion (i.e. ascends placing one foot on each step).
Will descend with two feet per step

Climbs nursery equipment easily, can turn around corners and obstacles when running

Can pedal a tricycle and steer it around wide corners

At 3 years a child can kick a ball forcefully. They can also throw and catch large balls

Age	Milestone	Description
	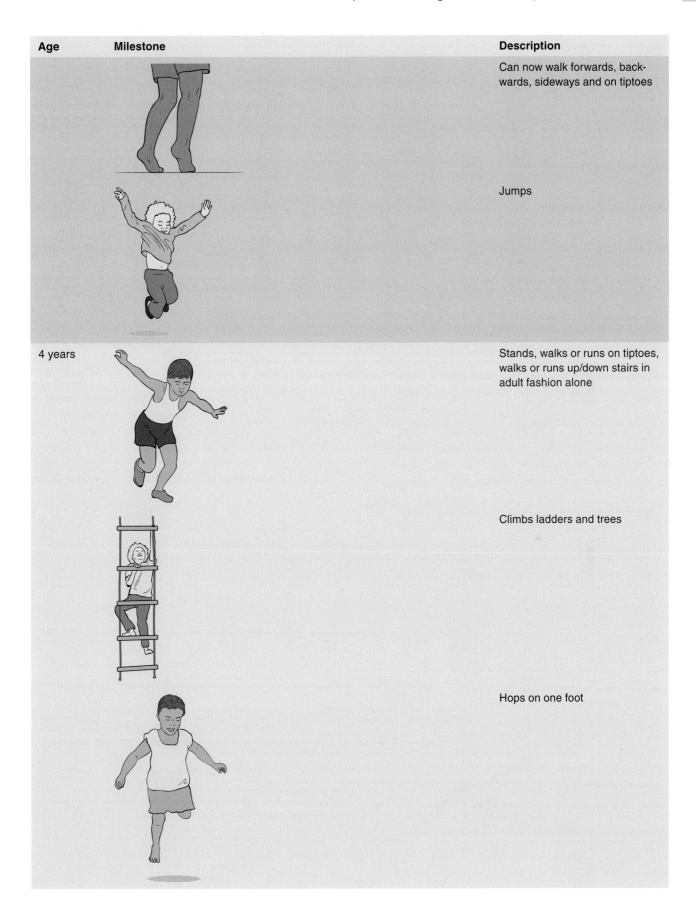	Can now walk forwards, backwards, sideways and on tiptoes
		Jumps
4 years		Stands, walks or runs on tiptoes, walks or runs up/down stairs in adult fashion alone
		Climbs ladders and trees
		Hops on one foot

(*continued*)

Age	Milestone	Description
	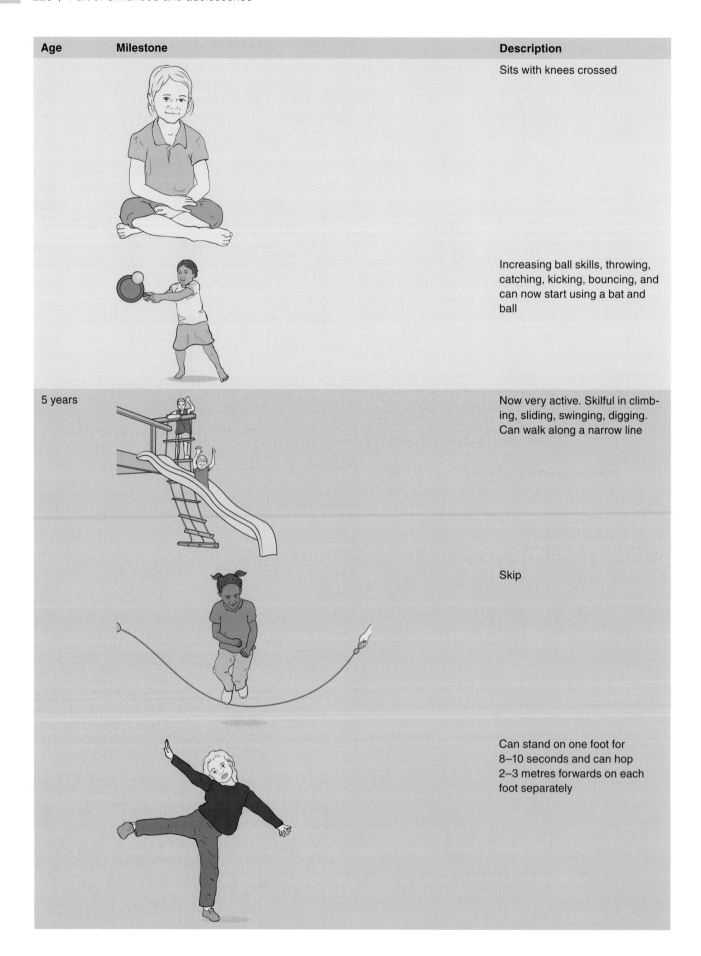	Sits with knees crossed
		Increasing ball skills, throwing, catching, kicking, bouncing, and can now start using a bat and ball
5 years		Now very active. Skilful in climbing, sliding, swinging, digging. Can walk along a narrow line
		Skip
		Can stand on one foot for 8–10 seconds and can hop 2–3 metres forwards on each foot separately

Age	Milestone	Description

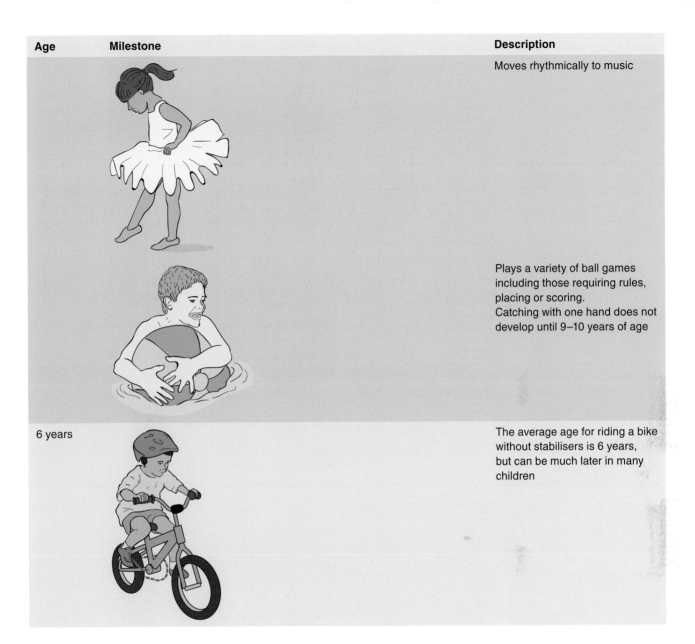

Moves rhythmically to music

Plays a variety of ball games including those requiring rules, placing or scoring.
Catching with one hand does not develop until 9–10 years of age

6 years — The average age for riding a bike without stabilisers is 6 years, but can be much later in many children

Table 27.4 Fine motor and vision skills.

Age	Milestone	Description
Newborn		Newborn infants will turn their eyes towards light and close their eyes to bright light. For a baby to show interest in an object it must be within 30 cm of their face
1 month		Pupils react to light. Will fix and follow a bright toy 15–25 cm from face in midline horizontally. Watches a familiar face when being talked to Defensive blink present by 6–8 weeks
3 months		Moves head purposely to look around. Shows hand regard when lying supine, opening and closing hands. Holds toys momentarily By 4 months starts reaching out for objects
6 months		Reaches out with both hands to grasp objects, with a palmar grasp. Passes toy from hand to hand. Watches when toy falls. Object permanence emerging
9 months		Pincer grip (can pick up small object between thumb and index finger)

Age	Milestone	Description
	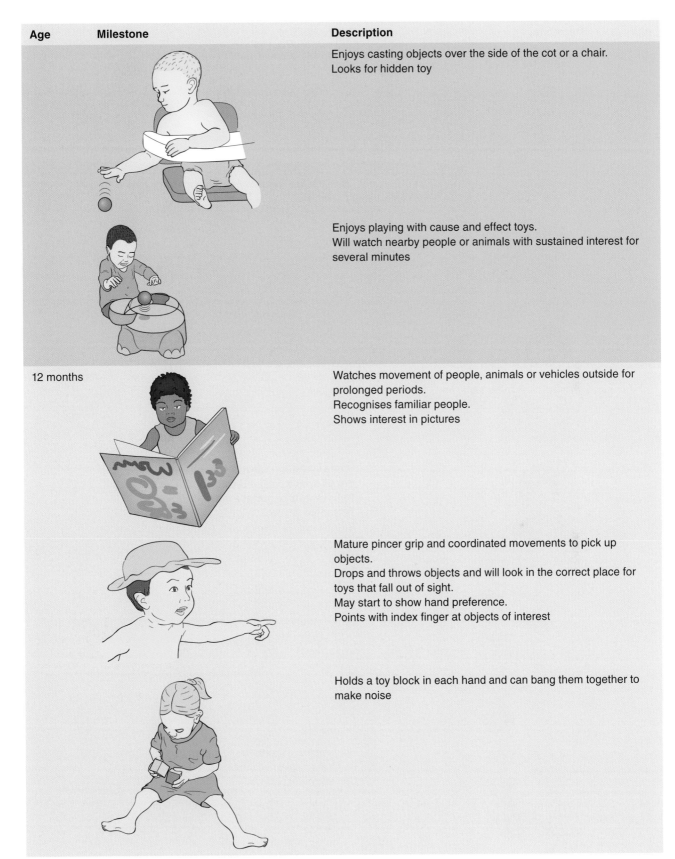	Enjoys casting objects over the side of the cot or a chair. Looks for hidden toy
		Enjoys playing with cause and effect toys. Will watch nearby people or animals with sustained interest for several minutes
12 months		Watches movement of people, animals or vehicles outside for prolonged periods. Recognises familiar people. Shows interest in pictures
		Mature pincer grip and coordinated movements to pick up objects. Drops and throws objects and will look in the correct place for toys that fall out of sight. May start to show hand preference. Points with index finger at objects of interest
		Holds a toy block in each hand and can bang them together to make noise

(*continued*)

Age	Milestone	Description
15 months		Builds a tower of two bricks
		Takes objects out of a container and replaces
		Palmar grasp of crayon
18 months		Points to distant objects of interest. Enjoys simple picture books. Turns several pages at a time. To-and-fro scribble. Builds tower of three bricks. Hand preference shown
2 years		Can match square, circle, and triangle shapes in simple jigsaw
		Holds pencil at bottom with immature tripod grip. Performs circular scribble. Can copy vertical line

Age	Milestone	Description
		Builds a tower of six bricks
2.5 years		Builds tower of 7+ bricks. Holds pencil with improved tripod grasp
3 years		Copies circle
		Builds bridge from three cubes
		Threads large beads
		Draws person with head and one or two other features. Enjoys painting. Knows colours.
		Cuts with toy scissors

(*continued*)

Age	Milestone	Description
4 years		Builds tower of 10+ bricks. Build three steps with six bricks Draws person with head, legs, trunk and usually arms and fingers. Draws recognisable house. Copies cross and square
5 years		Draws person with head, trunk, arms, legs and other features. Draws house with door, windows roof and chimney. Can write name. Copies triangle

Table 27.5 Speech and language skills.

Age	Milestone	Description
Newborn		Startles to loud noises
1 month		Startles to loud noises. May turn towards sound source but cannot localise sound yet. Cries loudly when hungry or upset
3 months		Calms to sound of familiar voice. Shows excitement. Vocalises and integrates this with smiles, eye contact and hand gestures
6 months		Turns to familiar voice. Turns to source when sounds heard at ear level. Vocalises tunefully, makes vowel sounds. Laughs. Screams in annoyance

Age	Milestone	Description
9 months		Localises sounds above and below ear level. Shouts to attract attention. Babbles in repetitive strings of syllables, e.g. 'dad-dad', 'mam-mam'. Responds to name
12 months		Tries to join in familiar tunes. Babbles in conversational cadences. Understands some words in context, e.g. cat, drink. Understands simple instructions, e.g. 'give it to daddy'. Vocalises to familiar songs
15 months		Says a few recognisable words (2–6 words). Enjoys looking at pictures in a book for 2 minutes or more. Obeys simple instructions, e.g. 'don't touch', 'give me the ball'. Points to familiar people, animals or toys when requested. Indicates needs by pointing and vocalising or screaming
18 months		Chatters to self during play with conversational intonation and emotional inflections. Uses 6–20 recognisable words and understands many more. Attempts to sing and joins in nursery rhymes. Points to body parts

(continued)

Age	Milestone	Description
2 years		Uses 50+ words. Puts two words together to make simple sentences. Refers to self by name. Echolalia (repeats words spoken by others). Carries out two-step commands, e.g. 'get your teddy and put it in the bag'
3 years		Uses 200+ words. Sentences grammatically immature and substitutes many letters (e.g. 'f' for 'th'). Uses pronouns correctly (I, me, you). Knows full name. Recognises family categories (mother, grandmother, sister). Constantly asking questions. Adds a running commentary to play. Identifies objects based on their function. Counts by rote up to 10 (but only understands number concept up to 2 or 3)
4 years		Speech grammatically correct. Gives full name, age and address. Tells long stories. Counts up to 20 or more
5 years		Fluent grammatically correct conversational speech. Understands time, e.g. 'first, then, last'. Enjoys jokes

Table 27.6 Social behaviour and self-care.

Age	Milestone	Description
Newborn to 3 months		Sucks well. Sleeps most of the time. Social smile by 6 weeks of age. Stops crying when picked up and spoken to, turns to look at speaker's face
3 months		Fixes on carer's face when feeding. Eager anticipation of feed; smiles and coos to familiar situations
6 months		Enthusiastic in rough and tumble play. Shakes rattle deliberately. Puts everything in mouth. Passes toys from hand to hand. Some stranger anxiety. Holds bottle (or breast) when being fed. Starts weaning to solids
9 months		Plays peek-a-boo. Offers food to familiar people. Offers toy to another but can't put it in the adult's hand. Watches toy being partially hidden then finds it – also referred to as 'object permanence'. Finger feeds
12 months		Will put objects in and out of box when shown. Waves bye-bye. Plays pat-a-cake. Demonstrates use of object, e.g. hair brush. Attempts to feed from spoon (but very messy). Helps with dressing by holding out arm for sleeve or foot for shoe

(continued)

Age	Milestone	Description
15 months	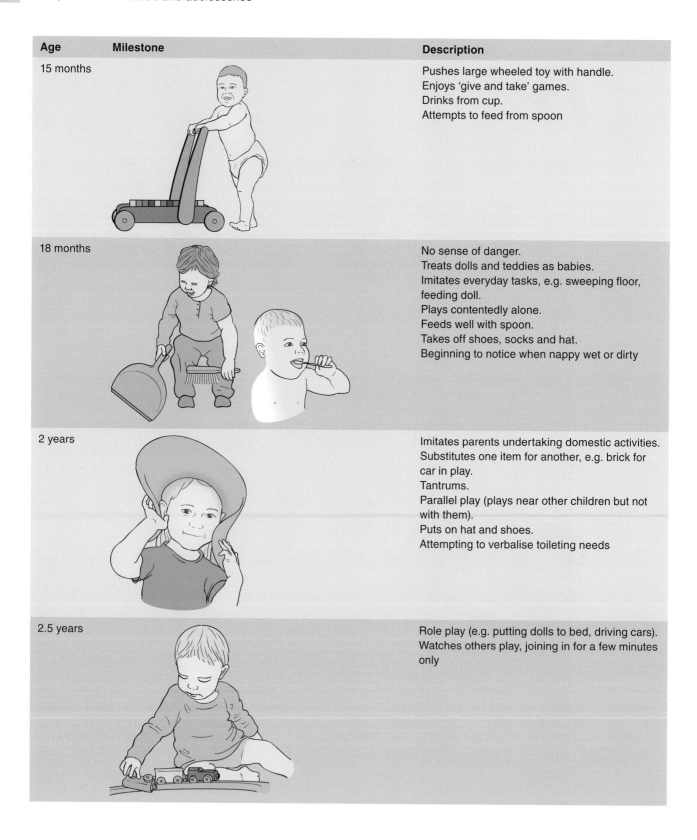	Pushes large wheeled toy with handle. Enjoys 'give and take' games. Drinks from cup. Attempts to feed from spoon
18 months		No sense of danger. Treats dolls and teddies as babies. Imitates everyday tasks, e.g. sweeping floor, feeding doll. Plays contentedly alone. Feeds well with spoon. Takes off shoes, socks and hat. Beginning to notice when nappy wet or dirty
2 years		Imitates parents undertaking domestic activities. Substitutes one item for another, e.g. brick for car in play. Tantrums. Parallel play (plays near other children but not with them). Puts on hat and shoes. Attempting to verbalise toileting needs
2.5 years		Role play (e.g. putting dolls to bed, driving cars). Watches others play, joining in for a few minutes only

Age	Milestone		Description
3 years	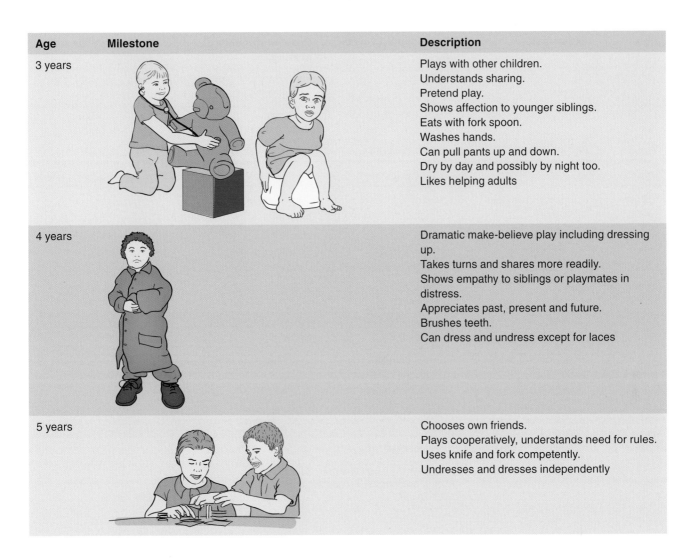		Plays with other children. Understands sharing. Pretend play. Shows affection to younger siblings. Eats with fork spoon. Washes hands. Can pull pants up and down. Dry by day and possibly by night too. Likes helping adults
4 years			Dramatic make-believe play including dressing up. Takes turns and shares more readily. Shows empathy to siblings or playmates in distress. Appreciates past, present and future. Brushes teeth. Can dress and undress except for laces
5 years			Chooses own friends. Plays cooperatively, understands need for rules. Uses knife and fork competently. Undresses and dresses independently

Table 27.7 Summary of key developmental milestones.

Age	Gross motor	Fine motor and vision	Speech, language and hearing	Social, behaviour and play
Newborn	Marked head lag	Follows face in midline	Startles to loud noises	
6–8 weeks	Raises head to 45°	Follows moving object by moving head	Calms to familiar voice	Smiles responsively
4 months	Rolls over	Reaches out for toys	Vocalises, coos	Fix on carer's face during feeding
6 months	Sits with rounded back	Transfers from one hand to another (palmer grasp)	Laughs	Some stranger anxiety
8 months	Sits with straight back			Puts food in mouth
9 months	Crawling		Localises sounds Shouts	Object permanence
10 months	Cruising furniture	Mature pincer grip	Says 'mama', 'dada'	Waves bye-bye Plays peek-a-boo
12 months	Walking unsteadily		Uses 2–3 words	Drinks from cup

(continued)

Age	Gross motor	Fine motor and vision	Speech, language and hearing	Social, behaviour and play
15 months	Walks steadily independently	Scribbles	Follows simple commands, e.g. 'give to Daddy'	Enjoys give and take games
18 months	Stoops and retrieves	Tower of three bricks	10 words Show four parts of body	Feeds with spoon Symbolic play
2 years	Ascends stairs in two feet per step fashion	Tower of six bricks	Two-word sentences Follows two-step commands	Dry by day Pulls off some clothing Parallel play
2.5 years	Jumps with both feet Kicks ball	Tower of eight bricks Train of four bricks	3–4-word sentences Echolalia	Role play
3 years	Pedals tricycle	Draws a circle Builds a bridge Threads beads	200+ words Knows full name Counts to 10	Interactive play Takes turns
4 years	Hops	Draws a cross Builds steps	Tells long stories	Make believe play
4.5 years	Climbs trees	Draws a square	Knows full name, age and address	Brushes teeth
5 years	Skips, dances, learning to ride bike	Draws a triangle	Understands time and tense	Dresses and undresses independently

Table 27.8 Primitive reflexes.

Reflex	Usual age to disappear	Description	
Sucking reflex	6–8 weeks	Baby will automatically suck if an object is placed in the mouth	
Rooting reflex	6–8 weeks	When a stimulus is near the mouth (e.g. stroking of cheek) the baby will open their mouth and turn towards the stimulus	
Palmar grasp	3–4 months	When an object is placed in the palm of the hand flexion of the hand and fingers occurs	
Plantar grasp	12–18 months	When the sole of the foot is stroked the baby curls its toes and feet.	

Reflex	Usual age to disappear	Description	
Moro reflex	4–5 months	Sudden head and neck extension causes extension and abduction of the arms followed by adduction of the arms, and flexion of the fingers, wrists and elbows	
Stepping reflex	2 months	When the baby is held vertically and the dorsum of the feet brought into contact with a surface the baby will lift one foot, then the other in a stepping fashion	
Asymmetric tonic neck reflex	6 months	When lying supine and the head is turned to one side, the arm and leg on the side the head is turned to extend, whilst the arm and leg opposite to the turn flex (the baby adopts a fencing or archer's position)	
Babinski reflex	Is initially up-going, but due to the plantar reflex can be difficult to elicit. By 1 year of age the reflex is down-going.		

Clinical case

Case investigations

Mary's health visitor reports that the family home is untidy and that attendance for vaccinations is erratic. In her opinion the parenting skills are suboptimal. Mary often appears unkempt, is often not in clean clothes, and Mary's mother does not own a cooker.

Mother reports that Mary does not like lumpy food and prefers to have commercial baby rice rather than fruit, vegetables or meat-based meals. Her mother typically lets Mary feed herself about twice a day.

Examination of Mary shows that she has excess skin folds around her buttocks and thighs, she is noticeably pale and somewhat withdrawn. Blood tests show that she has a microcytic anaemia and a low ferritin level. Anti-transglutaminase antibodies and IgA levels are both normal.

Case conclusions

It is likely that in Mary's case the cause of her suboptimal weight gain is inadequate nutrition. At this age she should be on a wide range of solid foods and efforts should be made to support Mary's mother to better understand Mary's nutritional needs. Mary will see a paediatric dietician who will be able to educate Mary's mother in regards to suitable weaning foods. The health visitor will be a key professional who will be able to find ways of supporting Mary's mother initially.

The situation will need to be monitored closely by monitoring Mary's weight on a regular basis. In this case there should be early recourse to involving social services should the situation not improve.

SUMMARY

Key learning points

- Growth and development are important indicators of health and can be assessed by measuring the length or height, and weight of the child, and by observing the development of skills and abilities. Growth charts and a knowledge of the ages at which half of children are able to perform skills associated with developmental milestones are helpful in determining whether or not a child is developing at the expected rate.

- Genetic, nutritional, environmental and endocrine factors all have roles to play in growth, and a limitation in one or more of these areas may limit the rate of growth or the final growth attainment of the child.

 Now visit **www.wileyessential.com/humandevelopment** to test yourself on this chapter.

CHAPTER 28
Developmental delay

Bethan Williams

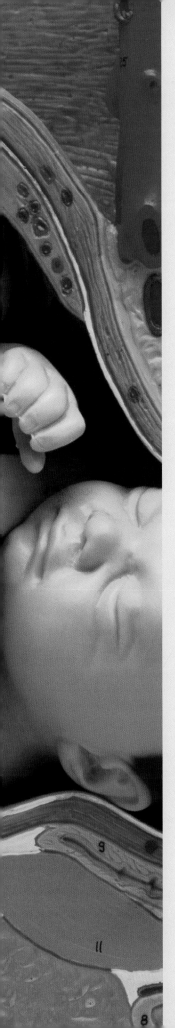

Case

An 18-month-old boy, Andy, presents because he is not yet walking. He was born at 30 weeks gestation and had meningitis in the neonatal period. He has just learned to crawl. He has shown left-sided hand preference since 10 months of age and does not use his right hand much at all. He has a vocabulary of 10 to 15 words and knows approximately four body parts. On examination his tone is increased on the right side and he also has brisk reflexes on this side.

Learning outcomes

- You should be able to describe the process involved in child health surveillance.

- You should be able to recall the difference between developmental delay and disordered development.

- You should be able to recognise the common causes of abnormal development and describe how these are investigated.

- You should appreciate the multidisciplinary approach to a child with additional needs.

Essential Human Development, First Edition. Edited by Samuel Webster, Geraint Morris and Euan Kevelighan
© 2018 John Wiley & Sons, Ltd. Published 2018 by John Wiley & Sons, Ltd.

Normal development

Normal development relies not only on genetic potential but also on the environment in which a child lives and the opportunities he or she is exposed to, highlighting the nature versus nurture phenomenon. Whilst there is a wide variation in the rate at which children acquire their developmental milestones (see Chapter 27) there are some important limit ages whereby if children have not acquired certain skills by these ages they should be referred for further assessment by a paediatrician. These can be found in Table 28.1.

Development can be abnormal in several ways. When a child is reaching their milestones later than the median ages (i.e. is slow to attain these skills) their development is said to be **delayed**. If the skills are being acquired in an unusual pattern or sequence, their development can be described as **disordered**. If a child loses a previously acquired skill, then this is known as **regression**.

Developmental delay

Developmental delay can be present in one modality only, indicating a specific developmental delay such as gross motor delay, or in more than one modality. When delay is present in two or more modalities it is referred to as **global developmental delay**. Developmental problems often present at an age when a specific area of development is most rapid and prominent. For example, gross motor delay usually presents prior to 18 months of age, whereas speech and language delay

Table 28.1 Limit ages of some developmental milestones.

Age	Warning sign
2 months	No social smile Poor eye contact Excessive head lag Silent baby (i.e. no cooing or gurgling)
6 months	Not reaching for objects
8–9 months	Poor interaction Not sitting without support Not babbling
12 months	Hand preference prior to the age of 12 months No pincer grip
18 months	Does not recognise own name Not walking Not using single words
2–2.5 years	Not giving or receiving affection Unable to build tower of three bricks Not linking two or three words
3 years	Unable to play Unsteady gait Not using more than 50 words

Table 28.2 Features that may suggest a neurodevelopmental disorder by age.

Age	Feature
Prenatal	Positive family history Antenatal screening test (e.g. trisomy 21, neural tube defect, chromosomal disorder)
Perinatal	Birth asphyxia/hypoxic ischaemic encephalopathy Prematurity with intraventricular haemorrhage, periventricular leucomalacia, post-haemorrhagic hydrocephalus Abnormal neurological behaviour, e.g. poor feeding, abnormal tone or movements, seizures
Infancy	Global developmental delay Delayed or asymmetric motor development Visual impairment Hearing impairment Neurocutaneous markers Dysmorphic features Early hand preference
Preschool	Speech and language delay Abnormal gait 'Clumsy' motor skills Poor social communication skills
School age	Balance or coordination difficulties, poor dexterity Learning difficulties (general or specific, e.g. dyslexia) Attention difficulties Hyperactivity Social communication difficulties
Any age	Acquired brain injury, traumatic or infective Neurodegenerative disorders

may present later, between the ages of 18 months and 3 years (Table 28.2). It is important to recognise that a child may appear to have a specific developmental delay but on detailed assessment this may prove to be part of a global developmental delay. Normal developmental progress may be disrupted by a neurological or neurodevelopmental disorder in the child that affects development directly, for example cerebral palsy, epilepsy or trisomy 21, or indirectly due to ill health, for example meningitis or cystic fibrosis, or be the result of poor environmental factors, for example neglect (Table 28.3). As children get older, the difference between normal and abnormal developmental progression becomes greater and therefore is more apparent.

Assessing development

At birth in the UK each parent is given a Personal Child Health Record, known popularly as the 'Red Book', wherein they may find useful information and support services; but it

Table 28.3 Conditions causing abnormal development and learning difficulties.

Age	Category	Condition
Prenatal	Genetic	Chromosome/DNA disorders, e.g. trisomy 21, fragile X syndrome, chromosomal microdeletions or duplications Cerebral dysgenesis, e.g. microcephaly, agenesis of the corpus callosum, hydrocephalus, neuronal migration disorder
	Vascular	Occlusions Haemorrhage
	Metabolic	Hypothyroidism Phenylketonuria
	Teratogenic	Alcohol Drug abuse Maternal prescribed medications
	Congenital infection	Toxoplasmosis Rubella Cytomegalovirus Human immunodeficiency virus
	Neurocutaneous syndromes	Tuberous sclerosis Neurofibromatosis
	Neuromuscular	Duchenne muscular dystrophy
Perinatal	Extreme prematurity	Intraventricular haemorrhage Periventricular leucomalacia
	Birth asphyxia	Hypoxic ischaemic encephalopathy
	Metabolic	Symptomatic hypoglycaemia Hyperbilirubinaemia
Postnatal	Infection	Meningitis Encephalitis
	Anoxia	Suffocation Near drowning Seizures
	Trauma	Head injury (accidental or non-accidental)
	Metabolic	Hypoglycaemia Inborn errors of metabolism
	Vascular	Stroke
Other	Unknown (25%)	

is also the place in which details about health checks, growth, development and immunisations are recorded. All children have regular health checks by their health visitors as part of the UK Healthy Child Programme. Assessments take place at the following ages for all children:

- neonatal examination (within the first 72 hours of life);
- new baby review (around 14 days of life);
- 6–8-week repeat examination;
- 12-month review;
- preschool review (between the ages of 2 and 2.5 years).

Health visitor contact is not limited to these ages, and additional support will be provided for families with difficulties at any time.

The developmental screening tool used by health visitors in the UK is the Schedule of Growing Skills (SOGS) Assessment. This assessment looks at nine skill areas: passive postural, active postural, locomotor, manipulative, visual, hearing and language, speech and language, interactive social and self-care social. A skills score is calculated for each area, which is then converted into a developmental age. A cognitive skills score is derived from selected items in the other nine areas. This screening takes approximately 20 minutes to complete and no formal training is required to undertake the assessment.

Should the SOGS Assessment highlight any area of concern then the health visitor should refer the child directly to a paediatrician, usually via the Child Development Team. A community paediatrician specialises in neurodevelopmental disorders and will arrange to meet with the child to undertake a full history and examination. The history should focus on the following aspects:

- pregnancy;
- birth history, including gestational age, mode of delivery, resuscitation, admission to the neonatal intensive care unit, risk factors for sepsis, birthweight;
- medical/surgical history including systems review and medications;
- developmental milestones (covering all modalities; see Chapter 27);
- sleep;
- behaviour and emotional development;
- immunisations;
- family history;
- social history;
- other professionals involved in the child's care.

During the consultation observations of the child's movements, behaviour, and play and interaction with relatives and the doctor will be noted. Using simple toys, paper, pencil, books and blocks an experienced paediatrician can carry out an informal assessment of development. This will give them a rough guide to the developmental age at which the child is functioning for each domain. Formal systemic examination should also be undertaken concentrating on the following areas as this may aid diagnosis and guide management:

- **Growth:** All parameters (height, weight and occipito-frontal head circumference) should be plotted on an appropriate growth chart (review of the 'Red Book' is also recommended in the UK).
- **Dysmorphic features:** Face, limbs, body proportions, genitalia.
- **Skin:** Neurocutaneous markers, injuries, cleanliness.
- **Central nervous system:**
  - Posture, symmetry, wasting, tone, power, reflexes, clonus, plantar responses, sensation, coordination, cranial nerves.
  - Gait.
- **Cardiovascular system:** Cardiac abnormalities are associated with many syndromes.
- **Respiratory system.**
- **Gastrointestinal system:** Organomegaly can be associated with certain metabolic conditions causing developmental delay.
- **ENT system.**
- **Musculoskeletal system**: Gross and fine motor skills.
- **Vision and hearing**.
- **Communication:** Social communication disorders (e.g. autism).
- **Sensory profile:** To include auditory, olfactory, visual, oral (both taste and texture), tactile, and proprioceptive aspects, as many children with developmental delay may have sensory seeking or sensory defensiveness.

It is sometimes necessary to undertake a more formal assessment of a child's development. In addition to the qualitative observations the clinician will make during the assessment, the tests are standardised and qualitative so therefore generate a test score. The most widely used assessment is the Ruth Griffiths Developmental Assessment. The test scores are available for the six individual developmental domains (locomotor, personal social, hearing and speech, eye and hand coordination, performance and practical reasoning) but can also be calculated to represent a general quotient reflecting the overall general abilities of the child. The results can be portrayed in age in months or in percentiles. The Ruth Griffiths Assessment must be carried out by individuals who have undergone specific training and takes approximately 1 to 1½ hours to complete. This test can be applied to children from 0 to 8 years of age.

Educational psychologists have a battery of other tools to assess children's cognitive ability – for example, the Weschler Intelligence Scale for Children (WISC), Weschler Preschool and Primary Scale of Development (WPPSI), British Ability Scales – all of which would evaluate the Intelligence Quotient (IQ). Whilst there is a high overlap between developmental delay and learning disability the two are not mutually exclusive. Developmental delay can be classified as mild, moderate or severe, but learning disability has specific criteria for classification, as outlined below:

Moderate: IQ 50–70
Severe: IQ 20–50
Profound: IQ <20

Investigations

The investigations required for a child with developmental delay will vary depending on whether the abnormality is specific to one modality or affecting global development. For global developmental delay current UK practice is to follow the Glasgow screening method (Box 28.1).

Other investigations such as an EEG will be arranged only if there is a suspicion of seizures.

These investigations will help establish the aetiology of the developmental delay, the most common of which are outlined in Box 28.2. More information about these common conditions can be found in other chapters in this book.

There are many phrases used to describe children with complex needs, such as disabled, handicapped and impaired. Whilst most families generally refer to their child as having special needs it is important to understand the meaning of impairment, disability and handicap. The definitions in Table 28.4 might help to clarify this confusing terminology.

It may also help to think how these terms can be applied to various conditions, as outlined in Table 28.5.

Managing a child with developmental difficulties is led by a multidisciplinary team of individuals providing therapy (Figure 28.1). The child may already be known to certain services and it is usually necessary to obtain further information from any other health professionals already involved in the

Box 28.1 The Glasgow screening method

First line

Full blood count	Urea and electrolytes	Thyroid function tests
Ferritin	Urate	Lead
Array CGH	Creatine kinase	Biotinidase

Second line
Metabolic

Family history, consanguinity, regression, organomegaly, coarse features

Blood	Urine
Lactate	Organic acids
Carnitine	Orotate
Amino acids	Glycosaminoglycans
Homocysteine	Oligosaccharides
Ammonia	
Disialotransferrin	
VLCFA	

Neuroimaging

Abnormal head size, seizures, focal neurological signs
MRI
CT

EEG

Speech regression, seizures, neurodegenerative disorder
Consider 24 hour EEG

Genetics

Dysmorphism, abnormal growth, sensory impairment, odd behaviour, family history

CGH, comparative genomic hybridisation; CT, computed tomography; EEG, electroencephalogram; MRI, magnetic resonance imaging; VLFCA, very long-chain fatty acids.

Box 28.2 The most common causes of developmental delay

- Autism
- Acquired brain injury (trauma or infection)
- Cerebral palsy
- Duchenne muscular dystrophy
- Epilepsy
- Fetal alcohol syndrome
- Fragile X
- Hearing impairment
- Neglect
- Prematurity
- Trisomy 21
- Visual impairment

Table 28.4 Definitions of terms associated with children with special needs.

Term	Definition
Disorder	Medically definable condition or disease
Impairment	Loss or abnormality of psychological, physiological or anatomical structure or function
Disability	Any restriction or lack of ability to perform an activity considered normal for a child of that age (usually due to an impairment)
Handicap	The impact of the impairment or disability

Table 28.5 The use of terms describing children with special needs in relation to some disorders.

Disorder	Impairment	Disability	Handicap
Cerebral palsy, e.g. spastic diplegia	Increased muscle tone in the lower limbs	Abnormal gait and delayed motor milestones	Difficulty joining in physical activities
Profound sensorineural hearing loss	Hearing loss secondary to a lesion in the cochlea and or neural pathways to the auditory cortex	Impaired hearing and delay in speech and language development	Inability to communicate with most strangers, difficulty understanding spoken conversation
Epilepsy	Tendency to recurrent seizures as a result of abnormal activity of cortical neurons	Recurrent seizures may prevent a child functioning normally at school	Restriction of certain activities, careers, etc.

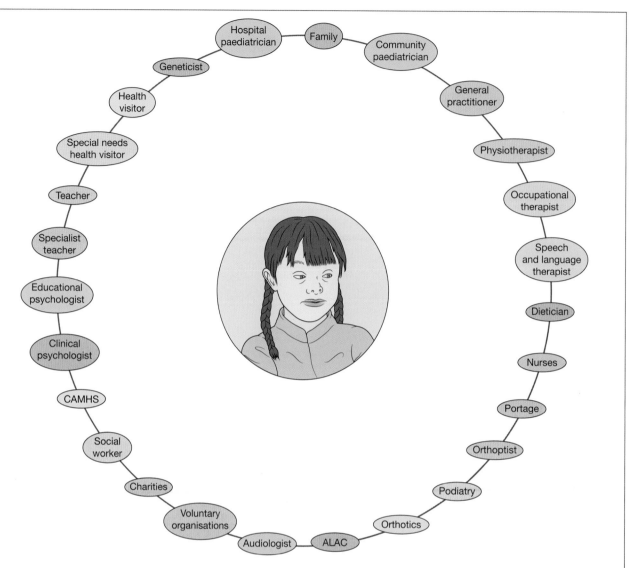

Figure 28.1 An example of a multidisciplinary team around a child with a neurodevelopmental disorder. ALAC, Artificial Limbs and Appliance Centre; CAMHS, Child and Adolescent Mental Health Services.

child's care, or to make referrals to these individuals both in terms of further assessment and for therapy.

Communication is the key to managing a child with special needs. As you can see from Figure 28.1, a single child could have over 20 specialists involved in their care. It is often necessary to appoint a key worker to a family so that care can be coordinated effectively. Multidisciplinary Team (MDT) meetings or Team Around the Child (TAC) meetings are an effective way of coordinating the health needs of children with complex needs.

Education

In addition to the medical support, children with additional needs require assistance at school. The Education Act 2002 in the UK defines a child with special educational needs as follows:

- A learning difficulty that calls for special educational provision.
- Has significantly greater difficulty learning than the majority of children his/her age.
- Has a disability that either prevents or hinders the child from making use of educational facilities of a kind generally provided for children of his/her age.

Under the Education Act, the Code of Practice must be followed for children with special needs. Under this Code of Practice every school must have a designated Special Educational Needs Coordinator (SENCO). This teacher will then be responsible for working with the child, the class teacher and education department so that the child's health and educational needs can be met at school. In order to do this all schools are allocated a budget to provide extra services to children to help meet their additional needs. This process is

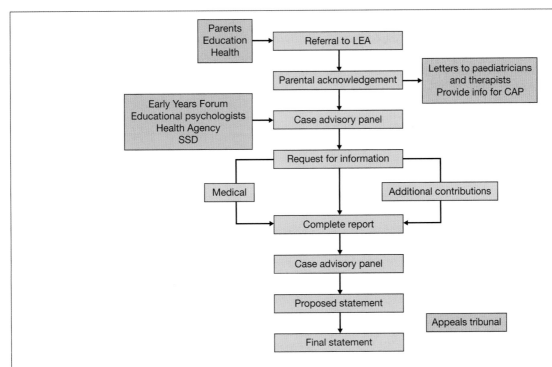

Figure 28.2 The process of application for a Statement of Special Educational Needs. CAP, Case Advisory Panel; LEA, Local Education Authority; SSD, Social Services Department.

known as 'School Action' and 'School Action Plus'. A child on School Action (and/or School Action Plus) will have an Individual Education Plan (IEP) that has very specific targets to help address their difficulties. The IEP is reviewed every term; if targets are met new ones are set, and if they are not met then new strategies to improve this can be employed.

Some children will require more support than can be delivered on School Action Plus and it may be necessary to issue a Statement of Special Educational Needs. This is a legally binding contract where the provision of support documented in the Statement must be adhered to. Statements are reviewed annually and the level of support adjusted according to need.

It may be necessary for some children to be placed in a specialist teaching facility. The Education Act 2002 in the UK defines Special Educational Provision as follows:

- In relation to a child who has attained the age of 2, educational provision which is additional to or otherwise different from, the educational provision made generally for children of his age in schools maintained by the local education authority.

All children placed in a special school will have a Statement of Special Educational Needs. Figure 28.2 outlines the process involved in applying for a Statement of Special Educational Needs.

Clinical case

Case investigations

Looking through Andy's neonatal notes it appears that apart from the meningitis his neonatal course was relatively uncomplicated. During his episode of meningitis he was noted to have a single seizure, which involved rhythmic jerking of the right arm and right leg. He passed his neonatal hearing screening test.

On observation Andy has a marked hand preference when playing with small objects and he is able to build a tower of three blocks. His right hand has reduced muscle

bulk and brisker tendon reflexes than the left. His lower limb reflexes are more difficult to elicit but his right leg seems stiffer than the left. His head circumference is normal and on a similar centile to his body length and weight, all corrected for his premature birth. He seems very sociable and willingly engages in conversation after some initial shyness.

Case conclusion

It is likely that Andy has had a neonatal brain injury, probably as a result of meningitis. This has resulted in a right

SUMMARY

hemiplegia with increased tone. His motor development is consequently delayed but his development in other areas seems normal so far.

In Andy's case it is important to avoid complications of hemiplegia such as joint contractures and stiffening, and to optimise the function of his right side. He will be referred to a paediatric physiotherapist initially but is likely to require the services of a wide range of professionals from various disciplines such as occupational therapy, and speech and language therapy as part of the disability team. His medical care is best led by a community paediatrician. It is difficult to tell at this stage what the extent of his disabilities might be and what the future might hold. Initial signs are promising in terms of his cognitive development, but his motor functioning is likely to be compromised to a certain extent.

Key learning points

- A child may display abnormal development by showing the ability to attain developmental milestones at a later age than most other children (delayed), may develop abilities in an unusual order (disordered) or lose an ability (regression). This may be noticed by assessing developmental milestones, but other formal tests are available and may be helpful in determining a cause.

- A thorough, formal, systemic examination will aid the diagnosis of developmental delay and guide management. Managing a child with developmental difficulties is led by a multidisciplinary team of individuals that may be extremely broad, providing therapy and support.

 Now visit **www.wileyessential.com/humandevelopment** to test yourself on this chapter.

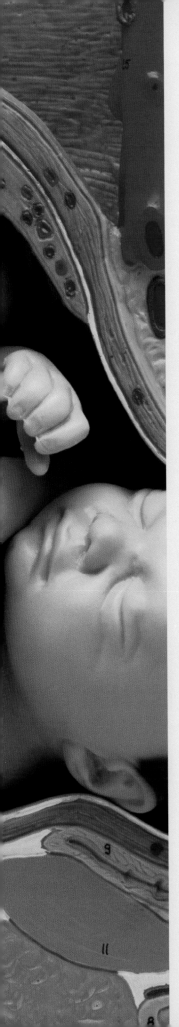

CHAPTER 29
Genetics

Dana Beasley

Case

Baby Daisy is the first child of a 25-year-old mother. She was born at term after an uncomplicated pregnancy. The 20-week ultrasound scan and antenatal clinic booking blood tests all showed normal results.

On the first day of life concerns are raised with regards to poor feeding and vomiting. The midwife also mentions some unusual facial features. On clinical assessment Daisy appears floppy, she is pink and well perfused with normal vital signs. Her weight and head circumference are just under the 50th centile. Her face appears flat with upslanting palpebral fissures, her chest is clear, and her abdomen soft. Cardiac examination reveals a systolic murmur.

Learning outcomes

- You should be able to describe types of genetic abnormalities.
- You should be able to recognise inheritance patterns of genetic abnormalities.
- You should be able to decide when to use genetic testing appropriately.

Essential Human Development, First Edition. Edited by Samuel Webster, Geraint Morris and Euan Kevelighan
© 2018 John Wiley & Sons, Ltd. Published 2018 by John Wiley & Sons, Ltd.

Introduction

Genetics is a rapidly advancing field of medicine. Over the last few decades enormous progress has been made in discovering the genetic backgrounds to many diseases leading to a better understanding and possible new treatment options. Genetic disorders are common; approximately 2% of all newborns are born with an underlying genetic defect. This has huge implications for patients, their families and society, and therefore knowledge of underlying principles is essential.

Clinical genetics and genetic tests

Most child health departments in the UK will have access to a clinical genetics department. The role of a clinical geneticist is to provide information with an overall aim of allowing patients, individuals, couples and families better choice in the management of a condition and reproductive decisions. Advice should always be non-directive but at the same time helpful for a decision making process. A clinical geneticist may confirm a clinically suspected diagnosis by taking a detailed history, drawing a family tree (pedigree), thorough clinical examination and then arranging appropriate tests. Geneticists help families to gain more insight into the condition and its prognosis. They also evaluate the risk of passing a disorder on to the next generation and explore options for management and prevention. Genetic counselling involves all the above as well as advice about recurrence risks and discussions about various reproductive options.

Prenatal testing enables identification of an at-risk fetus, may provide reassurance, and gives parents more information to make an informed choice. It also allows prompt medical treatment in some circumstances, for example a baby with an antenatally detected severe heart defect can have a planned birth in a cardiac centre to optimise treatment. Prenatal testing involves screening tests that give a probability of having a disease, such as nuchal ultrasound scanning at 11–14 weeks gestation, or fetal anomaly ultrasound scanning at 20–24 weeks gestation. Diagnostic tests like chorionic villus biopsy and amniocentesis enable DNA analysis, which can give a definitive diagnosis.

Genetic screening is another part of genetic testing that is suitable for frequently occurring mutations in populations. It looks for individuals who have a certain genotype and are therefore at risk of developing a disease. An example of population screening is the newborn screen (Box 29.1), which screens all babies born in the UK for rare but serious conditions and requires only a small blood sample. By detecting the disease early treatment can be instigated to prevent or minimise disabilities or death.

Genetic carrier testing looks at individuals at risk for a certain genotype associated with a disease in that family.

Chromosomal tests involve karyotype analysis (Figure 29.1) to look at the whole genome, or more targeted studies to look at submicroscopic defects via fluorescence in situ hybridisation

---

Box 29.1 The UK newborn screen

- Phenylketonuria
- Congenital hypothyroidism
- Sickle cell disease
- Cystic fibrosis
- MCADD (medium chain acyl CoA dehydrogenase deficiency)

Box 29.2 Indications for karyotyping

- Clinical suspicion of a syndrome
- Infertility screening
- Unexplained mental retardation
- Unexplained growth retardation
- Some forms of cancer
- To determine gender
- In pregnancy where maternal age is >35

(FISH). If a mutation is known analysis is fairly straightforward, but it can be very time consuming and expensive if entire genes need to be sequenced (Box 29.2).

Gene therapy is the treatment of a genetic disease involving the repair or suppression of abnormal genes, or the induction of healthy genetic information. Although this approach offers a hopeful outlook for the future it is only in experimental stages for most disorders. Many trials are currently in progress. There are encouraging results so far

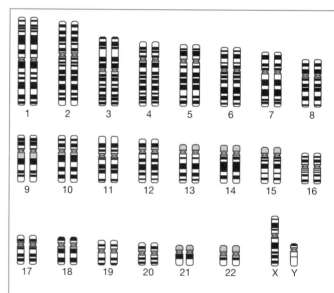

Figure 29.1 The human karyotype. (Source: S. Webster and R. de Wreede (2016) *Embryology at a Glance*, 2nd edn. Reproduced with permission of John Wiley & Sons, Ltd.)

for the treatment of cystic fibrosis and Duchenne muscular dystrophy. It is important to know that the current approach to gene therapy involves only the alteration of somatic cells and not germline cells.

Ethics

Before diagnostic testing is initiated careful genetic counselling should take place with regards to the impact a possible diagnosis might have on patients and their families. Some conditions are progressive and life-limiting, and others often affect children's ability to learn and communicate. There are a lot of ethical concerns around predictive testing. It is acceptable to test an asymptomatic child who is at risk for a condition that can be prevented, treated or even cured. It is also acceptable to test a child at risk for a genetic condition with paediatric onset even if there are no therapeutic measures available, but this should be done carefully under the guidance of a senior clinical geneticist. However, it is generally agreed not to test healthy children for disorders that have an onset in adulthood until an individual is able to give consent.

Dysmorphology

Dysmorphology is the recognition of unusual physical features that have an origin during embryogenesis and can be characteristic for a particular syndrome. Birth defects can be classified into single system defects, an association, a sequence or a syndrome. A **single system defect** results from a single congenital malformation, for example spina bifida or polydactyly. Causes are often multifactorial and have a fairly low recurrence rate.

An **association** is a group of malformations that usually occur together, for example CHARGE syndrome (**C**oloboma, **H**eart defects, **A**tresia of choanae, **R**etarded growth, **G**enital hypoplasia, **E**ar deformities) (Figure 29.2).

A **sequence** is a pattern of multiple abnormalities where secondary changes follow a primary defect. Renal agenesis is the primary defect in Potter's sequence, which results in severe oligohydramnios, facial abnormalities and pulmonary hypoplasia.

A **syndrome** is a consistently recurring pattern of several primary anomalies caused by a single aetiology, for example trisomy 21. Some syndromes can be recognised by their distinctive features.

Genetic mutations

A **genetic mutation** is a change in a DNA sequence that changes the function of the gene. In contrast, a simple variation in the sequence of a gene's DNA is called a **polymorphism** and is the reason for different genes amongst individuals. Differing sequences for the same gene are called **alleles** (see also Chapter 1). If the alleles on both pairs of chromosomes are the same a person is **homozygous** for that gene; if someone has a different genetic sequence in each allele the person is **heterozygous**.

Genetic mutations can occur due to:

- **Insertion** or **deletion** of one or more base pairs. The most common mutation in cystic fibrosis is D508, a three base-pair deletion at position 508 of the *CFTR* (cystic fibrosis transmembrane conductance regulator) gene.
- **Point mutation**, where one base pair is substituted for another. This can lead to a change in an amino acid that may alter a protein (missense mutation), or in the production of a stop codon (nonsense mutation).
- **Whole gene duplication**.
- **Expanded repeats**. In some genes the sequence is made out of a repetitive pattern of the same three base pairs. If those repeats increase in number it can cause an alteration in the gene product, for example as in fragile X syndrome.

All the above can occur naturally and are called spontaneous mutations. Others are induced by mutagens like UV light, chemicals or radiation.

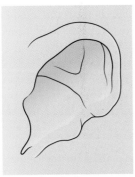
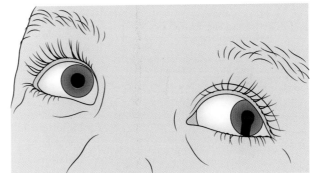

Dysplastic ear

Coloboma of the iris

Figure 29.2 Dysplastic ear and coloboma of the iris in CHARGE (Coloboma, Heart defects, Atresia of choanae, Retarded growth, Genital hypoplasia, Ear deformities) sequence.

Genetic disorders

Genetic abnormalities can be divided into:

- chromosomal disorders;
- single gene (Mendelian) defects;
- multifactorial inheritance;
- mitochondrial disorders;
- factors affecting inheritance patterns.

Chromosomal disorders

Chromosomal disorders can either be **numerical** or **structural** abnormalities. The phenotype of an affected individual is a result of too many or too few genes rather than a mutation in a specific gene. Numerical abnormalities are usually extra or missing individual chromosomes (**aneuploidy**) since an extra set of chromosomes (**polyploidy**) is usually not compatible with life. Numerical abnormalities are usually due to non-disjunction where chromosomes fail to separate during meiosis.

Down syndrome (trisomy 21) is the most common autosomal trisomy and also the most common genetic cause of severe learning difficulties. The risk of having a child with Down syndrome increases with maternal age. Incidence at all ages is approximately 1:650 although this number reduces with antenatal screening. Clinical features are hypotonia, distinctive facial features (Figure 29.3) with a round face, a flat nasal bridge, upslanting palpebral fissures, distinct epicanthic folds and a small mouth with protruding tongue. Affected patients also have a flat occiput, a single palmar crease and a sandal gap

Most common features:

Flat facial profile

Epicanthal fold

General hypotonia

Brushfield spots on iris

Variable features:
- Congenital heart defect (especially AV canal)
- Increased risk of leukaemia
- Duodenal atresia
- Hirschsprung disease
- Hypothyroidism

5th finger clinodactyly

Brachydactyly (short fingers)

Single transverse palmar crease

Large 'sandal' gap between 1st and 2nd toes

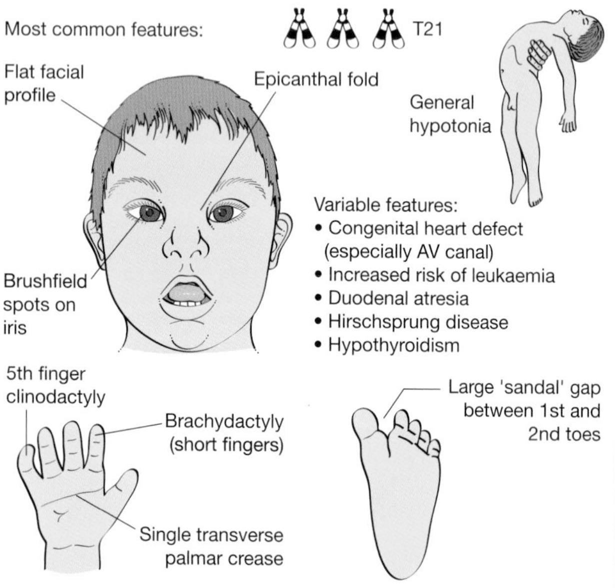

Figure 29.3 The distinctive features of Down syndrome. (Source: D. Pritchard and B. Korf (2013) *Medical Genetics at a Glance*, 3rd edn. Reproduced with permission of John Wiley & Sons, Ltd.)

(wide gap between the first and second toes). It is associated with congenital heart disease in 40% – atrioventricular septal defect (AVSD), ventricular septal defect (VSD), patent ductus arteriosus (PDA) and atrial septal defect (ASD) (see Chapter 36) – and increased incidence for Hirschsprung's disease, duodenal atresia, hypothyroidism, leukaemia and Alzheimer's disease.

Down syndrome is caused by an extra chromosome 21 or extra parts of it. There are four possible genetic mechanisms underlying this:

- **Non-disjunction** at meiosis is by far the most common cause of trisomy 21 (95%); the karyotype is 47+21.
- **Robertsonian translocation** is the cause in 3% of cases. The long arm of chromosome 21 is attached to either itself or to chromosome 14. The origin of the translocation can be either maternal or paternal and there is no maternal age effect. The common karyotype in this case is 46 t(14/21). Recurrence is less than 1% if neither parent has a translocation but is 100% if a parent has translocation 46 t(21/21).
- **Mosaicism** (2% of cases). Only a fraction of cells have trisomy 21 resulting from non-disjunction during meiosis after fertilisation. Depending on how many cells are normal or affected the phenotype varies.
- **Isochromosome 21** (<1%) is a duplication of a region of chromosome 21. The karyotype is 46 i(21).

It is difficult to predict the severity of learning difficulties and prognosis in general as Down syndrome can be highly variable.

Other examples of trisomies are Edward's syndrome (trisomy 18) and Patau syndrome (trisomy 13).

Gain or loss of a sex chromosome is relatively common. One example is Klinefelter syndrome, which is characterised by a gain of an X chromosome. The karyotype is 47, XXY and clinical features are variable. An estimated 1:500 males are affected.

The loss of an autosomal chromosome is usually not compatible with life but Turner syndrome is an exception. Usually the paternal sex chromosome is missing and the karyotype is 45, X0. This is generally caused by a sporadic event although underlying mosaicism is not uncommon. Hallmarks of Turner syndrome are congenital lymphoedema, a short, webbed neck, short stature and ovarian dysgenesis. It can also be associated with congenital heart disease, and 10% of patients have a coarctation of the aorta.

Structural abnormalities are characterised by a normal number of chromosomes that have partial defects as a result of chromosomal breakage or rearrangement. This is a common cause of spontaneous miscarriage, and acquired changes play an important role in carcinogenesis. There are several underlying mechanisms:

- **Deletions.** A partial deletion or microdeletion (detectable by FISH) of a chromosome can occur resulting in physical abnormalities and learning difficulties. For example cri du chat syndrome is caused by a deletion of the short arm of chromosome 5 leading to a combination of a cat-like cry, hypotonia and mental retardation. It can be associated with congenital heart defects. The karyotype is 46, XY (or XX) del5p. A loss of oncogenes results in development of malignancies; for example, deletion of the long arm of chromosome 13 is associated with development of retinoblastoma.

■ **Duplication.** A portion of the chromosome is duplicated. In Charcot–Marie–Tooth disease there are three copies of parts of the short arm of chromosome 17. This causes weakness and wasting of distal limb muscles.

■ **Translocation.** Genetic material is exchanged between two different chromosomes. In reciprocal translocation, two breaks on different chromosomes occur. If no genetic information is gained or lost this is a balanced translocation and the phenotype is normal as there is a normal chromosomal complement, but an offspring might have an unbalanced translocation with an incorrect amount of chromosomal material. This can cause dysmorphic features, developmental delay and learning difficulties. In a Robertsonian translocation occurs the long arms of two acrocentric chromosomes (namely chromosomes 13, 14, 15, 21 and 22 where the centromere is located near the end forming a long arm and a short arm) fuse together forming one long chromosome with loss of the short arm. This leads to an altered number of chromosomes.

■ **Inversion.** After a break the affected part of the chromosome rotates 180 degrees.

Single gene defects (Mendelian inheritance)

In the 19th century Gregor Mendel described patterns of inheritance based on the principle that genes occur in pairs (alleles). Only one allele is passed on from each parent to a child and an allele can be either dominant or recessive. Single gene defects are caused by a disturbance of the sequence of nucleotides in the DNA.

A pedigree of a family can help to understand the inheritance of a condition (Figure 29.4).

Autosomal dominant (AD) inheritance involves structural defects where an affected individual carries an affected gene on one pair of autosomes. This single defect allele exerts an effect and is vertically passed on to successive generations. Children of an affected parent have a 50% chance of inheriting the disease. This can be further complicated by variation of expression, meaning that some individuals in one family are more affected then others.

Another phenomenon is non-penetrance, where an individual with an abnormal gene does not display any clinical signs or symptoms. A lack of family history might be due to a new mutation or non-paternity. Generally major structural proteins, key enzymes or membrane receptors are changed as result of the defect. Examples of AD inheritance are Marfan syndrome, polyposis coli and achondroplasia.

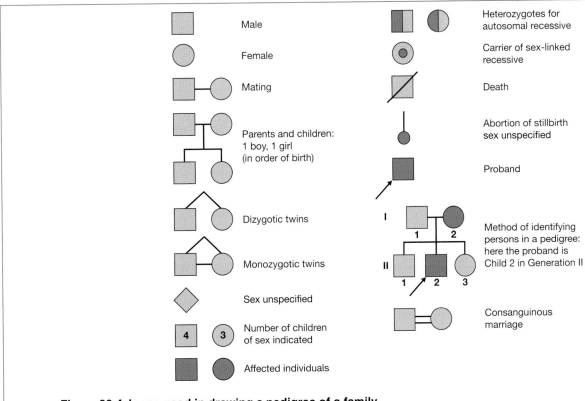

Figure 29.4 Icons used in drawing a pedigree of a family.

Autosomal recessive (AR) inheritance occurs with a phenotype that only manifests if both alleles are abnormal, which means an affected individual has inherited the abnormal gene from both parents. The parents are both heterozygous and therefore unaffected carriers but all of their children will be carriers, and one in four (25%) are at risk of being affected. The risk of AR inheritance is increased by consanguinity. In this mode of inheritance the defect often causes changes in enzymes for various pathways. Examples are cystic fibrosis, phenylketonuria and congenital adrenal hyperplasia.

X-linked recessive inheritance occurs when an abnormal gene is carried on the X chromosome. All daughters of affected males will be carriers whereas sons will be neither affected nor carriers. Females are usually healthy carriers and their sons have a 50% risk of being affected, whereas their daughters have a 50% risk of being a carrier. Examples of X-linked recessive disorders are Duchenne muscular dystrophy and haemophilia A.

X-linked dominant inheritance describes the inheritance of an abnormal gene carried on the X chromosome that has a dominant effect. It is rare and is usually only seen in females as it is lethal in affected males. Examples are Rett syndrome and incontinentia pigmenti.

Y-linked inheritance is extremely rare as the chromosome is very small and contains only a few known genes.

Multifactorial inheritance

Some disorders result from additive effects of genetic and environmental factors, many of which have not yet been identified. Some diseases are inherited in a multifactorial fashion, as are certain traits like height and blood pressure. The risk of recurrence is based on empirical data.

Examples of childhood multifactorial disorders are pyloric stenosis, atopy, obesity and epilepsy.

Characteristics of multifactorial inheritance include:
- common in populations;
- familial clustering that is not Mendelian;
- concordance in monozygote twins that is less than 100% but higher than in dizygote twins.

Mitochondrial disorders

Mitochondria contain their own chromosomes, and some diseases are the result of mutations in the mitochondrial genetic information. Mitochondrial DNA deletions generally occur de novo and thus cause disease in one family member only, with no significant risk to other family members. Only maternal transmission is seen. Some mitochondrial disorders affect only a single organ (e.g. the eye in Leber hereditary optic neuropathy, or LHON), but many involve multiple organ systems and often present with prominent neurological and myopathic features. An example is mitochondrial encephalomyopathy with lactic acidosis and stroke-like episodes (MELAS).

Factors affecting inheritance patterns

New mutations are frequently seen in some conditions and there is no previous family history.

Reduced penetrance describes an individual who has an abnormal gene but does not display any clinical signs or symptoms. They can transmit the gene to their children.

Variable expression means that some individuals in one family are more affected then others.

Non-paternity means that a lack of family history might be due to the fact that the apparent father is not the biological father.

Anticipation describes the observation of a more severe expression of symptoms in successive generations. Anticipation is often seen in disorders caused by trinucleotide expansion where the number of repeats increases through generations.

Premutation. Usually a number of three-base-pair repeats (triplet repeats) vary amongst individuals. However, if a certain threshold is reached the gene becomes unstable. An example of premutation is fragile X syndrome.

Imprinting means that some genes are only actively expressed if they are derived from a parent of a given sex. For example, in Prader–Willi syndrome (with patients displaying obesity, learning difficulties and neonatal hypotonia) only the paternal copy of the gene, located on the long arm of chromosome 15, is active. If the paternal copy of the gene is not inherited the child will be affected. This can happen either by a de novo deletion or by **uniparental disomy**, which means that an affected child inherits both genes from the same parent. Although the number of copies is normal there may be no active copies. The resulting syndrome depends on which copy is missing.

Techniques used for genetic testing

Chromosomal testing

A karyotype (see Figure 29.1) is a display of chromosomes during mitosis (see Chapter 1). By using staining techniques the chromosomal band can be analysed under a light microscope in order to outline the whole genome. The normal male karyotype is 46, XY and the normal female karyotype is 46, XX.

More targeted studies are possible with FISH. It is possible to detect submicroscopic deletions under a fluorescence microscope, for example in Angelman syndrome (15q; a deletion of the short arm of chromosome 15).

Recent advances allow detection of pathogenic chromosome gains and losses that cannot be seen in conventional karyotyping. The technique used is called array comparative genomic hybridisation (aCGH). It offers higher detection of underlying chromosomal imbalances with greater sensitivity compared to the use of light microscopy. It is particularly useful for patients with developmental delay or multiple congenital abnormalities.

Molecular techniques

Most genetic testing is undertaken by polymerase chain reaction (PRC). A specific DNA sequence is amplified by denaturating the DNA, adding a specific primer that binds within the region of interest and adding DNA polymerase. By repeating this cycle the amount of the specific segment of DNA increases to enable analysis of a small sample.

DNA sequencing can be undertaken after amplification of a specific region of DNA by adding fluorescent labels. This allows determination of the actual order of nucleotides and detection of mutations by comparison of the sequence with DNA of an unaffected individual.

Clinical case

Case investigations

In view of a suspicion of Down syndrome Daisy was admitted to the special care baby unit (SCBU) for further assessment and placement of a nasogastric tube. The parents were carefully counselled by a senior clinician, who provided information about Down syndrome and explained the process of confirming the diagnosis. A chest X-ray was unremarkable but an echocardiograph demonstrated a ventricular septal defect (VSD) that did not need any intervention at the time. An abdominal X-ray showed a 'double bubble', and Daisy underwent surgery to correct duodenal atresia. A blood test for rapid FISH looking for trisomy 21 revealed a karyotype 46, XX t(14,21).

Case conclusions

Further cytogenetic studies of both parents showed that the mother is carrier of a balanced translocation. The family was referred to a clinical geneticist for further counselling in view of the increased recurrence risk for Down syndrome in future pregnancies.

Key learning points

- Genetic conditions are common disorders that have a big impact on patients, families and society.
- There are a variety of genetic tests available but it is important to counsel patients and families carefully.

- A good understanding of the underlying principles of inheritance will help you to understand the presentations of genetic conditions.

 Now visit **www.wileyessential.com/humandevelopment** to test yourself on this chapter.

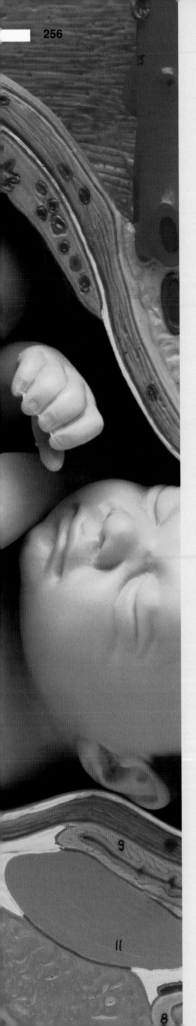

CHAPTER 30
Neurodevelopmental disorders

Surekha Tuohy

Case

A 3-year-old boy was referred to the community paediatric team by his health visitor. The concerns were that he had no speech, and he grunted and screamed to communicate. He randomly hummed. He was not interested in playing with his sisters aged 5 and 7 and preferred solitary play. His play was repetitive and consisted of lining up cars and toys and turning the light switches on and off. He did not point, to share or for his needs. His eye contact was poor and so was his response to his name being called. He flapped his hands when excited.

He was born at term after an uneventful pregnancy. His neonatal period was uneventful. He was slow with his feeding and needed hospital admission for faltering growth. Thereafter he thrived. He attained his motor milestones at appropriate ages. He was immunised. There was no family history of note. There were no positive findings on his examination and he was well nourished.

Learning outcomes

- You should be able to define, recognise and assess forms of learning and intellectual disabilities.
- You should be able to recommend investigations and management of learning and intellectual disabilities where appropriate.

Essential Human Development, First Edition. Edited by Samuel Webster, Geraint Morris and Euan Kevelighan
© 2018 John Wiley & Sons, Ltd. Published 2018 by John Wiley & Sons, Ltd.

Learning disability/intellectual disability (LD/ID)

Terminology

A myriad of terms have been used historically and globally to describe these disabilities. Mental retardation, mental handicap, intellectual handicap, learning disability, and intellectual disability are all terms used interchangeably. The preferred terminology is learning disability (UK) and intellectual disability (USA).

Global developmental delay/difficulties are the terms used to describe learning disabilities in children under 5 years of age.

Definition

Learning disability is a condition of arrested or incomplete development of the mind, which is especially characterised by impairment of skills. It is manifested during the developmental period, and affects the overall level of intelligence, that is, cognitive, language, motor and social abilities.

Learning disability is a descriptive term for significant sub-average intelligence, that is an IQ of less than 70 resulting in impaired adaptive functioning with an onset in the developmental period (before 18 years of age).

The individuals have difficulty in understanding new or complex information, learning new skills and coping independently.

Sub-classification and epidemiology of LD

- **Mild:** IQ of 50–69. Accounts for 80% of LD population and 1.5% of the whole population.
- **Moderate**: IQ of 35–49. Accounts for 12% of LD population and 0.5% of the whole population.
- **Severe:** IQ of 20–34. Accounts for 7% of LD population and 0.3% of the whole population.
- **Profound:** IQ less than 20. Accounts for 1% of LD population and 0.05% of the whole population.

The overall prevalence of LD is 1–3% of the population.

Aetiology

Learning disability results from any cause that interferes with the function of the central nervous system and can be considered in the following categories:

- **Genetic:** autosomal dominant (e.g. neurofibromatosis type 1), autosomal recessive (e.g. phenylketonuria), chromosomal abnormalities (e.g. Down syndrome), X-linked disorders (e.g. fragile X syndrome), polygenic factors, complex inheritance. The most common chromosomal abnormality in LD is Down syndrome, and the most common X-linked abnormality associated with LD is fragile X syndrome.
- **Prenatal:** infections, for example TORCH, intoxication (e.g. alcohol or teratogens) , endocrine and metabolic disorders.

- **Perinatal:** prematurity, hypoxic ischaemic encephalopathy (birth asphyxia), infections (e.g. meningitis), intracranial bleed.
- **Postnatal:** injury (accidental and non-accidental), infection, epilepsy, malnutrition, environmental (e.g. lead exposure), neglect.

Signs and symptoms

LD is a continuum of global developmental difficulties. LD can present at any time in childhood.

In preschool years developmental screenings through child health surveillance in primary care are in place for early recognition.

In school years children can present with language difficulties (one of the first signs), difficulties with self-care and self-help including toileting, self-feeding and dressing, immature behaviour, poor reading and understanding skills, and behavioural difficulties, for example inattention, temper tantrums and defiance. They can also have difficulties with memory, problem solving and practical reasoning.

Adults with LD struggle to adapt to the daily demands of the normal social environment.

The more severe the disability the earlier it presents.

Comorbidities

LD is often associated with other conditions that can complicate the clinical presentation. The recognised comorbidities are:

- autism spectrum disorder;
- attention deficit hyperactivity disorder;
- mental health problems;
- epilepsy;
- behaviour problems.

The prevalence of comorbidity varies with the severity of the disability.

Assessment of a child with LD

Early diagnosis ensures timely and appropriate interventions for the child. It also helps in genetic counselling and addressing anxieties of parents and carers.

Clinical evaluation should include a detailed history of pregnancy, birth, neonatal period, feeding difficulties, early development and family history with particular attention to a history of LD, consanguinity, miscarriages and stillbirths.

Examination should include examination of the skin for neurocutaneous stigmata, general examination for dysmorphic features, measurement of occipito-frontal circumference, height, weight and detailed neurological examination.

A formal assessment of the cognitive abilities is essential to make the diagnosis of LD. There are several assessment tools for preschool and school-aged children, for example Ruth

Griffiths' developmental assessment, the Bayley Scales of Infant and Toddler development, the British Ability Scales and the Wechsler Intelligence Scale for Children (WISC).

The type and depth of the assessment varies with the severity of the difficulties. A multidisciplinary team assessment is warranted in children with severe or profound and multiple learning difficulties. The team may include paediatric physiotherapists, paediatric occupational therapists, speech and language therapists, specialist health visitors, peripatetic teachers for sensory impairments and educational psychologists.

The assessment should include evaluation of the child's health and educational and social care needs to establish the support needed.

Investigations

The degree of LD and associated clinical signs and symptoms determine the investigations.

In current clinical practice most children with mild to moderate LD undergo array-based comparative genetic hybridisation (array CGH), fragile X testing, full blood count, ferritin, thyroid function tests, creatinine kinase, renal , bone and liver function tests. Some units undertake metabolic investigations. However, the clinical presentations can unfold over time, for example in case of developmental regression in autism spectrum disorder or Rett syndrome, therefore assessment and investigation can be an ongoing process.

Neuroimaging and complex genetic and metabolic tests are indicated in children with severe or profound and multiple learning difficulties.

For most cases of mild LD no specific abnormalities are found.

Management

Holistic care of the child with LD involves a multi-agency approach. It focuses on maximising the individual's participation and functioning in the community with optimal health.

In practice, after the diagnosis of LD is established and the needs are identified, educational authorities are informed. This initiates a formal assessment of the individual's special educational needs (SEN). This is a statutory process that takes into account the views of parents and professionals involved in the child's care and provides the formal 'Statement advice'.

The Statement advice is a comprehensive document that addresses the needs and outlines the provision for the individual in the educational setting.

Social care needs are met through the local 'child disability teams'. They assess and offer support, which includes financial support, adaptations for home, respite and transport.

Appropriate voluntary agencies also support the child and the family with recreational and community-based activities.

No treatments are available for cognitive deficiency.

Children with LD should be evaluated regularly to monitor their health needs, and mental health and social care needs.

Some of the conditions, such as Down syndrome, have established good practice guidelines for health maintenance. The level of support will depend on the severity of the difficulties.

Prognosis

Children with LD have considerable health needs and need easy access to healthcare services. Most children with mild to moderate LD transition to adults and are able to live in community settings. The outcome depends on the degree of LD, presence of comorbidities, support from the family and social settings.

Autism spectrum disorder (ASD)

Autism spectrum disorder (ASD) is a developmental disorder that affects the way a person communicates with and relates to other people and the world around them. Individuals are affected in a variety of ways and to different degrees. It is a lifelong condition that has a great impact on children, young people and their families. It can occur at any level of intelligence. Asperger's syndrome is included under this term.

The term ASD describes:
1. qualitative differences and impairments in social interaction and reciprocal communication behaviours;
2. restricted interests and rigid and repetitive behaviours.

This is the so-called 'dyad of impairment'. Onset is in early childhood impairing everyday functioning. Both components are required for the diagnosis.

Prevalence

The overall prevalence of ASD in children is around 1%, and recent epidemiological studies indicate increasing prevalence. Boys are more affected than girls at a ratio of 4:1. The presenting features of ASD vary with the age of the child and the associated comorbidities such as LD and attention deficit hyperactivity disorder (ADHD).

Aetiology

ASD causation is not known and is thought to be multifactorial. There is a strong genetic predisposition. There is no evidence to support vaccinations as causation.

Some medical conditions have an increased association with ASD, for example Down syndrome, fragile X syndrome and tuberous sclerosis.

Signs and symptoms of ASD

The clinical presentation in ASD can vary in different age groups but there is overlap between the ages. Signs and symptoms include:

Preschool children: Language delay, regression or loss of speech, frequent repetition of set words (echolalia), poor eye contact, absence of social smiling, poor response to name, lack of imaginative play, preference for solitary play, unusual attachment to toys, hand flapping and tip-toe walking.

Primary school children (5–11 years): Learnt speech, monotonous tone, reduced awareness of personal space, limited facial expressions and gestures, following own agenda, strong preference for routines and rituals, stereotypical movements and over-focused or unusual interests.

Secondary school children (older than 11 years): Odd intonation, taking things literally, difficulties with social situations and rules, preference for specific interests, lack of common sense, and an unusual profile of skills and deficits.

Comorbidities

The common comorbidities associated with ASD are LD (75%), epilepsy (35%), mental health problems, ADHD, sleep problems, coordination problems and tics.

Diagnosis

Early diagnosis is crucial for favourable outcomes. Some units use screening questionnaires in their child health surveillance programme, such as MCHAT (Modified Checklist for Autism in Toddlers) for early identification. There is no specific biomarker for the diagnosis of ASD. Diagnosis instead requires a structured approach and uses multidisciplinary team assessments and observations. There are set criteria for diagnosis formulated in the *Diagnostic and Statistical Manual of Mental Disorders* (5th edition; also known as DSM-5, the American Psychiatric Association's diagnostic text) and the World Health Organization's publication the *International Classification of Diseases* (11th revision; ICD 11). NICE guidance on 'Recognition, referral and diagnosis of children and young people on the autism spectrum' sets out the principles of diagnosing ASD.

Locally there should be an ASD referral pathway to access specialist ASD assessment teams. The pathway should outline the process of assessment to inform parents and professionals. The core autism assessment team consists of a community paediatrician, a child and adolescent psychiatrist, an educational psychologist, and a speech and language therapist, but may include others such as an occupational therapist based on the patient's need.

Typically, the work-up by the ASD assessment team includes:

- Information gathering from school and other settings through structured questionnaires.
- Detailed history from parents including their concerns, birth, development and family history.
- ASD-specific history using a semi-structured parental interview tool.
- Formal cognitive or developmental assessment and language assessment.

- Direct observation of the child's social communication in the clinic, at school and using tools such as the Autism Diagnostic Observation Schedule (ADOS).

The assessments are individually tailored, integrating reported and observed evidence.

No single assessment result gives a diagnosis. The final decision is a consensus of all the evidence.

Hearing difficulties also need to be ruled out.

Investigations

There are no routine investigations recommended for ASD. The clinical findings and comorbidities determine the tests. Genetic tests for fragile X syndrome and array CGH are used for children with ASD associated with LD.

Management

Behavioural and communication interventions are the approach to the management. Several approaches are used, which need to be individually tailored. Post-diagnostic support is offered to the families through programmes such as the 'Early Bird Programme' and through an ASD family support worker. Information and support is also provided through relevant charities, for example the National Autistic Society. Appropriate educational placement and support is central to the management of ASD.

There is no treatment for the core symptoms of ASD. Medications are used to treat associated conditions, for example melatonin for sleep disorders, antipsychotics for aggression, anxiety and self-injury, and stimulants if the ASD is associated with ADHD.

Prognosis

The outcome depends on the severity of the core symptoms, and if there are associated comorbidities, particularly learning difficulties. Independent living is achieved in fewer than one-quarter of adults with ASD.

Attention deficit hyperactivity disorder (ADHD)

Definition

ADHD is the most prevalent neurobehavioural disorder in children and is characterised by inattention, impulsivity and overactivity or a combination of the symptoms. It compromises everyday functioning such as learning and making friends.

To fulfil the diagnostic criteria the symptoms must have an onset from an early age (<7 years of age) and should manifest in at least two settings, that is home and school, and cause significant social and academic impairment.

Individuals with ADHD have difficulty in focusing on a task and in stopping their responses.

Prevalence

The prevalence varies in different countries and is estimated to be between 3 and 7% in school-aged children. Boys are more affected than girls, with a ratio of 2–4:1.

Aetiology

ADHD is a highly familial condition with a 3–5 times increased risk in children and siblings of an affected individual. The causation of ADHD is multifactorial and research supports interactions between genes and environment. The involved genes and chromosomes are not definitely known. Genes regulating dopamine and serotonin receptors are implicated.

There are several environmental factors that increase the risk of ADHD, such as low birthweight, exposure to toxins, brain disease and injuries, institutional rearing and deprivation. Factors that exacerbate the symptoms are poor parenting, and certain foods and food additives, but they are not causes of ADHD.

Clinical features

The symptoms of ADHD vary with age. Symptoms of inattention include failing to pay attention to detail, making careless mistakes with school work or other activities, difficulty sustaining attention to tasks, not listening to instructions, forgetfulness in daily activities and being easily distracted.

Symptoms of hyperactivity include fidgeting with hands and squirming in the seat, on the go all the time, running about and climbing excessively when inappropriate to the situation, leaving the seat in the classroom, and difficulty participating in leisure activities quietly.

Symptoms of impulsivity include difficulty in waiting one's turn, interrupting often and talking excessively.

The symptoms should be above what one would expect for the mental age of the child.

Comorbidities

Children with ADHD often have other associated neurodevelopmental or psychological problems. Some of the common associations are conduct disorders, depression, anxiety, developmental coordination disorder, tics, specific and global learning difficulties, autism spectrum disorder and substance abuse.

Assessment

ADHD has no biochemical marker and the diagnosis relies on behavioural symptoms. The assessment should be multidisciplinary. It is done by specialist child psychiatric or community paediatric teams using a structured and systematic approach, for example, by using an established ADHD pathway.

A full assessment involves the following:
- **Information gathering:**
  - Clinical interviews with parents and the child with specific questioning about the behaviours in different settings, family history, risk factors and symptoms of comorbid conditions.
  - Information from school gathered through reports and validated rating scales such as Connor's questionnaires, strengths and difficulties questionnaires, and so forth.
- **Observation:** observation of the child in the school setting and clinic.
- **Physical examination:**
  - This should include measurement of the weight, height and head circumference, cardiovascular examination including pulse and blood pressure, neurological examination and assessment of coordination.
- **Vision and hearing should also be assessed.**

Investigations are guided by the findings of the physical examination and the associated comorbidities.

Management

A comprehensive treatment plan includes psychological, behavioural and educational advice and interventions with or without pharmacological treatments. The approaches differ in preschool and school-aged children and also with the severity of impairment.

Post-diagnostic support and advice should be offered to the child and the family through ADHD support teams.

Non-pharmacological interventions

Parent-training/education programmes are the first-line treatment for both preschool and school-aged children. Individual psychological interventions such as cognitive behaviour therapy or social skills training are also offered as appropriate.

Information following the diagnosis should be shared with school personnel, and adequate support put in place if additional needs are identified. School-based behavioural interventions should be in place to support the child in the classroom setting.

Pharmacological interventions

There is clear evidence of benefits of psychostimulant medication in reducing ADHD symptoms. Psychostimulants such as methylphenidate and dexamphetamine are the first line of treatment. Atomoxetine, which is a non-stimulant, is also used widely. The choice of medication is based on a range of factors including the child's needs, preference, coexisting conditions and the side-effect profile.

All stimulants have similar side-effect profiles, the most common being weight loss and delayed onset of sleep. The medication use must be regularly and carefully monitored for efficacy and side effects.

Prognosis

Most children with ADHD have relatively good outcomes if there is adherence to the treatment and there are no associated comorbidities.

There is a decline in symptoms with age, but studies have shown that there is greater persistence of symptoms in females in adulthood. Individuals with ADHD have low self-esteem, which impacts on their academic careers, work and relationships. The diagnosis of ADHD is associated with a higher risk of conduct disorders, and of substance abuse into adolescence and adulthood.

Developmental coordination disorder

Definition

Developmental coordination disorder (DCD) is a condition characterised by impairment in fine and gross motor skills that impacts on a child's daily functioning, academic achievement, leisure and play. These children are frequently known as 'clumsy child' or 'physically awkward'. Other terminologies have been used such as 'developmental apraxia/dyspraxia'

DCD has four diagnostic criteria:
1. Motor skills below what would be expected for the chronological age of the child.
2. Onset of symptoms in the early developmental period.
3. Motor skills deficits not explained by learning disabilities or visual problems and not secondary to an underlying neurological cause.
4. Motor skills deficit significantly and persistently interferes with the activities of daily living and impacts on academic productivity.

Prevalence

DCD is fairly common disorder and is recognised usually between 6 and 12 years of age. Prevalence varies widely, ranging from 5 to 15%, but the estimate is around 5 to 8%. Boys are more commonly affected than girls, with a ratio of 3:1.

Aetiology

Several theories have been proposed regarding the aetiology of DCD, and environmental, intrauterine and genetic factors may all be responsible. It is felt that the damage responsible is from abnormalities at the level of neurotransmitter or receptor systems rather than structural problems. The risk factors for DCD are prematurity, antenatal exposure to drugs and alcohol, and family history.

Clinical features

Three main areas of function are affected:
Gross motor – poor balance, awkward running pattern, frequent falls and poor performance in physical activity and sports secondary to slow reaction and movement times.
Fine motor – difficulty with handwriting, dressing and undressing, using cutlery and gripping items.
Psychosocial - low self-esteem, anxiety, depression, school refusal, and children may become the class clown to gain recognition and friends.

Comorbidities

- ADHD
- Dyslexia
- ASD

Assessment

The assessment is multidisciplinary as with other neurodevelopmental conditions. Evidence from school is obtained prior to formal assessment. This should include information about the child's cognitive abilities, level of reading, and numeracy and language skills in comparison with their coordination skills.

Medical assessment – should include detailed history and examination to exclude underlying neurological conditions such as cerebral palsy causing coordination difficulties.
Motor tests – usually done by a physiotherapist and/or occupational therapist. Gross and fine motor assessments are done using standard tests. The scores are compared with standard scores. A score below the fifth centile would confirm DCD.

Management

Goals of the treatment should be to determine areas of difficulty and to design interventions that will promote adaptive functioning and minimise coordination difficulties.

Some of the treatment approaches used for DCD are as follows:
- CO-OP (cognitive orientation to daily occupational performance);
- GPDC framework: Goal-Plan-Do it-Check;
- task-specific interventions;
- sensory integration therapy.

Children with DCD benefit from advice on seating, work surface, modification to cutlery and writing materials. Following the exercise programme in school, extra time in examinations, IT support and provision of a scribe are some of the support measures that can be provided in educational settings.

Prognosis

The difficulties continue into adulthood. Early identification and appropriate support and interventions have good outcomes.

SUMMARY

Clinical case

Case conclusion

The history is highly suggestive of autism spectrum disorder (ASD). This boy will undergo formal developmental assessment and speech and language therapy assessment. A detailed ASD developmental history and an ADOS assessment will aid in establishing the diagnosis of ASD.

Following feedback of the diagnosis, the family are given 'Early Support' material on ASD and guided to the relevant websites. They are offered support through the local support programmes, such as the Early Bird Programme, and an ASD family support worker. Health needs such as poor sleep patterns and limited diets are addressed in the follow-up clinics if needed.

Key learning points

- Neurodevelopmental disorders are often discovered during childhood healthcare checks, and can be better defined and described by formal testing and investigation. Better understanding of the needs of the child helps ensure links are made to appropriate support services.

- A range of disorders occur, including attention deficit disorders, autism spectrum disorders, and learning and intellectual disabilities. Each child and their family can be affected in different ways, and better understanding of the individual's needs is key to optimising management and care.

 Now visit **www.wileyessential.com/humandevelopment** to test yourself on this chapter.

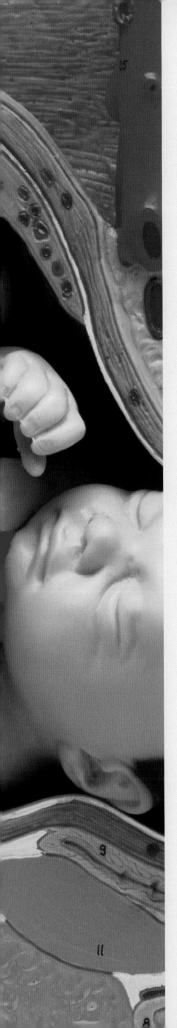

CHAPTER 31
Puberty

Christopher Bidder

Case history

A 13-year-old girl presents with concern about possible delayed onset of puberty. All of her friends are significantly more physically mature and she is self-conscious about her lack of development in comparison. She is otherwise well with no chronic disease symptoms, eats a normal diet and has not lost weight recently. She was born at term and had an uneventful neonatal period. She has a past medical history of glue ear and recurrent urinary tract infections when she was a young child. Both parents and her older siblings went through puberty at a normal age and there is no family history of note. Clinical examination shows she has relatively short stature (height on the second centile), normal weight for height (weight on the ninth centile), normal observations, normal cardiovascular, respiratory, abdominal and neurological examinations, and that she is prepubertal on Tanner staging. There is no goitre and she is euthyroid clinically. There are no neurocutaneous stigmata. You wonder if she has some dysmorphic features.

Learning outcomes

You should be able to:

- Describe the physiology of normal puberty.

- Recognise abnormal puberty, make a clinical assessment, interpret investigation results and formulate a differential diagnosis.

- Explain the psychological changes of adolescence and the changing health needs during this period of life.

Essential Human Development, First Edition. Edited by Samuel Webster, Geraint Morris and Euan Kevelighan
© 2018 John Wiley & Sons, Ltd. Published 2018 by John Wiley & Sons, Ltd.

Introduction

Puberty (from the Latin *puber*, mature or adult) and adolescence (from the Latin *adolescens*, growing up) are terms often used interchangeably to describe the changes that occur during the transition from childhood to an adult state. Physical changes include a growth spurt (followed by cessation of linear growth), the development of secondary sexual characteristics and achievement of reproductive capability. Psychological and emotional tasks include developing higher thinking skills (such as abstract reasoning, problem solving and decision making), forming mature relationships, developing self-identity and establishing a personal set of beliefs and values.

In both girls and boys, the physical changes of puberty follow a predictable sequence. Compliance with this pattern is called **consonance**. A good understanding of the physiology of normal puberty is essential to be able to recognise abnormal puberty and consider what the underlying diagnosis might be. A careful history and thorough physical examination will usually lead to a diagnosis, sometimes supported by a limited number of investigations.

Normal puberty

The hypothalamic-pituitary-gonadal (HPG) axis is shown in a simplified form in Figure 31.1. The axis is active in the fetal and early neonatal periods before becoming dormant in the first few months of postnatal life. The timing mechanism that controls the onset of puberty (in the hypothalamus) is not completely understood but has multifactorial influences, including genetic and environmental factors. The age of menarche has decreased significantly over the last 150 years, from a mean of around 17 years in 1850s' Norway to approximately age 13 years by 1960 in the UK. This change reflects improvements in socioeconomic conditions, particularly nutrition. This trend has slowed and possibly has reached a plateau.

At the onset of puberty, the GnRH secreting neurons of the hypothalamus begin producing increasing amounts of gonadotrophin-releasing hormone (GnRH) in a pulsatile fashion. GnRH moves down the pituitary stalk to the anterior pituitary where the gonadotrophic cells respond and produce the gonadotrophins luteinising hormone (LH) and follicle-stimulating hormone (FSH). These have a direct action on the gonads (ovaries in females, testes in males) with the end results being the growth of these tissues, the production of sex steroids (oestrogens and testosterone) and the achievement of fertility. The effects of sex steroids are listed in Table 31.1.

Independent of the above axis, the zona reticularis cells of the adrenal cortex produce androgen hormones such as androstenedione and dehydroepiandrosterone sulphate. These hormones may be detectable at the age of 6–8 years, rising through adolescence to peak in early adulthood. Their effects are also listed in Table 31.1.

The sequence of changes that occur in both sexes is predictable and represented in Figure 31.2. It is important to

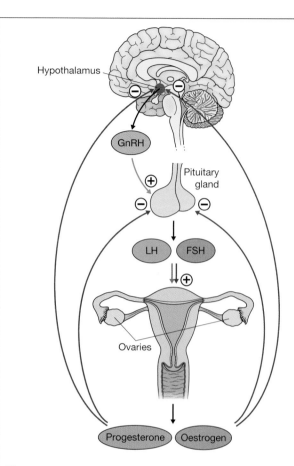

Figure 31.1 The female hypothalamo-pituitary-gonadal axis. FSH, follicle-stimulating hormone; LH, luteinising hormone

note that, on average, girls enter puberty approximately 18–24 months earlier than boys.

Assessment of puberty

Whenever there are concerns about puberty, a careful history is essential. This includes a family history, with attention to the timing of the parents' puberty. Mothers can usually remember how old they were when they achieved menarche; fathers more often have a vague sense of being an early, normal or late developer. A screen for chronic disease symptoms is important, along with medication history, birth and past medical history. Specific questions need to be asked about CNS symptoms (e.g. vision problems or headaches) and the presence of a normal sense of smell (Kallmann syndrome is a cause of delayed puberty associated with an absent sense of smell). The timing of any physical changes of puberty noted by the family and how those changes have progressed is vital. Asking the child or young person how they feel about the changes (or lack of them) is important.

Table 31.1 Effects of sex steroids and androgens.

Testosterone	Oestrogens	Adrenal androgens
Enlargement of the penis	Enlargement of the breasts	Growth of axillary, pubic, facial and body hair
Rapid skeletal growth and maturation (partly via conversion to oestrogens)	Rapid skeletal growth and maturation	Lesser contribution to skeletal growth and maturation
Increased muscle mass and strength	Change in body shape, increased fat mass	Greasy skin and hair, acne, development of body odour
Increased bone density	Increased bone density	
Growth of axillary, pubic, facial and body hair	Growth of the uterus	
Greasy skin and hair, acne, development of body odour	Development of the endometrium, culminating in menstruation	
Voice deepens		

Clinical examination will include careful measurement and plotting of height and weight, with comparison against earlier growth plots if available. The parental heights should be measured so that a target height range can be generated. In addition to a general systems examination, any dysmorphic features or birthmarks should be carefully noted. Visual fields and fundi should be checked, an assessment of thyroid status made and the neck should be examined for a goitre. Staging of puberty is performed using the somewhat subjective Tanner method (Figure 31.3). It is critical to manage this very personal examination sensitively, employing a chaperone when required.

In addition, in boys, the Prader orchidometer (Figure 31.4) allows the doctor to assess the testicular volume against a known reference. This can be a very helpful tool both at the initial assessment and on subsequent follow-up to chart progress.

Investigations are not always necessary as the diagnosis is often clinically apparent. When investigations are required, these may include blood tests for a general health screen or specific hormone levels, a bone age X-ray (comparing skeletal maturity against a known reference) and an ultrasound of the uterus and ovaries to assess size and morphology. Rarely, dynamic hormone tests are necessary, for example a GnRH stimulation test, when GnRH is given intravenously and serial measurements made of LH and FSH for 1 hour.

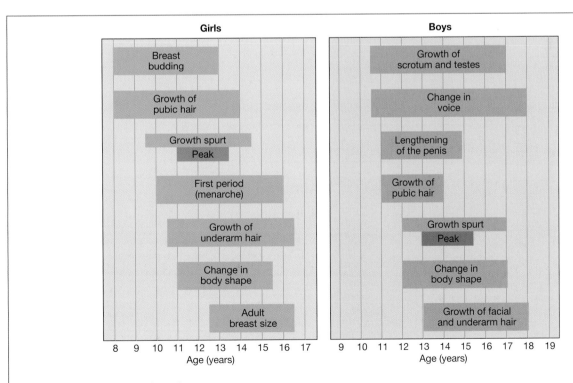

Figure 31.2 Milestones in puberty.

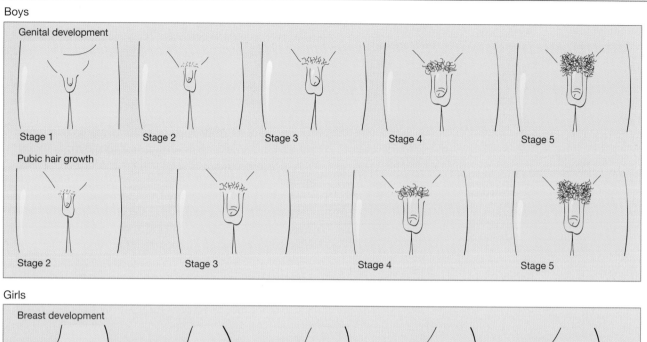

Boys

Genital development

Stage 1   Stage 2   Stage 3   Stage 4   Stage 5

Pubic hair growth

Stage 2   Stage 3   Stage 4   Stage 5

Girls

Breast development

Stage 1   Stage 2   Stage 3   Stage 4   Stage 5

Pubic hair growth

Stage 2   Stage 3   Stage 4   Stage 5

Figure 31.3 Line drawing representation of Tanner stages in boys and girls. (Source: L. Miall *et al.* (2012) *Paediatrics at a Glance*, 3rd edn. Reproduced with permission of John Wiley & Sons, Ltd.)

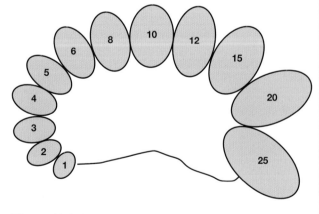

Figure 31.4 Prader orchidometer.

Abnormal puberty

Early puberty

In the UK, puberty is considered to be early if:
- In girls – there are breast changes before the age of 8 years, or – a first period occurs before the age of 9 years.
- In boys – there are any signs of puberty before the age of 9 years.

Exaggerated premature adrenarche

One of the commonest conditions causing concern is a variation of normal called exaggerated premature adrenarche. Typically the patient is a girl (occasionally a boy), aged between

6 and 8 years with limited pubertal changes due to production of adrenal androgens only. These include development of a limited amount of pubic or axillary hair, body odour and greasy skin but NOT other changes of puberty such as breast development, a significant growth spurt or menarche (i.e. **non-consonant** with normal puberty).

More often than not, investigations are not required and the diagnosis is confirmed by the continued absence of other pubertal signs on follow-up. Some authors advocate specific tests to exclude late-presenting congenital adrenal hyperplasia or an androgen-secreting tumour. No treatment is necessary and puberty occurs at a normal age. There is a limited amount of emerging evidence that some of these patients may have increased rates of polycystic ovarian syndrome as adults.

Isolated premature thelarche

Much less common, isolated premature thelarche describes the early onset of breast changes that are transient, isolated and not progressive. This occurs in very young girls (age <2 years) and can be very concerning for parents. Unlike true precocious puberty, there are no other signs of puberty (such as a growth spurt, pubic hair or menarche) and the breast changes are not progressive.

Investigations do not show advancement in bone age or pubertal development of the uterus and ovaries. Blood levels of FSH, LH and oestrogen are not elevated, although a small increase in FSH is occasionally observed.

Careful clinical follow-up is necessary to exclude progressive changes in keeping with true precocious puberty. In thelarche, the breast changes remain static and then regress, though this can take many months or years. Puberty occurs at a normal age. The cause is uncertain, though in some cases ovarian cysts are seen on ultrasound and may be implicated.

Central (gonadotrophin-dependent) precocious puberty (CPP)

CPP is uncommon; girls present more frequently than boys. Critical to the diagnosis of this condition is a history of consonant and progressive changes of puberty happening below the age limits above. Testicular volumes are increased (≥4 mL) in boys. A growth spurt is demonstrable on the growth chart. Tanner staging is advanced and progresses on follow-up.

Investigations show elevated levels of sex steroids and LH/FSH (either on random tests or after dynamic stimulation with GnRH), advanced bone age and, in girls, changes in the size and morphology of the ovaries and uterus. An MRI scan of the brain is necessary to exclude a structural lesion, though this is very often normal. Possible causes of CPP are listed in Box 31.1. It is important to note the majority of cases are idiopathic.

The adverse consequences of CPP include short stature as an adult (due to early closure of the growth plates) and the

> ### Box 31.1 Causes of central precocious puberty (CPP)
>
> - Idiopathic (90% of girls)
> - CNS structural lesion (e.g. hamartoma, optic glioma, neoplasm)
> - CNS radiotherapy
> - Previous CNS infection
> - Previous CNS trauma
> - Emotional trauma (e.g. adoption, child sex abuse)

significant psychological problems caused by the changes of puberty occurring in children this young.

Treatment is with a GnRH analogue to block the action of native GnRH on the pituitary. This is given by monthly injection, and continued until an age at which it is appropriate to stop treatment and allow puberty to occur normally.

Peripheral or pseudo (gonadotrophin-independent) precocious puberty (PPP)

This very rare condition mimics CPP with the exception that it is not possible to demonstrate high levels of LH or FSH either on baseline blood tests or after dynamic GnRH testing. The differential diagnosis includes sex steroid-secreting tumours and McCune–Albright syndrome (in which the ovaries are autonomously overactive).

Treatment is directed at the underlying cause but can be particularly challenging.

Delayed puberty

In the UK, puberty is considered to be delayed if:
- In girls – there are no breast changes by the age of 13 years or – a first period does not occur by the age of 16 years.
- In boys – there are no signs of puberty by the age of 14 years.

Boys present more often than girls to clinic, concerned about their lack of growth, lack of pubertal development and often a loss of sporting performance because of their relative short stature and decreased physical strength compared to their peers.

Constitutional delay of growth and puberty (CDGP)

This is a common cause of delayed puberty. There is often a family history of delayed puberty in one or both parents. An association with atopy may be elicited. Chronic disease symptoms are notably absent after careful questioning.

Clinical examination shows an otherwise well child who is prepubertal. In boys, testicular volumes are less than 4 mL.

Investigations show a degree of bone age delay (which can be helpful to reassure the patient about future growth potential), normal general health screen, normal thyroid function and prolactin, negative coeliac serology, low gonadotrophins and low testosterone levels.

Treatment is often unnecessary. If the young person is reassured and willing to be patient, clinic follow-up to ensure that spontaneous puberty occurs will often suffice. For some boys, this delay is not acceptable, and treatment can be given with low-dose testosterone injections for 4–6 months. Testosterone feedback onto the cells of the hypothalamus 'kick starts' spontaneous GnRH secretion and therefore progression through puberty, which can be confirmed by an increasing testicular volume on follow-up. Testosterone treatment can then be discontinued and progress monitored clinically.

Similar treatment with low-dose oestrogen can be given to girls, though this is less commonly necessary.

Chronic disease

Virtually any chronic disease can lead to delayed onset of puberty or arrest of progress through puberty. Common examples include eating disorders, inflammatory bowel disease, poorly controlled diabetes, hypothyroidism, chronic renal failure, cardiac disease, severe respiratory conditions such as cystic fibrosis and intense exercise.

This emphasises the importance of a careful history and examination to elicit symptoms of chronic disease. It is reasonable to do a limited number of investigations to screen for chronic disease (e.g. full blood count, inflammatory markers, liver, renal and thyroid function, prolactin levels, coeliac serology).

Treatment is directed at the underlying cause. For example, young girls with anorexia nervosa need to be supported to achieve and maintain a healthy weight to allow their body to go through puberty. Treatment with sex steroids is not indicated for this purpose.

Hypogonadotrophic hypogonadism (central cause)

This condition relates to the permanent failure of the anterior pituitary to produce LH and FSH. Often, this is anticipated, due to known pre-existing pituitary problems (e.g. a patient on multiple pituitary replacement hormones), or a past medical history of conditions that affect pituitary function (e.g. CNS radiotherapy).

Gonadotrophin deficiency as an isolated pituitary problem is not common. Kallmann syndrome is one example and is associated with an absent sense of smell. Hypogonadotrophic hypogonadism can be very difficult to distinguish from CDGP, and it is often only on follow-up and after further investigation that it becomes apparent that there is a permanent deficiency of LH and FSH.

Lifelong sex steroid treatment is necessary. Fertility is impaired.

Hypergonadotrophic hypogonadism (gonadal failure)

Primary gonadal failure is uncommon. The diagnosis is made when a child with delayed puberty has very high levels of gonadotrophins. The commonest cause in girls is Turner syndrome (45 XO chromosome complement) and in boys Klinefelter syndrome (47 XXY) or some form of injury to the testes earlier in life, such as maldescent, torsion or trauma. Less commonly, some girls go through a premature menopause, either before the onset of puberty or during puberty.

Treatment is with lifelong sex steroid replacement. Fertility is impaired.

The psychology of adolescence

Adolescence is also a time of profound psychological and emotional change that has been recognised for centuries. The World Health Organization (WHO) estimates that 1 in 5 of the world population are adolescents and defines adolescence to be:

> the period in human growth and development that occurs after childhood and before adulthood, from ages 10 to 19. It represents one of the critical transitions in the life span and is characterized by a tremendous pace in growth and change that is second only to that of infancy. Biological processes drive many aspects of this growth and development, with the onset of puberty marking the passage from childhood to adolescence. The biological determinants of adolescence are fairly universal; however, the duration and defining characteristics of this period may vary across time, cultures, and socioeconomic situations. This period has seen many changes over the past century namely the earlier onset of puberty, later age of marriage, urbanization, global communication, and changing sexual attitudes and behaviours.
> WHO (http://www.who.int/maternal_child_adolescent/topics/adolescence/dev/en)

A detailed discussion of adolescent psychology is beyond the scope of this text. Some brief notes are included below.

Tasks of adolescence

In order to develop a stable, independent identity as adults, the Raising Teens project identified 10 tasks adolescents need to undertake:

1. Adjust to sexually maturing bodies and feelings.
2. Develop and apply abstract thinking skills.
3. Develop and apply new perspectives on human relationships.
4. Develop and apply new coping skills in areas such as decision making, problem solving, and conflict resolution.

5. Identify meaningful moral standards, values and belief systems.
6. Understand and express more complex emotional experiences.
7. Form friendships that are mutually close and supportive.
8. Establish key aspects of identity (e.g. gender, sexual, spiritual, ethnic identity).
9. Meet the demands of increasingly mature roles and responsibilities.
10. Renegotiate relationships with adults in parenting roles.

Anatomy of the teenage brain

Advances in neuroimaging, particularly MRI and functional MRI, have helped us to understand that the human brain does not stop growing or developing in early childhood as some previously thought. The period of adolescence sees an initial substantial increase in the amount of grey matter (neurons and their synapses) followed by a gradual reduction in grey matter as these synapses are 'pruned'. This synaptic pruning (elimination of unwanted and underused connections) is partly influenced by the experience and environment of the individual; synapses that are used frequently are supported, strengthened and become permanent. Underused synapses are lost; a 'use it or lose it' principle is in effect.

Just like the external physical changes of puberty, this remodelling of the brain occurs later in boys than girls. Many of the characteristic behaviour patterns of adolescents are explainable by the neuroanatomical changes that are occurring, for example increased risk-taking behaviour (particularly when with peers) can be linked to different function of both the limbic system and prefrontal cortex when compared to adults.

Interested students can explore this topic further by watching a TED talk given by cognitive neuroscientist Sarah-Jayne Blakemore (https://www.ted.com/talks/sarah_jayne_blakemore_the_mysterious_workings_of_the_adolescent_brain).

Adolescent healthcare

Adolescent behaviour is often characterised by risk taking, poor impulse control and increased self-consciousness whilst an increasingly independent role in life, with decreased parental control, is sought.

This can have dramatic effects on health needs, whether it be with health problems directly linked to these behaviours (e.g. eating disorders, drug and alcohol intoxication, high-risk sexual activity, mood disorders, deliberate self-harm and suicide) or with effects on pre-existing chronic conditions (e.g. asthma, cystic fibrosis, epilepsy, heart disease, inflammatory bowel disease, diabetes), when compliance with the demands of treatment may well change, often for the worse.

Increasingly, adolescent healthcare is being recognised as an emerging subspeciality of paediatrics. It is clear that the health of adolescents needs special consideration in the light of our understanding of their specific needs.

Clinical case

Case conclusion

Because of the absence of any pubertal signs in this 13-year-old girl, you perform some investigations. These show normal general health screening blood tests, normal thyroid function, negative coeliac serology and undetectable levels of oestradiol. The LH and FSH levels are very high. A bone age X-ray shows significant bone age delay, and an ultrasound of the uterus and ovaries shows a prepubertal uterus with very small 'streak' ovaries. A karyotype is abnormal: 45 XO.

The diagnosis is primary ovarian failure due to Turner syndrome.

Case commentary

Girls with Turner syndrome do not always have characteristic phenotypic features and can present in this way. You will recognise that this diagnosis will be very upsetting for the girl and her parents, and sharing the information requires sensitive communication.

Further investigations are necessary to exclude problems associated with Turner syndrome (e.g. an echocardiogram and renal ultrasound). You offer support from the clinical nurse specialist on the team and provide information about local and national support groups.

You discuss the treatment options with the girl and her parents. Growth hormone is licensed for use in Turner syndrome, although the benefit is likely to be small when starting treatment in a child of this age. You consider deferring treatment to induce puberty (with ethinyloestradiol) to maximise the benefit of growth hormone but the girl elects to start both treatments simultaneously. Low-dose ethinyloestradiol is started and gradually increased over 2 years; secondary sexual characteristics develop at an appropriate, gradual rate with an associated growth spurt. Following menarche, you switch treatment to a low-dose oral contraceptive pill. Once final adult height is achieved you stop the growth hormone. You explain that fertility as an adult will require IVF treatment.

SUMMARY

Key learning points

- Normal puberty has a **consonant** pattern in both sexes. A good understanding of this process is essential to recognise and treat abnormal puberty.
- Abnormal puberty includes early, late and **non-consonant** pubertal changes.

- Good history taking and clinical examination skills are essential to make an accurate diagnosis. Investigations have a limited, supportive role.
- Adolescence is a time of profound psychological change. New health problems may emerge and chronic health conditions may change.

 Now visit **www.wileyessential.com/humandevelopment** to test yourself on this chapter.

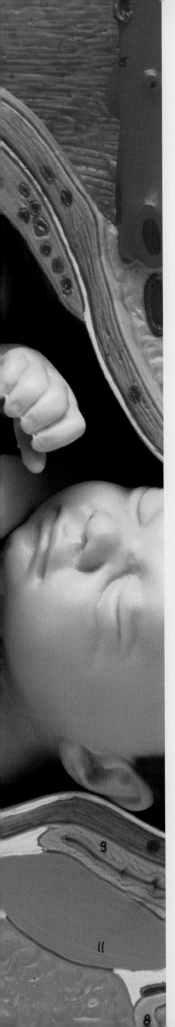

CHAPTER 32
Non-accidental injury and neglect

Catrin Simpson

Case

A 2-month-old baby is brought to the hospital via a 999 ambulance call. On arrival he is poorly responsive, with a bulging anterior fontanelle. His parents tell you that he has been unwell the past few days, taking fewer feeds and sleeping more than normal. He needs intubation to manage his airway, is stabilised and is then transferred for further management on the paediatric intensive care unit. On further examination on the ward a small 1 × 1 cm facial bruise is noted.

Learning outcomes

- You should be able to recognise signs of non-accidental injury, neglect and abuse in children.

- You should be able to describe the processes that can be used for safeguarding an at-risk child.

Essential Human Development, First Edition. Edited by Samuel Webster, Geraint Morris and Euan Kevelighan
© 2018 John Wiley & Sons, Ltd. Published 2018 by John Wiley & Sons, Ltd.

Introduction

According to the World Health Organization and International Society for Prevention of Child Abuse and Neglect (2006), child maltreatment refers to 'the physical and emotional mistreatment, sexual abuse, neglect and negligent treatment of children, as well as to their commercial or other exploitation'. Maltreatment of a child may occur in a number of environments including the home, school and within the looked-after system. Those inflicting abuse may include parents, friends, carers, teachers or other children.

Incidence

As of 2012, there were over 50 000 children in the UK on the child protection register or subject to a child protection plan. This number has increased dramatically over recent years. This increase may be a result of improved awareness of child maltreatment and better reporting to services.

Retrospective studies undertaken by the UK's National Society for the Prevention of Cruelty to Children (NSPCC, 2011) show that 25% of young adults in the UK report being severely maltreated during childhood, with 14% being maltreated by a parent or guardian. It is clear that safeguarding issues need to be at the forefront of our minds when seeing and assessing all children. Safeguarding children is everybody's responsibility, and therefore whatever speciality a medical career moves into, an awareness of child protection issues is paramount.

Important legislation

- The UK's Children's Act 2008 is government legislation that sets out the roles and responsibilities of agencies such as health, children's services and education with regard to safeguarding children. At the heart of this legal framework is the concept that the child's welfare is paramount.
- The United Nations Convention on the Rights of the Child (UNCRC) is an agreement that has been ratified by 193 countries across the world. It sets out 45 articles that stipulate children's rights that should be upheld by government. It covers a child's rights to be heard, to be with their family, to be able think and feel what they want, and practise a religion. It stresses that we have a duty to protect children from war, trafficking, exploitation and kidnapping. Children have a right to education. Importantly it states that all children have the right to be protected from 'all forms of physical or mental violence, injury or abuse, neglect, or negligent treatment, maltreatment or exploitation including sexual abuse' (UNICEF, no date).

The General Medical Council places a duty on all doctors to protect and promote the health and wellbeing of all children. This therefore means that all doctors have a duty to:

- keep up to date with relevant practice, laws and training;
- consider a child's wellbeing, even if he or she is not directly your patient;
- act on any concerns regarding the safety of a child;
- act in the child's best interests.

Vulnerable groups

Some groups of children are particularly vulnerable and need careful consideration. Children with disabilities may struggle to report maltreatment, and face higher rates of abuse. Children within the looked-after system may also be more vulnerable, and have often been victims of abuse prior to being placed in care. Children who are seeking asylum are often fleeing violence and difficult circumstances from their own country, and may be separated from their parents or caregivers. This may result in their being placed in temporary accommodation, facing frequent moves and struggling to access appropriate support and care.

Types of abuse

Child maltreatment is broadly divided into four main groups: physical abuse, sexual abuse, emotional abuse and neglect. It is rare that one type of abuse exists solely, and all have long-standing consequences for the child.

Physical abuse

Physical abuse may involve a number of different violent behaviours that result in the physical harm of a child. This may include hitting, shaking, burning, suffocating or drowning. Physical abuse also includes fabricated or induced illness of a child.

Physical abuse has a huge spectrum ranging from physical chastisement, sadly through to death or permanent disability. Signs may include injuries such as bruises, burns or fractures where the history does not fit the injury seen. Concerns should always be raised where injuries occur in non-mobile children. Consideration should also be given to the timings between when the injuries occurred and when help was sought. Delay in presentation is concerning. At all times an attempt should be made to gain a history of the injury from the child, although consideration must be made to the developmental ability of the child to do so.

Bruising

Bruising is very common in children and present in nearly every mobile child. It is therefore important to be aware of when bruising is of concern, so that children who are being abused can be differentiated. Normal childhood bruising is often in areas over bones, such as shins, elbows or forehead. Children will often tell you with pride about a fall or accident that caused an injury!

Bruising of concern may have the following features:

- Bruising in a non-mobile child.
- Bruises that are in relatively protected areas such as inner arms or thighs.
- Bruising not overlying bony areas, such as cheeks or buttocks.
- Bruising in clusters, or showing the outline of an implement or hand (Figure 32.1).
- Bruising that a child is trying to hide.

It is not possible to age a bruise accurately and therefore matching an injury with the history provided can at times be challenging. Investigations may be required to look for an underlying cause as to why a child might bruise more easily, but the presence of a blood clotting abnormality does not mean that physical abuse has not occurred.

Differential diagnosis may include:

- clotting disorder;
- birthmarks such as Mongolian blue spot;
- infections such as meningococcal disease;
- vasculitic conditions.

Fractures

Fractures again are very common in children but usually present with a clear history of causation. If there is any doubt it is important to consider the possibility of abuse and discuss with paediatrics, orthopaedics and radiology.

Concerning fractures may have the following features:

- fractures in a non-mobile child;
- fractures without adequate history;
- rib fractures without a clear history of bone disease or major trauma, such as a road traffic accident (Figure 32.2)
- occult fractures;

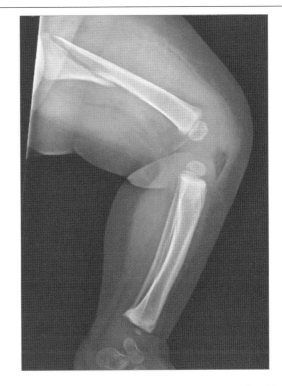

Figure 32.2 Fracture of the femur in a 4-month-old baby.

- multiple fractures, especially if of differing ages.
  Differential diagnosis may include:
- vitamin D deficiency;
- osteogenesis imperfecta;
- birth injury;
- malignancy.

Burns

Burns and scalds in children are a common presentation to emergency departments. Often there is a history of a child pulling an implement or container over themselves, resulting in injuries to the upper body and limb. Accidental scalds often show evidence of splash marking. Children touching hot objects tend to cause burns to their fingertips or palms of their hands.

Concerning burns may have the following features:

- Burns without an adequate history.
- Burns where there appears to be an element of neglect of the child's safety.
- Burns suggestive of immersion injury, i.e. showing a stocking or glove distribution, or involving the buttocks.
- Burns in areas that the child may not have been able to reach themselves such as the back or buttocks.
- Contact burns showing well-demarcated outlines of an implement.

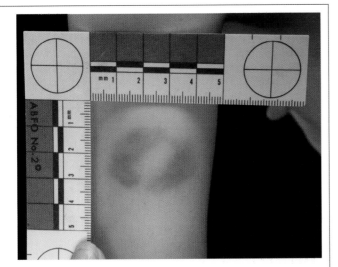

Figure 32.1 Bruising showing features of a bite mark.

Differentials to non-accidental burns may include:

- accidental burn or scald;
- staphylococcal skin infection.

Bites

Young children often bite each other resulting in marking. A bite mark in a child needs consideration as to the history and whether any incident has been witnessed. It can be difficult to differentiate between child and adult bites, and therefore an expert opinion from a forensic dentist is sometimes required. Where an animal bite is present consideration should be given to whether the child is receiving appropriate supervision.

Non-accidental head injury

Young children may present with non-specific symptoms either acutely or with delayed presentation. An acute head injury may present with altered consciousness, or shock. Delayed presentation of head injury may present with increasing head size, or neurological deficits. Neuroimaging may reveal intracranial bleeding. Head trauma may result from one forceful event, or from multiple repetitive movements such as in shaking.

Non-accidental head injuries may show the following features:

- inadequate history to explain the injury;
- subdural and subarachnoid haemorrhages;
- multiple bleeds;
- associated retinal haemorrhages;
- other skeletal injuries/ bruising.
  Differentials for non-accidental head injury may include:
- accidental injury such as road traffic accident or significant fall;
- metabolic diseases such as glutaric aciduria type 1;
- coagulation disorder;
- birth trauma.

Fabricated and induced illness (FII)

Physical abuse may also present as fabricated and induced illness, previously known as Munchausen syndrome by proxy. Caregivers may exaggerate or fabricate an illness in a child. This may involve withdrawal of nutrition, fabrication of rashes or fabrication of symptoms leading to multiple admissions and investigations. Often a child may have started with a genuine illness, and therefore it can be very difficult to gauge where the illness became fabricated. Investigations from a medical point of view need to be carefully considered, with clear indications of what needs to be ruled out medically whist being mindful of the potential harm to the child that may occur from unnecessary investigations. If there are concerns regarding FII the child should be discussed with social services and a paediatrician experienced in safeguarding. A chronology of

events, investigations and results is a useful way of organising information. In some cases the child will need to be observed without the parent/carer being allowed access in order to see whether symptoms persist. Multidisciplinary information sharing is essential for management.

Sexual abuse

Sexual abuse can be defined as forcing or enticing a child or young person to take part in sexual activities, whether or not the child is aware of what is happening. It may involve penetrative or non-penetrative contact, non-contact activities or encouraging children to behave in sexually inappropriate ways. Sexual activity in a child under 13 years of age is regarded as rape, regardless of the age of the partner.

An NSPCC retrospective study from 2012 reported that 24.1% of young people reported experiencing sexual abuse (contact and non-contact) by an adult or peer during their childhood. Worryingly, many children and young people report that they never told anyone about their abuse. Sexual abuse therefore needs to be considered by those working with children as it is likely that a child will not feel able to explain what is happening to them.

Sexual abuse may present with a disclosure of an event, either acute or historical. Regardless of whether a disclosure occurs sexual abuse needs to be considered where physical signs exist, such as localised trauma, sexually transmitted diseases or pregnancy. Children may present with emotional distress, behavioural issues or self-harm. Sexualised behaviour may be witnessed, raising concerns regarding what that child may have experienced or witnessed. Consideration needs to be given to sexual exploitation of young people, with expensive gifts, drugs or alcohol being used to gain trust. A young person may not feel that they are being abused at the time, and a sensitive enquiry about any mismatch in the power dynamics of a relationship may be required.

When concerns are raised about sexual abuse of a child, a medical examination will be required in parallel with discussions with social services and the police. Ideally, physical examination should be performed sensitively and by someone qualified to interpret signs. However, if a child presents acutely and there are concerns that they may require urgent medical attention, examination should not be delayed. In some areas Sexual Abuse Referral Centres (SARCs) exist that allow examination of the child in an environment that is equipped to deal with the physical examination and allows an appropriate child-friendly environment. Children and young people may need a forensic examination if there is indication that the abuse is recent, and children should be assessed as to whether post-exposure prophylaxis for HIV is required. When there are concerns regarding historical abuse, a physical examination is often still indicated to reassure the young person that no long-lasting physical damage has been done, to check for sexually transmitted diseases, and to risk assess any ongoing

Neglect

Neglect is the persistent failure to meet a child's basic physical or physiological needs. This may involve the parents or carer failing to provide adequate food or shelter, the failure to protect from physical or emotional harm, or ensure adequate supervision. It may also involve a failure to seek appropriate medical care, or delay in doing so.

Neglect is the most prevalent type of maltreatment reported in the family for all ages of children. According to the NSPCC (2011), 9% of children report that they have experienced severe neglect. Neglect can be life-threatening and needs to be treated with as much urgency as other forms of maltreatment. Neglect has been noted to have been present in 60% of serious case reviews where children have been seriously injured or died from safeguarding issues.

Neglect is likely to be under-reported to services as there is often no clear threshold event, such as a bruise or a fracture, to raise concerns. Concerns are likely to be more insidious, with a generalised feeling of unease amongst professionals. Neglect may be considered in children where a child presents as dirty or unkempt on a regular basis. The child may not be provided with a healthy diet, and may be failing to thrive (Figure 32.3),

needs such as hepatitis vaccination. SARC centres tend to have a safe and appropriate environment that allows children to be interviewed, and appropriate counselling and support can be provided.

or be obese. Children may be deprived of regular stimulation and may be falling behind with their development. A child may not be attending school regularly, or may not be taken for medical or dental appointments when required.

Consequences of neglect have been found to be longstanding and serious. Children experiencing serious early neglect have been found to have altered development with longstanding effects on educational achievement, emotional adjustment and behaviour, even after being removed from their neglectful environment. Neglect may also be considered in respect of the unborn child, if appropriate antenatal care is not sought, or where risky behaviour such as use of alcohol or drugs is continued despite advice.

Assessment of neglect requires multi-agency working in order to share concerns and to formulate a bigger picture of what is happening for a certain child.

Emotional abuse

Emotional abuse is the persistent emotional maltreatment of a child such as to cause severe and persistent adverse effects on the child's emotional development.

A study by the NSPCC (2011) found that 6.8% of children aged 11–17 years report having experienced emotional abuse. Emotional abuse will tend to accompany all other types of abuse but can occur solely and may be difficult to identify. Emotional abuse may involve being made to feel worthless or unloved. It may involve seeing or hearing the maltreatment of

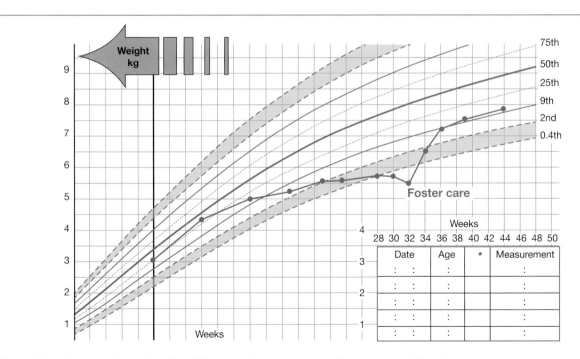

Figure 32.3 Growth chart showing failure to thrive, corrected by placement into foster care.

others, such as in domestic abuse. It may involve bullying or scapegoating, or putting inappropriate expectations upon the child.

A child may present with issues with behaviour, or be noted to be withdrawn. The child may have feelings of poor self-worth, which may lead to depressive symptoms and self-harm.

Actions required if you are concerned about a child

Safeguarding is everybody's responsibility.

If you have concerns regarding a child, at any stage of training or career, this should be discussed with a senior colleague and a decision taken as to whether a referral is made to social services. Local guidelines will be available as to how this referral is made. Consent is not required to make a referral where you feel the child is at risk of significant harm; however, it is good practice to discuss your concerns with the family. In many cases you are likely to have further involvement with the family in the future, and therefore having a good working relationship is preferable. Nonetheless, if you feel that discussing your concerns and plans for referral is likely to put the child, your staff or yourself in danger, it may be appropriate to refer prior to discussing with the family.

Children's services will assess whether further action is required. A strategy meeting may be held where people involved with that child, such as a health visitor, teacher or social worker, will share any concerns. The police will be present to see whether any legal avenues need to be pursued. A decision would then be made as to whether further investigations and actions are required in order to safeguard that child. This is known as a Section 47 enquiry.

A decision may be made that the child requires a safeguarding medical examination. This medical is performed by an experienced paediatrician (registrar level or consultant) and will document any clinical findings. A history should be gained from those involved, not forgetting to talk to the child where possible. Injuries will be assessed with respect to the child's developmental stage. Injuries should be documented on a body chart, and medical photography is also very useful to record findings. The examining paediatrician will be expected to provide an opinion on whether safeguarding concerns still persist.

Investigations may be required. These may include:
Physical abuse:
- Blood tests to look for any medical reason for easy bruising or fractures.
- Eye examination to look for any retinal haemorrhage.
- CT head scan to look for any intracranial injury.
- Skeletal survey and bone scan to look for occult fractures.

Neglect:
- Consideration of other differential diagnosis and tests as appropriate.

Sexual abuse:
- STI screening.
- Pregnancy testing.
- Hepatitis and HIV screening.

All cases:
- Consideration of the child's mental health.

A summary of medical findings should be collated into a report that is then shared with social services. It is imperative that documentation is clear, accurate and contemporaneous. Any history gained ideally should be documented as direct quotes. Injuries should be clearly documented on body charts. An opinion on a case may be required in court some considerable time after the event. Therefore making an effort to carefully document findings at the time may save a great deal of stress at a later point.

After completion of the Section 47 Enquiry

Once all information for all agencies has been gathered a decision will be made as to whether concerns have been substantiated, and whether the child is felt to be at risk of ongoing harm. A Case Conference will be held where agencies involved, including parents, will meet, share information and plan the continuing care of the child. If the child is felt to be at risk of significant harm a decision will be made to register that child on the Child Protection Register. A plan will be drawn up detailing further actions required to ensure the child's safety. A plan may involve the child being placed in alternative accommodation whilst further work is done with the family. It is also possible that the child may stay within the family environment, but with close supervision.

Once all information from the multi-agency team has been collated a decision may be made that the child is not at immediate risk or harm, but is in need of services in order to fulfil their potential.

Child in Need

Where a child is felt to be in need of additional help and support, but not felt to be at immediate risk of significant harm, in the UK a child may be referred to children's services as a Child in Need under Section 17 of the Children's Act. A Child in Need is a child who is unlikely to achieve or maintain a reasonable standard of health or development without the provision of services. A child with a disability is also a classified as being a Child in Need. Consent from the parent or carer is required prior to referring as a Child in Need. If consent is not given, consideration should be given to whether a Child Protection referral is therefore required.

Clinical case

Case discussion

What are the possible explanations for this scenario?

This is a case where a non-mobile child is presenting with indicators of significant head injury and a facial bruise. No clear history to explain the injuries has been given. The first differential in this case is non-accidental injury.

What further actions are required?

Once the child is medically stabilised consideration must be given to the safeguarding processes. The case must be discussed with your senior colleague and an urgent referral needs to be made to children's services. Someone experienced in safeguarding should sit with the family and take a full history of events plus a review of medical history, social history and family history. An explanation of concerns and processes should be given. At all times staff should be non-judgemental and sensitive to the fact that at this point it is unknown who a potential perpetrator may be. The child will need to undergo a careful physical examination and all findings documented, including using photography. The police are also likely to want to investigate the case and may also wish to interview the family.

What further investigations are required?

The child is likely to require blood investigations to rule out a clotting disorder. A CT head scan will give further information regarding the presence of any bleeds. Investigations may be required to rule out a metabolic condition that could cause a bleed. A skeletal survey +/− bone scan will give information regarding any occult injuries. An ophthalmology examination will provide information on whether retinal haemorrhages are present.

Key learning points

- Safeguarding children is the responsibility of everyone, not just those working in paediatrics.

- Guidelines and support structures are in place. If you have ANY concerns regarding a child's welfare discuss with a senior colleague or a named professional for safeguarding.

 Now visit **www.wileyessential.com/humandevelopment** to test yourself on this chapter.

FURTHER READING

See your local safeguarding procedures.

General Medical Council (GMC). Protecting children and young people: doctors' responsibilities (http://www.gmc-uk.org/guidance/ethical_guidance/13257.asp).

HM Government (2013) Working Together to Safeguard Children (https://media.education.gov.uk/assets/files/pdf/w/working%20together.pdf).

NSPCC website (https://www.nspcc.org.uk/).

RCPCH (Royal College of Paediatrics and Child Health) website (http://www.rcpch.ac.uk/), Child protection pages.

REFERENCES

NSPCC (2011) Child Abuse and Neglect Today. Available at: https://www.nspcc.org.uk/preventing-abuse/child-abuse-and-neglect (accessed 9 August 2017).

UNICEF. Overview of the United Nations Convention on the Rights of the Child. http://www.unicef.org/crc/files/Rights_overview.pdf (accessed 3 July 2017).

World Health Organization and International Society for Prevention of Child Abuse and Neglect (2006) Preventing child maltreatment: a guide to taking action and generating evidence. Available at: http://whqlibdoc.who.int/publications/2006/9241594365_eng.pdf (accessed 3 July 2017).

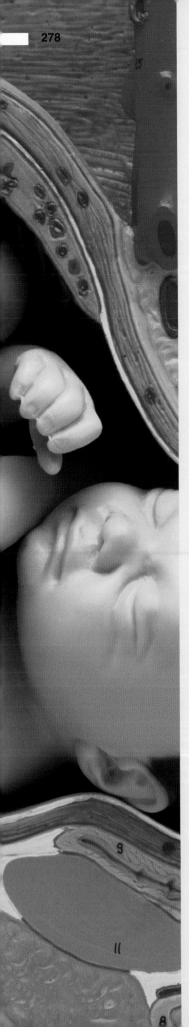

CHAPTER 33
Neurological problems

Cathy White

Case

A 13-year-old girl presents with a 9-month history of intermittent headaches. She describes bilateral throbbing headaches occurring once or twice a month lasting several hours. The pain is made worse by noise and relieved by sleep. Simple painkillers are not always helpful, perhaps because she often feels sick with the headaches. More recently she has had a number of episodes in school where she has collapsed to the floor and had some twitching. She recovers quickly from these episodes. Neurological examination, including fundoscopy was normal. Her blood pressure was within normal limits.

Learning outcomes

You should be able to:

- Understand the common causes of headache in children.
- Appreciate the range of paroxysmal events that occur in children and know how to distinguish them.
- Describe the main types of epileptic seizures.
- Recognise that children with one neurodisability are at high risk of having additional problems.
- Know the common developmental malformations of the central nervous system.

Essential Human Development, First Edition. Edited by Samuel Webster, Geraint Morris and Euan Kevelighan
© 2018 John Wiley & Sons, Ltd. Published 2018 by John Wiley & Sons, Ltd.

Headache

Contrary to popular belief, headaches are very common in children (2.5% in the under-12s rising to adult levels in teenagers). The primary headache disorders, which include migraine and tension-type headache, account for the majority of headaches, while secondary headache, that is those with underlying pathology, are much less common. The International Headache Society (IHS) classification is shown in Table 33.1. The cranial neuralgias are rare in children. Symptom overlap between the various headache syndromes is particularly common in children. Recurrent headaches, of whatever cause, are a cause of considerable morbidity, especially in terms of school loss.

Migraine headaches

The diagnostic criteria for migraine are broader in children as the headaches are often bilateral and last for a shorter time than in adults (see Table 33.2). They are frequently preceded by a behavioural prodrome with mood change or withdrawal from activity. Migraine with aura occurs in about 15% of children with migraine. Visual phenomena, for example flickering lines, spots or scotomata, are the commonest auras. Most children prefer to lie down in a quiet, darkened room and 'sleep it off'.

Uncommon forms of migraine include hemiplegic migraine (familial and sporadic), basilar-type migraine and the childhood periodic syndromes such as cyclical vomiting and benign paroxysmal vertigo.

Common triggering factors include stress, sleep deprivation, missing meals and hormonal changes. Migraine commonly 'runs in families', with approximately 70% of children having an affected first-degree relative.

Tension-type headaches

Tension-type headaches are more common in adults than children. The headache is usually bilateral and described as pressing or band-like. They can last for days and usually have no associated symptoms.

Secondary headaches

Secondary headaches are rare, and brain tumour as a cause of headache even rarer. For every child with a brain tumour there are around 5000 children with recurrent headaches, including 2000 children with migraine. For most secondary headaches the characteristics of the headache are poorly defined but there are features of the headache and, more importantly, of the examination that point towards the presence of a space-occupying lesion (Box 33.1).

Investigation

Careful history taking and examination should allow identification of the few children who require further investigation. As the diagnosis of a primary headache is clinical, diagnostic testing is only necessary when a secondary cause of the headache is suspected. Neuroimaging is rarely necessary, and of little value, unless the history or examination suggests a structural aetiology (see Box 33.1). The concept of red flag symptoms or signs as indicators of secondary headache, and therefore of the need for imaging, is well established in adult neurology but is not directly applicable to children. Magnetic resonance imaging is preferred to CT scanning.

Management

A thorough history and examination combined with explanation and advice is the most important means of reassuring the child and family that there is no serious cause for the headaches. Many parents are simply seeking reassurance that their child does not have a brain tumour. The same approach for all children with paroxysmal headaches who are well in between is often taken because of the overlap between the major headache types in children.

Table 33.1 The International Headache Society classification of headache disorders.

Primary headaches	Secondary headaches	Cranial neuralgias, facial pain and other headaches
• Migraine • Tension-type headache • Cluster headache and other trigeminal autonomic cephalgias • Other primary headaches	Headache attributed to: • Head and/or neck trauma • Cranial or cervical vascular disorder • Non-vascular intracranial disorder, e.g. IIH • A substance or its withdrawal • Infection • Homeostasis disorder • Disorder of facial or cranial structures, e.g. acute sinusitis • Psychiatric disorder	• Trigeminal and other cranial neuralgias • Other headaches

IIH, idiopathic intracranial hypertension.

Table 33.2 The International Headache Society (IHS) diagnostic criteria

Type of headache	Criteria
Migraine without aura	A. At least five attacks fulfilling B–D B. Duration between 1 and 72 hours C. At least two of the following: • Unilateral (or bilateral in younger children) • Pulsating • Moderate to severe in intensity • Aggravation by routine physical activity D. During the headache at least one of the following: • Nausea or vomiting • Photophobia or phonophobia E. Not attributable to another disorder
Migraine with aura	A. In addition to above criteria, at least two attacks fulfilling B B. At least three of the following: • One or more fully reversible aura symptoms indicating focal cortical or brainstem dysfunction • Aura developing gradually over minutes, or two or more symptoms occurring in succession • Aura lasts no more than 1 hour • Pain follows aura after less than 1 hour
Tension-type headache	A. At least 10 episodes occurring on <1 day per month average (<12 days per year) and fulfilling criteria B–D B. Headache lasting from 30 minutes to 7 days C. Headache has at least two of the following characteristics: • Bilateral location • Pressing/tightening (non-pulsating) quality • Mild or moderate intensity • Not aggravated by routine physical activity such walking or climbing stairs D. Both of the following: • No nausea or vomiting (anorexia may occur) • No more than one of photophobia or phonophobia E. Not attributed to another disorder

Box 33.1 Symptoms and signs suggestive of a space-occupying lesion

Symptoms

Headache history

Short history
• Recurrent severe headache(s) for a few weeks
Accelerated course
• Increasing frequency
• Worsening usual headache
Headache timing and posture
• Mainly from sleep, i.e. waking the child up
• Mainly or worse when lying down, relieved when upright
• Worse with bending, coughing, etc.

Associated symptoms
• Vomiting from sleep or before getting up
• Confusion, impaired consciousness

• Altered personality, behaviour or mood
• Worsening school performance
• Focal weakness
• Diplopia

Signs
• Visual field defects
• Cranial nerve abnormalities
• Abnormal gait
• Head tilt
• Papilloedema
• Other focal neurological signs
• Growth failure

Many children will have a lifelong tendency 'to take headaches' but, even so, will have long spells with no headaches. They (and their family) must learn to become 'experts in their own headaches'. Recognising triggers such as stress, sleep deprivation, sleep excess, missing meals and hormonal changes via a headache diary can help to give young people some control of their symptoms. Improving sleep patterns, maintaining hydration, eating sensibly and taking regular exercise are also helpful in reducing the frequency of headache. Relaxation exercises may help some children.

Simple painkillers, such as paracetamol or ibuprofen, should be taken as early as possible in an episode with or without an antiemetic (prochlorperazine or domperidone). Triptans are licensed for use in adolescents. Medication overuse headache is becoming an increasing problem, and painkillers should probably not be used on more than 2 days a week. Pizotifen, beta blockers and various anticonvulsants, for example topiramate or valproate, are used for prophylaxis when the headaches become too frequent or intrusive.

Fits, faints and funny turns

There are many childhood disorders that can be confused with 'epilepsy' (Table 33.3). A detailed account of what happened before, during and after the event from both the child and an eyewitness is the key to making a diagnosis. This can be difficult, but children are more likely than adults to bring their eyewitness along with them. The details of the early stages of the event are more likely to be informative than the late stages but least likely to have been observed. Asking the family to video any further events, as well as writing a contemporaneous account of the episode can be helpful. The eyewitness may also be able to mime the event. If you have no history you cannot make a diagnosis. Table 33.4 contains typical histories given for common events that are sometimes misdiagnosed as epileptic seizures.

The two commonest scenarios seen in outpatients are the child who has collapsed and the one who has blank spells.

Parents are usually worried that children who fall to the floor have had a generalised tonic clonic seizure (and therefore have epilepsy) but depending on their age they are more likely to have fainted (if older) or have breath-holding attacks or reflex anoxic seizures (when younger). Children with trances may have an absence epilepsy but are more likely to be daydreaming or engrossed.

Most of these events are benign but may cause considerable concern. Examination between events is rarely informative. Any child who collapses should have an ECG looking for cardiac abnormalities but otherwise investigations are rarely necessary.

The epilepsies

Recently the International League Against Epilepsy (ILAE) has developed a practical definition of epilepsy as a disease of the brain defined by at least two unprovoked seizures occurring more than 24 hours apart or, more controversially, a single seizure with a probability of further seizures of at least 60%. Previously it was defined as a neurological condition characterised by recurrent epileptic seizures unprovoked by any immediately identifiable cause.

It is more appropriate to think of the *epilepsies* as a whole group of conditions or disorders affecting children and young people, rather than a single condition.

Terms such as seizure, convulsion or fit are used in different ways by different people causing confusion and should probably be avoided unless clarified.

The epilepsies affect about 1 in 200 children in the UK and are the commonest chronic neurological condition.

Seizure types

There are many different types of epileptic seizure. Figure 33.1 outlines the latest ILAE classification. They can be divided into three groups: generalised, focal (previously known as partial) and unknown.

Table 33.3 Non-epileptic paroxysmal events by age.		
Infant	**Toddler**	**Older child**
Apnoea	Breath-holding attacks	Syncope
Hyperekplexia	Reflex anoxic seizures	Migraine and variants
Jitteriness	Paroxysmal dyskinesias	Panic attacks
Benign neonatal sleep myoclonus	Benign paroxysmal vertigo	Hyperventilation
Shuddering attacks	Stereotypies	Non-epileptic attack disorder
Sandifer syndrome	Self-gratification	Movement disorders
Self-gratification	Sleep disorders	Episodic ataxias
Cardiac arrhythmias	Cardiac arrhythmias	Tics
Cardiac lesions		Daydreaming
Metabolic disturbance		Parasomnias
		Narcolepsy
		Cardiac arrhythmias

Table 33.4 Typical histories of non-epileptic events.

Event	History
Syncope	A teenage girl feels dizzy, voices seem to come from far away and things go black before she finds herself on the floor. Eyewitnesses say she 'folded' to the ground and looked pale. Some twitching is common. Recovery is rapid
Breath-holding attacks	The child cries, holds his breath, may stiffen as he goes blue then limp. Recovery is swift
Reflex anoxic seizures (pallid syncopal attacks)	Following the trigger (usually minor head trauma) the child goes pale and collapses unconscious to the floor. Occasionally there is some stiffening and jerking before a rapid recovery
Non-epileptic attack disorder (NEAD)	An adolescent girl suddenly develops frequent daily, non-stereotyped episodes of variable length. Side-to-side head movements and asynchronous flailing movements are common. Recovery is rapid
Tics	A primary school age child develops stereotyped rapid repetitive movements, e.g. eye blinking, which are suppressible and compulsive
Daydreaming	The child has short-lived staring episodes where they are unresponsive to people calling them
Benign paroxysmal vertigo	A preschool child suddenly appears pale, unsteady and distressed. Consciousness is preserved in the episodes, which may last up to several hours. Nystagmus may be seen

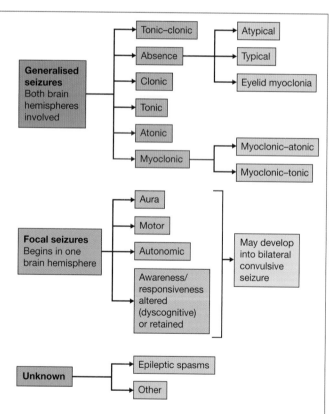

Figure 33.1 The International League Against Epilepsy (ILAE) Seizure Classification. (Source: ILAE Revised Terminology for Organisation of Seizures and Epilepsies 2011–2013.)

Generalised seizures are the result of abnormal activity in both hemispheres of the brain simultaneously; because of this, consciousness is lost at the onset of the seizure. There are many types of generalised seizures, as outlined in Table 33.5.

In focal seizures the abnormal activity starts in one area of the brain and may spread to other regions of the brain or remain localised. What happens in the seizure depends on the area of the brain involved. Awareness may be retained or altered but use of the older classification of simple (with retained awareness) and complex (altered awareness) is discouraged. The activity may spread throughout the brain causing the seizure to become secondary generalised. Examples of symptoms are:

- Sensory – numbness, tingling or burning sensation in a region of the body.
- Motor – jerking of a limb, twitching of the face.
- Autonomic – blushing, pallor, increased heart rate, nausea.
- Psychic – déjà vu, hallucinations (visual, sound, taste or smell), emotions such as fear.

There are epileptic seizures that cannot be diagnosed as either focal or generalised and are thus grouped as unknown, for example epileptic spasms.

Most people will only have one or two seizure types, which vary in frequency and severity. A person with severe epilepsy or significant other neurological disabilities may experience multiple different seizure types.

Epilepsy syndromes

An epilepsy syndrome is a complex of signs and symptoms commonly occurring together that define a distinctive,

Table 33.5 Generalised seizure types.

Tonic-clonic (GTC)	Often begin with a sudden cry, followed by stiffening (the tonic phase) then by jerking of all four limbs (clonic phase). They usually last less than 3 minutes and are followed by drowsiness. If standing, the person will fall to the ground as they lose consciousness. Breathing is irregular causing the lips and complexion to look grey/blue. Saliva (mixed with blood if the tongue has been bitten) may escape from the mouth, and incontinence may occur
Absence	Episodes of unresponsiveness lasting seconds. Eyelid flickering, hand or lip movements may occur. Ask about interruption of activities
Myoclonic	Brief isolated muscle jerks usually involving the upper body but can involve the lower or whole body
Atonic	A sudden, brief loss of muscle tone causing the child to suddenly drop to the floor
Tonic	Stiffening of the muscles of the whole body causes rigidity. Someone standing will fall to the ground, but they also occur in sleep. Recovery is swift, but injuries can occur
Clonic	Rhythmic jerking movements of the arms and legs without a tonic (stiff) phase

recognisable clinical disorder; these include seizure type(s), age of onset, EEG findings and natural history. The diagnosis of a particular epilepsy syndrome is important as it may guide anticonvulsant selection, and predict the outcome and the likelihood of finding an underlying cause and therefore the need for investigation.

Common epilepsy syndromes include childhood absence epilepsy (CAE) and benign epilepsy with centrotemporal spikes (BECTS).

Childhood absence epilepsy (CAE)

Frequent daily absences are the hallmark of this syndrome, which commonly starts between the ages of 5 and 7 years (range 4–12 years) in children who are otherwise neurodevelopmentally normal. Twenty percent of cases will have rare generalised tonic-clonic seizures as well. Hyperventilation can induce episodes in outpatients, and the EEG invariably shows 3-Hz generalised spike-and-wave discharges. Imaging is not necessary. Ninety percent of children are controlled with medication (usually valproate or ethosuximide) and are successfully withdrawn after two years of seizure freedom.

Benign epilepsy with centrotemporal spikes (BECTS)

This is the most common focal epilepsy of childhood (approximately 15% of all childhood epilepsies), characterised by infrequent seizures and an EEG showing frequent unilateral or bilateral diphasic sharp waves in the rolandic or centrotemporal area (hence the previous name 'benign rolandic epilepsy of childhood'). A sensory aura of paraesthesia or numbness of the tongue, lips, gums or cheek is followed by unilateral twitching of one side of the face. Consciousness is preserved but the child is unable to speak. Secondary generalisation may occur. The episodes commonly occur at night or on awakening. The seizures will cease by puberty and are often not treated with anticonvulsants. If the seizures are frequent or

cause significant distress carbamazepine is the first-choice anticonvulsant. Imaging is not needed.

Causes of epilepsy

The causes of epilepsy used to be divided into three – idiopathic (unknown), symptomatic (secondary to a known or presumed disorder of the brain) and presumed symptomatic, but the terms genetic, structural-metabolic and unknown are now recommended recognising the advances that have been made in identifying individual causes of epilepsy. Even so, no detectable underlying structural brain pathology is found in the majority of children with epilepsy, even after extensive investigation. It is thought that up to one-third of cases have a genetic basis.

Diagnosis of epilepsy

Epilepsy is a clinical diagnosis based on a detailed history from both the patient and the eyewitness. Replaying the event back to the witness is a good way of making sure you have an accurate account.

The diagnosis can be difficult as getting the history is not always easy, the events are rarely witnessed by professionals and there is no definitive diagnostic test. Investigations can even be misleading – funny events and an abnormal EEG do not equal epilepsy.

If there is any doubt do not diagnose epilepsy but watch and wait, and ask for video recordings. Retaking the history after further events often yields more information. Time is much more likely to clarify the diagnosis than performing lots of investigations.

Remember that the episodes not only have to be recurrent but also unprovoked (although there are reflex epilepsies where flashing lights, e.g., provoke seizures).

The misdiagnosis rate of epilepsy is up to 30%. The commonest reasons for this are failure to take an accurate history, failure to think of possible differential diagnoses and undue reliance on the EEG.

The examination is invariably normal but neurological signs may indicate an underlying pathology. Looking for the skin stigmata of the neurocutaneous syndromes (especially neurofibromatosis and tuberous sclerosis) is important.

An attempt should be made to identify the seizure type and epilepsy syndrome if possible.

Investigation of seizures

The history and examination will determine the need for further investigations. Only one in three children who have a generalised tonic-clonic (GTC) seizure will have a further GTC, and no further investigation is needed apart from an ECG.

Electroencephalogram (EEG)

Unless an episode is actually captured during the recording an EEG will not diagnose epilepsy but it may support the diagnosis or allow definition of the seizure type or syndrome. Many children with epilepsy (~50%) have a normal initial EEG, and some without epilepsy may have frankly epileptic features on their EEG (~5%). A sleep-deprived EEG may be helpful by bringing out abnormalities. Other techniques include 24-hour ambulatory EEG or videotelemetry.

Imaging

Imaging is not routinely needed. Guidance from the UK's National Institute for Health and Care Excellence (NICE) suggests that imaging should be considered in those:

- who develop epilepsy before the age of 2 years;
- who have any suggestion of a focal onset on history, examination or EEG (unless there is clear evidence of benign focal epilepsy);
- whose seizures continue in spite of first-line medication.

Neuroimaging should not be routinely requested when a diagnosis of an idiopathic generalised epilepsy has been made.

MRI is the preferred modality but in the acute situation CT is often more easily obtainable. Functional scanning techniques such as PET (positron emission tomography) and SPECT (single-photon emission computed tomography) are used to detect areas of abnormal metabolism suggestive of a seizure focus, usually as part of the work-up for epilepsy surgery.

Management

The aims of management are to stop the seizures whilst minimising the side effects of any drugs used, and to allow the child to lead a normal life. The psychosocial consequences of epilepsy can have more of an impact on the child's life than the seizure disorder itself.

Management is more than drug treatment. Specialist epilepsy nurses provide valuable education and support for families. Overprotection is understandable but unhelpful. There are few things that children with epilepsy cannot do but some activities will need more supervision, for example swimming. Adolescents need specific advice about driving, contraception, pregnancy and alcohol use. Lifestyle advice is important in certain syndromes; for example, teenagers with an idiopathic generalised epilepsy should try to avoid sleep deprivation. SUDEP (sudden unexpected death in epilepsy) is exceptionally rare in children but is associated with unwitnessed GTCs, especially those occurring at night.

Most children with epilepsy go to mainstream school although they do worse academically than would be predicted from their IQ. Schools need advice and support to ensure that the children participate fully in school life and achieve their full potential.

Not all children with epilepsy require drug treatment. Whether or not drug treatment is needed depends on the type, frequency and impact of the epileptic seizures. Defining the seizure type and epilepsy syndrome (if possible) often helps in deciding whether drug treatment is needed and which one to use. Monotherapy is best; starting on a low dose and building it up slowly tends to maximise compliance. The first-line treatment for generalised seizures is sodium valproate, with carbamazepine or lamotrigine used for focal seizures. About 60% of children become seizure free on the first drug; if this does not work the chances of the second drug being successful are only around 10%. Delay in starting treatment does not seem to have any adverse long-term consequences for the epilepsy. Anticonvulsant levels are not routinely needed, and are mostly used to assess compliance.

The parents of children who have had a GTC lasting longer than 5 minutes are often shown how to use buccal midazolam to stop the seizure at home. Parents also need to know the emergency treatment for their child's seizures and when to bring the child to hospital (rarely necessary).

A small number of children may be suitable for surgical treatment or respond to the ketogenic diet.

Prognosis

Many children 'grow out' of their epilepsy. Slow withdrawal of anticonvulsants is usually recommended if the child has been seizure free for 2 years.

Febrile convulsions

A febrile seizure is a seizure associated with a fever in the absence of an intracranial infection. These occur in 3% of children between the ages of 6 months and 6 years. It is the rate of rise of temperature that provokes the seizure in susceptible individuals. Most are brief generalised tonic-clonic seizures, that is simple febrile convulsions, but about 25% are complex, that is focal, prolonged (>15 min) or repeated in the same illness. Fifteen percent will have a parent who has had febrile convulsions.

About one in three children will have a further febrile seizure. If this was longer than 5 minutes buccal midazolam is prescribed for the parents to give at home if needed. Anticonvulsant prophylaxis has not been shown to significantly reduce the recurrence rate of febrile seizures or the subsequent development of epilepsy. An EEG is not necessary.

Children who have had febrile convulsions have a 1% risk of having established epilepsy at the age of 7 years – double that of other 7-year-olds who have not had febrile convulsions.

Cerebral palsy

Cerebral palsy (CP) is the most common cause of motor impairment in children, affecting about 2/1000 live births in developed countries. It describes a wide spectrum of motor problems, ranging from the child with minimal problems down one side that interfere with playing sports, to the child who is totally dependent on others for all their care needs with no voluntary movement or speech. The definition given (see Key facts 33.1) draws attention to the fact that these children often have additional problems. These additional difficulties (Table 33.6 may have a greater effect on the quality of life of the child and their family than the motor impairment itself.

It is important to recognise that although the underlying lesion does not change, the motor disorder evolves over time. The term is only used for insults occurring before the age of 2 years and does not apply to children with neurodegenerative diseases even if the clinical picture is the same.

Causation

There are very few known causes of cerebral palsy (CP) but there are many known risk factors associated with the development of CP (Table 33.7). Many children have more than one risk factor for CP and it is useful to consider causal pathways rather than single events.

Neuroimaging, in particular MRI, has helped clarify issues of cause and timing, shifting the debate away from

Table 33.6 Associated comorbidities of cerebral palsy.

Neurological	Epilepsy
	Hydrocephalus
	Cortical visual impairment
	Refractive errors and squint
	Hearing impairment
Behaviour and learning	Learning disability
	Specific learning difficulties
	Autistic spectrum disorders
	Communication difficulties
	Behavioural difficulties
	Sleep disturbance
	Depression
Gastrointestinal	Swallowing difficulties
	Reflux
	Constipation
	Drooling
Respiratory	Chest infections
	Aspiration
Skeletal	Osteoporosis
	Fractures
	Scoliosis
	Joint subluxation/dislocation
	Contractures
Skin	Pressure sores
	Poor healing
Dental	Caries

intrapartum events (particularly birth asphyxia), to an examination of prenatal factors.

Despite improvements in antenatal and perinatal care there has been little change in the overall numbers of children developing cerebral palsy in the last 40 years, although more extremely preterm children are surviving with more severe forms of cerebral palsy.

More recent classifications of CP emphasise the functional impact as well as the associated abnormalities; for example, the Gross Motor Function Classification System (GMFCS) is a functional classification in common use (Figure 33.2).

Clinical presentation

Cerebral palsy can present in a variety of ways (Box 33.2). The diagnosis is a clinical one, usually made at the end of the first year of life or later.

Children with a unilateral spastic cerebral palsy, that is hemiplegia, may present with an early hand preference, delayed walking or toe walking. Children with a bilateral spastic CP also present in a variety of ways. The most severely affected children (often said to have a spastic quadriplegia) may present with irritability, seizures and feeding difficulties before the severity of the motor difficulties is apparent. More mildly affected children (previously said to

> **① Key facts 33.1 Definition of cerebral palsy**
>
> Cerebral palsy describes a group of disorders of the development of movement and posture, causing activity limitation, that are attributed to non-progressive disturbances that occurred in the developing foetal or infant brain.
>
> The motor disorders of cerebral palsy are often accompanied by disturbances of sensation, cognition, communication, perception, and/or behaviour, and/or by a seizure disorder.
> Executive Committee for the Definition of Cerebral Palsy (2005)

Table 33.7 Risk factors associated with the development of cerebral palsy.

Prenatal (>80%)	Perinatal (~10%)	Postnatal (~5%)
Prematurity	Amnionitis	Meningitis
Multiple pregnancy	Antepartum haemorrhage	Traumatic head injury, including NAI
Small for gestational age	Neonatal meningitis	Hypoxic ischaemic events, e.g. near drowning
Placental insufficiency	Kernicterus	
Maternal infections	Hypoxic ischaemic	
Intrauterine infections, e.g. CMV	encephalopathy	
Cerebral malformations		

CMV, cytomegalovirus; NAI, non-accidental injury.

⬤	**Level I -**	Walks without limitations.
⬤	**Level II -**	Walks with limitations.
⬤	**Level III -**	Walks using a hand-held mobility device.
⬤	**Level IV -**	Self-mobility with limitations; may use powered mobility.
⬤	**Level V -**	Transported in a manual wheelchair

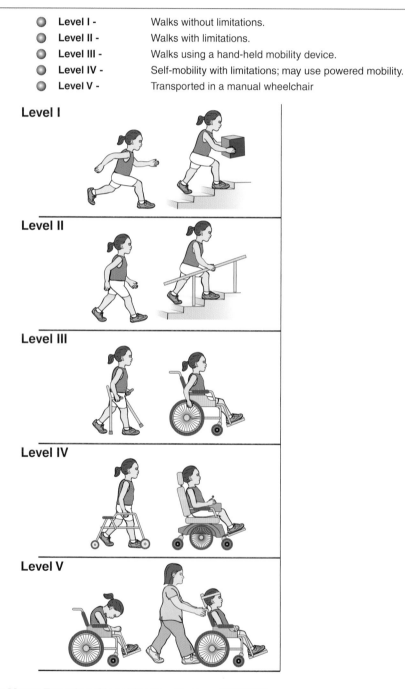

Figure 33.2 Gross Motor Function Classification System (GMFCS).

Box 33.2 Clinical presentations of cerebral palsy

- Delayed motor milestones
- Abnormal gait
- Early hand dominance (<12months)
- Reduced movements including sucking and feeding
- Persistence of primitive reflexes
- Other abnormalities of tone or posture
- Feeding difficulties
- Irritability
- Routine surveillance of at risk groups, e.g. severely asphyxiated infants, VLBW infants

have a spastic diplegia) may present with toe walking or an abnormal gait.

The clinical picture depends on the area of the brain involved. Damage to the upper motor neurone pathway causes spasticity, whereas damage to the cerebellum or its pathways causes ataxia; dyskinetic CP is a result of lesions to the basal ganglia or extrapyramidal pathways, for example in kernicterus.

Investigation

MRI is recommended in almost all cases of CP. Other investigation, if necessary, is usually determined by the findings on imaging. A normal MRI scan should prompt re-evaluation of the diagnosis as well as further investigation, although about 16% of children with agreed CP have normal imaging (Figure 33.3).

Management

There is no cure for cerebral palsy but there is much that can be done to improve the quality of life of the child and family. This needs a multidisciplinary team collaborating closely with the parents. The aims of management are to improve function in everyday life and increase participation and independence.

Medical management often centres on the reduction of muscle tone and the identification and management of comorbidities.

Outlook

Children who can sit independently before the age of 2 years and those who can crawl reciprocally before 30 months of age will achieve walking either independently or with aids. Almost all children with hemiplegia will walk independently compared with about 60% of children with other subtypes of CP.

Survival has increased and even the most profoundly handicapped children have a 50% chance of surviving to adult life. This is mostly due to improved nutrition and better management of chest infections.

Neuromuscular diseases in children

These comprise diseases of the muscle, anterior horn cell, peripheral nerve or neuromuscular junction (Table 33.8). Most neuromuscular disorders in children are individually rare. Although the identification of specific gene abnormalities in many muscle or nerve diseases has made diagnosis much easier, the history and examination still provide useful clues to direct investigations.

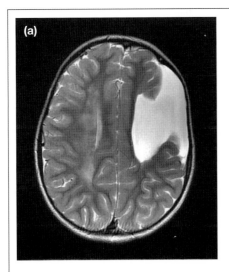
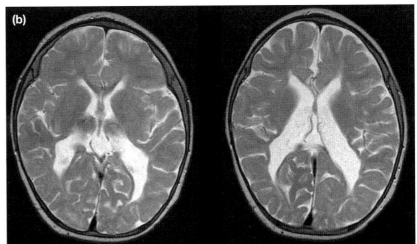

Figure 33.3 (a) MRI of child with unilateral spastic cerebral palsy (CP) showing a porencephalic cyst. (b) MRI of infant born prematurely with a spastic diplegia showing periventricular leucomalacia.

Table 33.8 Neuromuscular disorders classified according to anatomical site.

Anatomical site	Disorder
Anterior horn cell (AHC)	Spinal muscular atrophy Poliomyelitis
Peripheral nerve	Hereditary motor sensory neuropathy (type 1A = Charcot–Marie–Tooth disease)ç Guillain–Barré syndrome (acute post-infectious polyneuropathy)
Neuromuscular junction	Myasthenia gravis
Muscle	Muscular dystrophy • Duchenne • Becker • Congenital Congenital myopathies Myotonic disorders Metabolic myopathies Inflammatory myopathies • Dermatomyositis

Box 33.3 Symptoms of neuromuscular disease

- Floppiness in infancy
- Abnormal gait:
  - Waddling
  - Toe walking
  - High stepping
- Easy fatiguability
- Frequent falls
- Slow motor development
- Muscle cramps or stiffness
- Specific disability:
  - Elevating arms
  - Climbing stairs
  - Gripping objects
  - Rising from floor

Clinical features

The common presenting symptoms of neuromuscular disorders are given in Box 33.3. Many children with neuromuscular diseases are unable to walk as far as other children, cannot run as fast (if at all), fall over more than their peers, and struggle to get up and down stairs. They may also have chewing or swallowing difficulties, and respiratory problems.

Some key features of the history and examination are given in Table 33.9.

Gower's manoeuvre is used to pick up a proximal muscle weakness. Normal children over the age of 3 years can get straight up off the floor from lying supine. Children with a proximal lower limb weakness need to turn over onto their front first. As the weakness becomes more extreme they need to climb up their legs with their hands to stand up (Figure 33.4).

Investigations

Dystrophic muscles 'leak' creatine kinase (CK) so this is an important first test in the investigation of a child with suspected muscle disease; but it may be normal in other neuromuscular problems. Ultrasound and MRI of the muscles are increasingly used to identify the pattern of muscle involvement and to guide where the muscle biopsy would be best taken from. Increasingly, targeted genetic testing looking at the gene(s) specifically associated with the disease suggested by the clinical picture bypasses the need for muscle biopsy. Electromyography (EMG) can help in distinguishing myopathic from neuropathic conditions but is not well tolerated by children.

In the past nerve conduction studies (NCVs) were the only way of confirming the clinical suspicion of a neuropathy but most children are now diagnosed following genetic testing. Nerve biopsy is rarely needed.

Muscle disorders

Muscle disorders are divided up as shown in Table 33.8.

The muscular dystrophies

This group of disorders is associated with progressive muscle degeneration and therefore progressive weakness. The two most commonly seen in childhood are described below.

Duchenne muscular dystrophy (DMD)

This X-linked condition affects 1 in 3500 newborn boys, although about one in three cases are due to a new mutation in the dystrophin gene.

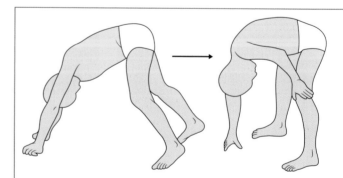

Figure 33.4 Gower's manoeuvre. (Source: H. Willmott (2015) *Trauma and Orthopaedics at a Glance*, 1st edn. Reproduced with permission of John Wiley & Sons, Ltd.)

Boys usually present with a waddling gait at about the age of 5 years. Some are identified because of their learning disability (this occurs in about 30% of boys) or even because of the serendipitous finding of an elevated alanine transaminase (ALT). Fifty percent will not be walking by 18 months and this offers an opportunity for earlier detection.

On examination the boys have calf (and occasionally deltoid) hypertrophy and usually cannot run, squat, hop or get off the floor without turning over. By definition, boys with Duchenne will have lost ambulation by their 13th birthday but with the use of steroids some boys are still walking, albeit with difficulty, into their mid-teens.

These boys have an elevated CK (at least 10 times normal), and dystrophin gene analysis usually confirms the diagnosis without the need for muscle biopsy.

Management

There is no cure for DMD but life expectancy has increased dramatically. Multidisciplinary management, surgery for scoliosis and the use of nocturnal non-invasive ventilation means these boys may live into their late 20s or early 30s. Steroid use and treatment of the associated cardiomyopathy is likely to increase the numbers surviving well into adulthood.

Becker muscular dystrophy

The in-frame abnormality in their dystrophin gene means these boys produce some functional dystrophin and are less severely affected than boys with DMD. They usually present with toe walking and an elevated CK. Muscle pain is a particular problem in teenagers. They remain ambulant well into adult life when they can develop cardiac problems.

Congenital muscular dystrophy

Increasing numbers of gene abnormalities have expanded the phenotype of this heterogeneous group of abnormalities that present with weakness and hypotonia at birth associated with an elevated CK. Many of them have associated brain and eye abnormalities.

Congenital myopathies

These static, or only slowly progressive, muscle diseases present in the early years with varying degrees of muscle weakness. They were initially characterised by the appearances seen in the muscle biopsy (hence central core disease, minicore disease, nemaline rod and centronuclear myopathy) but increasingly they are defined by the genetic abnormality found. CK is often normal or only minimally elevated.

Metabolic myopathies

Energy-depleting enzyme deficiencies or deposition of storage material cause dysfunction in the metabolic myopathies.

They commonly present in older children with exercise-related muscle cramps, myoglobinuria or as a floppy infant. Glycogen storage disorders, disorders of lipid metabolism or mitochondrial disorders are included in this group.

Inflammatory myopathies

Benign acute myositis

This is thought to be a self-limiting post-infectious phenomenon. Pain and symmetrical weakness follow an upper respiratory tract infection. CK is elevated and myoglobinuria may occur.

Dermatomyositis

This systemic illness presents insidiously in the primary school years with fever and misery. The symmetrical proximal weakness usually comes later. A heliotrope rash on the eyelids (and occasionally the extensor surfaces) with periorbital oedema is characteristic. CK and the inflammatory markers are usually raised, and muscle biopsy shows inflammatory changes and fibre necrosis. Initial immunosuppression is with steroids.

Myotonic disorders

Myotonia is slowed relaxation following muscle contraction. Patients do not complain of it, even when it is obvious clinically. When myotonia is present the child is unable to let go of your fingers quickly having gripped them firmly, and percussing the thenar eminence causes the thumb to abduct and then relax slowly. Percussion may also leave a depression in the muscle.

Myotonic dystrophy (DM1)

This is a multisystem disorder caused by a triplet repeat expansion in the *DMPK* gene on chromosome 19. Increased size of the expansion is associated with an earlier age of onset and more severe clinical phenotype.

It is a cause of hypotonia in neonates (and the reason for always examining the mother of a floppy infant). They may also have respiratory difficulties, poor feeding and joint deformities. Children can present with muscle cramps and a myopathic face but more commonly are diagnosed because they have an affected family member. Adults develop early cataracts, with men developing testicular atrophy and premature baldness. Women may only be picked up following the birth of an affected child. Cardiac conduction abnormalities are common in adults. Diagnosis is made genetically.

The floppy infant

Floppiness, or hypotonia, is diminished resistance to passive movement around a joint. The floppy infant tends to slip through your fingers when picked up or hang like a rag doll when held prone. When pulled to 'sit' there will be marked head lag.

It is an indication of low muscle tone and not a measure of strength, and is due to a variety of lesions of the central or peripheral nervous system (Tables 33.9 and 33.10). Other features of the examination are helpful in localising the cause. Determining whether the child is weak as well as hypotonic is crucial, but difficult. Weakness suggests a peripheral, neuromuscular cause. Central causes are by far the most common and are suggested by dysmorphic features, the presence of abnormalities in other organs and other signs of brain dysfunction.

Neural tube defects and hydrocephalus

Neural tube defects (NTDs) result from the failure of the neural plate to close (see Chapter 7). The birth prevalence has fallen dramatically in the UK for unknown natural reasons (possibly related to improved maternal nutrition) helped by antenatal screening.

Hydrocephalus

Hydrocephalus results from an imbalance between the intracranial cerebrospinal fluid (CSF) inflow and outflow. It is caused by obstruction of CSF circulation, by inadequate absorption of CSF, or (rarely) by overproduction of CSF. Regardless of the cause, the excessive volume of CSF causes increased ventricular pressure and leads to ventricular dilatation. In infants their head circumference may show an excessive rate of growth and cross lines on the centile chart as the skull sutures separate. A bulging fontanelle and prominent scalp veins may accompany irritability, lethargy and vomiting. Pressure on the tectal plate causes a downward fixed gaze or sun setting eyes (Figure 33.5). Older children present with the symptoms and signs of raised pressure.

Table 33.10 Causes of hypotonia in infancy.

Central	Peripheral
Cortical • HIE • Cortical malformations	Anterior horn cell • SMA
Genetic • Down syndrome • Prader–Willi syndrome	Peripheral nerve • Congenital neuropathy (rare)
Metabolic • Peroxisomal disorders • Acid maltase deficiency • Hypothyroidism • Hypocalcaemia	Neuromuscular junction • Congenital myasthenia • Botulism
Spinal cord injury	Muscle • Congenital myotonic dystrophy • Congenital myopathy • Metabolic myopathies

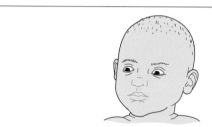

Figure 33.5. Infant with sun setting eyes.

Hydrocephalus is associated with open, not closed, dysraphic states.

The most common mechanism is anatomical or functional obstruction to CSF flow (known as obstructive or non-communicating hydrocephalus). The obstruction occurs at the

Table 33.9 Diagnostic pointers for neuromuscular disorders.

Disease	History	Examination
Anterior horn cell	Weakness	Signs of denervation: • Wasting • Fasciculation • Loss of reflexes • Weakness
Neuropathy	Heavy gait Unusually shaped feet	Clawed feet Tight Achilles tendons Distal weakness and wasting Absent reflexes
Neuromuscular junction	Fatiguability Swallowing difficulties	Ptosis Opthalmoplegia
Myopathy	Waddling gait	Weakness (often proximal)

foramen of Monro, the aqueduct, or the fourth ventricle and its outlets. Less commonly, hydrocephalus is caused by impaired absorption of CSF by the subarachnoid granulations, for example secondary to meningitis (communicating hydrocephalus). Cranial ultrasound, CT or MRI will show dilated ventricles. Treatment is with either the insertion of a ventriculoperitoneal shunt or a third ventriculostomy.

Clinical case

Case conclusion

She has migraine. No imaging was necessary even to reassure the parents that she didn't have a brain tumour.

As is common in teenagers she was going to sleep too late and couldn't get up in the morning so missed breakfast. Rectifying these and encouraging her to drink more significantly reduced the frequency of the events and she learned how to manage each individual episode with simple painkillers taken as early as possible, and sleep. Improving her lifestyle also made it less likely that she would faint.

Key learning points

- Headache is common in children.
- The diagnosis of epilepsy rests in a good eyewitness history not on investigations.
- Most cerebral palsy is prenatally determined.
- Multidisciplinary management is of paramount importance for children with disabilities and their families.

 Now visit **www.wileyessential.com/humandevelopment** to test yourself on this chapter.

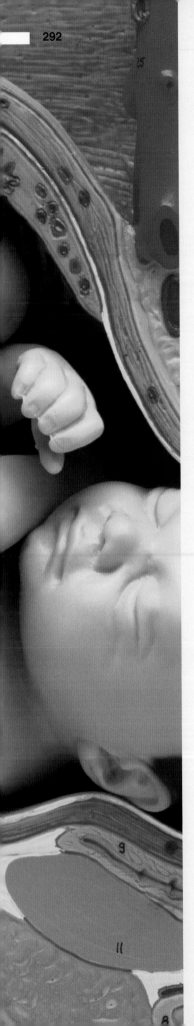

CHAPTER 34
Infections and immunodeficiency

Pramodh Vallabhaneni

Infection in children is a very common cause of illness, and as a group it is the commonest reason for admission to hospital in childhood. The pattern of infection varies across the world, depending on how developed the country is and other factors. This chapter gives you an overview of common infections in children. Please see Chapter 25 for infections in the perinatal period, Chapter 36 for infections affecting the cardiovascular system, Chapter 38 for respiratory infections and Chapter 39 for gastrointestinal infections.

Case

Sarah is a 2-year-old girl who presented with being generally unwell and having a high temperature. She had attended a birthday party 2 weeks previously, and it later transpired that a child who had attended the same party was unwell and had a rash. Her parents described an itchy rash that had appeared on her head and trunk.

On examination she looked miserable and flushed. There was a rash over her whole body but fewer lesions on her limbs than on her trunk and scalp. The rash consisted mainly of small 1–2 mm diameter vesicles. Other lesions were papules, which had a crusty appearance.

Learning outcomes

- You should be able to recognise rashes resulting from common infections in childhood.
- You should be able to recognise signs of serious infection in children.
- You should be able to describe empirical treatment of common infections in childhood.

Essential Human Development, First Edition. Edited by Samuel Webster, Geraint Morris and Euan Kevelighan
© 2018 John Wiley & Sons, Ltd. Published 2018 by John Wiley & Sons, Ltd.

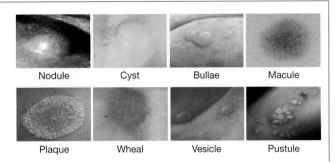

Figure 34.1 **Primary skin lesions resulting from infection.**

Nodule, Cyst, Bullae, Macule, Plaque, Wheal, Vesicle, Pustule

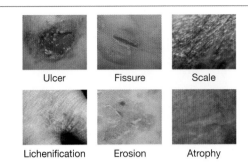

Figure 34.2 **Secondary skin lesions (not all of these lesions always result from infection).**

Ulcer, Fissure, Scale, Lichenification, Erosion, Atrophy

Table 34.1 Incubation period of common infections.	
Measles	10–14 days
Mumps	14–21 days
Rubella	14–21 days
Chickenpox	10–23 days
Enterovirus	3–5 days
Hand, foot and mouth	4–6 days
Scarlet fever	2–4 days

Paediatric rashes are common and can vary from simple viral rashes to serious bacterial infections (Figures 34.1 and 34.2). See also Chapter 41 (Dermatology) for an explanation of how to describe skin lesions.

The incubation period of an infection is the time elapsed between exposure to the infective agent and the appearance of the first symptoms or signs. This varies depending on the organism concerned, but also varies between individuals (Table 34.1).

Measles

Measles is an illness caused by a paramyxovirus and is spread by contact with respiratory secretions from an infected contact. It is highly contagious. It is characterised by high-grade fever, which peaks about day 4–5 after onset of coryzal (cold-like) symptoms, including cough, runny nose and conjunctivitis. The rash is a generalised maculopapular, erythematous rash that begins several days after the fever starts. It starts on the back of the ears and, after a few hours, spreads to the head and neck before spreading to cover most of the body. In the mouth, characteristic lesions are seen – Koplik spots, which resemble tiny grains of white sand surrounded by redness, usually seen on mucosa of the mouth opposite the first and second upper molar teeth.

Measles is generally self-limiting; however, it can be a severe illness and children affected are usually irritable and appear ill. It has a number of unusual, but well-described and serious complications, including secondary infection of the respiratory tract, manifesting as pneumonia, otitis media or tracheitis. Neurological sequelae include febrile convulsions and encephalitis. A rare but devastating complication is sub-acute sclerosing panencephalitis – a progressive encephalitis that causes neurological deterioration and eventually death in a matter of a few years.

Treatment

There is currently no treatment for measles, and supportive measures are taken, which may include analgesia and antipyretic treatment. Treatment of the complications such as pneumonia will require antibiotics.

Prevention

A measles/mumps/rubella (MMR) vaccine is currently given at 12–18 months of age followed by a booster dose at preschool age. The uptake for MMR vaccine has been relatively low since concerns were raised by the publication in 1998 of a paper linking MMR to autism. The paper caused a great deal of anxiety, which has diminished the uptake of the vaccine even many years later. The paper was subsequently discredited completely. The uptake has improved but there have been several outbreaks of measles in recent years.

Mumps

Mumps is a contagious illness spread by the mumps virus in respiratory droplets. It is characterised by swelling of one or both parotid glands (parotitis) (Figure 34.3), accompanied by fever, malaise and headache. Complications include viral meningitis and/or encephalitis, pancreatitis and orchitis (inflammation of the testicles) or oophoritis (inflammation of the ovaries). Orchitis may be associated with subsequent reduced fertility. The MMR vaccine is effective in providing immunity to the mumps virus.

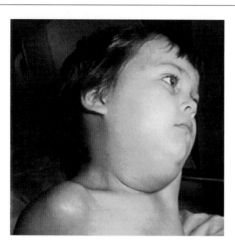

Figure 34.3 Swelling of the parotid gland. (Source: U.S. Centers for Disease Control and Prevention. Photo Credit: CDC/NIP/Barbara Rice.)

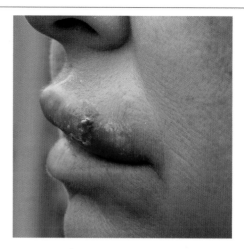

Figure 34.4 Cold sores. (Source: Ben Tillman, https://commons.wikimedia.org/wiki/File:Cold_sore.jpg. CC0-1.0 public domain)

Human herpes virus

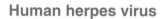

About eight herpes viruses are known. They have a characteristic tendency to become latent (to lie dormant in the body without causing any symptoms) and to reactivate (or proliferate) at a later stage. They are:

- Herpes simplex virus 1 and 2.
- Varicella zoster virus.
- Cytomegalovirus.
- Epstein–Barr virus.
- Human herpes viruses 6, 7 and 8.

Herpes simplex virus (HSV) usually enters via the mucous membranes or skin. The incubation period is usually 3–5 days. HSV1 is transmitted via body fluids especially saliva. HSV2 is transmitted through the transfer of genital secretions.

Gingivostomatitis

This is the most common form of primary HSV illness in children. It occurs in children between the ages of 1 and 3 years. Vesicular lesions appear on the lips, gums and the anterior surfaces of the tongue and palate. There may be a high fever and the children appear miserable. During the illness, food and fluids may feel painful in the mouth and oral intake may therefore reduce. Symptomatic management is usually indicated, with topical analgesia, antipyretics and encouragement to drink fluids.

Cold sores are recurrent HSV1 lesions on the lip margin (Figure 34.4). HSV may infect areas of skin affected by eczema (see Chapter 41).

Eye disease

Infection of the conjunctivae or eyelids may lead to ulceration of the cornea. Children with herpetic lesions around the eye will need ophthalmic review and may need treatment with topical antiviral agents (aciclovir or ganciclovir) and topical steroids.

Encephalitis

This is a rare but serious condition with high mortality if untreated. It is a severe viral infection of the central nervous system. It is usually caused by HSV1 and rarely by HSV 2, and is thought to result from the reactivation of the dormant virus. The presence of cold sores does not help in the diagnosis though it may draw the attention of the clinician to the possibility of encephalitis if there are neurological symptoms and/or signs. It is characterised by a wide spectrum of presentations including a flu-like illness with headache and fever followed by seizures, cognitive impairment, reduced consciousness, behavioural changes, and focal neurological signs such as limb weakness.

A definitive diagnosis can be made by demonstrating the presence of the virus in the cerebrospinal fluid (CSF) from a lumbar puncture. An MRI scan may show characteristic abnormalities, typically in the temporal lobes of the brain.

A high index of suspicion is required to treat encephalitis early and effectively – treatment is with high-dose intravenous aciclovir. Treatment can be commenced whilst waiting for definitive confirmation of the presence of the virus within the CSF.

Varicella zoster (chickenpox)

Chickenpox is an extremely common and highly contagious illness caused by the varicella zoster virus. It is characterised by pyrexia and a typical rash – a generalised vesicular rash appearing in crops for 3–5 days (Figure 34.5), usually on the

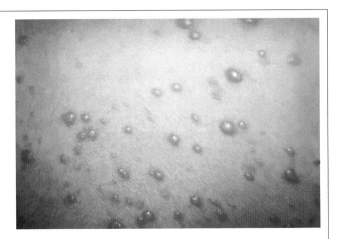

Figure 34.5 Characteristic chickenpox lesions.
(Source: U.S. Centers for Disease Control and Prevention. Photo Credit: Joe Miller.)

trunk and scalp with reducing density on the limbs. The vesicles go through phases starting as red papules, which then turn into vesicles filled with clear fluid. They then develop a more pustular appearance before finally crusting over. The lesions are typically very itchy.

Complications include secondary bacterial infections of the skin with staphylococci or streptococci, which may then lead to toxic shock syndrome or necrotising fasciitis. Central nervous system complications include cerebellitis, encephalitis and aseptic meningitis. The virus may also cause pneumonitis and secondary bacterial infection of the respiratory tract.

Treatment is symptomatic in healthy individuals; but the immunocompromised may become severely ill. In these cases systemic treatment with aciclovir or intravenous human varicella zoster immunoglobulin (ZIG) may be warranted (see also Chapter 25 for treatment of chickenpox in the perinatal period).

Vaccination for chickenpox is part of the routine immunisation schedule for some countries, and in others it is offered only to immunocompromised people or their relatives or carers.

Epstein–Barr virus (EBV)

EBV is the major cause of infectious mononucleosis syndrome; it is also implicated in the development of Burkitt's lymphoma, lymphoproliferative disease in immunocompromised hosts and nasopharyngeal carcinoma.

Infectious mononucleosis (glandular fever) is an unpleasant illness in children and presents with pyrexia, weakness, tonsillitis, pharyngitis and lymphadenopathy – mainly cervical but other lymph nodes may be involved as well. Other features include soft palate petechiae, splenomegaly, hepatomegaly, a rash and jaundice.

Typically there may be atypical lymphocytes seen on a blood film, and the monospot test (a rapid serological test for antibodies produced in response to EBV infection) is usually positive. Further serological tests may be useful in cases of doubt to demonstrate the production of IgM and IgG to EBV antigens.

Treatment is usually symptomatic. Ampicillin or amoxicillin may cause a florid maculopapular rash in children infected with EBV and should be avoided.

Parvovirus B19

This is a common viral infection in children and causes an illness characterised by intense redness of the cheeks – this has several names including erythema infectiosum, fifth disease or slapped cheek syndrome.

Symptoms include malaise, headache and myalgia followed by an erythematous rash on the face, which progresses to a maculopapular, lace-like rash on the trunk and limbs.

The parvovirus may cause a mild anaemia in healthy children, but in the fetus (following maternal infection – see Chapter 25) and in children who have chronic haemolytic anaemias, for example sickle cell disease or thalassaemia, it may cause a severe aplastic anaemia (aplastic crisis).

Meningitis and meningococcal septicaemia

Meningitis is usually a serious illness that results from inflammation of the meninges – the membranes that surround the brain and spinal cord. It usually results from infection of the meninges by microorganisms, including bacteria, viruses, fungi and parasites. The commonest organisms causing meningitis at various ages are shown in Table 34.2.

Presenting features in childhood include fever, headache, photophobia, nausea and vomiting. Other symptoms, particularly in younger infants and babies, include lethargy, poor feeding, irritability, hypotonia, drowsiness, loss of consciousness and seizures. In meningococcal disease, a typical non-blanching purpuric rash is also seen, which is due to

Table 34.2 Commonest causal organisms for meningitis at different age ranges.

Age range	Causal organisms
Newborn to 3 months	Group B streptococcus *E. coli* *Listeria monocytogenes*
1 month to 6 years	*Neisseria meningitidis* *Streptococcus pneumoniae* *Haemophilus influenzae*
>6 years	*Neisseria meningitidis* *Streptococcus pneumoniae*

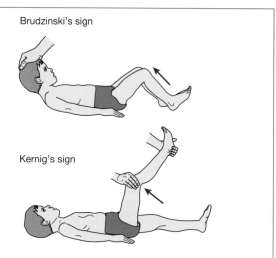

Figure 34.6 Brudzinski's sign and Kernig's sign.

vasculitis of the small vessels of the skin secondary to bacterial invasion of the vessel walls.

These children almost always look seriously ill, though in the early stages of the illness children may be surprisingly alert. Examine carefully for purpura (in meningococcal disease), fever, neck stiffness, signs of shock, focal neurological signs, altered consciousness level and papilloedema. There is a positive Brudzinski sign/Kernig sign (Figure 34.6). Brudinski's sign involves flexing the neck and is positive when the knees are involuntarily flexed. Kernig's sign is positive if, when the knee and hip are flexed to 90° and the knee then extended, the patient resists this movement and finds it painful.

Blood investigations may show raised inflammatory markers (high C-reactive protein, high white blood cell count), and characteristic CSF changes are seen depending on the infecting organism (Table 34.3). A lumbar puncture is diagnostic in the presence of typical abnormalities and bacterial growth on culture. In the presence of signs of raised intracranial pressure, lumbar puncture should be avoided, due to the possibility of sudden decompression of the spinal canal, which may then precipitate herniation of the brainstem into the foramen magnum.

In the presence of typical features of meningococcal septicaemia, many clinicians will not perform a lumber puncture as the treatment is the same whether there is meningitis present or not.

Management of bacterial meningitis and/or septicaemia requires prompt administration of intravenous antibiotics with supportive therapy, which may include fluid resuscitation to maintain the circulating volume, inotropic therapy, analgesia, intubation and admission to an intensive care unit. Careful monitoring is required as the disease may involve many organ systems. Renal failure due to underperfusion of the kidneys and subsequent tubular injury may require dialysis.

Without treatment, bacterial meningitis has a mortality of close to 100%, but with prompt and rigorous treatment, most cases of bacterial meningitis will do well; however. the mortality of bacterial meningitis still ranges from 2 to 20%. A low index of suspicion is therefore required, with early investigation and treatment.

Complications of meningitis include hearing loss, subdural effusion and localised brain injury. If meningococcal septicaemia results in significant vasculitis and ischaemia, then organ damage and loss of limbs may result.

Prevention

Effective vaccinations are now available against meningococcus A, C, W135 and Y. As yet there is no vaccination against meningococcus B as its proteins stimulate only a weak antibody response by the immune system. Vaccinations are also available against *Haemophilus influenzae* and *Pneumococcus*, and where the use of these vaccinations is common there have been dramatic falls in the incidence of meningitis and other infections caused by the corresponding organism.

Immune deficiencies in children

Primary immune deficiencies (PIDs) are disorders of the immune system that lead to increased susceptibility to infectious disease, autoimmunity and malignancy (Box 34.1 and Table 34.4).

Severe combined immunodeficiency (SCID)

This is a group of disorders characterised by profoundly defective cellular and humoral immunity. It presents in the first 6 months of life with unusual and severe infections and severe failure to thrive.

Table 34.3 Abnormalities of cerebrospinal fluid (CSF) in meningitis.

	Bacterial meningitis	Viral meningitis
Opening pressure	Usually elevated	Usually normal
WBC count/mm³	Elevated: 500–10 000+	Elevated: 6–1000
Differential count	Polymorphonuclear predominance	Lymphocytic predominance
Glucose level	Decreased: 0–40 mg/dL	Usually normal
Protein level	Elevated: >50 mg/dL	Normal or slightly elevated

Source: Adapted from Eric F. Reichman and Robert R. Simon (2004) *Emergency Medicine Procedures.* McGraw-Hill.

Box 34.1 When to suspect immune deficiency in children

- Four or more new ear infections within 1 year
- Two or more serious sinus infections within 1 year
- Two or more months of oral antibiotic treatment with little effect (possibly)
- Two or more episodes of pneumonia within 1 year (depending on organism)
- Failure of an infant to gain weight or grow normally
- Recurrent deep skin or organ abscesses
- Persistent thrush in mouth or fungal infection of skin
- Need for i.v. antibiotics to clear infections (possibly)
- Two or more deep-seated infections, including septicaemia
- A family history of primary immunodeficiency

Table 34.4 Examination findings that point to primary immune deficiencies (PIDs).

General appearance	Poor weight gain Short stature Dysmorphism (e.g. DiGeorge facies)
Ear, nose and throat	Chronically discharging ears Perforated tympanic membranes
Mouth	Severe gingivostomatitis Ulcers Recurrent or severe candidiasis Poor dentition
Lymphoid tissue	Excessive lymphadenopathy Absence of lymph nodes or tonsils Organomegaly
Skin	Severe eczema Neonatal erythroderma Severe BCG reaction Extensive warts or molluscum Albinism Telangiectasia Incontinentia pigmenti
Eyes	Retinal lesions Telangiectasia
Respiratory	Clubbing Signs of respiratory infection

Major immunoglobulin deficiencies

The most common example of a major immunoglobulin deficiency is X-linked agammaglobulinaemia, caused by abnormalities in the Bruton gene. It presents in the first 2 years of life with severe bacterial infections, particularly with sinopulmonary infections.

Chronic granulomatous disease

This is an inherited disorder in which phagocytic cells fail to produce superoxide after ingestion of microorganisms due to a lesion in a membrane-associated NADPH oxidase. Children present with recurrent bacterial and fungal infections.

Human immunodeficiency virus (HIV) infection in childhood

The incidence of childhood HIV is rising in the UK, with the major cities having the highest prevalence. Nearly 1 in 500 pregnant women is thought to be HIV positive. In childhood, HIV infection is almost always a result of maternal transmission during childbirth or breastfeeding, though a small number may be transmitted transplacentally. Direct infection in childhood from intravenous drug use, sexual abuse or sexual activity may also be rising.

The incidence of transmission to the offspring of HIV-infected mothers is around 25 to 40% without treatment, but with adequate treatment with antiretroviral medication and appropriate interventions, such as delivery by caesarean section and avoidance of breastfeeding, this transmission rate can be reduced to less than 1%.

HIV in childhood presents with frequent bacterial infection, which may be relatively minor (otitis media, urinary infection, sinusitis) or severe, such as meningitis, septicaemia and pneumonia. There may be evidence of unusual infections such as *Mycobacterium* or *Pneumocystis*, persistent oral candidiasis, severe viral infections such as cytomegalovirus (CMV) retinitis or shingles. Children also experience faltering growth with or without diarrhoea. Developmental delay and developmental regression with deteriorating school performance may result from HIV encephalopathy. Look out for unusual rashes such as dermatitis caused by herpes or *Candida*, and hepatosplenomegaly.

Prompt diagnosis of HIV infection is very important and should take place in all situations where the mother is HIV positive. Diagnosis is usually on the basis of viral polymerase chain reaction (PCR) in infants, as serological tests are unreliable – maternal IgG antibodies will have been transmitted across the placenta and will be found in the infant's blood.

Depending on the viral load in the newborn infant, newborns should be commenced soon after birth on antiretroviral treatment – usually zidovudine. Those with higher risk may be treated with a combination of drugs, as well as prophylactic anti-pneumocystis pneumonia therapy until confirmation is obtained of whether transmission has occurred.

Without treatment, HIV has a very high mortality, with 50% of children dying before they reach 2 years of age. The outlook is considerably worse if the child has been orphaned by the mother's or parents' HIV infection. Substantial improvements in outlook can still be made even if HIV has been transmitted to the child, but the prognosis is still variable, with some children having rapidly progressive disease.

SUMMARY

Clinical case

Case outcome

Sarah was diagnosed with chickenpox and was given supportive symptomatic management. She made a full recovery with no complications.

Key learning points

- Infections are common causes of illness in children.
- An awareness of common rashes helps make diagnoses.
- It is important to have an overview knowledge of warning signs that suggest immunodeficiency in children.

 Now visit **www.wileyessential.com/humandevelopment** to test yourself on this chapter.

CHAPTER 35
Haematology and oncology

Pramodh Vallabhaneni

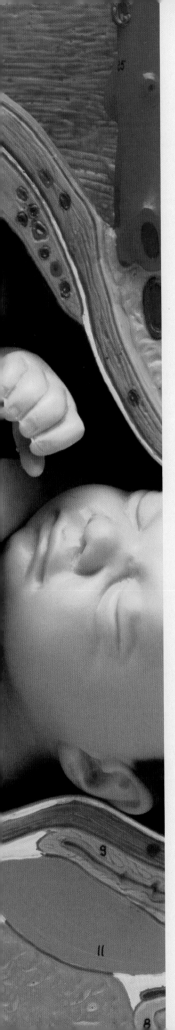

Case

Noah, aged 27 months, presented to the paediatric assessment unit with concerns of pallor for the last few weeks and right-sided hip pain since the previous day. He was previously well apart from an upper respiratory tract infection 2 weeks ago and a limited appetite. On examination he looked very pale, had a temperature of 37.3°C and mild tachycardia, but did not look seriously ill. There was mild cervical lymphadenopathy, and he had a palpable spleen. He was initially thought to have a viral infection with some arthritis of the hip and was admitted for further investigation.

Learning outcomes

- You should be able to recognise the signs and symptoms of paediatric diseases of the blood and recall what diagnostic tests are most appropriate for each.
- You should be able to recognise the signs and symptoms of the more common cancers of childhood.

Essential Human Development, First Edition. Edited by Samuel Webster, Geraint Morris and Euan Kevelighan
© 2018 John Wiley & Sons, Ltd. Published 2018 by John Wiley & Sons, Ltd.

Introduction

Haematopoiesis is the process by which immature precursor cells develop into mature blood cells. The currently accepted theory of how this process works is called the monophyletic theory, which simply means that a single type of stem cell gives rise to all the mature blood cells in the body. This stem cell is called the pluripotent stem cell.

Erythrocytes, or red blood cells (Figure 35.1), are the most common cells within blood. They contain haemoglobin (Hb), a molecule with a high affinity for oxygen. Hb contains iron and gives the erythrocytes their red colour. There are a number of different types of haemoglobin. Red blood cells survive for around 120 days before they are recycled.

Haematological changes after birth

Following birth Hb levels are high (14–21.5 g/dL); they then fall over the first weeks of life, and reach their lowest at around 8–10 weeks of life. Fetal Hb (Hb F) is gradually replaced by adult forms of Hb (Hb A and Hb A2) during infancy.

Anaemia in children

Childhood anaemia is a relatively common problem. Anaemia is a condition in which the number of red blood cells (and consequently their oxygen-carrying capacity) is insufficient to meet the body's physiological needs. Normal ranges vary with age. Anaemia can be defined as:
- Hb <14 g/dL during the neonatal period;
- Hb <10 g/dL at 1–12 months of age;
- Hb <11 g/dL at 1–12 years of age.
  Causes of anaemia can be categorised as follows:
  1. Reduced production:
     - nutrient deficiency (iron, folate, etc.);
     - aplasia/hypoplasia;
     - marrow infiltration;
     - renal failure (reduced erythropoietin production);
     - anaemia of chronic disease.
  2. Increased loss:
     - bleeding (e.g. gastrointestinal bleeding, menstruation).
  3. Increased destruction:
     - haemolysis;
     - hypersplenism (e.g. portal hypertension).

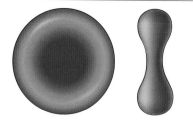

Figure 35.1 Erythrocytes are flattened, round or oval cells with a concavity on either side.

Associated features and clues to diagnosis

- Fever (suggests leukaemia, aplastic anaemia).
- Bleeding diathesis (leukaemia, aplastic anaemia).
- Gastrointestinal bleeding (cow's milk hypersensitivity, Meckel's diverticulum/gastric ectopia).
- Diarrhoea (malabsorption).
- Peripheral oedema (malabsorption).
- Jaundice (haemolysis).
- Failure to thrive (chronic disease, e.g. renal failure).
- Dysmorphic features (e.g. Fanconi's anaemia).
- Purpura (leukaemia, aplastic anaemia).
- Organomegaly of liver or spleen (leukaemia, portal hypertension).

Iron deficiency anaemia (IDA)

Iron deficiency is a common problem amongst children, believed to affect 43% of children worldwide. Iron is distributed around the body, stored as ferritin and then transported to the bone marrow where it is incorporated into haemoglobin for red blood cell production.

The main causes of iron deficiency anaemia are:
- poor intake of iron;
- malabsorption;
- blood loss.

The main sources of iron are red meat, meat products, offal, shellfish and oily fish, leafy green vegetables, grains, pulses, beans and dairy products. Breakfast cereals are fortified with extra iron. Iron is added to white and brown flour to replace that lost in the milling process. Standard infant milk formulas, follow-on formulas and growing-up milks are fortified with iron. Excessive intake of cow's milk can lead to iron deficiency anaemia in toddlers. Breast milk contains low levels of iron but it is readily absorbed.

How do children with IDA present?

Most children remain asymptomatic until Hb levels drop below 7 g/dL. Children present with fatigue and tiredness. They may appear pale, and some toddlers may have feeding problems. Some children present with 'pica' (inappropriate eating of non-food material such as soil, chalk or paper). If left untreated iron deficiency can lead to behavioural problems.

Diagnosis

A blood film from a child with IDA shows microcytic hypochromic anaemia with low mean corpuscular volume (MCV) and mean corpuscular haemoglobin (MCH) along with low serum ferritin levels. Other causes that should be included in differential diagnosis of a microcytic hypochromic picture include thalassaemia traits (alpha and beta), sideroblastic anaemia and lead poisoning.

Treatment

Management includes both dietary and therapeutic approaches. Oral preparations of iron should be introduced gradually as they occasionally can cause local bowel irritation. Hb levels are usually checked 10–12 weeks after treatment. Compliance should be stressed whilst the child is on treatment.

Megaloblastic anaemia

This is a macrocytic anaemia caused by deficiency of cobalamin (vitamin B_{12}), folic acid or both. Cobalamin deficiency due to dietary insufficiency may occur in infants who are breastfed by mothers who are strict vegetarians or who have pernicious anaemia. Intestinal malabsorption occurs in children with Crohn's disease (inflammatory bowel disease), surgical resection of the terminal ileum or rare deficiency of intrinsic factor.

Typical features

- Pallor and fatigue.
- Nutritional deficiency or intestinal malabsorption.
- Macrocytic anaemia.
- Megaloblastic bone marrow changes.

Treatment

In mild deficiency oral replacement of cobalamin may be sufficient .In severe cases parenteral treatment may be required.

Other rare causes in the category of inefficient production include rare conditions like Diamond–Blackfan anaemia (red cell aplasia) and transient erythroblastopenia of childhood.

Anaemia caused by increased red cell destruction (haemolytic anaemia)

Haemolysis from increased red blood cell breakdown leads to anaemia, hepatomegaly and splenomegaly. Tests show elevated bilirubin levels in the blood and urinary urobilinogen.

Conditions of haemolytic anaemia include:
- Red cell membrane disorders, including hereditary spherocytosis.
- Red cell enzyme disorders, e.g. glucose-6-phosphate dehydrogenase (G6PD) deficiency.
- Haemoglobinopathies, including thalassaemia and sickle cell disease.
- Immune response pathologies, such as haemolytic disease of the newborn and autoimmune haemolytic anaemia.

Hereditary spherocytosis

Hereditary spherocytosis is a red cell membrane disorder occurring in 1 in 5000 births of Caucasian families. It is autosomal dominant in inheritance. Children present with jaundice and anaemia with associated splenomegaly. Complications include aplastic crisis and gallstones.

Typical features

- Anaemia and jaundice.
- Splenomegaly.
- Family history of anaemia, jaundice or gallstones.
- Spherocytosis and increased reticulocyte count.
- Increased osmotic fragility.
- Negative direct Coombs' test.

Treatment

Treatment of hereditary spherocytosis includes supplementary dietary folic acid to prevent the development of red cell hypoplasia because of folate deficiency. Splenectomy is beneficial in children with poor growth or severe features of anaemia. Post-splenectomy lifelong penicillin prophylaxis is advised.

Glucose-6-phosphate dehydrogenase (G6PD) deficiency

G6PD deficiency is the most common red cell enzyme defect that causes haemolytic anaemia. The disorder has an X-linked recessive inheritance and occurs with high frequency among persons of African, Mediterranean and Asian ancestry. In most cases the deficiency is due to enzyme instability thus older red cells are more deficient than younger ones and unable to generate sufficient nicotinamide adenine dinucleotide phosphate to maintain the levels of reduced glutathione necessary to protect the red cells against oxidant stress.

Presenting features

- Neonatal jaundice.
- Haemolytic episodes triggered by infection or drugs such as antimalarials and sulphonamide antibiotics.
- Ingestion of fava beans may trigger haemolysis in children of Mediterranean and Asian ancestry.

Treatment

Drugs known to cause haemolysis should be avoided. Infections must be treated promptly and antibiotics given when appropriate.

Haemoglobinopathies

Haemoglobinopathies are an extremely heterogeneous group of congenital disorders that occur in many different ethnic groups. They are classified into two major groups. The first group is the thalassaemias, which are caused by quantitative deficiencies in the production of globin chains. The second group are caused by structural abnormalities of globin chains (Table 35.1).

Table 35.1 Types of haemoglobinopathies detectable by electrophoresis of blood samples.

	Hb indication on electrophoresis
Birth	Hb A2 1%, Hb F 74%, Hb A 25%
Normal adult	Hb A2 2%, Hb F 0%, Hb A 97%
Beta-thalassaemia trait	Hb A2 raised
Beta-thalassaemia major	Hb A2 and Hb F raised, no Hb A
Sickle cell trait	Hb S, Hb F and Hb A
Sickle cell disease	Hb S and Hb F, no Hb A

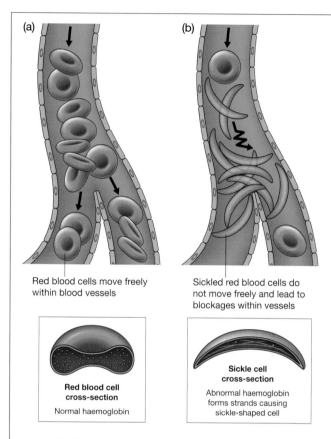

Figure 35.2 Normal red blood cells and sickle cells, with the normal and abnormal haemoglobin within.

Red blood cells move freely within blood vessels

Sickled red blood cells do not move freely and lead to blockages within vessels

Red blood cell cross-section
Normal haemoglobin

Sickle cell cross-section
Abnormal haemoglobin forms strands causing sickle-shaped cell

Sickle cell disease

This is a collective name given to haemoglobinopathies in which Hb S (the sickle cell haemoglobin type) is inherited. It results because of a mutation in codon 6 of the beta-globin gene causing a change in the encoded amino acid from glutamine to valine. The haemoglobin molecule that results is malformed and causes the red blood cells to lose their elasticity, and narrow and curve into sickle shapes when in a low oxygen tension environment. These sickle-shaped red blood cells do not pass easily through capillaries causing occlusion and ischaemia (Figure 35.2). Sickle cell disease is most commonly seen in Afro-Caribbean and Middle Eastern populations.

Three main forms of sickle cell disease are well recognised:
- sickle cell anaemia;
- sickle cell disease;
- sickle beta-thalassaemia.

Typical features

- Positive neonatal screening test for abnormal haemoglobins.
- African, Mediterranean, Middle Eastern, Indian or Caribbean ancestry.
- Anaemia, elevated reticulocyte count, jaundice.
- Recurrent episodes of musculoskeletal or abdominal pain.
- Splenomegaly in early childhood with later disappearance.
- High risk of bacterial sepsis.

Management

Prophylaxis with oral penicillin is given to prevent pneumococcal infection, plus immunisation against pneumococcus. Oral folic acid is also given. Exposure to cold should be minimised and maintainenance of adequate hydration is important.

Acute sickle cell crisis

Occlusion of small blood vessels causes acute sickle cell crises. Rapid treatment measures should be initiated; these include analgesia and intravenous hydration. Antibiotics are usually given during an acute crisis. Exchange transfusion is indicated for acute chest syndrome, stroke and priapism.

Thalassaemia

General considerations

Adult haemoglobin contains two alpha chains and two beta chains. Thalassaemia is a genetic disorder in which one of the two protein chains that make up haemoglobin is deficient. The different types of thalassaemia refer to the affected protein globin chain (Figure 35.3).

Alpha thalassaemia

Four gene loci code for the production of the alpha chain. Deletions of these genes are prevalent in certain populations (see below). The greater the number of genes affected or deleted, the more severe the disease.

Typical features

- African, Mediterranean, Middle Eastern, Chinese or Southeast Asian ancestry.

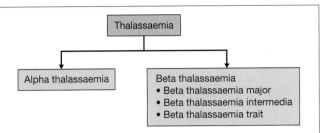

Figure 35.3 Forms of thalassaemia.

- Microcytic, hypochromic anaemia of variable severity.
- Barts haemoglobin (Hb Barts) detected by neonatal screening.

Treatment
Patients who are silent carriers (one gene affected) or who have alpha-thalassaemia trait (two genes affected) require no treatment. Those with haemoglobin H disease (three genes affected) should receive supplemental folic acid and avoid the same oxidant drugs that cause haemolysis in G6PD deficiency. Anaemia may be exacerbated in periods of infections and transfusions may be required. Hypersplenism may develop in childhood and require splenectomy. Fetuses with severe alpha thalassaemia (all four genes affected) have severe oedema (hydrops fetalis) and rarely live beyond birth.

Beta thalassaemia

Beta thalassaemia occurs with a mutation of the beta-globin gene that results in an inability to produce adult haemoglobin.

Typical features
Beta thalassaemia minor:
- Normal neonatal screening test.
- African, Mediterranean, Middle Eastern or Asian ancestry.
- Mild microcytic, hypochromic anaemia.
- No response to iron therapy.
- Elevated level of haemoglobin A2.

Beta thalassaemia major:
- Neonatal screening test shows haemoglobin F only.
- Mediterranean, Middle Eastern or Asian ancestry.
- Severe microcytic, hypochromic anaemia with marked hepatosplenomegaly.
- Extramedullary haematopoiesis, causing bone marrow expansion leading to classical facies with maxillary overgrowth and skull bossing.

Treatment
Beta thalassaemia minor requires no specific treatment but may have genetic implications for the family. For children with beta thalassaemia major chronic transfusion with iron chelation forms a mainstay. In children who have a HLA-identical sibling donor the probability of haematological cure is greater than 90% with bone marrow or umbilical cord blood transplantation.

Bleeding disorders

Bleeding disorders occur as a result of:
1. Quantitative or qualitative abnormalities of platelets.
2. Quantitative or qualitative abnormalities in plasma procoagulant factors.
3. Vascular abnormalities.
4. Accelerated fibrinolysis.

The coagulation cascade and fibrinolytic system are shown in Figure 35.4.

Acquired disorders of coagulation include haemorrhagic disease of the newborn due to a vitamin K deficiency, liver disease, immune thrombocytopenia and DIC (disseminated intravascular coagulation).

General considerations

Vitamin K is essential for the production of active forms of coagulation factors II, VII, IX, X, protein C and protein S. Vitamin K deficiency causes reduced levels of all these factors.

Thrombocytopenia

Thrombocytopenia is defined as a platelet count of less than 150×10^9 platelets/L (normal range is $150–400 \times 10^9$ platelets/L). The causes of thrombocytopenia in children are either

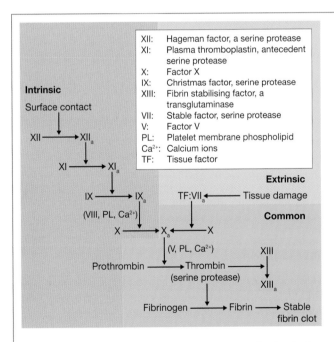

Figure 35.4 The coagulation cascade and fibrinolytic system. (Source: Dr Graham Beards, https://commons.wikimedia.org/wiki/File:Classical_blood_coagulation_pathway.png. Used under CC-BY -SA 3..0.)

a decreased production rate of platelets or an increased rate of destruction of platelets.

Thrombocytopenia arising from decreased platelet production can be due to:

1. Congenital causes, including Fanconi anaemia, Wiskott–Aldrich syndrome, thrombocytopenia with absent radii, metabolic disorders and osteopetrosis.
2. Acquired causes, including aplastic anaemia, leukaemia and other malignancies, and vitamin B_{12} and folate deficiencies.

Thrombocytopenia due to increased platelet destruction can be the result of:

1. Antibody-mediated causes, including immune (idiopathic) thrombocytopenia, infection and immune system diseases.
2. Coagulopathy causes, including DIC and sepsis.

Typical features in children

- Bruising.
- Petechiae.
- Purpura.
- Mucosal bleeding (e.g. epistaxis, bleeding from gums when brushing teeth).
- Haematuria.
- Intracranial bleeding (rare).

Immune thrombocytopenic purpura (ITP)

Immune thrombocytopenic purpura is the most common bleeding disorder of childhood. It occurs most frequently in children aged 2–5 years and often follows infection with viruses such as rubella, varicella, measles, parvovirus, influenza or Epstein–Barr virus (EBV). Most children recover spontaneously within a few months. Chronic ITP (>6 months duration) occurs in 10–20% of affected patients.

ITP results from clearance of circulating IgM- or IgG-coated platelets by the reticuloendothelial system.

Typical features in children

Principal features are usually acute, multiple petechiae and ecchymoses. Epistaxis is also common.

Investigations

In blood analysis platelet concentrations are usually less than 50×10^9 platelets/L (normal 150–400 $\times 10^9$ platelets/L). White blood cell counts and Hb levels are usually normal.

Complications

Complications of ITP include severe haemorrhage and bleeding into vital organs. Intracranial haemorrhage is the most serious but rarely seen complication (less than 1% of affected children).

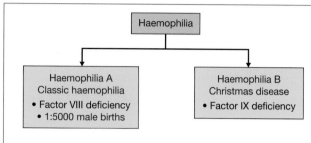

Figure 35.5 Forms of haemophilia.

Treatment

In about 80% of children the disease is self-limiting and results in spontaneous recovery after 6–8 weeks. Treatment with oral steroids and/or intravenous immunoglobulin remains controversial. Platelet transfusions are reserved for life-threatening haemorrhage.

Inherited disorders of coagulation

Inherited disorders of coagulation seen in children include haemophilia and von Willebrand's disease (vWD).

Haemophilia

The most common severe inherited coagulation disorders are haemophilia A and haemophilia B (Figure 35.5). Both occur with an X-linked recessive inheritance pattern. Haemophilia A occurs because of a genetic defect in the gene for coagulation factor VIII, and haemophilia B results from a mutation in the gene for factor IX.

Typical features in children

There are frequent spontaneous bleeding episodes involving skin, mucous membranes, joints, muscles and viscera. The most crippling aspect of factor VIII deficiency is recurrent haemarthroses that incite joint destruction.

Investigations

- Activated partial thromboplastin time (APTT) is prolonged.
- Prothrombin time (PT) is normal.
- Decreased factor VIII:C.
- Normal levels of von Willebrand factor (vWF) antigen.
- Ristocetin-induced platelet aggregation (RIPA) is normal.

Management

Recombinant factor VIII concentrate for haemophilia A or recombinant factor IX concentrate for haemophilia B is given by prompt intravenous infusion whenever there is any bleeding. Appropriate levels need to be maintained prior to surgery.

von Willebrand's disease

von Willebrand's disease (vWD) is a commonly inherited bleeding disorder in Caucasian people with a population prevalence of around 1%. von Willebrand factor facilitates platelet adhesion to damaged endothelium and acts as the carrier protein for factor VIII:C, protecting it from inactivation and clearance. The disease results from either a quantitative or qualitative deficiency of von Willebrand factor; there are a number of different types of vWD.

Types I and 3 vWD have quantitative deficiencies in von Willebrand factor, and type 2 has qualitative deficiencies. Inheritance of type I vWD typically follows an autosomal dominant pattern, as do most of the type 2 forms, but type 3 vWD is inherited in an autosomal recessive manner.

Typical features in children
- Bruising.
- Excessive prolonged bleeding after surgery.
- Epistaxis.

Investigations
- APTT is prolonged or normal.
- PT is normal.
- Decreased or normal levels of factor VIII:C.
- Decreased vWF antigen levels.
- Ristocetin-induced platelet aggregation is abnormal.

Management
Treatment is varied depending upon the type and severity of the disease. DDAVP (or desmopressin, a synthetic version of vasopressin) causes secretion of both factor VIII and vWF into blood plasma and can be used to treat type 1 vWD. More severe types need to be treated with plasma-derived factor VIII concentrate.

Oncology

Cancer in children is not a common diagnosis. Annually about 1500 children are diagnosed with cancer in the UK. The survival rate for many tumours has increased over the last decades, and the overall 5-year survival rate is about 75%.

Specific types of childhood cancers occurring in the UK as a proportion of total childhood cancers include:
- leukaemia, 32%;
- brain and spinal tumours, 24%;
- lymphomas, 10%;
- neuroblastoma, 7%;
- soft tissue sarcomas, 7%;
- Wilms' tumour, 6%;
- bone tumours, 4%;
- retinoblastoma, 3%;
- other, 7%.

Leukaemia

Leukaemia is a bone marrow cell cancer resulting in unusually high numbers of immature leucocytes. Acute lymphoblastic leukaemia (ALL) accounts for 80% of all types of leukaemia in children. The majority of the remaining cases are of acute myeloid or acute non-lymphocytic (AML/ANLL) leukaemia.

Typical features in children presenting with ALL
- Pallor.
- Petechiae.
- Purpura, abnormal bruising.
- Bone pain.
- Hepatosplenomegaly.
- Lymphadenopathy.

Investigations

A full blood count with a differential test that counts and compares the proportions of different types of cells is the most useful test because 95% of patients with ALL have a decreased count in at least one cell type (single cytopenia): neutropenia, thrombocytopenia or anaemia. Most patients will have a decrease in at least two cell lines.

A bone marrow biopsy examination is diagnostic for ALL, showing an infiltration of leukaemic blasts replacing normal bone marrow elements. Histochemical stains specific for myeloblastic and monoblastic leukaemias distinguish between types of leukaemia.

Treatment

The intensity of treatment is determined by specific prognostic features present at diagnosis, the patient's response to therapy, and specific biological features of the leukaemia cells. The initial phase involves induction of remission with drugs like vincristine, methotrexate and steroids.

Tumour lysis syndrome should be anticipated when treatment is started because of rapid cell lysis. Additional hydration and treatment with oral allopurinol are given to prevent this.

Due to the immunocompromised state of the patient during treatment they are prone to having bacterial, fungal and viral infections. Febrile neutropenia needs prompt assessment and treatment.

Lymphomas

A lymphoma is a B- or T-lymphocyte cancer that may form tumours that often arise within a lymph node or another lymphatic organ. Lymphomas can be divided into Hodgkin lymphoma and non-Hodgkin lymphoma (NHL). NHL is more common in childhood, while Hodgkin lymphoma is seen more frequently in adolescence.

Non-Hodgkin lymphomas are a diverse group of cancers accounting for 5–10% of malignancies in children less than 15 years old. There is a male predominance of approximately 3:1. Presentation depends on the site of the disease; A-cell malignancies present as ALL or NHL, with both being characterised by mediastinal mass with varying degrees of bone marrow infiltration. B-cell malignancies present more commonly as

NHL, with localised lymph node disease. Treatment is via chemotherapy.

Hodgkin lymphoma is relatively uncommon in prepubertal children. It usually presents as painless lymphadenopathy, most frequently in the neck. Clinical history is often long-standing with systemic symptoms. Treatment is via chemotherapy, possibly in combination with radiotherapy.

Brain tumours

Brain tumours in children are almost always primary tumours and the majority of them are infratentorial (60%).

Typical features in children

- Headache.
- Vomiting.
- Papilloedema.
- Squint secondary to cranial nerve VI nerve palsy.
- Nystagmus.
- Ataxia.
- Personality or behavioural change.

Astrocytomas are the most common brain tumour type, occurring in 40% of brain tumour cases; they originate from the astrocyte population of glial cells in the central nervous system. Juvenile astrocytomas are cystic, often slow growing, and the results of treatment with surgery are excellent. Non-juvenile astrocytoma occurs at all sites but more frequently in the cerebral hemispheres. Treatment options involve surgery and chemotherapy.

Medulloblastomas usually arise in the midline of the posterior cranial fossa and account for roughly 20% of brain tumour cases. Presentation is with ataxia as well as headache and vomiting. Treatment options involve surgery and chemotherapy.

Neuroblastomas and related tumours arise from neural crest tissue in the adrenal medulla and sympathetic nervous system. Neuroblastomas occur most commonly before the age of 5 years. The usual mode of presentation is with an abdominal mass, but they can arise anywhere from the ganglia of the sympathetic chain (neck to pelvis).

Children with neuroblastoma present with bone pain, abdominal pain, anorexia, weight loss, fever and irritability. Examination findings may include abdominal mass(es), adenopathy, proptosis, periorbital ecchymosis, skull masses, subcutaneous nodules, hepatomegaly and spinal cord compression. CT scanning provides useful diagnostic information, including the extent of the primary tumour and effects on surrounding structures. The main treatment is surgical resection coupled with chemotherapy.

Wilms' tumour (or nephroblastoma) originates from embryonic renal tissue and is the commonest renal tumour of childhood. It most commonly occurs between the ages of 2 and 5 years. Children may present with an asymptomatic abdominal mass or swelling. The mass is usually smooth and firm, well demarcated and rarely crosses the midline. Twenty-five percent of patients will be hypertensive at presentation.

Ultrasound or CT abdomen scanning should establish the presence of an intrarenal mass. It is also essential to evaluate the contralateral kidney for presence and function.

Treatment of Wilms' tumour is initially chemotherapy followed by nephrectomy when indicated. Occasionally children may require radiotherapy. Overall the prognosis is good, with a 5-year survival rate of more than 80% of all patients.

SUMMARY

Clinical case

Case investigations

Blood tests showed a haemoglobin concentration of 77 g/L (normal range 120–140 g/L) and platelets at 84 × 10⁹/L (normal range 150–400 × 10⁹/L). A blood film was reported as showing blast cells and raised the possibility of acute lymphoblastic leukaemia (ALL). Noah was transferred to a tertiary oncology centre where the diagnosis was confirmed. Further investigations included a bone marrow biopsy, chest X-ray and lumbar puncture. There was no evidence of central nervous system involvement.

Case conclusions

A diagnosis of acute lymphoblastic leukaemia was made. Noah underwent treatment with chemotherapy and went into remission quickly. Three years later following a complete course of treatment, Noah was well and free of any evidence of leukaemia.

Key learning points

- Anaemia is somewhat common in children and is generally caused by changes in the rates of production or destruction of erythrocytes, or by blood loss.
- It is helpful to understand the normal pathway of coagulation as problems associated with clotting mechanisms tend to occur with abnormalities of platelets or plasma procoagulant factors, vascular abnormalities or increased fibrinolysis.
- Paediatric malignances are uncommon but these can be serious conditions.

 Now visit **www.wileyessential.com/humandevelopment** to test yourself on this chapter.

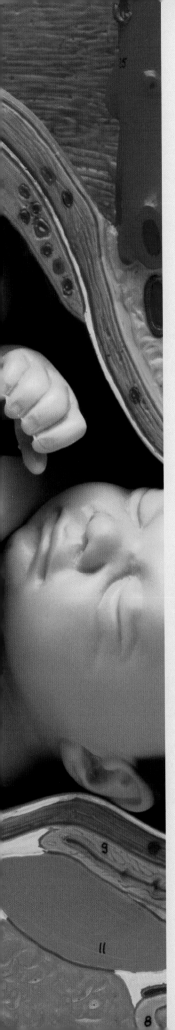

CHAPTER 36
Congenital and acquired heart disease

Geraint Morris

Case

A 2-month-old child presents to her local GP with shortness of breath and faltering growth. She failed to attend for her routine 6-week check. She has a history of drinking small amounts of milk then either sleeping or becoming breathless. These symptoms started when she was around 3 to 4 weeks old. Her health visitor visited the family at home and became concerned that the baby looked small and thin. Her weight was 200 g less than the 0.4th centile whereas her length was on the 25th centile and her head circumference on the 10th centile.

On examination the baby appears pale and undernourished. She has a respiratory rate of 55 per minute and has mild intercostal recession. Her capillary refill time is 2 seconds, her femoral pulses are very easy to palpate, her heart rate is 165 per minute, and her precordial impulse feels prominent. Her liver is palpable at 2 cm below the right costal margin. She has a loud second heart sound and a harsh grade 3/6 continuous murmur at the left upper sternal border.

Learning outcomes

- You should be able to describe how the commoner congenital and acquired heart diseases in childhood result in clinical symptoms and signs.
- You should be able to recognise the common ways in which heart abnormalities present in children.

Essential Human Development, First Edition. Edited by Samuel Webster, Geraint Morris and Euan Kevelighan
© 2018 John Wiley & Sons, Ltd. Published 2018 by John Wiley & Sons, Ltd.

The fetal circulation

The priority for the fetal heart before birth is not only to pump blood around the body (the systemic circulation) but to get blood to the placenta, the source of all nutrients and oxygen before birth (Figure 36.1). The fetal lungs do not take part in gas exchange, so pumping blood around the lungs (the pulmonary circulation) is not a priority. The heart is therefore specifically designed to meet these demands before birth and to enable the dramatic change from placental to pulmonary gas exchange that takes place immediately after birth.

In the fetal circulation, blood gets to the placenta via the umbilical cord in the umbilical arteries – these are branches of the iliac arteries. The blood is oxygenated by the placenta and returns to the fetus in the umbilical vein. The blood then flows along the ductus venosus on the inferior aspect of the liver. The blood enters the right atrium and most is directed by a sheet of tissue attached to the posterior wall of the right atrium (the Eustachian valve) through an opening in the atrial septum (the foramen ovale) into the left atrium. Here it is joined by the small amount of venous return from the lungs coming into the left atrium via the pulmonary veins. The blood is still rich in oxygen as it then goes into the left ventricle and is ejected into the aorta to supply the upper half of the body especially the brain. As the remaining blood reaches the descending aortic arch it is joined by blood from the ductus arteriosus, which has been pumped out of the right ventricle. This blood then flows down the descending aorta towards the lower body and the placenta.

The venous return from the head and upper body flows through the superior vena cava into the right atrium and most flows anteriorly over the Eustachian valve into the right ventricle. The remainder joins the blood coming up from the inferior vena cava and flows through the foramen ovale. From the right ventricle blood is pumped into the pulmonary artery, where most flows across the ductus arteriosus into the descending aorta, with a small amount entering the pulmonary artery to supply the lungs. In order to ensure that most of the blood goes into the descending aorta (and hence the placenta), the vascular resistance is kept high in the pulmonary artery by the constriction of pulmonary arterioles in the lungs throughout fetal life.

Changes at birth

The first breath after birth marks a dramatic change in the circulation. The lungs expand and fill with air as the lung fluid is expelled and absorbed. There is a fall in pulmonary vascular resistance as the pulmonary arterioles vasodilate within the oxygen-rich environment. This leads to an increase in the flow of blood into the pulmonary vasculature and a fall in the pulmonary artery pressure. The blood is then oxygenated in the lungs and flows into the left atrium, where it increases the pressure in the left atrium, which closes the foramen ovale. It then flows to the left ventricle and the aorta. Because the pressure in the pulmonary artery has dropped, the flow in the ductus arteriosus reverses, and the blood in the aorta, which is now rich in oxygen, passes through the ductus. This stimulates the

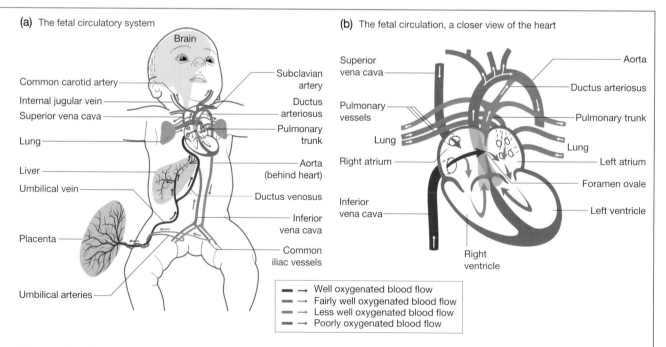

(a) The fetal circulatory system

Brain

Common carotid artery
Internal jugular vein
Superior vena cava
Lung
Liver
Umbilical vein
Placenta
Umbilical arteries

Subclavian artery
Ductus arteriosus
Pulmonary trunk
Aorta (behind heart)
Ductus venosus
Inferior vena cava
Common iliac vessels

(b) The fetal circulation, a closer view of the heart

Superior vena cava
Pulmonary vessels
Lung
Right atrium
Inferior vena cava
Right ventricle

Aorta
Ductus arteriosus
Pulmonary trunk
Lung
Left atrium
Foramen ovale
Left ventricle

→ Well oxygenated blood flow
→ Fairly well oxygenated blood flow
→ Less well oxygenated blood flow
→ Poorly oxygenated blood flow

Figure 36.1 The fetal circulatory system. (Source: S. Webster and R. de Wreede (2012) *Embryology at a Glance*. Reproduced with permission of John Wiley & Sons, Ltd.)

smooth muscle of the ductus to close. The oxygenated blood flows into the umbilical arteries, which vasoconstrict, taking out the placenta from the circulation. The circulation thus becomes the standard lung-heart-body-heart circulation that exists in the normal postnatal cardiovascular system.

Heart disease in children

With a few notable exceptions, most heart problems in childhood result from congenital heart disease. This is almost invariably a result of structural malformations of the heart that arise in early fetal life.

Ventricular septal defect (VSD).

This is the commonest structural heart lesion and results from incomplete septation of the ventricles during the fifth and sixth weeks of gestation (Figure 36.2). As the pressure in the left ventricle is higher than that in the right ventricle, as long as there are no other abnormalities, blood will flow across a VSD from left to right – this is known as 'shunting', so a VSD is a 'left-to-right shunt'. If the VSD is large, this causes two problems: firstly too much blood enters the pulmonary circulation, and secondly less blood gets into the aorta and the systemic circulation.

As a consequence of increased pulmonary blood flow, the lungs become engorged with blood and less compliant. All the additional lung blood flow comes back to the left side of the heart, which becomes both dilated (due to increased volume, or 'preload') and hypertrophied (due to the added work of

pumping extra blood, or 'afterload'). There is also increased pressure in the left atrium and this causes a back pressure in the pulmonary veins and capillaries. When the hydrostatic pressure in the capillaries exceeds the oncotic pressure, fluid leaks out into the interstitial spaces and air spaces in the lungs – pulmonary oedema. As a result of these events, the child becomes breathless.

The reduced systemic output of the heart results in an increased secretion of catecholamines, which causes a compensatory increase in heart rate, peripheral vasoconstriction and increased metabolic rate.

Presentation

In the case of a large VSD, this will present in the newborn period, though not necessarily at birth. At birth, and for up to a few weeks afterwards, the vascular resistance in the pulmonary circulation remains high but decreases gradually to normal levels as the pulmonary arterioles continue to grow and vasodilate. This means that the difference between the pressures in both ventricles may not be large enough to cause significant flow across the VSD initially. Thus the newborn baby may not present with any symptoms or signs, and routine examination in the first 24 hours or so may not detect a VSD.

When the pulmonary vascular resistance falls, pulmonary congestion and oedema cause breathlessness, which becomes most obvious when the baby feeds, as feeding involves exertion as well as coordination of breathing, suckling and swallowing. The increased metabolic demand associated with increased catecholamine release causes a diversion of energy resources away from growth and the infant may show faltering growth.

The age and severity of symptoms depends very much on the size of the VSD. Moderately sized VSDs may present later and with mild symptoms (e.g. breathlessness just on exertion) and small VSDs may not produce any symptoms at all, presenting as incidental murmurs on routine examinations.

Examination findings

In the case of a large VSD, the general examination may reveal tachypnoea with signs of increased work of breathing (sternal recession, subcostal recession), pallor, sweating and cold peripheries. Pulses may be thready and reveal tachycardia. The cardiac impulse may be prominent resulting from hypertrophy and dilatation of the ventricles. The liver may be congested due to high pressure in the systemic veins and consequently may be enlarged. This constellation of symptoms and signs is often termed 'heart failure'. Auscultation reveals a pansystolic murmur caused by the turbulent jet of blood crossing the VSD throughout systole. There is little flow across the VSD in diastole. The murmur may be quiet in the case of a very large VSD. This is because the VSD is not small enough to restrict the flow of blood from left to right ventricles and the flow is therefore smooth and not turbulent. If the murmur is loud, particularly if it is accompanied by a thrill, the VSD is likely

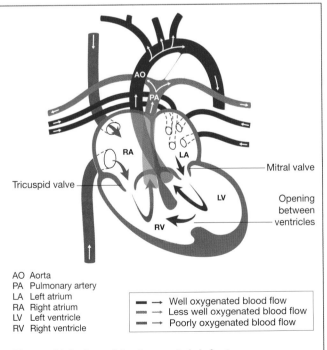

AO Aorta
PA Pulmonary artery
LA Left atrium
RA Right atrium
LV Left ventricle
RV Right ventricle

- ━ → Well oxygenated blood flow
- ━ → Less well oxygenated blood flow
- ━ → Poorly oxygenated blood flow

Tricuspid valve
Mitral valve
Opening between ventricles

Figure 36.2 A ventricular septal defect.

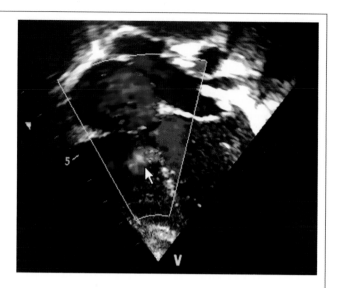

Figure 36.3 Cardiac echogram in a child with a ventricular septal defect.

to be small. In the case of a very small VSD, the murmur may again be quiet due to the very small quantity of flow across it. The location of the murmur is at the left lower sternal edge, consistent with the usual position of the ventricular septum.

Investigation findings in a child with a VSD

The investigations that are helpful in a child with cardiac pathology are an ECG, a chest X-ray and an echocardiogram (Figure 36.3).

In the case of a VSD, the ECG shows both left and right ventricular hypertrophy and the enlargement of the heart is evident on a chest X-ray. Increased blood flow around the lungs also shows as prominent vascular markings ('pulmonary plethora'), and pulmonary oedema may also be evident.

The definitive investigation is an echocardiogram, which can describe the abnormality very accurately including its haemodynamic significance, and can detect any complication such as pulmonary hypertension. Most children who require cardiac surgery need no other investigations, but some children with more complicated lesions may require further investigation with cardiac catheterisation. This can allow blood sampling and pressure measurement inside the cardiac chambers.

Pulmonary hypertension

The extra blood flow in the lungs resulting from a large VSD will cause pulmonary arteriolar vasoconstriction, which, if it persists over a long time, may cause smooth muscle hypertrophy in the arterioles and eventually fibrosis of the arteriolar walls. These changes cause an increase in the vascular resistance of the pulmonary circulation and added work for the

right ventricle. The right ventricle becomes hypertrophied and the pressure in the pulmonary arteries increases. The longer this situation continues, the higher the pressure becomes and eventually the pressure in the right ventricle may exceed that of the left and the VSD shunt reverses, becoming right to left. This causes cyanosis and is known as Eisenmenger's syndrome. Fibrosis of the pulmonary arterioles is irreversible and the only definitive treatment may be a heart-lung transplant. The treatment of VSDs and all other left-to-right shunt lesions is aimed at avoiding this situation as well as to relieve symptoms and other complications such as bacterial endocarditis.

Treatment

VSDs tend either to stay the same size or get smaller over time. Large VSDs are less likely to close spontaneously and so may require eventual surgical closure.

If there are signs of heart failure this can be treated pharmacologically with diuretics, angiotensin-converting enzyme (ACE) inhibitors and digoxin. Poor feeding and faltering growth can be treated with the use of high-energy formula feeds, nasogastric tube feeding and overnight feeding. Pharmacological therapy can improve symptoms and hence buy some time for lesions to get smaller, or to address nutritional issues so that the child is in a better condition for surgery.

Paediatric cardiologists and surgeons generally discuss individual cases together to decide on the most appropriate form of surgery as well as the timing of surgery. Modern cardiac surgery has become safer at young ages and it is now commonplace for children to have surgery to repair large VSDs at around 3 to 4 months old, as the risk of pulmonary hypertension increases after this. In general, most children currently undergo open heart surgery for VSD repairs, but some VSDs have been successfully closed by a 'cardiac catheter' inserted through the large vessels of the groin or the neck, by which a device can be inserted into a defect, or a balloon can be inflated to dilate a narrow valve or vessel.

If, for some reason, the VSD cannot be closed safely until the child is older, a band may be inserted around the pulmonary artery to induce a narrowing of the artery. This protects the pulmonary circulation from the development of pulmonary hypertension until the defect can be definitively repaired.

Endocarditis

This is an uncommon disease, but children with haemodynamically significant heart lesions who have not yet undergone cardiac surgery are at increased risk.

It is a serious disease presenting with persistent fever, lethargy and signs such as a changing murmur, splinter haemorrhages, clubbing and subcutaneous nodules in the finger tips (Osler's nodes) or in the palms and soles (Janeway lesions), and retinal lesions (Roth spots). Septal defects and abnormal heart valves are a common site of infection, and vegetations may be seen near these structures on echocardiography. Heart structures may be seriously damaged by the invasive infection. The treatment is a prolonged course of intravenous antibiotics, and, in some cases, cardiac surgery to remove vegetations and repair damaged tissue.

In the past it was common practice to prescribe antibiotic prophylaxis for surgical procedures (especially dental extractions) that were thought to induce streptococcal or staphylococcal bacteraemia in these children. In the UK this practice is now much less prevalent as there is little evidence to support its use. However, it is still considered important to advise good dental hygiene, as the bacteria that often cause endocarditis may originate from the oral cavity.

Other 'left-to-right' heart lesions

Patent ductus arteriosus (PDA)

The ductus arteriosus may remain open after birth and cause problems similar to those of a VSD (Figure 36.4). Because the pressure in the aorta is greater than that in the pulmonary artery, blood flow in a PDA is left to right. This causes excess pulmonary blood flow and reduced systemic flow to the lower body. The pathophysiology, clinical presentation, investigation findings and complications of a PDA are similar to those of the VSD with a few notable differences.

PDAs are a very common abnormality in preterm infants, as the smooth muscle responsible for the closure of the ductus is not so well developed. The presenting problem in a preterm infant is often failure to wean from a ventilator and/or supplemental oxygen.

In the case of a PDA, the flow is diastolic as well as systolic, as there is still a large diastolic difference in pressure between the two arteries. The murmur is therefore a continuous harsh ('machinery type') noise throughout the cardiac cycle, with some increase in volume during systole. It is heard best high on the left sternal border in keeping with the usual anatomical position of the PDA.

PDAs can be treated pharmacologically in the neonatal period with indometacin or ibuprofen. Those that do not respond to this, or present outside of the neonatal period, usually require surgical closure. This can be done either through a thoracotomy incision with a clip or ligature applied to the PDA, or via the transcatheter route with an occlusion device being inserted into the PDA.

Atrial septal defect (ASD)

If the foramen ovale does not close after birth, a defect in the atrial septum may result (Figure 36.5). If the defect is not thought to be large enough to have any significant haemodynamic effect then it is simply called a 'patent foramen ovale' (PFO). This is very common and is often identified as an incidental finding on an echocardiogram or on postmortem examination. It may be relevant to deep-sea divers; if nitrogen bubbles form within the systemic veins during decompression as the diver surfaces, the bubbles could then pass through the PFO and cause systemic nitrogen emboli.

If the defect left by the failure of the foramen to close is large, or if there has been inadequate septation of the septum secundum during early fetal life, the defect may be significant,

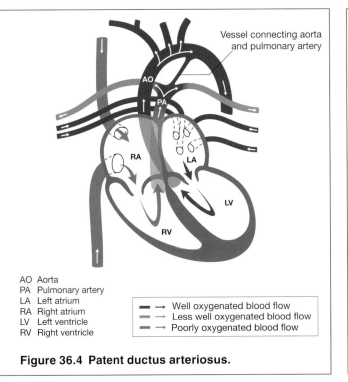

Vessel connecting aorta and pulmonary artery

AO Aorta
PA Pulmonary artery
LA Left atrium
RA Right atrium
LV Left ventricle
RV Right ventricle

- → Well oxygenated blood flow
- → Less well oxygenated blood flow
- → Poorly oxygenated blood flow

Figure 36.4 Patent ductus arteriosus.

Atrial septal defect

AO Aorta
PA Pulmonary artery
LA Left atrium
RA Right atrium
LV Left ventricle
RV Right ventricle

- → Well oxygenated blood flow
- → Poorly oxygenated blood flow

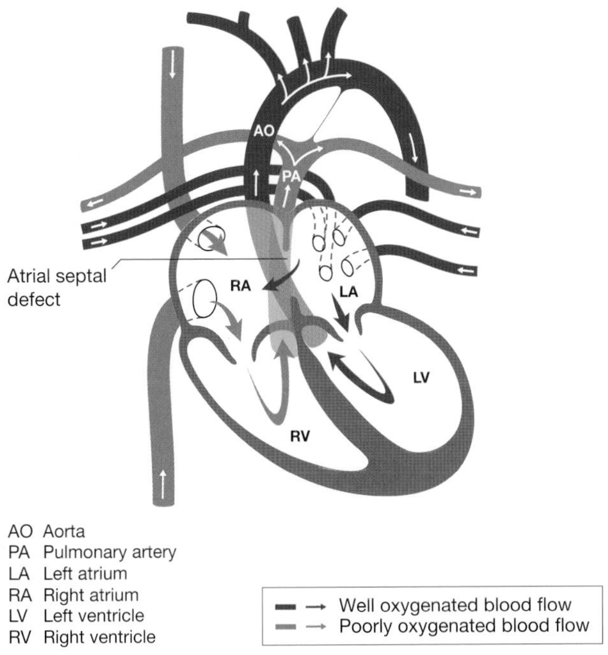

Figure 36.5 Atrial septal defect.

in which case it is called an atrial septal defect (ASD). Even though the pressure is usually greater in the left atrium than the right, the pressure difference between the two atria is low. Therefore the blood flow across ASDs is usually not great enough to cause clinical problems in the newborn or infant period. Children are usually asymptomatic, but older children and adults with large ASDs may experience shortness of breath especially on exertion.

The principal pathophysiological mechanisms are the same as those of a VSD with excess pulmonary blood flow. There is dilatation of the right atrium and ventricle due to extra blood coming from the left atrium through the ASD, but there is no dilatation of the left ventricle, as the excess pulmonary venous return to the left atrium does not pass into the left ventricle but is diverted through the ASD.

The murmur that signifies an ASD does not come directly from the ASD itself but arises from the pulmonary valve. The excess blood flow through the right side of the heart passes through the pulmonary valve, causing a flow murmur. This is generally a smooth, relatively soft murmur heard best at the upper left sternal border. Because of the added volume of blood entering the right ventricle, the pulmonary valve takes longer to close than the aortic valve. This delayed closure of the pulmonary component of the second heart sound causes a wide splitting of the sound. The splitting does not vary with respiration ('fixed splitting'). This is because the normal changes in systemic venous return to the heart, which are responsible for the variation in splitting that is heard in normal individuals, are cancelled out by changes in flow across the ASD with respiration.

The dilatation of the right ventricle causes a conduction delay across the myocardium, which shows up on an ECG as right bundle branch block pattern. Otherwise ECG and chest X-ray changes are similar to those in the case of a VSD.

Pulmonary hypertension is still a risk though this tends to take many years to develop rather than months. There is therefore no need to correct an ASD in infancy. Most children found to have an ASD undergo repair at around school age. This is usually done by the transcatheter route with an occlusion device, though if there is inadequate septum around the defect to site the device, open repair can be performed.

Atrioventricular septal defect (AVSD)

AVSDs are the commonest cardiac defect in children with Down syndrome. They result from the incomplete formation of that part of the atrioventricular septum (Figure 36.6) that is formed by the endocardial cushions in early fetal life (the septum primum, the atrioventricular valves and the upper ventricular septum). In terms of the development of symptoms and signs, the physiology is similar to that of the VSD; however, there are some important exceptions.

The endocardial cushions are integral to the formation of the atrioventricular (mitral and tricuspid) valves. In an AVSD these valves do not form properly and the resulting

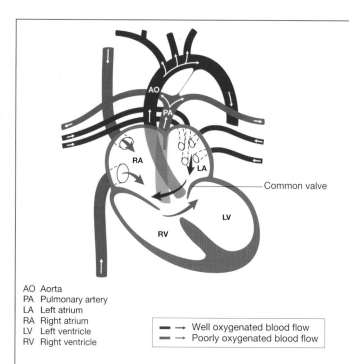

AO Aorta
PA Pulmonary artery
LA Left atrium
RA Right atrium
LV Left ventricle
RV Right ventricle

■ → Well oxygenated blood flow
■ → Poorly oxygenated blood flow

Figure 36.6 Atrioventricular septal defect.

atrioventricular (AV) valves are highly abnormal. They do not resemble separate mitral and tricuspid valves, and are therefore generally called right and left AV valves. Because of the absence of the septum to which the tricuspid valve would normally attach, the AV valves in an AVSD are attached only around the perimeter of the heart. Their function is impaired and there is usually some degree of regurgitation. AVSDs vary in size and, as the name suggests, can straddle both the atria and the ventricles. There may be a larger ventricular component than an atrial component, and vice versa. Perhaps somewhat confusingly, an AVSD may have no ventricular component at all. It is called a 'partial AVSD' rather than an ASD. This is because the term ASD is reserved for defects higher up, in the secundum portion of the atrial septum. In an ASD, the AV valves are not involved and so are generally normal. In a partial AVSD, there is no atrial septum below it and the valves are abnormal.

AVSDs do not close spontaneously and are likely to need surgical intervention. Surgery may or may not involve a repair of the AV valves depending on how regurgitant they are.

In addition to the ECG abnormalities found in a VSD, the ECG in an AVSD shows extreme left axis deviation above the horizontal ('superior axis') due to inferior displacement of the AV node.

Pulmonary stenosis (PS)

This term covers narrowing of the pulmonary valve and/or artery/arteries. Most children are asymptomatic, but if the stenosis is very severe, exertional tiredness and syncope may occur. Stenosis of the branch pulmonary arteries is a common cause of a murmur in the newborn period.

Signs include a prominent cardiac impulse due to right ventricular hypertrophy, and a harsh ejection-type systolic murmur at the upper left sternal border, which is occasionally loud enough to be associated with a thrill at the same location.

The ECG may show right ventricular hypertrophy, and the chest X-ray may show cardiomegaly with post-stenotic dilatation of the pulmonary artery.

Echocardiography may show thickening of the pulmonary valve leaflets and turbulence in the pulmonary artery and/or its branches depending on the location of the stenosis. The velocity of blood flow through the stenotic segment will indicate its severity. Severe stenosis is an indication for intervention – usually transcatheter balloon dilatation; surgical valvotomy is reserved for those who are unsuitable for balloon dilatation or in whom balloon dilatation is unsuccessful.

Coarctation of the aorta

This is a narrowing of the aorta usually at the distal part of the aortic arch where the ductus arteriosus is joined to it. Coarctation can present at any age depending on how severe it is. In severe coarctation in the newborn period, infants may present with cardiovascular collapse when the duct closes, with symptoms such as breathlessness, lethargy, sweating, tachycardia and poor perfusion. In this case, the distal aorta is supplied only by blood from the pulmonary artery. Infants, children and even adults with milder degrees of coarctation may present with asymptomatic hypertension or an incidental finding of difficulty palpating the femoral pulses during a medical examination.

Specific signs on examination are cyanosis in the lower half of the body (only in severe neonatal coarctation – can be confirmed by finding lower oxygen saturation on the feet compared to the hands), inability or difficulty palpating the femoral pulse, a prominent cardiac impulse due to left ventricular hypertrophy, and an ejection-type systolic or continuous murmur between the scapulae. The blood pressure may be a lot higher in the arms than the legs.

An ECG may show left ventricular hypertrophy and a chest X-ray may show cardiomegaly. There may be 'rib notching' (a scalloped appearance to the surface of the ribs) secondary to the development of collateral arteries close to the ribs in older children.

An echocardiogram will show the extent and location of the coarctation turbulent blood flow at the site of narrowing, and increased diastolic flow due to the backlog of blood in the aortic arch in systole working its way through the narrow segment in diastole.

In severe neonatal coarctation the duct must be kept open with a prostaglandin infusion until more definitive treatment can be given in a cardiac surgical unit. Most coarctations will require intervention either with balloon dilatation or with surgical resection. The narrow segment is removed and either an

end-to-end anastomosis is performed or a flap is formed from the proximal part of the left subclavian artery and used to bridge the gap. In the latter case the left brachial and radial pulses may disappear or become difficult to palpate.

Severe neonatal coarctation resembles another aortic arch abnormality – **interruption of the aortic arch**. This is a complete gap in the aortic arch, which is bridged only by the duct. When the duct closes in the first few days of life, the infant can become severely ill. There is usually a VSD present, which is usually repaired at the same time. Treatment is similar to that for neonatal coarctation. This abnormality is associated with microdeletions of the long arm of chromosome 22 (22q11) – which may give rise to DiGeorge syndrome with absent thymus, palatal defects, immunodeficiency and hypoparathyroidism.

Aortic stenosis

This refers to a narrowing below, at or above the aortic valve. The presentation depends on its severity. Severe (or 'critical') aortic stenosis may present in the neonatal period with severe shock when the duct closes. Mild aortic stenosis may be asymptomatic and present only as an incidentally found heart murmur. Intermediate degrees of stenosis may present as exertional tiredness, chest pain and/or syncope. In these infants and children, the pulses may be difficult to feel generally, there may be a prominent cardiac impulse due to left ventricular hypertrophy, and an ejection-type systolic murmur at the upper right sternal border in keeping with the anatomical position of the aortic valve. The murmur may radiate to the neck and be palpable as a thrill in the suprasternal notch.

An ECG may show left ventricular hypertrophy, and a chest X-ray may show cardiomegaly with post-stenotic dilatation of the ascending aorta visible as a bulge to the right in the upper mediastinum.

An echocardiogram will show turbulent blood flow through the narrow segment with left ventricular hypertrophy in significant stenosis. The velocity of blood flow through the stenosis will indicate its severity.

Severe aortic stenosis will need intervention; some patients will benefit from balloon dilatation but surgical treatment is frequently required, either to open the valve or to replace it.

Cyanotic heart lesions

Cyanosis develops when the concentration of deoxygenated haemoglobin in the skin circulation rises to about 3–5 g/dL. Peripheral cyanosis generally results from slow blood flow in capillary beds of the skin as result of vasoconstriction, for example in cold environments or sepsis. Central cyanosis, on the other hand, results from either inadequate oxygenation (e.g. severe respiratory disease) or from deoxygenated blood getting into the systemic arterial circulation. The flow of deoxygenated blood into the systemic circulation is called a 'right-to-left' shunt and this is what occurs in cyanotic heart lesions.

In addition, cyanosis may be worsened in some of these conditions by inadequate delivery of oxygenated blood into the systemic circulation, or by inadequate blood flow to the lungs.

Many of these lesions are becoming easier to detect on antenatal ultrasound scans – especially if there is a discrepancy in the size of the heart chambers. If it is anticipated that the abnormality will cause problems in the immediate newborn period, the birth can then be planned in a cardiac surgical unit.

Tetralogy of Fallot

There are four abnormalities that occur together in this condition; hence the name 'tetralogy':

- Large VSD.
- Overriding aorta – this describes the aortic valve placed on top of the VSD such that it straddles both right and left ventricles.
- Right ventricular outflow tract (RVOT) obstruction – this means a narrowing, usually of the pulmonary valve and the muscular infundibulum of the right ventricle just below the pulmonary valve.
- Right ventricular hypertrophy.

The combination of these abnormalities results in deoxygenated blood from the right ventricle flowing through the VSD into the aorta, rather than passing through the stenosed RVOT (Figure 36.7).

The presentation of this condition depends very much on the severity of the RVOT stenosis. If very severe, the condition may present in the newborn period with severe cyanosis. In this case, the pulmonary blood flow may be dependent on the patency of the duct. Newborns may also present with mild cyanosis detected incidentally on measuring their oxygen saturation. In most cases, however, presentation is later with the discovery of a heart murmur. When detected the condition can be treated early but if left untreated, older infants may develop 'hypercyanotic episodes' or 'spells'. These are caused by the infundibular stenosis suddenly worsening. These are now fortunately rare, as they can result in myocardial and cerebral ischaemia. Symptoms are severe cyanosis, irritability, ischaemic pain, breathlessness resulting from acidosis and squatting (which increases the vascular resistance through the arteries of the legs and help to divert blood into the pulmonary artery rather than the aorta).

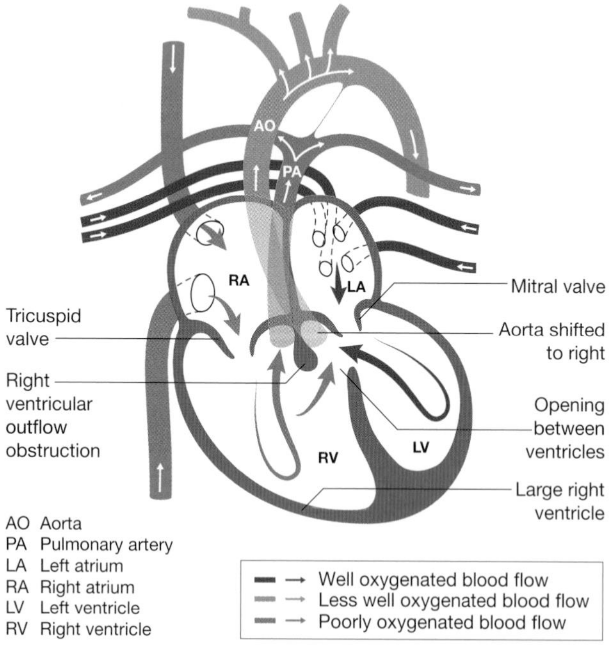

Clubbing of the fingernails may occur in older children due to chronic cyanosis, and an ejection systolic murmur will be heard at the upper left sternal border. The VSD tends not to cause a murmur.

The ECG shows signs of right ventricular hypertrophy, and the chest X-ray shows reduced pulmonary vascular markings consistent with reduced lung blood flow ('pulmonary oligaemia') and an upturned apex to the heart.

Echocardiography will demonstrate the abnormalities very well; the most important assessment is gauging the severity of the stenosis of the RVOT as well as the pulmonary arteries, which can all be small.

Treatment

If the child has a hypercyanotic spell, treatment is symptomatic until the spell resolves. Pain relief, sedation, occasionally intubation and muscle relaxation, and correction of acidosis may all need to be given. Propranolol may also help reduce the infundibular stenosis. Newborn infants with severe RVOT stenosis may be too small and immature for a complete repair, in which case the pulmonary circulation is protected by giving prostaglandin intravenously to keep the duct open. This may then be followed by the creation of a tube between the subclavian artery and the pulmonary artery to bypass the obstructed RVOT (Blalock–Taussig shunt) and secure the lung blood flow. A full repair an then be performed a few months later consisting of closing the VSD and enlarging the infundibulum and the pulmonary artery.

Transposition of the great arteries (TGA)

In this condition the arterial connections of the heart are abnormal, resulting from the failure of normal septation of the truncus arteriosus in fetal life, with failure of the new aorta and pulmonary arteries to connect to the correct ventricle. In TGA the aorta arises from the right ventricle and the pulmonary artery arises from the left ventricle. This creates a situation where there are two separate circulations – from the right ventricle to the body and back again, and from the left ventricle to the lungs and back again. This is not an arrangement

Tricuspid valve

Right ventricular outflow obstruction

Mitral valve

Aorta shifted to right

Opening between ventricles

Large right ventricle

AO Aorta
PA Pulmonary artery
LA Left atrium
RA Right atrium
LV Left ventricle
RV Right ventricle

━━ → Well oxygenated blood flow
━━ → Less well oxygenated blood flow
━━ → Poorly oxygenated blood flow

Figure 36.7 The heart of tetralogy of Fallot.

that is compatible with life unless blood returning from the lungs can somehow get into the systemic circulation, and the venous return from the body can somehow get into the lungs.

TGA presents in the first few days of life with severe cyanosis that worsens as the duct and the foramen ovale close. There may also be an associated VSD. If these channels that connect the two circulations can be kept open the infant can survive so that a full repair can be performed.

Except for cyanosis, the cardiovascular examination may be normal. The ECG is generally normal. The chest X-ray, however, usually shows a narrow mediastinum (as the great arteries have lost their usual spiral configuration and arise vertically from the heart with the pulmonary artery lying directly behind the aorta). The heart may have the appearance of an 'egg on its side'.

An echocardiogram is able to differentiate the aorta from the pulmonary artery by its appearance, and shows the aorta lying anterior and parallel to the pulmonary artery. Their origins from the wrong ventricles can be demonstrated. The patency of the ductus arteriosus and the foramen ovale can also be checked.

The PDA will enable blood that has returned from the systemic veins to be directed to the lungs. This can be kept open with an infusion of prostaglandin. The blood flow across the patent foramen ovale (PFO) will enable oxygenated blood in the left atrium to be directed to the right atrium then the right ventricle and then the systemic circulation. The PFO is therefore crucial to the oxygenation of the body. If the PFO is thought to be small, or 'restrictive', this can be enlarged by performing a 'septostomy'. A cardiac catheter is passed through the femoral or umbilical vein, into the right atrium and across the PFO into the left atrium. A balloon at the end of the catheter is then inflated and pulled back forcefully through the PFO causing the atrial septum to tear thus allowing more of the oxygenated blood in the left atrium to flow into the systemic side of the circulation.

A full corrective surgical procedure to restore the normal connections can then be performed within the first few weeks of life. This is called an 'arterial switch' procedure and involves disconnecting the aorta and the pulmonary arteries from their origins, then connecting them to the correct ventricles. The procedure also requires disconnecting and reconnecting the coronary arteries to the newly positioned aorta.

This operation did have high mortality when it was first introduced, but surgical mortality is now very low.

Total anomalous pulmonary venous connection

In this condition the pulmonary veins are connected to the right atrium rather than the left. The pulmonary veins come together and form a connection to one of the systemic veins – typically the superior vena cava, the coronary sinus or the hepatic vein. There is usually a PFO through which there is a right-to-left shunt causing cyanosis. The condition presents with breathlessness as the pulmonary venous pressure may be raised causing pulmonary congestion and oedema. Treatment is usually immediate surgical repair.

Tricuspid atresia

If the tricuspid valve has not formed at all, the right ventricle becomes small and non-functional. All the blood from the right atrium crosses the PFO into the left atrium, and the only way the lungs can receive blood is from the PDA. The condition presents with cyanosis in the newborn period and must be treated with prostaglandin to maintain ductal patency in the first instance. The blood flow to the lungs is then secured by the insertion of a Blalock–Taussig shunt. A full repair is not possible in this condition as the right ventricle is non-functional. The only way the cyanosis can be relieved is through the creation of a Fontan circulation. This involves disconnecting first the superior vena cava, and later the inferior vena cava, then connecting them both directly to the pulmonary artery. The pulmonary artery is separated from the heart. This means that the heart pumps blood to the systemic circulation as usual, but the blood flow around the pulmonary circulation is driven only by the systemic veins.

Hypoplastic left heart syndrome

In this condition, as the name implies, all the structures of the left side of the heart are abnormally formed. The mitral valve, left ventricle, aortic valve and ascending aorta are small and underdeveloped. The left ventricle cannot sustain the systemic circulation and most of the blood returning from the lungs into the left atrium will pass through the PFO into the right atrium. There is excess blood flow through the right side of the heart, which then flows through a PDA ('right-to-left shunt') into the systemic circulation. The condition presents in the neonatal period with cyanosis and shock as the duct closes. These babies can be severely ill and need a prostaglandin infusion to keep the duct open. In the past this condition was considered inoperable but in recent years, surgery has become a much more realistic option. The surgical approach involves a complex sequence of operations resulting in a Fontan circulation (see 'Tricuspid atresia' above) with the right ventricle pumping blood around the body and the systemic veins draining directly into the pulmonary artery.

Truncus arteriosus

Here the pulmonary arteries remain joined to the truncus arteriosus in embryonic life and there is complete failure of aorto-pulmonary septation. The end result is that there is one artery (truncus arteriosus) leaving the heart, which then gives rise to the pulmonary arteries (Figure 36.8). The truncus straddles the two ventricles between which there is a VSD. The condition presents with cyanosis (due to the flow of blood from

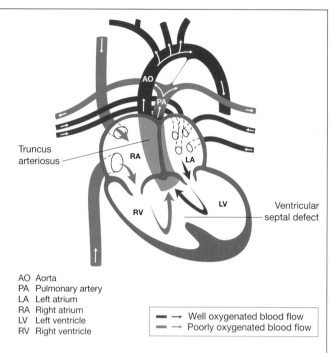

AO Aorta
PA Pulmonary artery
LA Left atrium
RA Right atrium
LV Left ventricle
RV Right ventricle

- - → Well oxygenated blood flow
- - → Poorly oxygenated blood flow

Figure 36.8 Truncus arteriosus.

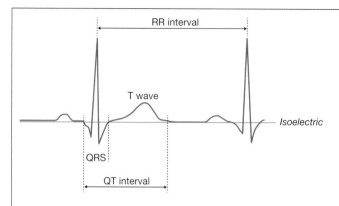

Figure 36.9 The ECG pattern of long QT syndrome.

the right ventricle into the truncus – a right-to-left shunt) and breathlessness (due to high blood flow into the pulmonary circulation from the truncus into the pulmonary arteries causing pulmonary congestion and oedema). The condition is strongly associated with chromosome 22q11 microdeletion. Treatment is with surgery in the neonatal period to join the pulmonary arteries to the right ventricle and close the VSD.

Arrhythmias

Supraventricular tachycardia

The most common arrhythmia in childhood is supraventricular tachycardia (SVT). It can occur at any age, including during fetal life. In the fetus it may cause cardiac failure and hydrops fetalis if it persists, and it is normally treated by giving the mother anti-arrhythmic treatment.

SVT can be asymptomatic especially in younger children, unless it is so prolonged that it causes heart failure. In older children rapid palpitations can occur with sudden onset and often, sudden resolution. Other symptoms are more unusual but can include dizziness, nausea, breathlessness and chest pain. SVT may be due to an accessory pathway (a pathway of conducting tissue between the atria and the ventricles in addition to the atrioventricular node) causing a re-entry circuit and uncontrolled activation of atria and ventricles.

The heart rate is typically between 250 and 300/min with narrow QRS complexes and no beat-to-beat variation on the ECG. The P wave tends to get obscured or may be inverted.

Treatment includes vagal manoeuvres (drinking a glass of cold drink quickly, performing a Valsalva manoeuvre, carotid sinus massage), intravenous adenosine, or, in severe cases, DC shock.

Preventative treatment can be tried with various anti-arrhythmic medications, but definitive treatment is now increasingly performed by destruction of the abnormal pathway by electrophysiological studies and radio frequency ablation. This can be performed via a cardiac catheter.

Long QT syndrome

Long QT syndrome is increasingly being recognised as a cause of lethal arrhythmias particularly *torsade de points*. It tends to run in families and is caused by ion channel abnormalities within the myocardium. A family history of sudden death at an early age may be elicited, and the ECG shows a corrected QT interval in excess of 0.45 seconds (Figure 36.9). The corrected QT (QTc) interval is the QT corrected for heart rate (RR interval). It can be calculated using Bazett's formula:

$$QTc = QT/\sqrt{RR} \text{ interval}$$

The condition may be exacerbated or caused by certain drugs that prolong the QT interval such as macrolide antibiotics, antifungal agents and antipsychotic agents. Treatment with anti-arrhythmic medication and an implantable defibrillator may be indicated.

Congenital complete heart block

There is a well-known association between congenital complete heart block (CCHB) and maternal systemic lupus erythematosis. Usually this is detected incidentally by finding a bradycardia, but symptoms may include reduced exercise tolerance and syncope. The ECG shows complete dissociation between the P waves and the QRS complexes. Treatment is with pacemaker insertion if symptomatic or if there is severe bradycardia.

The innocent heart murmur

Whilst many of the conditions described above may give rise to a heart murmur, most children who are found to have a heart murmur are not symptomatic, and the murmur is not a sign of any abnormality at all. In these children the murmur is called an 'innocent murmur'. It may also be called a 'flow' murmur or a 'physiological' murmur. Innocent heart murmurs may arise from structures within the heart or its major vessels. Well over 50% of children may have a heart murmur at any one time, and it is a common reason for children to be referred to specialists. The following are examples of innocent heart murmurs:

Still's murmur

This is best heard between the apex and the left lower sternal border typically in slim preschool children. It is a soft, smooth, ejection systolic murmur. It has a peculiar musical quality and tends to get louder on lying flat. It is not clear which heart structures give rise to the murmur.

Venous hum

This is a noise generated by turbulent flow in the venous confluence of the major veins draining into the superior vena cava at the base of the neck and the infraclavicular area at both sides of the upper sternum. It can be heard most easily with the child sitting or standing upright. It usually disappears completely, or becomes much softer, with the child lying flat – this is due to the increase in the size of the lumen of the large veins when lying flat. It is continuous (present throughout systole and diastole) and therefore may be confused with a PDA. There is some systolic accentuation.

Aortic and pulmonary flow murmurs

These are ejection murmurs produced at the aortic and pulmonary valves by the blood flow through these structures. They are heard in the relevant areas of the precordium and may warrant further investigation given the difficulty in distinguishing them from pathological lesions of these valves.

Branch pulmonary artery stenosis

This is a common but innocent murmur in babies, whose branch pulmonary arteries have not yet grown in proportion to the increased flow in them that occurs from birth. The murmur is an ejection systolic murmur heard best in the axillae and at the back of the chest, and may continue into diastole. This usually disappears by the age of 12 to 18 months.

Diagnosis of innocent murmurs

This can be difficult, and there is a tendency to investigate all murmurs regardless of clinical features. Nevertheless the diagnosis may still be made without any investigations if the clinical features are obvious. All innocent murmurs tend to be louder during high-output states such as anaemia, fever and acute illness, so it is always worth reviewing the child again when these have resolved before undertaking further investigation (Box 36.1).

> ## Box 36.1 Features of innocent heart murmurs
>
> - Soft
> - Systolic, or continuous
> - Asymptomatic
> - Not accompanied by other abnormal cardiovascular abnormalities
> - Variable over time
> - Variable with postural change
> - Not associated with abnormality on investigation

Clinical case

Case investigations

This infant has presented at around the time that significant left-to-right shunt lesions cause symptoms. Such lesions are often not symptomatic at birth as the pulmonary vascular resistance is still high. This means that the right ventricular and pulmonary artery pressures are also high so there is little difference between right and left sides 'driving' blood flow across the left-to-right shunt.

The history of drinking only small amounts of milk is typical of a lesion causing breathlessness; feeding is the most demanding activity this infant would undertake at this age. As breathing is more difficult due to the increased pulmonary blood flow, the congestion of the lungs and the development of pulmonary oedema, she is getting tired after only a small volume of milk has been taken. The poor weight gain results from both the restricted intake and the increased metabolic demand imposed by the added work of breathing, and the undernourished appearance of the baby is consistent with this.

Her capillary refill time is at the upper limit of normal – this implies vasoconstriction. Assuming the environment is

SUMMARY

warm, this is due to vasoconstriction due to the release of catecholamine in response to the reduced output of the heart. The ease with which the femoral pulse can be palpated suggests that the lesion may be a patent ductus arteriosus. With this lesion there is diastolic flow of blood out of the aorta into the pulmonary artery, thus reducing the diastolic pressure. The systolic pulsation of the artery therefore becomes easier to palpate as the difference between the systolic and diastolic pressure (the 'pulse pressure') is increased.

The heart rate is higher than the normal resting heart rate at this age and this again suggests that there is an excess of catecholamine release as a result of low cardiac output.

In left-to-right shunts the pulmonary blood flow is increased. This increases the pulmonary vascular resistance and increases pulmonary arterial pressure. This in turn leads to right ventricular hypertrophy. Consequently the right ventricle may not be able to relax fully during diastole and the left atrial pressure may rise. This causes the systemic venous pressure to rise and this in turn causes enlargement of the liver, which has a rich blood supply and is easily palpable in the abdomen of a baby when enlarged.

The hypertrophied right ventricle in combination with the tachycardia causes a prominent cardiac impulse on palpation of the precordium. The pulmonary valve tends to snap shut more forcefully due to the higher pressure in the pulmonary artery, leading to a loud second heart sound.

Finally, the murmur heard is consistent with that of a patent ductus arteriosus (PDA); it is heard loudest high up at the left sternal border and is present throughout the cardiac cycle, as the pressure in the aorta still exceeds that of the pulmonary artery in both systole and diastole. The blood flow is usually quite high velocity and turbulent in a PDA as it is driven by the aortic pressure and the jet is directed anteriorly into the pulmonary artery. The murmur is therefore loud, harsh and continuous.

Case conclusion

The diagnosis is a PDA. It requires surgical closure at an age that allows the surgery to be undertaken safely and in time to prevent the onset of pulmonary hypertension. In most cases closure can be achieved with a cardiac catheter by inserting an occlusion device within the PDA to block the flow of blood through it.

Key learning points

- The majority of heart problems in childhood result from congenital, structural heart lesions, which may present at any age depending on their severity and how they affect the function of the heart.

- Understanding the physiology of each abnormality helps us understand how they present.
- Acquired heart diseases are uncommon in the paediatric age group but these can be serious conditions.

 Now visit **www.wileyessential.com/humandevelopment** to test yourself on this chapter.

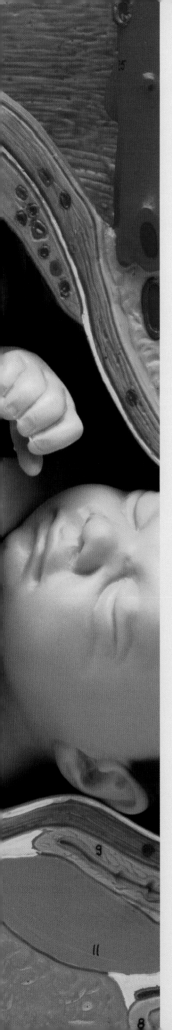

CHAPTER 37
Metabolic and endocrine disorders

Shabeena Webster

Case

Megan is a 4-week-old female infant born to non-consanguineous parents. She presents with a 2-day history of refusal of feeds, persistent vomiting, loose stools, excessive crying and anuria since 12 hours. She was delivered normally with a birthweight of 3.5 kg at full term without any antenatal or postnatal complications. She is exclusively breastfed and has three elder siblings with no significant medical history other than that they are all recovering from viral gastroenteritis over the preceding week.

On examination, she has a temperature of 35.6°C, she has a dry mouth, skin that has lost its elasticity, a depressed fontanelle and muscle wasting. She has clitoromegaly but no other abnormality of the genitalia. She weighs 3.1 kg. The rest of the systemic examination is normal. Subsequent biochemical investigations reveal hyponatraemia, hyperkalaemia and hypochloraemia.

Learning outcomes

- You should be able to recognise the signs and symptoms of common and less common endocrine diseases and metabolic disorders, and recommend appropriate treatment plans.

- You should be able to describe the causes of diabetes, differentiate between type 1 and type 2 diabetes, and describe the management of both types.

Essential Human Development, First Edition. Edited by Samuel Webster, Geraint Morris and Euan Kevelighan
© 2018 John Wiley & Sons, Ltd. Published 2018 by John Wiley & Sons, Ltd.

Introduction to endocrinology

In this chapter the basic physiology and pathology of hormone disorders will be discussed. The hypothalamo-pituitary axis (Figure 37.1) plays a key role in the regulation of the endocrine system. The hypothalamus is situated directly above the pituitary gland and has connections both to the cerebral cortex and pituitary. Functionally, it controls the endocrine system via the secretion of several hormones: corticotrophin-releasing hormone (CRH), thyrotropin-releasing hormone (TRH), gonadotrophin-releasing hormone (GnRH) and growth hormone-releasing hormone (GHRH). These act on the pituitary gland to regulate the production of several essential hormones. Somatostatin and dopamine are also released from the hypothalamus.

The pituitary gland lies within the sella turcica and consists of two lobes. Functionally, it connects signals from feedback mechanisms from the hypothalamus to the various peripheral endocrine organs. Under the control of the hypothalamic hormones, the anterior pituitary produces six main hormones:

- growth hormone (GH);
- thyroid-stimulating hormone (TSH);
- adrenocorticotrophin (ACTH);
- luteinising hormone (LH);
- follicle-stimulating hormone (FSH); and
- prolactin (PRL).

The posterior lobe of the pituitary releases antidiuretic hormone, vasopressin and oxytocin.

Obesity

Obesity is an important and increasing public health issue, and in the UK approximately 20% of children and adolescents are obese. Obesity is an important risk factor for later

Table 37.1 Causes of obesity.	
Endocrine causes	**Genetic causes**
• Hypothyroidism • Cushing's syndrome/disease • Growth hormone deficiency • Pseudohypoparathyroidism • Polycystic ovarian syndrome • Acquired hypothalamic injury, i.e. CNS tumour	• Prader–Willi syndrome • Bardet–Biedl syndrome • Monogenic causes, i.e. leptin deficiency

life-threatening diseases including type 2 diabetes, hypertension, cardiovascular disease and cancer. The definition of obesity is an increased central fat mass that is quantified using the body mass index (BMI), calculated by the weight (in kg) divided by the square of the patient's height (in metres). A BMI between the 91st and 98th centile is classified as overweight, and a BMI above the 98th centile is classified as obese.

Obesity is idiopathic in 95% of cases and has multifactorial causation, including a genetic predisposition, an increasingly sedentary lifestyle and a trend towards increasing consumption of high-energy foods. Pathological conditions resulting in obesity include genetic and endocrine causes and are listed in Table 37.1.

Evaluation and investigations

In the evaluation of obesity a detailed clinical and family history is essential, and features such as birthweight, feeding habits, growth pattern, physical activity and comorbidities must be assessed. In the family history features of obesity, diabetes and cardiovascular disease are important. Significant comorbid conditions to be aware of include: psychological issues (especially low self-esteem or depression), ENT or respiratory

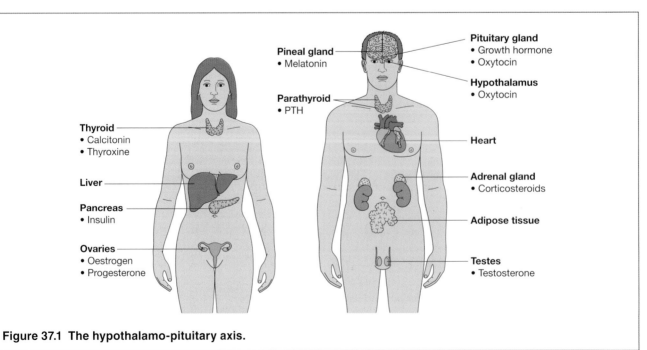

Figure 37.1 The hypothalamo-pituitary axis.

pathology (such as obstructive sleep apnoea), orthopaedic problems (slipped femoral epiphysis or osteoarthritis) and metabolic issues (principally impaired glucose tolerance or type 2 diabetes, hypertension and polycystic ovarian syndrome).

The investigation of obesity may include an oral glucose tolerance test (OGTT), a thyroid function test, a liver function test, determination of cortisol levels and a fasting lipid profile.

The management of obesity is difficult, but is best done through a multidisciplinary approach based on making significant changes to the patient's nutritional intake and lifestyle. Behaviour modifications and family therapy have also shown positive effects whilst medication and bariatric surgery are rarely required.

Diabetes mellitus

The incidence of diabetes has increased steadily and has a prevalence of around two cases per 1000 children. Diabetes in children is almost exclusively insulin-dependent (type 1) diabetes although the rate of non-insulin-dependent (type 2) is increasing due to the increasing rates of childhood obesity.

- Insulin-dependent (type 1) diabetes: This is an autoimmune disorder characterised by T-cell-mediated destruction and progressive loss of pancreatic B cells resulting in insulin deficiency.
- Non-insulin-dependent (type 2) diabetes: This is a multifactorial condition in which the balance between insulin secretion and insulin sensitivity is impaired, with a relative insulin insufficiency unable to overcome an underlying high tissue insulin resistance (Figure 37.2).

Insulin-dependent (type 1) diabetes

Aetiology

Type 1 diabetes is thought to be caused by the interaction of genetic predisposition and environmental precipitants. The co-twins of children with type 1 diabetes and children whose parents have type 1 diabetes all have an increased risk of the disease. Studies have shown an association between human leucocyte antigen (HLA) classes DR3 or DR4 and an increased risk of developing type 1 diabetes.

Pathophysiology

Insulin-dependent diabetes is a chronic autoimmune condition characterised by the development of autoantibodies against specific pancreatic B cell antigens. This causes T-cell activation, inflammation and pancreatic B cell destruction resulting in the characteristic insulin deficiency.

Clinical features

Diabetes is uncommon before the age of 1 year and reaches a peak incidence between 12 and 13 years, more commonly occurring at the onset of puberty. The clinical features include

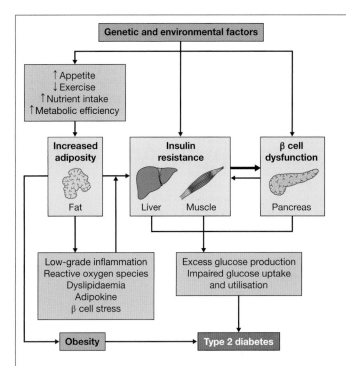

Figure 37.2 Factors that can cause type 2 diabetes. (Source: C.J. Bailey, BMJ (2011, p.342). Reproduced with permission of BMJ Publishing Ltd.)

polyuria, polydipsia and weight loss. Less common presenting features include skin infection, typically with *Candida*, and other persistent infections.

Uncommonly, children can present with the life-threatening complication of diabetic ketoacidosis (DKA). The symptoms of DKA include vomiting, dehydration, abdominal pain, a characteristic smell of ketones on the breath and hyperventilation due to acidosis. If untreated, continued deterioration leads to hypovolaemic shock, drowsiness and coma, which can be fatal.

Diagnosis of diabetes

A typical history and single blood glucose level measurement above 11.1 mmol/L will establish a diagnosis without the need of additional investigations such as an oral glucose tolerance test in childhood.

A blood glucose level greater than 11.1 mmol/L taken 2 hours after an oral glucose tolerance test, glycosuria and ketonuria, or a fasting blood glucose of greater than 7.0 mmol/L are also diagnostic indicators. Raised glycosylated haemoglobin (Hb A1C) levels can also be a helpful marker of persistently raised glucose levels.

Initial management

Most children who present as a new case of diabetes will be clinically stable, are able to eat and drink, and can be managed with subcutaneous insulin. The management of these patients can be entirely outpatient-based once the initial diagnosis is made. Children who present as an emergency with DKA require urgent admission and aggressive treatment with intravenous fluids and infusion of insulin.

Children and the parents of children with newly diagnosed diabetes will require intensive education based around the following important areas:

- Understanding of the basic pathophysiology of diabetes.
- Dietary changes, including carbohydrate counting and healthy eating.
- The injection of insulin; techniques and sites.
- Prevention of DKA.
- Monitoring, including blood glucose, urine glucose and ketones.
- The recognition and treatment of hypoglycaemia.

Families also require contact information for the multidisciplinary diabetic team, typically consisting of a paediatrician, a specialist nurse, a dietician, a clinical psychologist and a social worker.

Liaison with school and the primary care team is essential, as is coordination with the adult diabetic services at the time of transition from paediatric care. Information and contact numbers for support groups locally and nationally, such as Diabetes UK, are also a great source of help to many families with a child with diabetes.

Insulin administration

Insulin is a protein consisting of two peptide chains linked by two sulphide bonds. It is available for the treatment of diabetes in short-, intermediate- and long-acting formulations. There are also a number of preparations with premixed amounts of short- and intermediate-acting insulin.

Insulin is given by injection using a variety of 'pen and needle' devices. It is injected into the subcutaneous tissues of the upper arm, anterolateral upper thighs, buttocks and abdomen. Rotation of the injection site to prevent the complications of lipohypertrophy or lipoatrophy is essential.

The amount of insulin a child requires varies with age and can range from 0.5 IU/kg/day in infants to 1–2 IU/kg/day in adolescents. Long-acting insulin is usually given in the morning for younger children and in the evening with older children. Short-acting insulin is typically given three times a day around mealtimes. Although this varies significantly, the regime of injections is chosen depending on the ease of administration and effectiveness for the individual child. Some patients choose a continuous subcutaneous infusion of insulin via a pump device. Other common regimens include two or three dose mixes of short- and rapid-acting insulin plus an intermediate-acting insulin. The amount of insulin administered at mealtimes can be matched to the amount of carbohydrate consumed, a method known as 'carb counting'.

In the initial period after diagnosis there is often a so-called 'honeymoon' period where the insulin requirement of the child appears to be minimal. This is due to residual pancreatic function and is usually short lived.

Diet

The diet of a child with diabetes needs to be well controlled and adapted to the patient's insulin regime, with the overall goals of optimising metabolic control, reducing the risk of long-term complications from the disease and maintaining normal growth parameters. Food is required to avoid hypoglycaemia as well as to provide nutrition. The diet should be high in fibre with a high proportion of complex carbohydrates, which is essential to ensuring the release of steady levels of glucose into the circulation.

Blood glucose monitoring and management

Initially, blood glucose levels may need to be frequently checked until the body has adjusted to the new routine. Patients are encouraged to keep a diary of blood glucose measurements and to aim to maintain levels as near as possible to normal (4–6 mmol/L). The avoidance of hypoglycaemic episodes is important whilst an effective and tolerable treatment regime is established. In very young children it may be preferable to use urine glucose testing rather than subject the child to frequent distressing capillary glucose tests. Adherence to monitoring and compliance can be assessed through the measurement of glycosylated haemoglobin (Hb A1c), reflecting the level of glucose control over the previous 6 weeks.

Sick day management

During illnesses and in periods of increased physiological stress the insulin requirements of a child significantly increase. Counterintuitively, despite the reduced oral intake of food and fluids that is common during coincident illness, insulin treatment must be continued at all times and occasionally needs to be increased. Closer monitoring of urinary or blood glucose and ketones to prevent gross hyperglycaemia is essential during intercurrent illnesses and can help to avoid DKA.

Diabetic ketoacidosis (DKA)

Illness or other periods of heightened physiological stress result in increases in levels of stress hormones, including cortisol and catecholamines. These stress response hormones counter-regulate the effect of insulin, resulting in a relative increase in insulin requirements. If patients and caregivers are unaware of this physiological response the intuitive reaction to the typical poor appetite during illness or stress is to cut insulin doses to match the decreased oral intake, compounding the acute relative insulin deficiency.

The result of an acute relative shortage of circulating insulin is increased blood glucose levels, resulting in hyperosmolality and an increase in lipolysis as a compensatory metabolic response to decreased cellular glucose uptake, resulting in ketonaemia and metabolic acidosis. The outcome is an osmotic diuresis, dehydration, loss of electrolytes, acidosis and ketonaemia, which can result in ileus, nausea and vomiting. If untreated continued deterioration leads to hypovolaemic shock, drowsiness and coma. These patients need urgent hospital admission for careful correction of dehydration and electrolyte imbalances with intravenous fluids, and correction of the underlying metabolic disturbance with intravenous infusion of insulin.

Long-term management

The objective of the longer term management of patients with diabetes is normal growth and development, maintenance of a normal home and school life, and good diabetic control by encouraging the child to take control of their disease over time, so reducing the risk of long-term complications.

Adolescence and puberty are a particularly challenging stage in the management of children with diabetes. The rapid growth spurt and normal psychological changes of adolescence frequently cause disruption in previously stable disease control. Poorly controlled diabetes can delay sexual maturation and social stigma is commonly associated with the administration of insulin. These factors can result in impaired body image. Close involvement of the multidisciplinary team and parents in every aspect of day-to-day life can also be an issue for a teenager as they become more autonomous and make decisions for themselves. In these circumstances liaison with a child psychiatrist or psychologist may be helpful. It may also be helpful for the multidisciplinary team to set clear short-term goals fully involving the patient in key decisions. Key aspects to successful management during this period are ongoing education and the gradual development in the adolescent of self-reliance and the longer-term self-management of their condition.

The prevention of long-term complications

Long-term complications of poorly controlled diabetes mellitus can be divided into microvascular and macrovascular complications. Damage to small blood vessels results in retinopathy, nephropathy and peripheral neuropathy. The less common macrovascular complications include hypertension and coronary heart disease, which are unusual in the paediatric age group.

A multidisciplinary approach is essential, with focus on the encouragement of maintaining a healthy diet and appropriate blood glucose testing with good documentation in order to monitor control. As mentioned above, measuring the levels of Hb A1c helps to monitor control over the previous 6 weeks. Annual clinical review includes an assessment of growth and pubertal development, blood pressure measurement, screening for microalbuminuria, and an ophthalmological examination to screen for retinopathy or cataract formation, which although rare should be checked for. The feet should be examined and assessed for the development of peripheral neuropathy, and foot injuries and infections should be treated early. As diabetes is associated with other autoimmune conditions, others illnesses that should be screened for include thyroid disease and coeliac disease.

Type 2 diabetes mellitus

This condition is not an autoimmune disease, but has a strong genetic link thought to be polygenic in nature. Significant risk factors include obesity, family history, ethnic origin, polycystic ovary disease and a history of being small for gestational age. The condition may present as incidentally discovered hyperglycaemia through to the symptoms and signs of type 1 diabetes as described above, although DKA is rare as a presentation.

The management of type 2 diabetes is based on the same multidisciplinary approach as described above, focusing on lifestyle and nutritional education in mild cases. If this fails, oral hypoglycaemic medication with metformin or even insulin may be required.

Hypoglycaemia

Children may become symptomatic if blood glucose levels fall below 4 mmol/L. Symptoms may vary from abdominal pain and hunger to sweatiness and dizziness, and if left untreated this may progress to seizures or coma, and can even be fatal.

Severe hypoglycaemia is defined as a plasma glucose level of less then 2.6 mmol/L. Symptoms include sweating, pallor, irritability, seizures and coma. If left untreated the neurological sequelae may be permanent, and in the long term may include epilepsy, learning delay and microcephaly. Infants especially have a high energy requirement and because they have low glucose reserves from gluconeogenesis, and poor glycogenesis, they should not be starved for more than 4 hours. This can occur clinically, for example preoperatively, or in real-life situations such as when an infant has been on a long car journey. If the cause of hypoglycaemia is uncertain a screen should be conducted to look for specific triggers. A hypoglycaemic 'screen' includes formal assessment of blood glucose, growth hormone, cortisol, insulin C peptide levels, fatty acids, acetoacetate, β-hydroxybutyrate (ketone bodies), glycerol, branched-chain amino acids, lactate, pyruvate, and assessment of the urine for the presence of carnitine.

Fasting causes of hypoglycaemia

Hypoglycaemia with insulin excess

This can include excess exogenous insulin, persistent hypoglycaemic hyperinsulinism of infancy or an insulinoma. Other causes include ingestion of sulphonylurea medication, autoimmune diseases and Beckwith syndrome.

Hypoglycaemia without hyperinsulinaemia

Causes include liver disease, ketotic hypoglycaemia of childhood, inborn errors of metabolism such as glycogen storage disorders, hormonal deficiency such as decreased growth hormone, adrenocorticotrophic hormone (ACTH), Addison's disease or congenital adrenal hyperplasia (CAH).

Non-fasting causes of hypoglycaemia

Galactosaemia, leucine sensitivity, fructose intolerance, maternal diabetes, hormone deficiency and aspirin/alcohol poisoning all belong to this category of causes.

Treatment

Hypoglycaemia can be corrected with an intravenous infusion of 10% dextrose; alternatively, an intramuscular injection of glucagon can be used. Corticosteroids may be useful if hypopituitarism or hypoadrenalism is the cause, and diazoxide has a role in hyperinsulinism.

The thyroid gland

Thyrotropin-releasing hormone (TRH) is secreted by the hypothalamus, and in turn stimulates the production of thyroid-stimulating hormone (TSH, or thyrotropin) from the anterior pituitary gland. TSH, after release into the circulation from the pituitary, binds to specific receptors on thyroid cells, regulating the synthesis of thyroid hormones (Figure 37.3). These hormones are released into the bloodstream bound to thyroid-binding globulin, before being released as free hormone at target tissues.

Congenital hypothyroidism

After birth there is a surge in TSH. This is accompanied by a rise in thyroid hormones T3 (triiodothyronine) and T4 (thyroxine). Over the next week the TSH levels fall to the normal adult range. Of note, preterm infants may have a low level of T4 within the first few weeks after delivery, whilst the TSH level is in the normal range.

Clinical features

A child with hypothyroidism can present with a wide spectrum of clinical signs, including jaundice, macroglossia, umbilical hernia, wide posterior fontanelle or hypotonia (Figure 37.4). Alternatively, early symptoms may have a more subtle manifestation of altered metabolic regulation, and may include problems such as poor feeding, lethargy, sleepiness and constipation.

Hypothyroidism is a relatively common paediatric condition, occurring in approximately 1:4000 births, and is also one of the few preventable causes of severe learning difficulties.

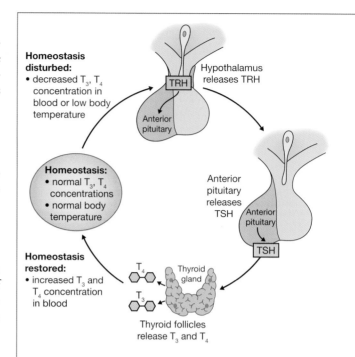

Figure 37.3 Regulation of thyroid hormones. T3, triiodothyronine; T4, thyroxine; TRH, thyrotropin-releasing hormone; TSH, thyroid-stimulating hormone.

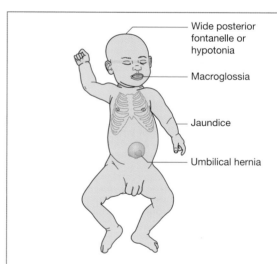

Figure 37.4 Features of hypothyroidism seen shortly after birth.

Causes include maldescent of the thyroid gland during development, or athyrosis as a result of failure of the lingual thyroid to descend during development and remaining as a lingual mass or thyroglossal cyst. Dyshormonogenesis, an inborn error of thyroid hormone synthesis, may be a common cause of hypothyroidism in particular ethnic groups. TSH deficiency can also be a result of panhypopituitarism, along with accompanying growth hormone and ACTH deficiency.

Diagnosis and management

Most children are identified via the newborn Guthrie (heel prick) screening test performed by midwives in the second week of life. A raised TSH level of greater than 10 mU/L is indicative of the condition, and treatment with lifelong oral levothyroxine is subsequently commenced within 3 weeks of age. Early treatment prevents learning difficulties.

Acquired hypothyroidism

Iodine is essential in the synthesis of thyroid hormones, and dietary deficiency is the most common cause of acquired hypothyroidism worldwide. Autoimmune conditions (e.g. Hashimoto's thyroiditis) are more common in the more developed Western world. Hypothyroidism can also be acquired following damage to the pituitary gland or hypothalamus, by diverse causes such as tumours, cranial surgery or radiotherapy.

In later childhood the signs of hypothyroidism include a goitre, obesity or short stature. Symptoms may present in the form of weight gain, decreased growth or delayed puberty, fatigue, cold intolerance or constipation.

Once biochemical abnormalities have been confirmed, oral hormone replacement can begin.

Hyperthyroidism

Graves' disease, an autoimmune thyroiditis secondary to the production of thyroid-stimulating antibodies (TSi), is the most common cause of hyperthyroidism.

Clinical features

Signs of hyperthyroidism include a diffusely enlarged thyroid gland, thyroid bruits, tachycardia, exophthalmos, and warm hands with fine tremor or restlessness. Symptoms may present as heat intolerance, anxiety, palpitations, weight loss, deteriorating school performance and behaviour, or rapid growth.

This condition is more common in girls than boys. Biochemically, the level(s) of T4 or/and T3 are elevated and TSH levels are low. The first-line treatment is usually with oral medication to block the overproduction of thyroid hormones using carbimazole or propylthiouracil. Beta-blockers can be used for symptom relief.

Many patients respond to a course of anti-thyroid hormone medication, although relapse occurs and usually requires definitive treatment typically with a small oral dose of radioactive iodine, which partially ablates the thyroid gland and reduces the production of thyroid hormones. Many patients may need subsequent oral thyroxine replacement following radioiodine treatment.

Neonatal hyperthyroidism can occur in infants of mothers with Graves' disease as thyroid-stimulating immunoglobulins can cross the placenta in utero. Urgent treatment is required as the infant is at risk of arrhythmias and heart failure.

Calcium homeostasis

Vitamin D is obtained from the diet and by synthesis in the skin when exposed to sunlight. Circulating vitamin D is metabolised in the liver to 25-hydroxyvitamin D_3, which is further hydroxylated in the kidney to the active form of 1,25-dihydroxyvitamin D_3 (Figure 37.5). Vitamin D mainly

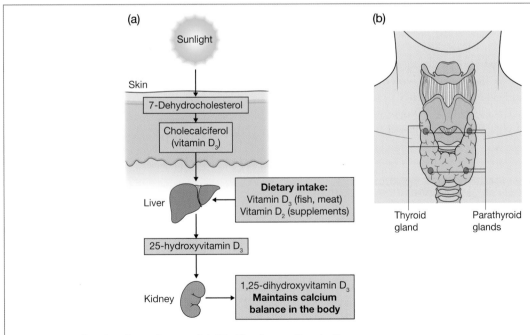

Figure 37.5 Synthesis pathway of 1,25-dihydroxyvitamin D_3.

acts to increase absorption from the diet of calcium and phosphate and maintain their blood plasma levels, and results in bone mineralisation.

Parathyroid hormone

The four parathyroid glands are found posterior to the thyroid gland and develop from the third and fourth pharyngeal pouches during embryogenesis. They function to maintain calcium levels by secreting parathyroid hormone (PTH) in response to low circulating levels of calcium. PTH increases the 1-hydroxylation of vitamin D resulting in increased renal calcium absorption, and also mobilises calcium and phosphate stored in bone.

Hypocalcaemia

In most cases, hypocalcaemia is due either to impaired kidney function, or to abnormalities in the vitamin D and PTH systems (Table 37.2). It typically presents in infants with jitteriness, vomiting, seizures and apnoeic episodes. In older children typical clinical features include neuromuscular irritability such as tetany, paraesthesiae and seizures, or cardiac conduction abnormalities such as long QT ECG changes or ventricular arrhythmias.

In order to diagnose hypocalcaemia biochemical markers need to be evaluated. The serum levels of calcium, phosphate, parathyroid hormone and vitamin D are the basic tests required. Once the diagnosis has been established treatment can begin, dependent on whether the cause is acute or chronic. In acute cases calcium supplements or possible infusions may be warranted, whereas in chronic cases calcium replacement may be supplemented by oral vitamin D replacement.

Rickets

Rickets is a disorder of the growing skeleton due to inadequate mineralisation of the bone at the epiphyseal growth plates. It may be due to calcium and vitamin D deficiency, or defects in vitamin D metabolism and action (vitamin D-dependent rickets types 1 and 2 respectively). Other causes include phosphate

deficiency such as renal tubular loss, Fanconi syndrome, renal tubular acidosis and nephrotoxic drug induction.

Clinical features include growth delay, bone pain, muscle weakness and skeletal deformities, namely swelling of the wrists, rachitic rosary (swelling of the costochondral joints around the sternum giving the impression of a ring of beads under the skin), bowing of the long bones (Figure 37.6), frontal bossing and craniotabes (an easily compressible skull bone that recoils back into shape when pressure is removed).

Hypercalcaemia

Causes of elevated serum calcium levels include Williams syndrome, idiopathic infantile hypercalcaemia, hyperparathyroidism, vitamin D intoxication and familial hypocalciuric hypercalcaemia. Other secondary causes include sarcoidosis, renal failure, hyperthyroidism, Addison's disease and thiazide diuretics.

Clinical features

Presentation may consist of non-specific pains, polyuria and polydipsia, depression, drowsiness and often constipation.

Parathyroid disorders

Hypoparathyroidism is rare. Parathyroid hormone is essential for the mobilisation of calcium from bone via osteoclasts and for the excretion of phosphate in the urine. Low serum

Table 37.2 Causes of hypocalcaemia.	
Infants	**Childhood**
• Prematurity	• Vitamin D deficiency
• Maternal vitamin D deficiency	• Hypoparathyroidism
• Maternal hyperparathyroidism	• Renal disease
• Hypomagnesaemia	
• High milk phosphate	
• Congenital hypoparathyroidism	

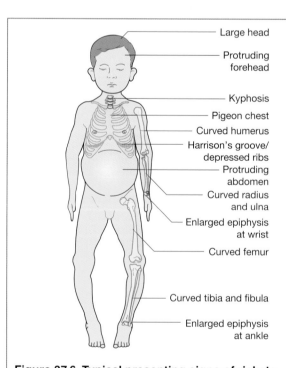

Figure 37.6 Typical presenting signs of rickets.

calcium, raised phosphate and normal alkaline phosphate levels suggest hypoparathyroidism. The hormone level itself is very low. In infants it is usually due to a congenital abnormality such as DiGeorge syndrome. In older children it can be associated with an autoimmune disorder such as Addison's disease. In **pseudohypoparathyroidism** there is end organ resistance to parathyroid hormone. Calcium and phosphate levels are abnormal but the PTH level can be normal. This condition is associated with short stature, obesity, subcutaneous nodules, short fourth metacarpal bones and mild learning difficulties.

Pseudopseudohypoparathryoidism has a similar phenotype but the biochemical markers are within normal limits.

Treatment of the hypocalcaemia, if symptomatic, is with intravenous calcium gluconate. Chronic hypocalcaemia is treated with oral supplements of vitamin D analogues and calcium. Urinary calcium excretion must be monitored to avoid hypercalciuria and associated nephrocalcinosis.

In contrast, **hyperparathyroidism** is uncommon in children. It may be caused primarily by pituitary adenoma or multiple endocrine neoplasia, or secondarily by rickets or renal failure.

Multiple endocrine neoplasias

Multiple endocrine neoplasias (MEN) are a family of endocrine neoplasia syndromes with autosomal dominant inheritance patterns. Genetic screening is available for this condition and can be subtyped as below:
- MEN type 1 is associated with hyperparathyroidism, pancreatic endocrine tumours (typically multifocal pancreatic islet cell tumours), pituitary adenomas and thyroid adenoma.
- MEN type 2 has two subtypes. Type 2a is associated with medullary thyroid cancer, phaeochromocytoma and parathyroid adenomas. Type 2b differs slightly in its association with medullary thyroid cancer, phaeochromocytoma and intestinal ganglioneuromas, marfanoid features and Hirschsprung's disease.

von Hippel–Lindau syndrome

Due to a mutation in the VHL gene located on chromosome 3, von Hippel–Lindau syndrome is characterised by retinal and CNS haemangioblastomas, phaeochromocytomas and renal cysts.

McCune–Albright syndrome is another closely associated condition. It is defined by its triad of clinical features:
- Hyperpigmented skin macules, classically on one side of the body with a 'coast of Maine' (i.e. jagged edge) appearance.
- Polyostotic fibrous dysplasia.
- Autonomous endocrine gland hyperfunction, particularly ovarian, thyroid, adrenal, pituitary and parathyroid organ involvement.

The adrenal gland

The adrenal gland is located adjacent to the upper pole of the kidney. The outer cortex synthesises steroid hormones and the inner medulla synthesises catecholamines.

The adrenal cortex can be divided into three zones:
- The zona glomerulosa on the outside, which produces aldosterone.
- The zona fasciculata, which secretes glucocorticoids.
- The zona reticularis, which secretes adrenal androgens, predominantly during puberty.

Adrenocortical insufficiency

Congenital adrenal hyperplasia (CAH) is the commonest non-iatrogenic cause of insufficient cortisol and mineralocorticoid secretion. Enzyme defects in the steroidogenic pathways lead to abnormal biosynthesis of cortisol, aldosterone and androgens.

Acquired adrenocortical insufficiency is rare in children. The most common cause is autoimmune Addison's disease, but adrenal damage can occur as a result of haemorrhage or infarction (e.g. during meningococcal septicaemia), adrenoleukodystrophy or tuberculosis. Insufficiency may also be secondary to hypopituitarism or hypothalamo-pituitary-adrenal axis suppression following long-term corticosteroid therapy.

Presentation

CAH can present in the newborn by causing virilisation of female genitalia due to excess androgen synthesis in the adrenal glands. Newborn girls may have ambiguous genitalia, with clitoromegaly giving the appearance of a penis with hypospadias and a scrotum, but with no palpable testes. Such cases usually prompt investigation for adrenal hormone abnormalities. In the absence of genital abnormality, the child with CAH may present acutely with dehydration, a salt-losing crisis, hypotension and/or hypoglycaemia. There may be excess pigmentation on a background of chronic ill health. Pigmentation of gums, scars and skin creases is said to be a classical feature.

Diagnosis

Diagnosis is made through biochemical findings of hyponatraemia, hyperkalaemia and metabolic acidosis with associated hypoglycaemia. Cortisol is low and the plasma ACTH is high, except in pituitary causes. An ACTH or Synacthen test shows cortisol levels remaining low and a normal response excludes adrenocortical insufficiency. In CAH elevated 17-OH, 21-OH and increased adrenocorticosteroid metabolites in the urine help to confirm diagnosis.

Management

The management of an adrenal crisis involves intravenous saline, glucose and hydrocortisone. The long-term treatment is with glucocorticoid and mineralocorticoid replacement. During illness or surgery (i.e. periods of heightened physiological stress) the dose of glucocorticoid may need to be increased as much as three-fold. Parents are shown how to inject hydrocortisone intramuscularly for use in an emergency situation.

Cushing's syndrome

Glucocorticoid excess can result from long-term steroid administration, and may cause growth suppression and clinical features of Cushing's syndrome (Figure 37.7). Other causes include a pituitary adenoma or an ectopic ACTH-producing tumour. The midnight concentration of cortisol is abnormally high and the normal diurnal variation can be lost. Adrenal tumours are identified on neuroimaging and can be treated by radiotherapy and surgery.

Hypopituitarism

Growth hormone deficiency can be inherited due to mutations in the genes regulating growth or can be caused by developmental defects in the pituitary gland. Mutations in pituitary transcription factor genes are associated with septo-optic

dysplasia (optic nerve hypoplasia, absent septum pellucidum, pituitary gland hypoplasia).

Hypopituitarism can be acquired due to intracranial tumours and/or their surgical treatment, pituitary irradiation, infection or infarction.

History and examination, accompanied by basal hormone levels – LH:FSH ratio, thyroid function tests, cortisol, insulin-like growth factor 1 (IGF-1) and prolactin levels – will usually lead to a diagnosis. Further investigations include X-rays to calculate bone age, and an MRI scan of the brain. These are followed by treatment, which typically involves hormone replacement and management of the underlying cause.

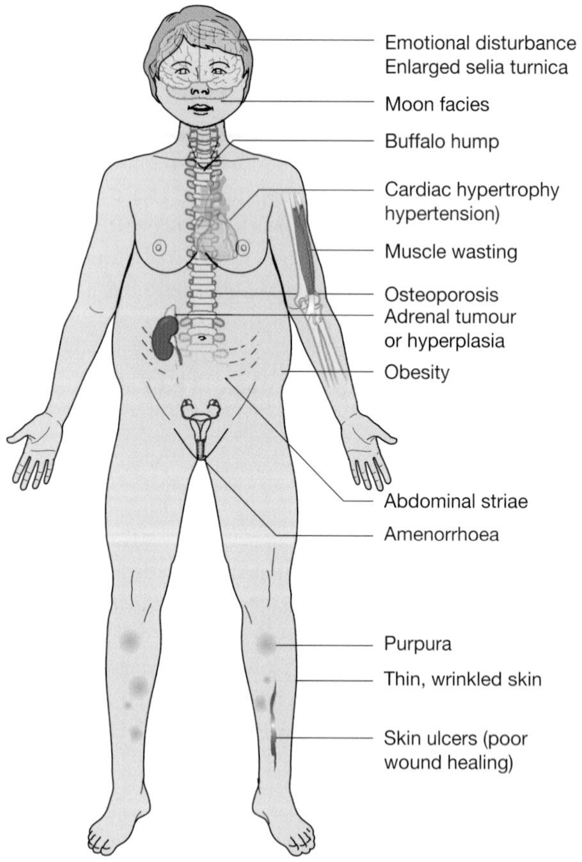

Diabetes insipidus

Diabetes insipidus (DI) is defined as the inappropriate passage of dilute urine of less than 300 mOsm/L due to deficient antidiuretic hormone (ADH), also known as vasopressin, or end organ resistance (nephrogenic DI). Cranial DI usually results from mechanical damage or infiltrative disease. Nephrogenic DI is usually inherited (Table 37.3). The presentation of DI includes polydipsia, polyuria and dehydration.

In order to obtain a diagnosis, measurement of 24-hour urinary volume and paired serum and urine osmolality levels are required. If blood hypertonicity (osmolality >300 mOsm/L) with inappropriate urine hypotonicity is the result of investigations, this is followed up by performing a water deprivation test with the administration of antidiuretic hormone to distinguish the subtype of DI. Once this is established the appropriate treatment can be provided. For cranial DI the ADH analogue desmopressin is administered. In the case of nephrogenic DI the underlying cause needs to be sought and corrected alongside the temporary administration of diuretics.

Figure 37.7 Clinical features of Cushing's syndrome.

Emotional disturbance
Enlarged selia turnica

Moon facies

Buffalo hump

Cardiac hypertrophy hypertension)

Muscle wasting

Osteoporosis
Adrenal tumour or hyperplasia

Obesity

Abdominal striae

Amenorrhoea

Purpura

Thin, wrinkled skin

Skin ulcers (poor wound healing)

Table 37.3 Classifications of diabetes insipidus (DI).

Cranial DI	Nephrogenic DI
Inherited/familial: • AD, AR, XLR, Wolfram syndrome	Inherited/familial: • AD, AR, XLR
Congenital: • Midline craniofacial defects • Holoprosencephaly	
Acquired: • Intracranial tumours • Traumatic brain injury • Infiltrative/inflammation • CNS infection	Acquired: • Idiopathic • Drugs (lithium, cisplatin) • Metabolic (hypercalcaemia)

AD, autosomal dominant; AR, autosomal recessive; XLR, X-linked recessive.

Syndrome of inappropriate ADH

The syndrome of inappropriate antidiuretic hormone (ADH) secretion results in hypotonic hyponatraemia and impaired urinary dilution. There may be elevated levels of ADH, or it may be inadequately suppressed.

Causes include brain trauma and tumours, infections and common respiratory conditions such as asthma.

Diagnosis can be obtained through biochemical findings of hyponatraemia, hypotonic plasma (osmolality <270 mOsm/L), reduced urine output, renal sodium loss (urinary sodium >20 mmol/L) and increased ADH levels. Management consists of fluid restriction and treating the underlying cause.

Metabolic disease

Inborn errors of metabolism

Inborn errors of metabolism are individually rare but collectively represent a very important group of conditions. Most are due to mutations in genes responsible for coding enzyme proteins. When enzymes are missing or deficient, metabolites may accumulate and produce toxic effects on a wide range of tissues and organ systems. Most, though by no means all, are inherited in an autosomal recessive manner. Many have serious complications and may be treated effectively if suspected early. In the neonatal period infants with metabolic disorders may become severely unwell with poor feeding and failure to thrive, jaundice or hepatomegaly, seizures or vomiting. There may be a severe metabolic acidosis, ketosis or raised ammonia levels. Older children may present with similar symptoms with learning difficulties and abnormal growth or facial appearance. There may be a positive family history or previous unexplained deaths in early life.

There is a large spectrum of clinical presentations. Some may have a mild and transient abnormality, whereas others may have a devastating and progressive course resulting in early death. It is important to have a low index of suspicion in any child who presents with the above symptoms and if there are any other unusual symptoms. In many cases, diagnosis can be established or suspected from requesting a basic set of metabolic investigations, which may include:

- Blood tests for glucose, urea, electrolytes, liver function, lactate, ammonia, ketones, free fatty acids and blood spot acylcarnitine profile.
- Urine tests for organic and amino acids, ketones, glycosaminoglycans.

Disorders of amino acid metabolism

Phenylketonuria

Phenylketonuria can be due to a deficiency of the enzyme phenylalanine hydroxylase or of its biopterin cofactor. Untreated it is associated with developmental delay, learning difficulties and seizures. Those affected typically have a musty odour due to the metabolite phenylacetic acid, fair hair, blue eyes and eczema. The Guthrie test, a heel-prick blood spot screening test performed in the first week of life, is designed to detect this abnormality so that treatment can be started early. Treatment thereafter is with restriction of dietary phenylalanine for at least 10 years. The outlook is excellent if detected early.

Homocystinuria

Homocystinuria is caused by a deficiency of cystothionine synthase resulting in increased levels of homocysteine in blood plasma and urine. The child presents with failure to thrive, developmental delay and ectopia lentis (dislocation of the lens of the eye). This progresses to psychiatric disorders and convulsions. Skeletal manifestations resemble Marfan's syndrome. The treatment may include administering the coenzyme pyridoxine or a low-methionine diet supplemented with cysteine.

Albinism

Albinism reflects a defect in melanin. It may be oculocutaneous, ocular or partial dependent on the distribution of depigmentation in the eye or skin. Lack of pigment in the eye results in pendular nystagmus and photophobia. Treatment consists of correcting refractive errors and limiting exposure to direct sunlight.

Tyrosinaemia

Tyrosinaemia refers to a group of conditions with severity ranging from mild and transient to life-threatening. It is mainly caused by deficiency of the enzyme fumarylacetoacetase, an enzyme involved in the catabolism of tyrosine. The resultant accumulation of toxic metabolites results in kidney and liver damage. Treatment involves specific medical therapy, treating complications and a low-tyrosine and low-phenylalanine diet.

Disorders of organic acid metabolism

Disorders of organic acid metabolism involve deficiencies of enzymes in the catabolic pathways of several amino acids including leucine, isoleucine, valine and threonine. They cause maple syrup urine disease, methylmalonic acidaemia and propionic acidaemia to name a few. Maple syrup urine disease presents in the neonatal period with severe metabolic acidosis, hypoglycaemia and seizures. The increased excretion of the branched-chain amino acids gives a characteristic smell to the urine. Delay in diagnosis leads to learning difficulties and neurological dysfunction.

Organic acidaemias are managed through the restriction of dietary protein, with specific therapy to treat metabolic disturbances such as acidosis and hyperammonaemia.

Urea cycle disorders

Urea cycle disorders (Box 37.1) tend to cause neonatal encephalopathies due to high blood ammonia. Ornithine transcarbamylase deficiency is an X-linked recessive disorder but most have autosomal recessive inheritance patterns.

Diagnosis involves determination of plasma and urine amino acid profiles, and treatment is with dietary provision of essential amino acids and protein restriction to suppress ammonia formation.

Disorders of carbohydrate metabolism

Galactosaemia

Galactosaemia is a rare, recessively inherited disorder resulting from galactose-1-phosphate uridylyltransferase (GALT) deficiency. This may result in hypoglycaemia, and infants may also present with vomiting, jaundice and hepatomegaly, which when untreated progresses to chronic liver failure, cataracts and developmental delay. Management of this condition is with a lactose- and galactose-free diet.

Glycogen storage disorders

Glycogen storage disorders (GSDs) are mostly inherited in recessive patterns and have specific enzyme defects that prevent mobilisation of glucose from glycogen (Table 37.4). Clinical features include muscle weakness, cardiomyopathy, hepatomegaly and hypoglycaemia, with long-term complications including hyperlipidaemia and the development of hepatic adenomas and cardiovascular disease. The outlook varies from mild problems to life-limiting disease, depending on the specific enzyme deficiency. Treatment involves dietary measures to maintain normal blood glucose levels, with enzyme replacement and liver transplant in severe cases.

Lysosomal storage diseases

Mucopolysaccharidoses

Mucopolysaccharidosis results from deficiency in the lysosomal enzymes needed to break down glycosaminoglycans

Box 37.1 Urea cycle disorders

- *N*-acetylglutamate synthetase deficiency (NAGS)
- Carbamyl phosphate synthetase deficiency (CPS)
- Ornithine transcarbamylase deficiency (OTC)
- Argininosuccinic acid synthetase deficiency (AS)
- Argininosuccinase acid lyase deficiency (argininosuccinic aciduria; AL/ASA)
- Arginase deficiency (AL/ASA)

(GAGS). The accumulation of these GAGS progresses to tissue damage. Clinical features include neuropathy, developmental delay, visual loss, coarse features, short stature and valvular heart disease. Examples include Hurler syndrome, Hunter syndrome and Sanfilippo syndrome. All of these disorders are inherited in an autosomal fashion except Hunter syndrome, which is X linked.

Sphingolipidoses

Sphingolipidoses are a group of progressive peripheral and central nervous system diseases caused by the accumulation of lipid metabolites within the brain and other tissues. They are characterised by psychomotor retardation, myoclonus, weakness and spasticity. They include Fabry disease, Gaucher's disease, Tay–Sachs disease, gangliosidosis, Krabbe disease, Niemann–Pick disease and metachromatic leucodystrophy

Disorders of fatty acid oxidation

Deficiencies in the acyl-CoA dehydrogenase enzyme complex, in carnitine, or a defect in the carnitine transport process lead to disorders of fatty acid oxidation. Medium-chain acyl-CoA dehydrogenase deficiency (MCAD) is the most common condition. Clinical features consist of acute encephalopathies precipitated by prolonged fasts, hypoglycaemia and hepatomegaly.

The diagnosis is confirmed by biochemical assessment of urinary organic acid and plasma acylcarnitine profiles. Treatment involves carnitine supplements, a high-carbohydrate

Table 37.4 Glycogen storage disorders (GSDs).

GSD type	Enzyme defect	Tissue	Clinical features
I. von Gierke	Glucose-6-phosphatase	Liver	Poor growth, hypoglycaemia, hepatomegaly
II. Pompe	Lysosomal α-glucosidase	Liver, muscle	Cardiac failure, hypotonia
III. Cori	Glycogen debrancher	Liver, muscle	Poor growth, muscle weakness, hypoglycaemia
IV. Andersen	Glycogen branching	Liver, muscle	Liver failure, muscle weakness, poor growth
V. McCardle	Phosphorylase	Muscle	Muscle weakness, cramps

diet and avoidance of prolonged fasts. Provided treatment is started early, the outlook is good and the treatment relatively straightforward. Because of this, screening is now routinely undertaken in the UK as part of the Guthrie blood spot screening test.

Mitochondrial disorders

Mitochondrial disorders represent a wide range of conditions resulting from mitochondrial dysfunction. They cause abnormalities such as lactic acidosis, muscle weakness, hypotonia, poor growth, seizures and neurodevelopmental delay. They may be inherited either by mutations in nuclear DNA encoding mitochondrial functions, or by mutations in the mitochondrial DNA, which is inherited from the mother. Diagnosis may require a muscle biopsy. Examples include Leigh syndrome (encephalopathy, lactic acidosis, seizures, cardiomyopathy, hepatic and renal dysfunction) and Pearson syndrome (failure to thrive, lactic acidosis, sideroblastic anaemia, hypoparathyroidism and diabetes mellitus).

Peroxisomal disorders

Peroxisomal disorders result in defective lipid metabolism. Common features include neurodevelopmental delay, weakness, seizure, hepatic dysfunction, and impaired hearing and vision. Diagnosis is made with a liver biopsy, and analysis for very-long-chain fatty acid and phytanic acid abnormalities. Examples include Zellweger syndrome and infantile Refsum disease. Life expectancy is poor in these conditions.

Disorders of nucleotide metabolism

Disorders of nucleotide metabolism result from abnormalities in enzymes responsible for metabolism and removal of purine and pyrimidine components of amino acids and proteins.

Lesch–Nyhan syndrome, for example, is an X-linked recessive disorder with a deficiency in hypoxanthine-guanine phosphoribosyltransferase that leads to excessive accumulation of uric acid. Features include neurodevelopmental delay, self-mutilative behaviour, spastic cerebral palsy, choreoathetosis and renal stones.

Disorders of porphyrin metabolism

The porphyrins are the main precursors of haem, and an accumulation of porphyrins leads to tissue toxicity. Patients present with neurological and skin problems including seizure, neuropathy, psychosis, pain and light sensitivity. Precipitants include drugs (including the oral contraceptive pill and various antibiotics), foods or other chemicals. Porphyrin metabolite profiles in urine and stools are required for diagnosis.

Disorders of metal metabolism

Wilson's disease

Wilson's disease is an autosomal recessive disorder caused by a mutation in the *ATP7B* gene that encodes for a copper-transporting pump protein. An accumulation of hepatic copper leads to abnormalities that include liver dysfunction, neurological disturbance with similarities to parkinsonism, renal tubular acidosis, renal stones, cardiomyopathy and Kayser–Fleischer rings (dark rings that encircle the iris). Diagnosis is made by demonstrating low caeruloplasmin levels and increased urinary copper excretion. Treatment is with lifelong D-penicillamine to bind excess copper, and liver transplant if severe.

Menkes syndrome

Menkes syndrome is an X-linked recessive disorder whereby a mutation in a copper-transporting alpha peptide leads to a characteristic phenotype. Growth retardation, kinked sparse hair, cerebral and cerebellar degeneration leading to seizures and hypotonia are the main features. Low caeruplasmin and copper levels are diagnostic.

Haemochromatosis

Haemochromatosis is an iron overload disorder that is inherited in an autosomal recessive manner. It is caused by gene mutations that result in excess iron absorption.

The clinical features of haemochromatosis include hepatomegaly, splenomegaly, cirrhosis of the liver, hypermelanotic pigmentation of the skin, heart failure, arthritis, diabetes mellitus and hypopituitarism. Diagnostic markers are increased iron and ferritin levels, and diagnosis is confirmed with a liver biopsy. Treatment is by repeated phlebotomy.

Clinical case

Case investigations

The immediate medical treatment involves administering fluids and electrolytes intravenously to treat dehydration and to correct electrolyte disturbance. The suspicion here is of congenital adrenal hyperplasia (21-hydroxylase deficiency), as Megan has presented with severe fluid and salt loss with clitoromegaly. A serum 17-hydroxyprogesterone test showed elevated levels, confirming the diagnosis. Megan needs to be treated with fludrocortisone and hydrocortisone, which should improve her symptoms. Hormone replacement will be needed for the rest of her life. The deficiency of the enzyme 21-hydroxylase leads to cortisol deficiency and high levels of androgenic metabolites.

SUMMARY

These then cause clitoromegaly, which, in severe cases, may cause ambiguous genitalia.

Case conclusions

The diagnosis is congenital adrenal hyperplasia.

Key learning points

- The endocrine system has many functions including regulation of tissue function, development and growth of the body, metabolism, mood regulation and reproductive processes.
- Children with metabolic disorders can present at any age with single organ involvement or more generalised developmental delay. Early detection and treatment is vital to prevent the progression of the disease.

- The incidence of diabetes and obesity is increasing in the paediatric population, emphasising the need to educate families about healthy lifestyles in order to prevent complications previously typically seen in adult populations.

 Now visit **www.wileyessential.com/humandevelopment** to test yourself on this chapter.

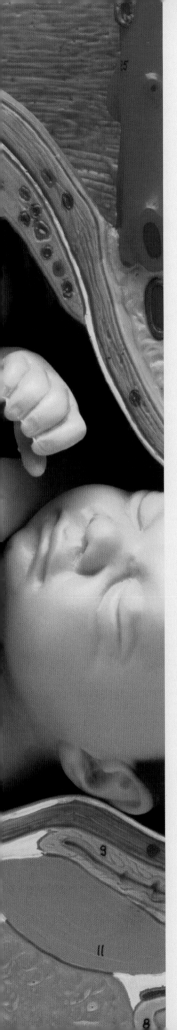

CHAPTER 38
Respiratory problems

Toni Williams

Case

A 7-year-old boy is referred to the children's assessment unit with a 3-day history of cough and coryza and a 24-hour history of worsening breathlessness and wheeze. Parents describe that Jack is usually well with no previous admissions. He had mild eczema as a baby and has had one prior episode of wheeze at 4 years of age. He lives at home with his parents and 8-year-old sister. There is a family history of atopy, with Jack's father suffering from hayfever and childhood asthma and Jack's sister having asthma. Both parents are smokers and there are no pets. On examination, Jack has a respiratory rate of 40/minute, heart rate of 138 beats per minute and oxygen saturations of 91% in air. He is unable to talk in sentences and you note subcostal and intercostal recessions on inspection of his chest. On auscultation there is widespread expiratory wheeze. The rest of his examination is normal and his growth is appropriate.

In view of his low oxygen saturations and respiratory distress Jack is admitted to the ward. He receives supplementary oxygen at 2 L/minute, which maintains his oxygen levels above 95%. He is given regular salbutamol by inhaler with spacer and commenced on a 3-day course of oral prednisolone. Jack responds well to these treatments and after 48 hours he is discharged home. Jack's parents are advised to give him salbutamol via a spacer if required and provided with smoking cessation advice.

Learning outcomes

- You should be able to recognise signs and symptoms of common respiratory disorders of childhood.

- You should be able to describe the causes of common respiratory disorders of childhood and recommend appropriate treatment options.

Essential Human Development, First Edition. Edited by Samuel Webster, Geraint Morris and Euan Kevelighan
© 2018 John Wiley & Sons, Ltd. Published 2018 by John Wiley & Sons, Ltd.

Introduction

Respiratory disorders are the most frequent causes of illness amongst children, accounting for around 30% of acute paediatric admissions.

Why children are different

It is important to realise that a child's respiratory system differs immensely from adults and this must be considered when evaluating a child with a possible respiratory illness.

- Children's airways are smaller; this means that they are more likely to become obstructed with foreign bodies, secretions and mucosal inflammation.
- Their respiratory muscles are relatively inefficient so they are more prone to becoming tired.
- A child's chest wall is more compliant and recesses more readily (e.g. intercostal and sternal recessions).

Assessment of the respiratory system in children

When assessing a child with possible respiratory disease it is important to consider whether they have respiratory distress. The child with a breathing problem may have symptoms of breathlessness with difficulty feeding and be too breathless to talk. They may have a wheeze or be sweating. On examination, there may be tachypnoea with chest recessions, use of accessory muscles and tachycardia (see Chapter 28).

Upper airway disorders

Upper respiratory tract infections

Upper respiratory tract infections (URTIs) are the most common infections seen in children and account for around 80% of all respiratory infections. These include the common cold, pharyngitis, tonsillitis, acute otitis media and sinusitis.

The common cold

This is an extremely common infection and children can have between five and eight colds per year. They are frequently caused by rhinoviruses, respiratory syncytial virus (RSV) and coronaviruses, and typically cause symptoms of sneezing, blocked nose and nasal discharge. Associated symptoms include headache, pyrexia, malaise and sore throat. The cold is a self-limiting condition requiring supportive measures with simple analgesics. There is no role for antibiotics.

Pharyngitis

Pharyngitis is usually viral in origin (adenoviruses, enteroviruses and rhinoviruses) and occasionally due to group A beta-haemolytic *Streptococcus* in the older child. There is inflammation of the pharynx and soft palate accompanied by cervical lymphadenopathy.

Tonsillitis

In tonsillitis there is acute inflammation of the tonsils, sometimes with a purulent exudate. Most episodes of tonsillitis are caused by viruses and especially in younger children. Bacterial tonsillitis (usually group A beta-haemolytic *Streptococcus*) accounts for up to one-third of tonsillitis cases. However, it is difficult to distinguish between a viral and bacterial cause clinically. Bacterial tonsillitis is more likely if there are systemic symptoms such as headache, abdominal pain and cervical lymphadenopathy with exudative tonsils. A throat swab can help identify the pathogen. Bacterial tonsillitis should be treated with antibiotics, with penicillin V as a first-line treatment. Severe cases may require hospital admission for intravenous fluids and antibiotics. Quinsy (peritonsillar abscess) can occur secondary to tonsillitis and requires surgical drainage. Infectious mononucleosis is caused by Epstein–Barr virus and can present in a similar way although this tends to have more marked malaise and may have splenomegaly. There can be associated hepatitis, and a blood count would show increased monocytes and lymphocytes. Amoxicillin, if given in the context of glandular fever, can cause a maculopapular rash.

Croup

Croup, or acute laryngotracheobronchitis, is the commonest cause of acute stridor in children and is a frequent cause of admission to A&E. It is caused by a viral infection, most commonly parainfluenza virus but also rhinovirus, influenza and RSV. The infection causes mucosal inflammation leading to oedema and increased secretions both of which result in narrowing of the subglottic area. Croup tends to occur from the age of 6 months to 6 years with peak incidence in the second year of life. The illness begins with a low-grade pyrexia and coryza (acute nasal mucous membrane inflammation) and then the child develops a barking, 'seal-like' cough with hoarse voice and harsh stridor – this is a high-pitched, usually inspiratory noise caused by turbulent airflow in the upper airway.

Symptoms are typically worse at night. In most children the upper airway obstruction is mild, evident by stridor and recessions, which are present only on exertion or when the child is upset. However, in some cases symptoms can be much more severe, with marked recessions and biphasic stridor. It is important to disturb the child with severe acute stridor as little as possible to minimise symptoms. The throat should not be examined since this could provoke laryngeal spasm and complete airway obstruction.

Children under 12 months (with a narrower airway) and those with an underlying abnormality of the upper airway are particularly at risk of severe croup.

Treatment of croup is with steroids, either orally as dexamethasone or nebulised as budesonide. In the child with very severe symptoms nebulised adrenaline can provide transient improvement. However, symptoms can rebound within an hour and so the child must be closely monitored. Most children with croup can be managed at home with parental advice, but those with severe symptoms or the very young will require admission and observation. A few (<1%) may have symptoms severe enough to need intubation and ventilation

Epiglottitis

Epiglottitis is usually caused by infection of the epiglottis by *Haemophilus influenzae* b and is now rare since the introduction of the Hib vaccination. It usually occurs in children between the ages of 1 and 7 years. Children present acutely with rapidly progressing upper airway obstruction. In contrast to croup the child usually has a very high fever and looks unwell. On examination there is stridor, a muffled cough with tachypnoea and tracheal tug. The child sits upright with open mouth and extended neck. There is drooling since swallowing of secretions is difficult. If epiglottitis is suspected a senior anaesthetist and ENT surgeon should be involved immediately. It is important not to upset the child until the airway is secure. At intubation the characteristic is a cherry red epiglottis. Management involves intubation and ventilation and intravenous antibiotics (usually cefotaxime).

Bacterial tracheitis (pseudomembranous croup)

This is a rare condition that is similar to viral croup. The child typically looks unwell with a high fever but symptoms usually develop less acutely than epiglottitis over 2–3 days. On examination, there is hoarseness of the voice, quiet cough and a soft stridor. The child is at risk of developing a rapidly progressive upper airways obstruction and may require intubation and ventilation. Bacterial tracheitis is usually caused by *Staphylococcus aureus*, and treatment with intravenous antibiotics is required.

Spasmodic croup

In spasmodic croup there are recurrent episodes of sudden onset of inspiratory stridor with barking cough. Symptoms begin at night and subside quickly.

Wheeze in childhood

Wheeze is a polyphonic wheeze noise that primarily occurs on expiration. Causes of wheeze in childhood include:
- viral-induced wheeze;
- non-atopic asthma;
- atopic asthma;
- recurrent feed aspiration;
- inhaled foreign body;
- cystic fibrosis;
- anaphylaxis;
- congenital abnormality of lung, airway or heart.

Viral-induced wheeze

Intermittent acute episodes of wheezing are seen in preschool children between the ages of 1 and 4 years in association with viral infections. There is no link with atopy but a history of prematurity or maternal smoking is associated with an increased risk of viral-induced wheeze. The condition is managed in the same way as acute asthma, with bronchodilators given via a spacer, and steroids for moderate to severe attacks. Most will grow out of the condition by the age of 5 years.

Asthma

Asthma is a chronic condition affecting up to 1 in 10 children. It is characterised by reversible bronchoconstriction, mucosal oedema and excessive mucus production. The severity of disease can vary considerably, and children can suffer with acute exacerbations and chronic symptoms of cough and wheeze. In some children 'triggers' can be identified such as animal dander, house dust mites and viral infections.

Asthma is known as an atopic (IgE-mediated) condition, and children with asthma may have a history of other atopic conditions. Other features of atopy are eczema, allergic rhinitis and allergic conjunctivitis. The child may have a raised IgE level and positive skin prick test to common allergens. There is frequently a positive family history.

Clinical features

The diagnosis of asthma can be difficult to make especially in young children, and the diagnosis is often retrospective. Common reported symptoms are wheeze, difficulty in breathing, cough and chest tightness. Parents may use the term 'wheeze' for a variety of noises such as stridor or noisy breathing so it is important to clarify what they mean by 'wheeze'. The British Thoracic Society guidelines advise that the diagnosis of asthma is more likely if the above symptoms are frequent and recurrent, worse at night and in early morning, or worse after 'triggers' such as exercise, exposure to pets, cold or damp air, or emotions. Children have a high likelihood of asthma if they have a history of an atopic disorder or a family history of atopy. Their symptoms and lung function improve with appropriate therapy.

Management of asthma

The management of asthma should be considered in terms of both long-term treatments and interventions of acute exacerbations.

Chronic management
Children with asthma should be seen every 3–6 months to monitor interval symptoms, frequency of exacerbations and compliance with prescribed treatment. The aim is to provide control, described as no daytime symptoms, no nocturnal

Table 38.1 British Thoracic Society (BTS) guidelines on chronic management of asthma. See the full guidelines on the BTS website (www.brit-thoracic.org.uk) for more information.

Symptoms	Treatment
Mild intermittent asthma	Inhaled, short-acting β_2-agonist as needed
Regular preventer therapy	Inhaled steroid or leukotriene receptor antagonist
Add-on therapy	Inhaled steroid and leukotriene receptor antagonist. If the child is under 2 years old consider referring to respiratory paediatrician
Persistent poor control	Refer to respiratory paediatrician

symptoms, no exacerbations, no use of reliever inhaler, no limitations in activity and minimal side effects from medication (Table 38.1). The British Thoracic Society guidelines are available from www.brit-thoracic.org.uk.

Important questions to address include:

- Presence of nocturnal cough (number of nights per week).
- Frequency of interval symptoms (e.g. cough/wheeze) and triggers (exercise, animal dander, etc.).
- Number of exacerbations (triggers, severity, hospital admission, courses of steroids).
- Number of school days missed.
- Number of times reliever medication required.
- Compliance with preventative medications.
- Household smokers.

The British Thoracic Society (BTS) advocates a step-wise approach to management, and children should be on the least medication possible to control symptoms. Treatment should be escalated if necessary but should be reduced when possible with gradual reduction in medications if symptoms have been stable for 3 months.

Peak expiratory flow rate (PEFR)

PEFR can be a useful measure for the severity of asthma, and most children over the age of 5 years can use a peak flow meter.

The child places their mouth firmly around the mouthpiece of the meter and, following inspiration, blows out as hard and fast as they can. The best of three successive readings is usually taken and can be compared to the best expected value based on the child's height. Families should be encouraged to keep a diary of their peak flow readings, which can be examined at clinic visits as a guide to control. In those with poor control there is greater day-to-day variability in PEFR, and values are lower in the morning than the evening. PEFR can also be used to assess response to treatment, with an expected increase of more than 10–15% following a bronchodilator. Peak flow can also be useful during an acute attack.

Acute management

Acute exacerbations of asthma frequently occur secondary to a trigger such as a viral infection. The child is breathless, often with a cough and wheeze. On examination, there is a tachycardia with tachypnoea, and there may be signs of respiratory distress with recessions. On auscultation there is frequently widespread wheeze heard bilaterally. In a severe exacerbation air entry can be reduced and wheeze therefore may not be appreciated.

The British Thoracic Society has produced guidelines for the management of asthma (2011). It considers management in terms of the severity of the exacerbation (Tables 38.1–38.3): moderate, severe and life-threatening. Children with acute symptoms require admission to hospital if symptoms have not improved after 10 puffs of a β2-agonist.

Inhalers

There are a variety of different devices available for administration of medications used acutely and in long-term treatments. The most suitable inhaler will depend on the medication prescribed and the age of the child. The device must also be acceptable for the patient. Spacer devices improve deposition of the drug in the airways, but are bulky to carry around and may not be acceptable to some patients (Figure 38.1). A key principle is that the technique of the child should be adequate to ensure good delivery of the drug into the lungs. It is therefore very important that the technique is explained and checked by a health professional skilled in the use of inhalers.

Table 38.2 Assessment of acute exacerbation of asthma.

Mild/moderate	Severe	Life-threatening
• Oxygen saturations >92% • PEFR >50% of predicted or best value • No clinical features of severe asthma	• Too breathless to talk or feed • Use of accessory neck muscles • Oxygen saturations <92% • Respiratory rate >50/min (2–5 years) or >30/min (over 5 years) • Heart rate >130/min (2–5years) or >120/min (over 5 years) • PEFR <50% of predicted or best	• Silent chest • Poor respiratory effort • Altered consciousness • Cyanosis • Oxygen saturation <92% • PEFR <33% of predicted or best

Source: Adapted from British Thoracic Society guidelines (www.brit-thoracic.org.uk).
PEFR, peak expiratory flow rate.

Table 38.3 Management of acute exacerbation of asthma.

Moderate	Severe	Life-threatening
• Short-acting β₂-agonist via spacer, 2–4 puffs, increasing by 2 puffs every 2 min to maximum of 10 puffs • Consider oral prednisolone Reassess within 1 hour	• Oxygen to achieve normal saturations • Short-acting β₂-agonist 10 puffs via spacer or nebulised (2.5–5 mg salbutamol, 5–10 mg terbutaline) • Oral prednisolone (20 mg if 2–5years, 30–40 mg if >5years) or i.v. hydrocortisone (4 mg/kg) • Nebulised ipratropium bromide (250 µg) if poor response • Repeat bronchodilators every 20–30 min as needed	• Oxygen to achieve normal saturations • Nebulised β₂-agonist plus ipratropium bromide • i.v. hydrocortisone • Repeat bronchodilators every 20–30 min

REGULAR ASSESSMENT

• Respiratory rate, heart rate, oxygen saturation, PEFR

If responding	If not responding
• Continue bronchodilators 1–4-hourly as required • Continue oral prednisolone for 3 days • Discharge when stable on 4-hourly treatment	• Transfer to high-dependency or intensive care • Consider chest X-ray and blood gas • i.v. salbutamol or aminophylline (caution if on regular theophyllines) • Bolus of i.v. magnesium sulphate

Source: Adapted from British Thoracic Society guidelines (www.brit-thoracic.org.uk).
PEFR, peak expiratory flow rate.

Bronchiolitis

Bronchiolitis is the most common lower respiratory infection seen in infancy, with peak incidence between 3 and 6 months. It tends to occur in seasonal peaks, most commonly between October and March. The causative organism is respiratory syncytial virus (RSV) in 75–80% of cases, with other viruses such as human metapneumovirus, rhinovirus, adenovirus and influenza viruses being largely responsible for the remaining cases.

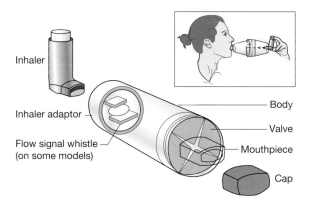

Figure 38.1 Inhaler with spacer device.

Clinical features

The first symptom of bronchiolitis is typically rhinorrhoea followed by a dry cough and worsening breathlessness. Affected infants often present with feeding difficulties secondary to breathlessness. Young infants are at risk of recurrent episodes of apnoea (stopping breathing). The natural history of bronchiolitis is for symptoms to worsen over the first 2–5 days with the cough persisting for 2 weeks or more. The characteristic findings on examination are dry cough, tachypnoea, tachycardia, subcostal and intercostal recessions, and cyanosis or pallor. On auscultation the hallmark findings are fine inspiratory crackles often with wheeze.

Those at increased risk of severe disease include infants:

- less than 6 weeks of age;
- born prematurely;
- with chronic lung disease (CLD), especially CLD of prematurity;
- with congenital heart disease;
- with neuromuscular abnormalities;
- with immunodeficiency.

Diagnosis of bronchiolitis

The diagnosis of bronchiolitis is clinical and based on the described history and classical examination findings. Pulse oximetry should be performed in all cases. The causative virus can be isolated from nasopharyngeal secretions with rapid antigen testing. This confirms the diagnosis and can help with cohorting. Further investigations are not indicated in uncomplicated bronchiolitis. A chest X-ray would show hyperinflation with small airways obstruction and air trapping.

Management

Management of bronchiolitis is supportive. Oxygen should be administered in infants with oxygen saturations of less than 92% in air. This can be delivered via nasal cannula or headbox. Feeding may need to be supported with nasogastric feeding, and a small number of infants require intravenous fluids. Respiratory support such as continuous positive airway pressure (CPAP) and mechanical ventilation is required in those with severe disease. There is no role for antibiotics, steroids or bronchodilators in the treatment of bronchiolitis.

In 50% of infants recovery from the acute illness occurs within 2 weeks. However, 50% will have recurrent episodes of wheeze over the next 3–5 years. Rarely, bronchiolitis obliterans can occur with permanent destruction of the airways.

Those at high risk of severe bronchiolitis can be given palivizumab (a monoclonal antibody) as prophylaxis against severe disease. This is given by monthly intramuscular injection during the bronchiolitis season and reduces the need for hospitalisation.

Pneumonia

Pneumonia (lower respiratory tract infection or chest infection) is a common childhood infection that can occur at any age but is commoner in younger children.

Causes

A number of different viruses and bacteria are responsible for pneumonia but the causative agent varies according to the age of the patient.

In the newborn period pneumonia may be caused by organisms from the maternal genital tract, most commonly group B *Streptococcus*, but others include *Escherichia coli*, *Listeria monocytogenes*, *Klebsiella pneumoniae*, *Chlamydia trachomatis* and cytomegalovirus (CMV).

In infants and children less than 5 years old pneumonia is most often caused by viruses, with RSV being the most common. Other viruses isolated include influenza, parainfluenza and adenovirus. *Streptococcus pneumoniae* is the commonest bacterium to cause pneumonia, accounting for up to 40% of children hospitalised, with *Haemophilus influenzae*, *Strep. pyogenes* and more rarely *Staphylococcus aureus* implicated in other cases.

In children over 5 years old *Mycoplasma pneumoniae*, *Streptococcus pneumoniae* and *Chlamydia pneumoniae* are the most frequent causative organisms.

The pathogen is isolated in less than 50% of cases and it is difficult to distinguish between viral and bacteria pneumonia clinically. Tuberculosis should be considered in all age groups.

Clinical features

Children may present with a cough, fever and difficulty breathing. Presentation can be non-specific especially in younger children, with lethargy, poor feeding and being generally unwell as signs. Pleuritic irritation may cause neck pain or stiffness, abdominal pain or chest pain. It is not unusual for a child thought to have an acute abdomen and possible appendicitis to turn out to have pneumonia. On assessment the child is often flushed with a temperature above 38.5°C. Tachypnoea is the commonest clinical finding but there may be other signs of respiratory distress such as grunting, nasal flaring, and subcostal and intercostal recessions. On auscultation over the site of infection you may hear crackles, reduced breath sounds or bronchial breathing. These signs may not be apparent in all cases.

Investigations

Pneumonia is a clinical diagnosis, and current British Thoracic Society guidelines suggest that investigations may not be necessary in a child thought to have an uncomplicated community acquired pneumonia that does not require admission to hospital. If performed, a chest X-ray may show patchy consolidation suggesting bronchopneumonia or a lobar pneumonia with a more localised consolidation. A lobar pneumonia is characteristic of *Streptococcus pneumoniae* but otherwise a chest X-ray is unable to distinguish between viral and bacterial infection. Nasopharyngeal aspirates can be taken to look for a viral cause, and if the child has a productive cough then sputum can be sent for microscopy, culture and sensitivities.

Treatment

All children suspected of having pneumonia should be treated with antibiotics since it is difficult to distinguish between a viral and bacterial cause clinically. In most cases oral amoxicillin should be used as a first-line treatment with co-amoxiclav, cefaclor, erythromycin, azithromycin and clarithromycin as alternatives. Young babies should receive intravenous antibiotics. Most children with an uncomplicated pneumonia do not require admission. Reasons for admission include a supplemental oxygen requirement to maintain oxygen saturations above 92%, severe respiratory distress, history of apnoea or poor feeding.

Complications of pneumonia

A small number of children with pneumonia can develop a pleural effusion, which will usually resolve with antibiotics. However, some of these will develop into an empyema in which there is a collection of pus within the pleural cavity. These will usually require drainage. This can be achieved by two methods: either a chest drain (sometimes with a fibrinolytic agent) or with surgery. Other complications include bronchiectasis and lung abscess with staphylococcal pneumonia.

Prognosis

The vast majority of children with pneumonia make a full recovery. A repeat chest X-ray after 4–6 weeks is sometimes indicated, for example in cases with lobar collapse, atelectasis or empyema.

Cystic fibrosis

Cystic fibrosis is the commonest autosomal recessive genetic condition in the UK, with an incidence of 1 in 2500 live births. Amongst northern Europeans the carrier rate is 1 in 25. The condition is caused by a mutation in the gene encoding for the cystic fibrosis transmembrane regulator (CFTR) protein located on chromosome 7. There are over 1000 known mutations but the commonest is delta 508, responsible for over 80% of UK cases. CFTR is a cAMP chloride channel blocker and the defect results in abnormal salt and water transport causing thick viscid secretions in the lungs and from exocrine glands. Cystic fibrosis is a multi-system disorder but the most common problems involve the respiratory tract and pancreatic insufficiency.

Presentation of cystic fibrosis

In the UK the majority of children with CF are detected via newborn screening (Guthrie test) of a capillary blood sample taken around day 7 of life. This screening test detects a raised immunoreactive trypsin (IRT) level. Infants with an abnormal screening result will then need further investigations to confirm the diagnosis.

Approximately 10–20% of infants with CF present in the first few days of life with meconium ileus. This occurs when the viscid meconium causes bowel obstruction. Affected babies present in the neonatal period with vomiting, abdominal distension and failure to pass meconium. The obstruction is relieved with either Gastrografin® enemas or surgery.

Outside of the neonatal period children with CF can present with failure to thrive, malabsorption or recurrent chest infections. Over 90% of children with CF have pancreatic exocrine insufficiency with deficiency of lipase, amylase and proteases. This is caused by pancreatic duct blockage secondary to thick secretions and results in malabsorption and hence failure to thrive. Stools are large, pale, greasy and offensive (termed steatorrhoea), and testing will show a low faecal elastase. Recurrent chest infections can occur with pathogens such as *Staphylococcus aureus*, *Haemophilus influenzae* and *Pseudomonas aeruginosa* leading to chronic lung damage and bronchiectasis.

Diagnosis of cystic fibrosis

The gold standard for diagnosis of CF is the sweat test. This relies on the excessive concentrations of sodium and chloride that are present in the sweat of those with CF as a result of abnormal sweat gland function. Sweating is stimulated by pilocarpine iontophoresis, and the resulting sweat is collected and analysed. The concentration of chloride is markedly elevated in children with CF (>60 mmol/L compared with 10–40 mmol/L in normal children). Confirmation of the diagnosis can be made by gene analysis for the common CF mutations. Since it is an autosomal recessive condition those with CF will have two abnormal alleles. Clinical features of cystic fibrosis are shown in Table 38.4.

Management of cystic fibrosis

CF is a multi-system disorder and requires a multidisciplinary approach where all aspects of the disease are considered and anticipated. Regular follow-up is essential with a team consisting of paediatricians, physiotherapists, dieticians and specialist nurses. It is recommended that children with CF should be seen at least annually in a specialist centre. Management aims to ensure optimum growth and nutrition whilst preventing progression of the lung disease.

Table 38.4 Clinical features of cystic fibrosis.

System	Features
Respiratory	Recurrent respiratory infections Chronic lung damage: bronchiectasis, lobar collapse, pneumothorax, respiratory failure Hyperinflation, scoliosis
Cardiovascular	Right-sided heart failure (secondary to severe lung disease)
Pancreas	Pancreatic exocrine insufficiency in 90% presenting as steatorrhoea CF-related diabetes: incidence increases with age
Gastrointestinal	Meconium ileus as neonate DIOS (distal intestinal obstruction syndrome, meconium ileus equivalent) Rectal prolapse Intussusception Constipation
Liver	Fatty infiltrate Cholesterol gallstones Pericholangitis Cirrhosis Portal hypertension
ENT	Nasal polyps Sinusitis
Joints	CF-related arthropathy
Fertility	Infertility in males (absent vas deferens)

SUMMARY

Clinical case

Case investigations

Four weeks after discharge Jack was reviewed by the paediatric nurse specialist. He had been well since discharge. His technique with the inhaler and spacer device was checked and found to be good. He was also taught how to measure peak expiratory flow rate (PEFR) and advised to keep a diary of his recordings. His best PEFR in clinic was 200.

Four months later Jack is admitted again with signs of respiratory distress and wheeze. His parents report that since discharge, Jack has required salbutamol 1–2 times per week, usually at times of exertion. They have also noticed a persistent nocturnal cough occurring five nights out of seven per week. The family had been regularly recording his PEFR, with a highest value of 170 over the last 6 weeks.

On admission, Jack has signs of respiratory distress with widespread wheeze on auscultation. His PEFR measures 140, increasing to 160 following salbutamol. He again responds well to regular bronchodilators (salbutamol) and

a short course of oral steroids and is discharged home after 24 hours. Prior to discharge inhaler technique was assessed. In view of a further acute wheezy episode, nocturnal cough and salbutamol use twice per week, Jack was commenced on regular preventer therapy, beclometasone dipropionate at 100 μg to be given twice daily using a spacer device.

The diagnosis in this case is asthma. Jack has had acute wheezy episodes and also regular interval symptoms with persistent nocturnal cough and wheeze with exertion. There is also a personal history of atopy (eczema) as well as family history of atopy. In view of his recurrent symptoms, Jack would be likely benefit from the addition of regular low-dose inhaled corticosteroids as per step 2 of the BTS guidelines on the management of chronic asthma.

Jack was reviewed in outpatient clinic 3 months later. Since commencing a regular inhaled corticosteroid he has had no further acute exacerbations. His nocturnal cough has also subsided and his salbutamol use has decreased markedly to once per month. His PEFR is 210 suggesting good response to the preventer therapy.

Key learning points

- There are a number of important differences between the respiratory systems of adults and children. These include relatively inefficient respiratory muscles, more compliant chest wall and smaller airways in children.
- Acute respiratory diseases are among the commonest reasons for illness in paediatrics, most frequently occurring as a result of a bacterial or viral infection.

- Cystic fibrosis is the commonest autosomal recessive inherited condition in the UK. It is a multi-system disease that causes recurrent respiratory infections and chronic lung damage.

 Now visit **www.wileyessential.com/humandevelopment** to test yourself on this chapter.

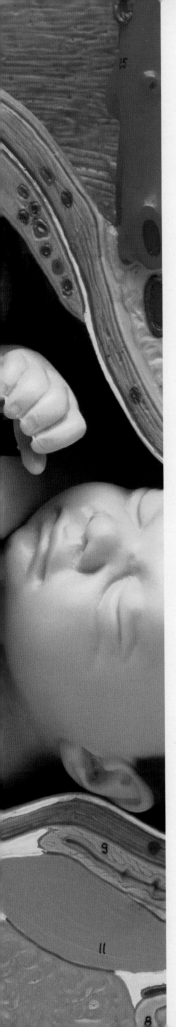

CHAPTER 39

Gastroenterology, nutrition and faltering growth

Lakshmipriya Selvarajan

Case

Hannah is a 14-year-old girl who presented to her GP with a 6-month history of weight loss and intermittent abdominal pain. She is otherwise healthy and has no past medical history of note. She and her family have tended to put down her abdominal pain to nervousness, as she is quite timid and tends to worry about her schoolwork. She is a conscientious student at her school and is a keen netball player, though she has missed a few games recently because of pains in her knees, which have now got better. She visited her dentist a few weeks ago because of a tendency to have ulcers in her mouth. She has always been fair skinned but several family members have commented on how pale she looks. Others have said that she seems 'run down'. Her appetite is not as good as it used to be.

Her GP noted that she looked pale and unwell. Her height was on the 25th centile for her age, which the GP thought was lower than expected as both her parents are relatively tall. Her temperature was 37.4°C. Her abdomen was slightly distended and a little tender especially in the right lower quadrant. Examination of her knees was normal. The GP requested some blood tests and organised a referral to a paediatric gastroenterologist.

Learning outcomes

- You should be able to recognise the symptoms of common gastrointestinal (GI) problems in children.
- You should be able to describe how to begin investigating children with common presentations of GI disease in childhood.
- You should be able to list common causes of abdominal pain.

Essential Human Development, First Edition. Edited by Samuel Webster, Geraint Morris and Euan Kevelighan
© 2018 John Wiley & Sons, Ltd. Published 2018 by John Wiley & Sons, Ltd.

Introduction

Children commonly present with symptoms arising from the gastrointestinal tract, the most common of which are:

- vomiting;
- diarrhoea;
- constipation;
- abdominal pain;
- gastrointestinal bleeding;
- faltering growth.

Vomiting

Posseting

In the newborn period, small, insignificant amounts of milk may be regurgitated with no harmful effects. The baby remains well, no discomfort or pain is evident, and growth and weight gain are normal. This generally improves over the first few months of life, and it needs no investigation or treatment other than reassurance.

Gastro-oesophageal reflux disease (GORD)

Occasionally vomiting results from an incompetent, inappropriately relaxed, or immature lower oesophageal sphincter (Figure 39.1). This may cause pain (due to oesophagitis), faltering growth (due to the large quantity vomited), poor feeding, aspiration with coughing and recurrent chest infections, apnoea and dystonic neck movements. GORD is particularly common in preterm infants, especially those with chronic lung disease, children with cerebral palsy and neurodevelopmental disorders, and children who have had surgery for oesophageal atresia or diaphragmatic hernia.

In most children it usually resolves with age and with the introduction of solid food.

Investigations

Taking a careful history, noting amount and frequency, with monitoring of growth is all that is usually needed (Table 39.1). The majority of cases remain well and free of complications such as faltering growth, haematemesis or oesophageal stricture. Further investigations are necessary only if symptoms fail to resolve with simple measures (see below) or if complications develop.

Oesophageal pH measurement can be useful to confirm a diagnosis. It involves placing a pH probe in the lower oesophagus and measuring the percentage of time that the pH is less than 4 in a 24-hour period. A barium swallow and meal (upper gastrointestinal contrast study) is used to look for anatomical abnormalities like malrotation, hiatus hernia and oesophageal stricture. Endoscopy for older children may be needed in some situations, for example to look for oesophagitis or to treat strictures of the oesophagus.

Management

Uncomplicated reflux has an excellent prognosis. To manage the condition the baby should be nursed head-up after a feed. Feed thickeners like Carobel® can be added to feeds or pre-thickened feeds used. Drugs to neutralise or reduce the secretion of acid can be tried (e.g. Gaviscon®, ranitidine or omeprazole). If a child fails to respond to these measures, it is possible that they may have a specific intolerance to cow's milk protein; changing feeds to a protein hydrolysate formula may be worth trying.

Surgery involving wrapping part of the fundus of the stomach around the lower oesophagus (Nissen fundoplication) is reserved for complicated reflux and patients not responding to medical management.

Pyloric stenosis

This is a condition caused by hypertrophy and spasm of the pyloric muscle, resulting in gastric outlet obstruction

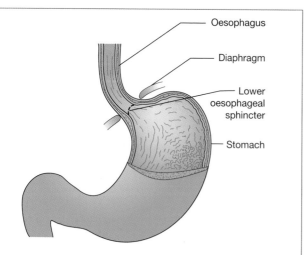

Figure 39.1 The lower oesophageal sphincter.

Oesophagus

Diaphragm

Lower oesophageal sphincter

Stomach

Table 39.1 Important points in the history of gastro-oesophageal reflux.	
Growth chart	Length, weight, head circumference
Feeding history	Frequency and amount, type of foods, positioning and burping
Pattern of vomiting	Frequency and amount, painful, forceful
Past medical history	Growth and development, prematurity, surgery, etc.
Psychosocial history	Stress
Family history	Significant illness, GI problems, metabolic or allergies

(Figure 39.2). It has a 4:1 male predominance and is common in first-born children. The cause is unknown.

Clinical features

Pyloric stenosis presents with persistent, projectile, non-bilious vomiting between 2 and 7 weeks of age. The gastric outlet obstruction is proximal to the duodenum and hence the vomiting is non-bilious. Affected infants are typically very hungry after vomiting, until dehydration leads to loss of interest in food. Repetitive vomiting of pure gastric contents, which contains a lot of hydrochloric acid, results in hypochloraemic metabolic alkalosis with loss of sodium and potassium.

Diagnosis

If clinically well, the baby is given a test milk feed. The stomach becomes enlarged with retained food and secretions, and gastric peristalsis may be seen as a wave moving from left to right across the abdomen. The hypertrophied pylorus may be felt like an olive on gentle deep palpation. Ultrasound examination shows marked elongation and thickening of the pylorus.

Management

Correction of fluid and electrolytes is vital. Hypochloraemic alkalosis is corrected by infusions of saline and dextrose with potassium chloride. Fluid status and urine output should be monitored closely. When hydration and electrolytes are

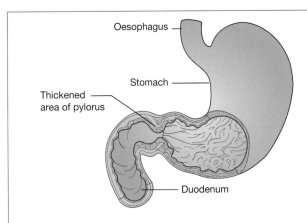

Figure 39.2 Pyloric stenosis.

normal, surgical pyloromyotomy can be performed. A small incision is made on the pyloric muscle longitudinally to release the constriction. Care is taken not to cut the mucosa itself. Recovery is usually very good with no long-term complications.

Warning signs in a vomiting child (Table 39.2):
- Bilious or blood-stained vomiting.
- Severe abdominal pain.
- Projectile vomiting, in the first few weeks of life.
- Abdominal distension, tenderness.
- High fever.
- Persistent tachycardia or hypotension.
- Neck stiffness and/or photophobia.

Table 39.2 Other causes of vomiting in childhood.		
	Newborns/infants	**Childhood**
Mechanical	Gastro-oesophageal reflux Intussusception Malrotation with volvulus Obstructed hernia Duodenal atresia	Adhesions from previous surgery
Infection and inflammation	Necrotising enterocolitis Gastroenteritis Any infection (e.g. meningitis, urinary tract infection, pneumonia, septicaemia)	Gastroenteritis Appendicitis Pancreatitis Cholecystitis Meningitis
CNS	Intracranial haemorrhage Non-accidental injury Hydrocephalus	Intracranial haemorrhage Intracranial tumour Migraine Head injury
Metabolic	Diabetic ketoacidosis Inborn errors of metabolism Congenital adrenal hyperplasia Poisoning	Diabetic ketoacidosis Overdoses
Others	Diabetic ketoacidosis	Diabetic ketoacidosis

Malabsorption

Malabsorption may result from either a generalised mucosal abnormality affecting the absorption of multiple nutrients, or from abnormalities of specific transport mechanisms or deficient enzymes. In children, malabsorption may present with faltering growth and/or diarrhoea. The key to a successful evaluation is careful history taking and the application of physiology. Examination of the stool will also provide valuable information. The severity of symptoms and the impact on nutritional status and hydration will determine the urgency with which evaluation needs to proceed. There are four main elements to small intestinal absorption of nutrients:

1. Digestive enzymes from the pancreas.
2. Bile acids from the liver.
3. Large surface area formed by mucosal folds and villi.
4. Digestive enzymes produced by the mucosa of the gut.

Coeliac disease

Coeliac disease is an autoimmune disorder that involves a heightened immunological response to dietary gluten in genetically susceptible people. The gliadin fraction of gluten in food causes immune-mediated damage to the mucosa of the proximal small intestine with subsequent atrophy of villi and loss of absorptive surface (Figure 39.3). It is associated with HLA antigens DQ2 and DQ8, insulin-dependent diabetes mellitus, Down syndrome and hypothyroidism. The prevalence of coeliac disease is estimated to be 1:100 in the UK.

Clinical features

Symptoms manifest when gluten-containing foods made from wheat, rye, barley (and occasionally oats) are eaten. Typically, steatorrhoea (malabsorption of fat) occurs with bulky, offensive, light-coloured stools. There may be accompanying poor weight gain, abdominal distension and muscle wasting.

Other presentations include faltering growth, irritability, abdominal pain, rectal prolapse, anaemia due to iron or folate deficiency, clubbing and dermatitis herpetiformis (itchy vesicles on extensor surfaces of limbs), which improve on a gluten-free diet.

Diagnosis

Testing for coeliac disease should be done when the child is still taking gluten. Total IgA and IgA anti-tTG (tissue transglutaminase) antibodies are measured in the blood. If there is a raised level of anti-tTG antibody (or if there is IgA deficiency) this requires further diagnostic testing, usually a small bowel biopsy. Alternatively, in the case of IgA deficiency, a second blood test for IgG anti-tTG, IgG EMA (endomysial antibody) and HLA DQ typing may help to decide on the need for biopsy. Confirmation is usually by mucosal biopsy of small intestine to demonstrate the histological abnormalities. Villous atrophy with crypt hyperplasia and increased intraepithelial lymphocytes is characteristic of coeliac disease (Figure 39.4).

ESPGHAN (European Society for Paediatric Gastroenterology, Hepatology, and Nutrition) has suggested that diagnosis can be made without duodenal biopsy if the anti-TTG levels are more than 10 times normal. However, further testing of anti-endomysial antibody and HLA typing is needed to reinforce the diagnosis.

Management

Treatment is lifelong elimination of gluten (wheat, rye and barley) from the diet. Consultation with a dietician is essential. Resources are available on the internet to help the family cope with large changes in diet and cooking. Gluten-free products are now readily available in supermarkets. A gluten challenge may be necessary in children in whom the initial biopsy is ambiguous, or the response to gluten withdrawal is unclear, or when diagnosis is made before the age of 2 years. Most patients respond within a few weeks, with weight gain, improved appetite and an improved sense of wellbeing.

Cow's milk protein allergy (CMPA)

Cow's milk protein is the leading cause of food allergy in infants and children younger than 3 years. The immune reaction may be IgE-mediated, non-IgE-mediated or mixed. In infants, it may be difficult to distinguish CMPA from

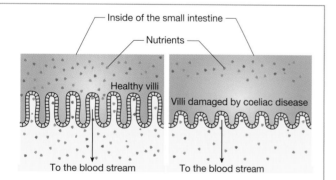

Figure 39.3 Subtotal villous atrophy in coeliac disease.

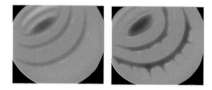

Figure 39.4 Macroscopic appearance of normal jejunum and jejunum in coeliac disease.

gastro-oesophageal reflux disease. A correct diagnosis allows the appropriate diet to be given to affected infants, thus supporting normal growth and development.

Clinical features

Usually infants present with gastrointestinal symptoms, notably diarrhoea, vomiting, refusal to feed, blood in the stool and constipation. Other manifestations include atopic dermatitis, persistent distress or colic, and respiratory symptoms such as runny nose, chronic cough and wheeze. In severe cases there may be iron deficiency anaemia and faltering growth.

Investigations

To establish the diagnosis, a trial of a cow's milk protein-free diet using extensively hydrolysed formula for at least 2–4 weeks is needed. If symptoms improve, a cow's milk challenge can be undertaken with clinical supervision. If symptoms recur an elimination diet will need to be continued. Measurement of total IgE and specific IgE (RAST. or radioallergoabsorbent test) for CMP and skin-prick test for CMP may be helpful.

Management

A diet free of cow's milk using specialised formula milk containing extensively hydrolysed protein will usually be needed for at least 6 months. In cases of severe CMPA, an amino acid-based formula is used. Breastfeeding mothers may need to avoid cow's milk and soya protein (due to cross-sensitivity). Fifty percent of children recover within 1 year and the rest by 2 years.

Post-gastroenteritis syndrome

Children often develop temporary lactose intolerance after an episode of diarrhoeal illness. The stools give a positive Clinitest® result due to the presence of reducing sugar. In such cases, a temporary diet free of lactose may be needed for a brief period of time.

Inflammatory bowel disease (IBD)

The incidence of IBD is increasing. It includes Crohn's disease, which can involve the entire gut, and ulcerative colitis, which affects only the colon. Genetic factors play a role in susceptibility, with a significantly higher risk if there is a family history of IBD.

Ulcerative colitis (UC)

As the name suggests, UC is a chronic relapsing inflammatory condition of the colon, extending from the rectum proximally to a varying degree (Figure 39.5). UC is suspected in a patient

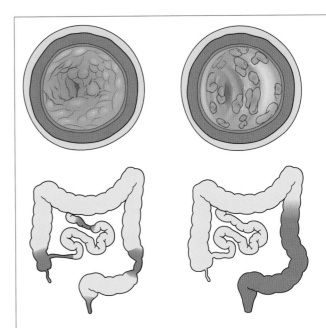

Figure 39.5 Comparison of bowel wall abnormalities in Crohn's disease and ulcerative colitis.

presenting with bloody diarrhoea, tenesmus (a sensation of incomplete emptying after defecation) and abdominal pain (Table 39.3). When symptoms become severe there is weight loss, fatigue, vomiting, anaemia and growth retardation.

Extraintestinal manifestations such as primary sclerosing cholangitis, arthritis, uveitis and pyoderma gangrenosum are common in UC compared to Crohn's disease. Anaemia, fever, pancreatitis, and renal and hepatobiliary conditions may also be associated.

Table 39.3 Comparison of symptoms and signs in Crohn's disease and ulcerative colitis.

Symptoms/signs	Crohn's disease	Ulcerative colitis
Rectal bleeding	++	++++
Abdominal pain	++++	+++
Diarrhoea	++	++++
Weight loss	++++	++
Growth failure	+++	+
Perianal disease	++	
Mouth ulcers	++	+
Erythema nodosum	+	+
Fevers	++	+
Anaemia	+++	+++
Arthritis	+	+

Toxic megacolon is a life-threatening complication characterised by fever, abdominal distension, pain, massively dilated colon, anaemia and low serum albumin due to faecal protein loss.

There is frequent overlap of symptoms between UC and Crohn's disease.

Investigation

Anaemia, elevated platelet counts, and raised inflammatory indicators such as ESR (erythrocyte sedimentation rate) and CRP (C-reactive protein) are typical, and if there is a strong suspicion of UC the following tests are undertaken:

- Ileo-colonoscopy with biopsy. Ninety percent of children show pancolitis, with mucosal inflammation, crypt damage and ulceration.
- Upper gastrointestinal contrast study with small bowel follow-through to rule out small bowel involvement typical of Crohn's disease.

Management

Oral aminosalicylates like sulfasalazine and mesalazine are used for treatment of mild cases. Topical steroids may be indicated for disease confined to the rectum and sigmoid colon, and systemic steroids may be required to treat acute exacerbations and/or extensive disease. Immunomodulatory therapy with azathioprine, ciclosporin and other treatments may be required either alone or in combination with steroids. Severe fulminating disease may require fluid resuscitation and intravenous steroids. Surgical colectomy with ileostomy or ileorectal pouch is an option for unresponsive severe disease, or electively to end chronic symptoms to reduce the risk of adenocarcinoma, which has a higher incidence in patients with UC.

Crohn's disease

Also known as 'regional enteritis', this is a transmural inflammation that can involve any part of the GI tract from mouth to anus, most commonly the distal ileum and proximal colon (see Figure 39.5). Initially the affected bowel is inflamed and thickened. Subsequently, strictures of the bowel and fistulous tracts may be formed. Skin tags and perianal fistulae are distinguishing features. Symptoms can be subtle and hence there may be a delay in diagnosis. Many of the symptoms overlap with UC (see Table 39.3). The histological hallmark is transmural inflammation with skip lesions and non-caseating granulomas. Arthritis, erythema nodosum, uveitis and iritis are extraintestinal manifestations that are commonly seen. The differential diagnosis includes chronic bacterial or parasitic infection such as giardiasis and *Yersinia enterocolitica*. Features are compared between Crohn's disease and ulcerative colitis in Table 39.4.

Table 39.4 Summary of features of Crohn's disease and ulcerative colitis.

Crohn's disease	Ulcerative colitis
Any part of GI tract	Colon
Discontinuous	Continuous
Rectal sparing	No rectal sparing
Non-caseating granulomas	No granulomas
Transmural inflammation	Muscosal inflammation
Abscesses and fistulae	Abscesses very rare
Strictures	Strictures rare
Ileum commonly involved	
Perianal disease	

Diagnosis

As in UC, raised inflammatory indicators may be seen. Because the terminal ileum is often affected as well as other parts of the intestine, anaemia may occur due to vitamin B_{12}, folate or iron deficiency, or due to anemia of chronic disease.

An array of investigations may be needed as the disease can affect any part of the GI tract, including colonoscopy with biopsy, wireless capsule endoscopy (a disposable capsule that transmits images to a recording device), computed tomography with contrast, magnetic resonance imaging and a small bowel contrast study.

Management

Elemental diets can be used for 6–8 weeks orally or via nasogastric tube, and may improve symptoms markedly. Specialised feed is given in which the individual components are present in simple forms, including glucose, electrolytes, amino acids, vitamins and lipids.

Oral or intravenous steroids may be required to induce remission, and immunosuppressant therapy with azathioprine, methotrexate or mercaptopurine may be required to maintain remission.

Anti-tumour necrosis factor agents (e.g. infliximab and adalimumab) may be tried when conventional treatment has failed. Relapse is common, though the long-term prognosis is good and most patients lead a relatively normal life. Surgery may be necessary as a last resort to treat fistulae, abscesses and strictures.

Gastroenteritis

Gastroenteritis is a common disease and is responsible for a large proportion of hospital admissions. It is caused by infection of the gastrointestinal tract, usually by viruses, and presents with vomiting and diarrhoea. The severity is variable; in the UK most children do not require admission. Rotavirus is responsible for most cases. A history of recent travel abroad, or severe symptoms, may prompt consideration of other organisms (Table 39.5).

Dehydration due to fluid loss in the stool is the main danger of this condition, and young infants and babies are at particularly at risk, especially if there is history of frequent watery stools (six or more per day), frequent vomiting (three or more vomits per day), and if the infant takes little/no feeds (Table 39.6).

Treatment

The mainstay of treatment is the restoration and maintenance of normal fluid status. If there is no sign of dehydration, breast or formula milk feeds should continue until the child recovers. If there is mild dehydration, the child should be monitored for the 'red flag' symptoms and oral rehydration solution used in addition to milk. A nasogastric tube may be used if the child cannot drink fluid. If signs of severe dehydration develop, then intravenous fluids may be needed, with careful replacement of losses and maintance of normal fluid balance. Hypovolaemic shock is rare, but should be treated as an emergency with rapid intravenous fluid replacement and, if necessary, admission to an intensive care unit.

Investigation

No investigations are needed in most cases. However, further investigations, including stool culture, serum electrolytes, urea, creatinine and glucose, should be considered in children who have a history of travel abroad, severe disease, features of septicaemia, blood in the stool, symptoms lasting more than 7 days, or who are immunocompromised.

Role of antidiarrhoeal drugs and antibiotics

Oral rehydration is the main aim of management. Antidiarrhoeal drugs should not be used in this condition as they may prolong the retention of bacteria in stool and may be associated with side effects. Antibiotics are rarely indicated except for specific bacterial infections such as invasive salmonellosis, *Campylobacter*, *Clostridium difficile* associated with pseudomembranous colitis, giardiasis or amoebiasis.

Other causes of diarrhoea

Diarrhoea may be osmotic or secretory or both. It may also be secondary to motility disorders.

Osmotic diarrhoea

This involves damage to the villous brush border of the intestine and/or enzyme deficiency leading to malabsorption of intestinal contents and osmotic diarrhoea.

Examples of this form of diarrhoea include lactase deficiency, Crohn's disease and cystic fibrosis. Diarrhoea stops or improves when feeding is discontinued. Reducing substances are present in the stool and stool sodium levels are low (<50 mEq/L).

Secretory diarrhoea

The release of toxins that bind to specific enterocyte receptors causes the release of chloride ions into intestinal lumen leading to secretory diarrhoea.

Examples of this form of diarrhoea include cholera, enterotoxigenic *E. coli* and congenital chloride diarrhoea. Diarrhoea does not stop when feeding is discontinued. Stool is very watery with increased stool sodium levels (>90 mEq/L).

Table 39.5 Age-related pattern of the most common enteropathogens.

<1 year	1–4 years	>5 years
Rotavirus	Rotavirus	*Campylobacter*
Norovirus	Norovirus	*Salmonella*
Adenovirus	Adenovirus	Rotavirus
Salmonella	Salmonella	
	Campylobacter	
	Yersinia	

Table 39.6 Assessment of children for dehydration. Signs and symptoms of clinical dehydration and clinical shock, derived from NICE guidance. Bold italic text signifies item with a high risk of progression to hypovolaemic shock.

Clinical dehydration	Clinical shock
Appears unwell or to be deteriorating	
Altered responsiveness, e.g. irritable or lethargic	Decreased level of consciousness
Decreased urine output	
Sunken eyes	
Dry mucous membranes (unless a 'mouth breather')	
Tachycardia	Tachycardia
Tachypnoea	Tachypnoea
Reduced skin turgor	
	Pale or mottled skin
	Cold extremities
	Weak peripheral pulses
	Prolonged capillary refill time
	Hypotension (indicated decompensated shock)

Motility disorders

Irritable bowel syndrome, post-vagotomy and dumping syndrome cause decreased transit time with increased gut motility resulting in diarrhoea.

Certain conditions like intestinal pseudo-obstruction result in diarrhoea due to bacterial overgrowth secondary to decreased motility.

Immunisation

From July 2013, a vaccine immunisation programme was introduced in the UK to protect infants against rotavirus. It provides two doses of the vaccine to babies before they are 6 months of age. The vaccine is given as an oral liquid at the same time as other routine childhood immunisations.

Toddler diarrhoea

This is also known as chronic non-specific diarrhoea of childhood, or 'peas and carrots diarrhoea'. It usually affects children from 6 months to 5 years of age. Diarrhoea typically occurs during the day when the child is awake, and is of varying consistency. The stool is frequently watery and may have undigested food particles in it. Despite the diarrhoea, the child thrives well, is active and has a normal appetite.

The cause isn't exactly known but intestinal contents most probably move more quickly through the colon, which decreases the amount of fluid that can be absorbed.

Most children grow out of symptoms by 5 years of age.

Constipation

Constipation is extremely common in childhood and affects at least 5–30% of the paediatric population. It is the infrequent passage of dry, hard and painful stool. Usually the children have fewer than three complete stools per week (type 3 or 4 of Bristol stool chart in Figure 39.6). It results in a cycle of holding stools, forming a larger and harder stool, followed by a painful bowel movement and reinforcement of the need to hold stools.

The most common causes are a low-fibre diet including excess milk, inadequate fluid intake, lack of exercise and obesity. Organic causes are less common but include Hirschsprung's disease, cystic fibrosis, hypothyroidism, hypercalcaemia, a neurological disability (e.g. cerebral palsy), anorectal anomalies and many drugs (e.g. antihistamines, anticonvulsants, iron supplements and analgesics). Constipation may also be a symptom of sexual abuse.

Examination often reveals a palpable abdominal mass in a well looking child. Investigations are not routinely needed to diagnose idiopathic constipation. Digital rectal examination should be done only if a pathological cause is suspected.

In more longstanding constipation, the rectum becomes dilated with a loss of the feeling to defecate resulting in

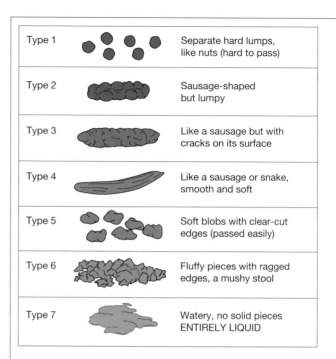

Type 1		Separate hard lumps, like nuts (hard to pass)
Type 2		Sausage-shaped but lumpy
Type 3		Like a sausage but with cracks on its surface
Type 4		Like a sausage or snake, smooth and soft
Type 5		Soft blobs with clear-cut edges (passed easily)
Type 6		Fluffy pieces with ragged edges, a mushy stool
Type 7		Watery, no solid pieces ENTIRELY LIQUID

Figure 39.6 The Bristol stool chart. (Source: S.J. Lewis and K.W. Heaton (1997) Stool form scale as a useful guide to intestinal transit time. *Scandinavian Journal of Gastroenterology* 32: 920–4. Reproduced with permission of Taylor & Francis Group.)

involuntary soiling. The fear of defecation and embarrassment of overflow leads to secondary behaviour problems in children.

Management

If the faecal mass is palpable a disimpaction regime of a macrogol laxative is often used for 2 weeks. If there is no result, then a stimulant laxative (senna/picosulfate) +/<minus> osmotic laxative (lactulose) is added. It should be followed by a maintenance laxative, preferably polyethylene glycol. Children need encouragement and positive reinforcement. Stress the need for a balanced diet and sufficient fluid intake. Occasionally the faecal retention is so severe that evacuation is only possible using enemas or manual evacuation under an anaesthetic. The key principles of treatment are to instigate a regular pattern of bowel movements, maintaining a soft, non-painful stool, overcoming the fear of bowel actions, and allowing the bowel to regain its sensitivity and the sensation of needing a bowel action.

Hirschsprung's disease

This disease is due to the absence of ganglion cells from the myenteric and submucosal plexuses of part of large bowel extending from the rectum to a variable distance proximally. Its incidence is 1 in 5000 babies. The condition should be suspected in all infants who have not passed meconium within 48 hours of birth and in all infants with signs of bowel obstruction. In older children it presents with chronic constipation and abdominal distension that does not respond to laxatives.

Diagnosis

A suction rectal biopsy is needed to confirm the diagnosis. This shows the absence of ganglion cells, together with the presence of large, acetylcholinesterase-positive nerve trunks. If confirmed, surgery is usually required.

Management

Management is usually surgical with an immediate definitive repair or a temporary colostomy followed by anastomosis of normally innervated bowel to anus 3–6 months later.

Abdominal pain

No specific diagnosis will be found in up to half of children who attend hospital with abdominal pain (Table 39.7). The challenge is to swiftly identify and treat the child with a more serious cause of pain. A thorough history and examination will help distinguish these, including hernial orifices, testes, hips and lung bases. Some investigations may also be required. (See Chapter 43 for surgical causes of abdominal pain.)

Investigations

Always check urine for the presence of infection and glycosuria in younger children. Inflammatory markers are non-specific and do not help to distinguish one cause from another. Urea and electrolyte levels should be measured if dehydration, for example from vomiting and diarrhoea, is suspected. Liver function tests are required in the presence of jaundice, and other tests may be required based on the history, for example amylase in the presence of severe abdominal pain in a severely ill child. Ultrasound is of most use in intussusception but may also be useful when there is an abdominal mass and/or abscess.

Chronic abdominal pain

Chronic or recurrent abdominal pain is common in childhood and often causes significant disruption to daily life. It is most often due to a non-organic or functional gastrointestinal disorder. A thorough history and examination together with an event diary, recognition of 'alarm' symptoms and signs, and appropriate investigation will assist in identifying patients with organic disease.

A diagnosis of functional abdominal pain allows both the physician and family to focus on understanding the brain–gut interaction, avoid unnecessary investigations and implement appropriate pain management. Abdominal symptoms may be a manifestation of psychological or emotional problems, and it is always worth asking about bullying or others stressful events/factors in the child's day-to-day life.

Alarm symptoms when a child presents with chronic abdominal pain

- Involuntary weight loss.
- Deceleration of linear growth.
- Gastrointestinal blood loss.
- Significant vomiting.
- Chronic severe diarrhoea.
- Unexplained fever.
- Persistent right upper or right lower quadrant pain.
- Family history of inflammatory bowel disease.

Gastrointestinal bleeding

Gastrointestinal bleeding can be an emergency when a large volume of bleeding is present. On seeing blood in the child's stool/vomitus, the caregiver and child may become extremely anxious, fearing a devastating diagnosis. Whilst it is rare for children to lose a significant quantity of blood, evaluation should include confirmation that blood is truly present, an estimate of the amount of bleeding, restoring the patient's intravascular volume, locating the source of bleeding, and appropriate treatment of the underlying cause (Table 39.8).

Table 39.7 Causes of abdominal pain at various ages.

Birth to 1 year	2–5 years	6–11 years	12–18 years
Infantile colic	Gastroenteritis	Gastroenteritis	Gastroenteritis
Gastroenteritis	Appendicitis	Appendicitis	Appendicitis
Constipation	Constipation	Constipation	Constipation
Urinary tract infection	Urinary tract infection	Functional pain	Dysmenorrhoea
Intussusception	Intussusception	Urinary tract infection	Mittelschmerz
Volvulus	Volvulus	Trauma	Pelvic inflammatory disease
Incarcerated hernia	Trauma	Pharyngitis	Threatened abortion
Hirschsprung's disease	Pharyngitis	Pneumonia	Ectopic pregnancy
	Sickle cell crisis	Sickle cell crisis	Ovarian/testicular torsion
	Henoch–Schönlein purpura	Henoch–Schönlein purpura	
	Mesenteric lymphadenitis	Mesenteric lymphadenitis	

Table 39.8 Causes of gastrointestinal bleeding in the upper and lower GI tract at various ages.

Age group	Upper gastrointestinal bleeding	Lower gastrointestinal bleeding
Neonates	Haemorrhagic disease of the newborn Swallowed maternal blood Stress gastritis Coagulopathy	Anal fissure Necrotising enterocolitis Malrotation with volvulus
Infants aged 1 month to 1 year	Oesophagitis Gastritis	Anal fissure Intussusception Malrotation with volvulus Milk protein allergy
Infants aged 1–2 years	Peptic ulcer disease Gastritis	Polyps Meckel's diverticulum
Children older than 2 years	Oesophageal varices Gastric varices	Polyps Inflammatory bowel disease Infectious diarrhoea Vascular lesions of the bowel

Meckel's diverticulum

This is a congenital abnormality of the small intestine, caused by incomplete obliteration of the vitello-intestinal duct. It is present in 1–2% of the population and is usually asymptomatic. It is usually 5 cm long and is 60 cm proximal to the ileocaecal valve (the 'rule of 2s' describes this as being 2 inches long and 2 feet proximal to the valve). Some Meckel's diverticula may cause profuse painless GI bleeding. It may be a lead point of intussusception and volvulus.

It is diagnosed by a technetium scan (Meckel scan), which labels the acid-producing mucosa. Treatment is surgical excision.

Other surgical conditions involving the gastrointestinal tract are dealt with in Chapter 43.

Faltering growth

Faltering growth is a failure to gain adequate weight or achieve adequate growth during infancy at a normal rate for age. It is thought to affect 5% of children below age 2 years.

Most children with faltering growth have weights that lie below the second centile. Remember, however, that if a child's weight falls through two or more standard centile lines (see Chapter 27), this may also be a sign of faltering growth. This is likely to be picked up by the child's health visitor or GP as part of the child health surveillance programme in the UK. The parent-held Child Health Record ('red book') gives invaluable information about growth.

Children do not all grow at exactly the same rate, and there is a wide variation in what is considered as 'normal' growth. Centile charts can give the impression that children should grow exactly along certain centile lines, whereas in practice this rarely happens; serial measurements of weight and height can fluctuate quite markedly. Many children who do not grow well simply eat a poor diet, and can be helped by simple nutritional advice. It is important, however, not to overlook the child who has a serious medical cause for faltering growth or the child who is suffering neglect.

Most children who present with concerns about their growth will fall within normal limits, or may be constitutionally small. Hence it is very important to see the child within the context of his/her family.

Causes of faltering growth

Causes of faltering growth can be classified as follows:
1. Inadequate food intake
   A. Organic causes:
      - mechanical problems, e.g. cleft palate;
      - oro-motor dysfunction, neurological disorder, e.g. cerebral palsy;
      - chronic illness leading to anorexia.
   B. Non-organic/ environmental:
      - parental depression;
      - food aversion;
      - chaotic meal times;
      - neglect.
2. Vomiting
   - Gastro-oesophageal reflux, pyloric stenosis.
   - Feeding problems.
   - Food intolerance.
3. Defects of digestion or absorption
   - Cystic fibrosis.
   - Inflammatory bowel disease.
   - Coeliac disease.
   - Chronic infective diarrhoea.
4. Failure of utilisation
   - Chronic disease.
   - Syndromes, chromosomal disorders.
   - Metabolic disorders, e.g. congenital hypothyroidism, storage disorders.

5. Increased requirements
  - Thyrotoxicosis, cystic fibrosis, malignancy.
  - Congenital heart disease, chronic renal failure.
  - Chronic infection (HIV, immunodeficiency).

Investigation and management

The investigation and management of faltering growth are guided by clues from the history and examination findings. It is important to ask about birth gestation, birthweight, family history including heights of parents and siblings, dietary habits and any symptoms that may be a sign of a gastrointestinal abnormality or a chronic illness of any kind. On examination, check height, weight, head circumference, general appearance and developmental assessment. Look out for signs of muscle wasting, loss of subcutaneous fat, neglect or abuse as well signs of chronic disease, for example heart failure, respiratory disease, malabsorption and specific nutritional deficiencies.

For an otherwise healthy and normally developing child with no worrying features in the history or examination, no investigations are necessary at first, and the family can be reassured. Continued monitoring may be indicated. For a child with clues in the history or examination that are suggestive of a particular diagnosis, investigate accordingly. For a child where there is significant concern but no specific pointers to a medical cause, simple investigations may be appropriate. These include:

- Full blood count with differential white cell count and blood film.
- Acute phase reactants like CRP.
- Urea, electrolytes, renal function test and bone profile.
- Liver function test.
- Ferritin.
- Urine for microscopy, dipstick and culture.
- Coeliac screen if on solid feeds containing gluten.
- Stool for microscopy, culture and elastase.

For all groups, consider a follow-up appointment to confirm the growth pattern of the child and to allow a further opportunity to investigate or give reassurance, but avoid weighing the child too frequently. Keep in mind the normal fluctuations in weight velocity to avoid unnecessary anxiety.

Treatment

If an underlying medical reason is found, then treatment should be directed to that condition, but further help to improve parenting, diet and general care may require help from a multidisciplinary approach involving the general practitioner, health visitor, dietician, breastfeeding coordinator, speech and language therapist, clinical psychologist and social services.

Malnutrition

Malnutrition in children is generally related to poor quality or insufficient quantity of nutrient intake, absorption or utilisation. The assessment of nutritional status involves a clinical assessment, specific anthropometric measurements (weight, height, mid-arm circumference, and skin fold thickness), dietary history and laboratory tests (e.g. haemoglobin, ferritin and albumin levels, lymphocyte count, vitamin and mineral levels). Short-term malnutrition causes weight loss by loss of fat and muscle mass, but may not affect linear growth. However, chronic malnutrition will cause stunting of growth.

Traditionally malnutrition is classified into marasmus, kwashiorkor and marasmic kwashiorkor.

Marasmus

This is a mixed deficiency of both protein and calories, resulting in non-oedematous malnutrition. It manifests as severe weight loss and a wasted appearance (Figure 39.7).

Clinical features

Clinical features include extreme wasting and extremely low weight, low levels of subcutaneous fat giving the appearance of an old person's face, hunger, a 'pot belly', irritability and fretfulness.

Kwashiorkor

Kwashiorkor is a form of malnutrition characterised by a disproportionately low protein intake compared to calorie intake. It presents with pitting oedema due to hypoalbuminaemia that starts in the lower extremities and ascends with increasing severity. Weight may not be severely reduced because of oedema (see Figure 39.7).

Clinical features

Clinical features include growth failure, wasting and anaemia, like marasmus, but unlike marasmus the child is likely to have

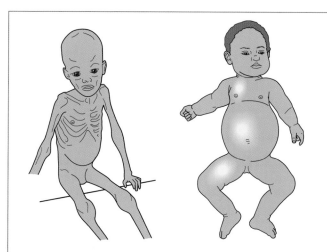

Figure 39.7 Child with marasmus (left) and kwashiorkor (right).

poor appetite, oedema, dermatosis and hair changes. The child will have reduced subcutaneous fat but is likely to have an oedematous face, giving a contrasting appearance to a child with marasmus (see Figure 39.7).

Complications of malnutrition

Malnourished children are susceptible to infection, especially sepsis, gastroenteritis and pneumonia. Hypothermia and bradycardia signify a decreased metabolic rate to conserve energy. Bradycardia and poor cardiac output predispose malnourished children to cardiac failure. Depending on the age of onset and the duration of malnutrition, these children may have permanent stunting (from in utero or infancy) and delayed development.

Management

It is important that the commencement of adequate nutrition is done with care after a prolonged period of starvation. Severe electrolyte abnormalities can follow if refeeding is done too rapidly, and this may result in arrhythmias, cardiac failure, seizures and coma ('refeeding syndrome'). The gut may not tolerate large volumes of food and fluids. Hence nutritional rehabilitation should be initiated and advanced slowly. Specialised feeds are available for this purpose.

Vitamin D deficiency

See Chapter 37.

Vitamin A deficiency

Vitamin A deficiency is the commonest cause of blindness in developing countries. Because vitamin A is a fat-soluble vitamin, deficiency is caused by any condition that causes fat malabsorption. The eye disease progresses from impaired dark adaptation (night blindness) to corneal ulceration followed by scarring. It increases the susceptibility to infection, especially measles.

Zinc deficiency

Zinc deficiency may be due to inadequate intake, malabsorption, excessive loss or a combination of these factors. If treated early most of the symptoms are reversible and usually cause no sequelae.

Mild zinc deficiency causes anorexia, faltering growth and immune impairment. Acrodermatitis enteropathica is an autosomal recessive disorder that begins within 2 to 4 weeks of weaning the child off breast milk. It is characterised by perioral and perianal dermatitis, alopecia and failure to thrive. Treatment is with zinc supplementation.

SUMMARY

Clinical case

Case investigations

Hannah's blood tests showed a macrocytic anaemia with a total haemoglobin concentration of 89 g/L (the normal range is 120–150 g/L), an elevated platelet count and ESR, and normal renal and liver function tests.

She was seen by a paediatric gastroenterologist, who noted in addition to the examination findings described by the GP, two perianal skin tags.

MRI enterography was undertaken, which showed enhancement, fissuring and thickening in the wall of the terminal ileum. A colonoscopy with biopsy of the terminal ileum was undertaken. This showed patchy ulceration of the terminal ileum with a 'cobblestone' appearance. Histological examination showed extensive mucosal inflammation with crypt abscess formation.

Hannah was started on an elemental diet, which she tolerated well. She began to feel better after 3 weeks and her inflammatory indices improved. She started to put on some weight.

Case conclusions

Based on the presentation, the examination findings and the investigation findings the likely diagnosis is Crohn's disease.

Key learning points

- Careful history taking and thorough examination usually helps with diagnosing GI problems in children.
- We should be well aware of extraintestinal manifestations of GI illness.
- A child's height should be plotted on a growth chart regularly to pick up faltering growth.

 Now visit **www.wileyessential.com/humandevelopment** to test yourself on this chapter.

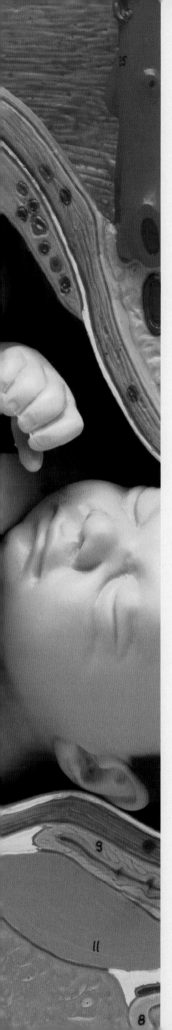

CHAPTER 40
Renal and urinary problems

Dana Beasley

Case

Connor was born at term with a birthweight of 3.6 kg. He was breastfed and his weight gain was satisfactory. From the age of 7 weeks Connor was not feeding well, he seemed irritable and had occasional vomiting. During the following week he had intermittent fevers, stopped gaining weight and was referred to the local hospital by the GP. On clinical examination he was tachycardic, febrile and appeared septic.

Learning outcomes

- You should be able to describe common presentations of renal and urinary problems in childhood.

- You should be able to recommend appropriate investigations and management options of diseases of the urinary tract in children.

Essential Human Development, First Edition. Edited by Samuel Webster, Geraint Morris and Euan Kevelighan
© 2018 John Wiley & Sons, Ltd. Published 2018 by John Wiley & Sons, Ltd.

Urinary tract infections

Urinary tract infections (UTIs) represent the second most common bacterial infection during childhood. They can involve the bladder only (cystitis or lower UTI) or the kidneys (pyelonephritis or upper UTI). The latter is usually associated with systemic illness and fever. An underlying UTI is present in 20–30% of febrile infants presenting to A&E. By the age of 7 years, 2% of boys and 8% of girls will have had symptoms of a UTI at some time. Before the age of 1 year more boys are affected than girls. Complications include septicaemia, possible kidney damage or chronic ill health, which can lead to faltering growth. UTIs can be difficult to diagnose, especially in infants and children under the age of 3.

Clinical features

Presentation varies widely with age (Table 40.1). Infants usually have non-specific symptoms including fever, vomiting and jaundice and may become unwell rapidly. The preschool child might complain of abdominal pain, frequency and wetting. Classical presentation with dysuria, frequency, fever and flank pain is usually seen in older children.

Urine analysis and microscopy

To establish the diagnosis of a UTI urine should be collected for dipstick testing and culture. Often this is done by applying a plastic bag to the perineum. However, contamination with skin flora is very likely despite cleaning of the area. This can lead to false positive results. Similar problems occur with sterile cotton wool pads. Neither of these methods is therefore recommended. Obtaining a 'clean catch' sample after cleaning is a recommended method of urine collection but might be time consuming. To avoid delays, especially in the unwell infant, catheter samples or ultrasound-guided suprapubic aspiration (SPA) should be undertaken. Collection of midstream urine is a good method of obtaining urine in the older child.

A positive dipstick for leucocyte esterase is quite a sensitive test for UTI, and a positive result for urinary nitrite is quite specific for UTI. Although detection rate is high if both are positive, a significant number of infants with a UTI are missed by these tests. A negative dipstick test for leucocytes

and nitrites is useful in older children. Urinary nitrite testing is also used in monitoring children with recurrent urinary tract infections. Weekly nitrite testing of early morning urine has been reported to detect UTIs in asymptomatic children enabling early treatment. Urine microscopy can give further clues: a leucocyte count of more than 10 cells/µL is suggestive of a UTI but this is not a reliable test as white cells might lyse during storage or give a false positive result, for example if there is balanitis or vulvovaginitis. Therefore urine culture is the gold standard for diagnosing UTI. If urine cannot be cultured within 4 hours of collection, the sample should be refrigerated or preserved with boric acid immediately. A bacterial culture of greater than 10^5 colony-forming units of a single organism/mL in a well collected sample gives 90% probability of infection. This rises to 95% if the same result is found in a second sample. Any bacterial single organism growth in a catheter or SPA specimen is diagnostic.

Organisms

With an 80–90% incidence in UTIs, *Escherichia coli* is the commonest organism, followed by *Proteus* and *Pseudomonas*. The latter might indicate a structural abnormality. *Klebsiella* is commonly found in neonates whereas coagulase-negative *Staphylococcus* (CONS) is commonly found in teenagers.

Predisposing factors

A UTI is often caused by bowel flora entering the urinary tract via the urethra. In the neonate, infection is more likely to be haematogenous. Incomplete bladder emptying due to infrequent voiding, constipation or neuropathic bladder is a contributing factor as are structural abnormalities of the urinary tract and the retrograde flow of urine from the bladder along the ureters to the kidneys, namely vesicoureteric reflux (VUR).

Management and prevention

Prompt treatment of UTIs, especially in infants, can prevent renal damage. Infants under 3 months of age and systemically unwell children (dehydrated or with signs of septic shock) require intravenous antibiotics such as cefotaxime and an aminoglycoside (e.g. gentamicin) for 48 hours or until clinically improved. Most other cases can be treated with oral antibiotics (e.g. cephalosporin or co-amoxiclav), adjusting according to the sensitivity on urine culture, for 5–10 days.

Several measures have been shown to be effective in preventing or reducing recurrence of a UTI such as regular voiding and high fluid intake. Constipation should be avoided and treated. Antibiotic prophylaxis is a controversial issue but is frequently used in infants and children under 2 years of age. Trimethoprim or nitrofurantoin are commonly used agents because of their excretion in the urine and high urinary concentration. They are usually well tolerated over a long period

Table 40.1 Presenting symptoms and signs in infants and children with UTIs.

Infants	Children
• Fever/febrile convulsions	• Dysuria/frequency
• Lethargy/irritability	• Fever +/– rigors
• Vomiting	• Abdominal/loin pain
• Reduced oral intake	• Recurrence of enuresis
• Prolonged jaundice	• Lethargy
• Faltering growth	• Vomiting
• Sepsis	• Cloudy urine

of time. Antibiotic prophylaxis for asymptomatic bacteriuria or following a first-time UTI in children is not recommended.

Investigations

The question of when to investigate and which investigations should be done after a UTI is a controversial issue. At the moment there is no evidence that outcome is improved by extensive investigations. The aim should be to detect obstruction or underlying urinary tract malformations. Most centres would investigate children who are at risk of significant renal damage.

Risk factors are :

- antenatally detected renal malformations;
- UTI in infancy;
- UTI in boys;
- recurrent UTI;
- prolonged clinical course and septicaemia at presentation;
- family history of VUR;
- unusual organisms.

A renal ultrasound gives information about the presence, site, size and shape of the kidneys but generally ureters cannot be visualised unless significantly enlarged. Post-voidal volumes can be measured to roughly assess bladder function. Depending on results from the ultrasound scan further radiological tests might be required. If urethral obstruction is suspected a micturating cystourethrogram (MCUG) should be performed to identify structural problems of the urethra and bladder, and to look for VUR. Nuclear medicine investigations with technetium labelled isotopes are used to obtain further information on the renal tract. A MAG3 scan can identify obstruction of urinary flow from the kidney to the bladder and determine the differential renal function between right and left kidneys. A DMSA (dimercaptosuccinic acid) scan can demonstrate damaged or absent renal tissue also known as 'scarring'. Functional studies after a UTI should be deferred for 3–6 months in order to allow detection of a newly developing scar and avoid detection of transient impairment after pyelonephritis.

Abnormalities of the urinary tract

Vesicoureteric reflux (VUR)

This is a common structural abnormality at the vesicoureteric junction (of the bladder and ureter) in which urine passes in a retrograde direction from the bladder into the ureter (Figure 40.1). Instead of entering the bladder at an angle, ureters may be displaced laterally and have less muscle in their walls. In some cases, VUR is associated with renal malformations and abnormalities of bladder function. VUR can be familial affecting 30–50% of first-degree relatives. More severe cases

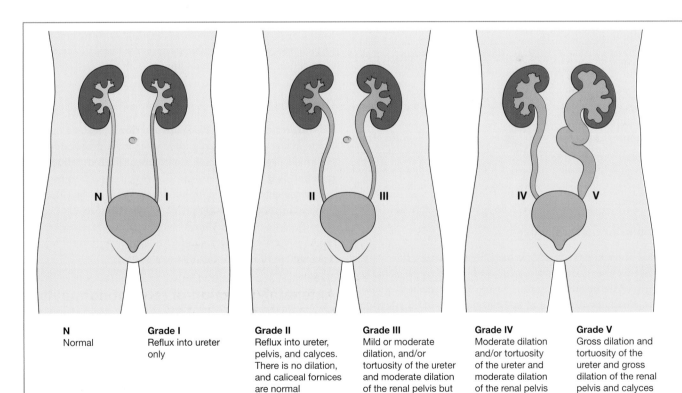

| **N** Normal | **Grade I** Reflux into ureter only | **Grade II** Reflux into ureter, pelvis, and calyces. There is no dilation, and caliceal fornices are normal | **Grade III** Mild or moderate dilation, and/or tortuosity of the ureter and moderate dilation of the renal pelvis but little or no blunting of the fornices | **Grade IV** Moderate dilation and/or tortuosity of the ureter and moderate dilation of the renal pelvis and calyces | **Grade V** Gross dilation and tortuosity of the ureter and gross dilation of the renal pelvis and calyces |

Figure 40.1 Grades of vesicoureteric reflux.

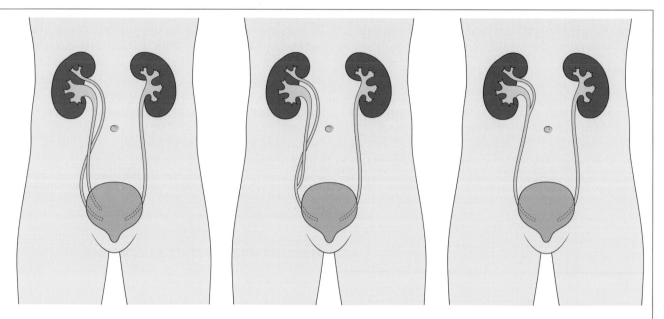

Figure 40.2 Variants of the duplex kidney: duplicated ureter (left), ureter fissus (middle) and bifid renal pelvis (right).

are associated with a high recurrence rate of UTI. Diagnosis is made by micturating cystourethrogram (MCUG).

Previously higher grades of VUR were managed with anti-reflux surgery. Recent studies, however, have not shown any advantage of surgery over antibiotic therapy in the prevention of UTI, hypertension or renal damage. The aim should be to prevent urinary tract infection by avoiding precipitating factors for UTIs, early use of antibiotics and selective surgery. Often VUR can resolve spontaneously although UTIs can still be expected for affected females, especially when teenagers become sexual active.

Approximately 10% of patients with VUR suffer from reflux-associated nephropathy. This can lead to the development of hypertension in early adulthood. If reflux-associated nephropathy is bilateral and extensive, renal failure may occur in childhood.

Posterior urethral valves

This abnormality causes obstruction of urinary flow in the posterior urethra. It affects males only and may be associated with VUR in 50% of cases. Severe cases can be diagnosed antenatally by detection of hydronephrosis and oligohydramnios, with a thickened bladder wall. Less severe cases present commonly in early infancy with urinary infection. Some children may present later in childhood with dribbling and wetting. PUV can also be seen in association with other congenital anomalies like Down syndrome, bowel atresia or craniospinal defects.

An ultrasound shows a thick-walled bladder and in most cases hydronephrotic kidneys. MCUG and cystoscopy are used for diagnosis. Treatment is transurethral ablation.

Bladder abnormalities

Abnormalities of the bladder are often associated with urinary tract infections.

Duplex kidney means the presence of two separate collecting systems (Figure 40.2). Depending on how ureters are formed and where they enter the urinary tract, incontinence, obstruction or reflux can be found.

Other obstructions

Pelviureteric junction (PUJ) obstruction is most commonly found as a result of work-up after antenatally detected hydronephrosis. Most cases resolve spontaneously and periodic ultrasound is used for follow-up. If a PUJ obstruction presents with renal colic in later childhood surgery might be required.

Vesicoureteric junction (VUJ) obstruction causes delayed passage of urine from the ureter into the bladder. Enlarged ureters are detected on ultrasound scanning. Surgical reimplantation is the treatment of choice.

Antenatal detection of renal abnormalities

Routine antenatal scanning at around 20 weeks gestation has led to increased detection (1:200) of kidney and urinary malformations. Early treatment may prevent or reduce progressive renal damage.

Bilateral renal agenesis (absence of both kidneys) can be detected on ultrasound. The frequency of this condition is 1:4000 births, and the risk of recurrence is 3%. The aetiology is variable and may include chromosomal or genetic disorders. There is severe oligohydramnios, which causes the fetus to be

Table 40.2 Causes of cystic kidney disease.

Cystic renal disease	Incidence	Genetics	Clinical features
Autosomal dominant polycystic kidney disease	1–2 in 1000	Three genes involved 50% risk in subsequent children	Renal failure in later life Family history
Autosomal recessive polycystic kidney disease	1–2 in 10 000	One gene involved 25% risk in subsequent children	Present in infancy with enlarged polycystic kidneys Associated with hepatic fibrosis causing portal hypertension Progression to hypertension and renal impairment
Cystic renal dysplasia	Common	Polygenic	Often asymptomatic, associated with VUR, may be bilateral
Multicystic dysplastic kidney	Uncommon	Unknown, low risk of recurrence	Enlarged, cystic non-functioning kidney, other kidney usually not affected but might be associated with VUR

VUR, vesicoureteric reflux.

compressed in the uterus. This leads to pulmonary hypoplasia and misshapen head and limbs (Potter's syndrome). Prognosis is extremely poor; around 40% are stillborn and the others live only for a short time after birth.

If an increased renal pelvis diameter is detected at the anomaly scan, ultrasound should be repeated during the third trimester. Bilateral hydronephrosis and an enlarged bladder in a boy are suggestive of posterior urethral valves. After birth the infant should be given prophylactic trimethoprim. If the baby is well, renal ultrasound can be deferred until a few weeks of life. However, if severe abnormalities are suspected or the infant appears unwell investigations should be performed sooner.

Cystic renal disease

Multicystic dysplastic kidney (MCDK) is the most severe form of cystic renal dysplasia (Table 40.2). It consists of numerous non-communicating cysts with no identifiable renal tissue. The diagnosis is most frequently made by antenatal ultrasound, with an overall incidence of 0.3 to 1 per 1000 live births (Figure 40.3). Management consists of serial renal ultrasounds to monitor contralateral kidney growth, evidence of renal scarring and involution of the affected kidney. In addition, routine follow-up includes blood pressure measurements to detect hypertension, urinalysis to detect proteinuria, and renal function studies.

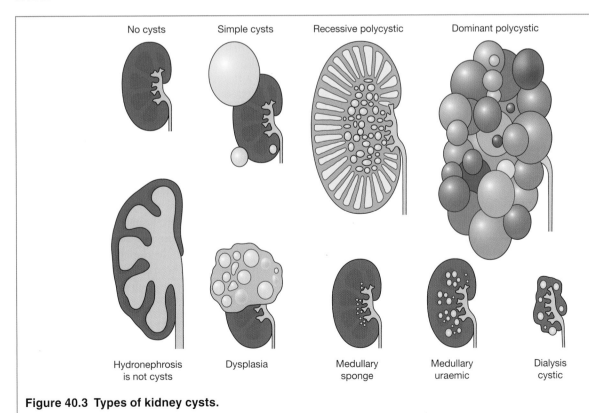

Figure 40.3 Types of kidney cysts.

Table 40.3 Causes of haematuria.

Non-glomerular	Glomerular
• Infection (bacterial, viral, TB) • Trauma • Kidney stones • Tumour • Sickle cell disease • Bleeding disorders • Renal vein thrombosis	• Acute glomerulonephritis • Chronic glomerulonephritis • IgA nephropathy • Familial nephritis

Haematuria

Haematuria is the presence of red cells in the urine. It can be an important sign of renal tract disease. Red-coloured urine should be investigated with a dipstick, microscopy and culture. Urinary tract infection is the most common cause for haematuria in children. Other causes are outlined in Table 40.3.

Renal biopsy may be required if there is recurrent macroscopic haematuria, abnormal renal function and proteinuria.

Glomerulonephritis

Glomerulonephritis (GN) refers to a group of conditions affecting both kidneys in which there is immune-mediated damage to the glomerulus. Causes include:

- post-infectious GN;
- Henoch–Schönlein purpura;
- IgA nephropathy;
- membrano-proliferative GN;
- vasculitis;
- lupus erythematosus.
  Clinical features of GN are:
- macroscopic haematuria;
- proteinuria;
- acute fluid overload (oedema, pulmonary oedema or congestive cardiac failure);
- hypertension;
- renal impairment (oliguria).

Post-streptococcal GN

Most cases of GN have an insidious onset; a more acute onset suggests post-streptococcal GN. This is seen usually 7–14 days after throat infection with Group A haemolytic streptococcus or 3–6 weeks after a streptococcal skin infection. Streptococcal antigen is deposited in the glomeruli and activates complement proteins, which can be seen with immunofluorescence microscopy.

Patients are usually of school age and present with macroscopic haematuria, oedema and hypertension. Fever and loin pain may also occur. Urine analysis shows red blood cell casts or dysmorphic red cells. Serum urea, creatinine and potassium levels are elevated as well as antistreptolysin O titre (ASOT) and antistreptococcal DNAse B. Due to the activation of the complement pathway, serum levels of C3 and C4 are low.

Management

Acute renal failure and hypertension need to be managed carefully. Mild hypertension can be treated with fluid restriction and furosemide. Moderate or severe hypertension requires management with antihypertensive agents, such as nifedipine. Oral penicillin should be given for 10 days to eradicate any streptococcal infection but does not alter the course of GN. Diet should be low in salt, potassium and protein (1 g/kg/day).

Complications

Major complications are hypertensive encephalopathy, left ventricular failure, acute renal failure and convulsions due to hypertension. Convulsions can be associated with papilloedema and temporary cortical blindness; this requires emergency antihypertensive treatment. Oliguria can last up to 10 days. Dialysis is required when serum urea, potassium and pulmonary oedema are difficult to control.

Prognosis is excellent, with only 1% developing chronic renal failure. Proteinuria should clear within 6 months whereas microscopic haematuria might continue for 2 years. Renal biopsy is usually not required unless oliguria persists for more than 3 weeks, or there is uncertainty about the diagnosis. Other organisms like staphylococci, pneumococci, Epstein–Barr virus (EBV) or coxsackievirus can cause a similar illness to post-streptococcal GN.

Henoch–Schönlein purpura (HSP)

HSP is a vasculitis of the small vessels in the skin, large joints and gastrointestinal tract. It is usually seen in children between 3 and 10 years of age and affects more boys than girls. There is often a history of recent upper respiratory chest infection and therefore HSP is more common in the winter. Affected children present with fever and a typically symmetrical, palpable petechial rash over the buttocks and the extensor surfaces of the arms and legs. In addition to the characteristic petechial rash, arthritis, abdominal pain and mild nephritis are seen in 50–70% of patients. Whilst microscopic haematuria and proteinuria are commonly seen, hypertension and a rise in serum creatinine are rare. Other complications include intussusception, ileus or protein-losing enteropathy. In general HSP is a self-limiting, benign illness. Prognosis is good, with less than 5% of children developing chronic symptoms and less than 1% developing chronic renal failure. All children with renal involvement need follow-up as hypertension might develop some years after the illness.

Proteinuria

Proteinuria is commonly defined as more than 4 mg protein/h/m² in a 24-hour urine collection, or a protein/creatinine ratio of more than 20 mg/mmol in an early morning sample. There are many causes (Box 40.1), some of which are benign like

Box 40.1 Causes of proteinuria

- Orthostatic proteinuria
- Glomerular abnormalities (glomerulonephritis, minimal change disease)
- Hypertension
- Renal mass
- Tubular proteinuria

transient proteinuria during febrile illness and don't require further investigations.

Nephrotic syndrome

Nephrotic syndrome is defined as heavy proteinuria leading to oedema, hypoalbuminaemia and hyperlipidaemia. It is the result of massive renal protein loss due to glomerular diseases. Depending on the histological picture after renal biopsy, nephrotic syndrome can be classified as:

- minimal change disease;
- focal segmental glomerulosclerosis;
- membranoproliferative glomerulonephritis;
- membranous glomerulopathy;
- congenital nephrotic syndrome.

Presentation

The earliest sign of nephrotic syndrome is periorbital oedema. Other features are generalised oedema, scrotal and ankle oedema, ascites or breathing difficulties due to abdominal distension or pleural effusions.

Relevant investigations include urine for dipstick analysis, protein/creatinine ratio, microscopy and culture, throat swab and blood tests including serum complement. Heavy proteinuria and low plasma albumin are diagnostic. There is no established cause for this disease but some cases present after infections, especially viral upper respiratory tract infection (URTI), systemic vasculitis or exposure to certain allergens.

Management

Children with significant oedema will benefit from mild fluid restriction, which must be balanced against the risk of hypovolaemia. Nephrotic syndrome can also be divided according to the response to steroids into steroid-sensitive, steroid-dependent and steroid-resistant nephrotic syndrome. About 90% of cases respond to treatment with prednisolone but approximately 70% of children have relapses. Steroids given on alternate days, cyclophosphamide and ciclosporin are used to prevent or reduce further relapses. Most of the children who relapse will relapse less frequently as they become older. Even if relapse continues into adult life the nephrotic syndrome usually remains steroid-sensitive. Progress to chronic renal failure is rare.

Steroid-sensitive nephrotic syndrome comprises 80% of cases of nephrotic syndrome in childhood; suggestive features are:

- age 1–10 years;
- normal blood pressure;
- normal renal function;
- no macroscopic haematuria;
- normal complement.

There are three major complications of nephrotic syndrome: infections, hypovolaemia and thromboembolism. Peritonitis and septicaemia occur due to loss of immunoglobulins. Antibiotic treatment should cover Gram-positive and Gram-negative organisms until culture and sensitivity are available. Loss of fluid into tissues causes a fall in the circulating blood volume and consequently hypovolaemia. The patient develops abdominal pain, tachycardia with poor peripheral perfusion and oliguria. High haematocrit and low urinary sodium confirm this complication, which is treated with infusions of 20% albumin and intravenous furosemide. Although rare, renal vein thrombosis and pulmonary embolism can occur due to haemoconcentration and loss of antithrombin in the urine. Prompt treatment with anticoagulants is required.

Steroid-resistant glomerulopathy is found in 5–10% of children with nephrotic syndrome. Renal biopsy shows focal segmental glomerulosclerosis. Treatment consists of diuretics, mild fluid restriction and low-salt diet. About 60% will progress to end-stage renal failure over 10 years. There is a 30% recurrence risk in a kidney transplant.

Congenital nephrotic syndrome presents during the first 3 months of life with oedema and is inherited in an autosomal recessive fashion. Treatment is supportive. Kidney transplant is an option when renal failure occurs but proteinuria might recur.

Acute renal failure (ARF)

Acute renal failure is an abrupt reduction or loss of kidney function. There are many underlying causes for acute renal failure, which are dived into pre-renal, renal and post-renal problems (Table 40.4).

Management

Management of acute renal failure consists of the assessment of circulation, strict monitoring of fluid balance and treatment of the underlying cause.

Pre-renal failure is the most common cause of ARF in childhood. Hypovolaemia needs to be corrected with fluid replacement and circulatory support as indicated.

Renal failure might respond to fluid restriction and diuretics if fluid overload is present. A high-calorie and low-protein diet will reduce uraemia, catabolism and hyperkalaemia. Metabolic abnormalities need to be monitored and treated, for example metabolic acidosis with administration of sodium bicarbonate. A renal biopsy may be indicated if no cause for the

Table 40.4 Causes of acute renal failure.

Pre-renal	Renal	Post-renal
Hypovolaemia	Kidney disease	Posterior urethral valves
• Gastroenteritis	• Glomerulonephritis	Neurogenic bladder
• Haemorrhage	• Acute tubular necrosis	Calculi
• Burns	• Pyelonephritis	Tumours
• Hypoalbuminaemia	Nephrotoxic drugs	
Vasodilatation	Vascular	
• Sepsis	• Haemolytic uraemic syndrome	
Congestive cardiac failure	• Embolus	
	• Renal vein thrombosis	

acute renal failure is identified. The commonest renal causes for ARF in childhood in the Western world are acute tubular necrosis, usually in very unwell patients, and haemolytic-uraemic syndrome (HUS).

Post-renal failure is caused by urinary obstruction. An ultrasound scan can help to identify the site of the obstruction, and temporary treatment options are bladder catheterisation or nephrostomy. When electrolyte abnormalities and fluid balance have been normalised surgery can be performed.

Indications for dialysis in acute renal failure:
- hyperkalaemia;
- severe hypo- or hypernatraemia;
- severe metabolic acidosis;
- pulmonary oedema;
- multi-organ failure.

Prognosis for return of renal function in children is generally good.

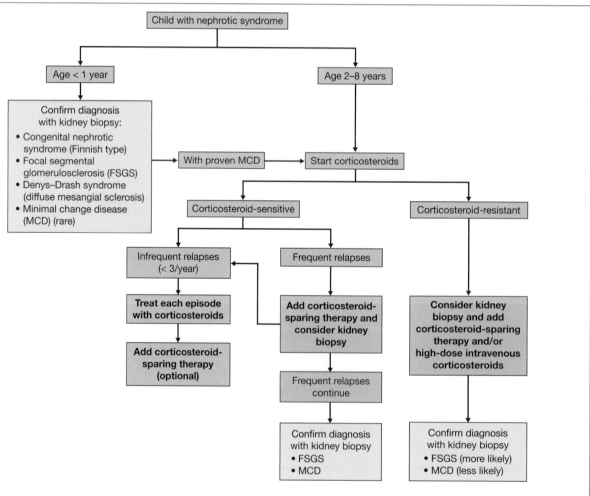

Figure 40.4 Management of nephrotic syndrome.

Haemolytic-uraemic syndrome (HUS)

Classical features of haemolytic-uraemic syndrome at presentation are:

- haemolytic anaemia;
- thrombocytopenia;
- acute renal insufficiency.

HUS is more common under the age of 3 years, often preceded by gastroenteritis with blood-stained diarrhoea. The affected child becomes unwell, with pallor, oliguria and hypertension. Urine analysis shows haematuria and proteinuria. Blood tests show increased serum creatinine, thrombocytopenia and fragmented red cells on a blood film.

The pathogen is typically a verotoxin-producing *E. coli*, usually serotype 0157 although other serotypes can also cause HUS. The toxin penetrates the damaged gut mucosa into endothelium of arterioles. Some cases might follow a pneumococcal pneumonia. This is classified as atypical or sporadic (D – HUS) compared to the diarrhoea-associated (D+) type.

Management of HUS is challenging and patients should be referred to a paediatric nephrologist as dialysis is often required. Although about 90% of children recover fully, prognosis is poor when the onset of HUS is beyond the age of 5 years, with oliguria lasting for more then 2 weeks. Atypical HUS carries a high risk of developing hypertension, chronic renal failure and has a high mortality rate.

Chronic renal failure (CRF)

Chronic renal failure is a rare condition in childhood. Congenital causes outnumber acquired causes. Common causes for CRF include:

- chronic glomerulonephritis;
- reflux nephropathy;
- obstructive uropathy;
- medullary cystic disease.

A variety of clinical features can be found. Children may present with anorexia and lethargy, polydipsia, polyuria, faltering growth, anaemia, hypertension or bony deformities. Often there is a history of an antenatally detected anomaly or known renal disease.

Management should aim for prevention of metabolic abnormalities and preservation of renal function. It should also allow for normal growth and development and is based on the following principles:

1. Prevent and treat hypertension.
2. Improve nutrition; in order to delay progression of renal failure but maintain growth, the diet should be adequate in protein, low in phosphates and high in calories. Nasogastric or gastrostomy feeding might be indicated.
3. Prevention of renal osteodystrophy; hyperphosphataemia should be treated with a low-phosphate diet and phosphate binders to prevent secondary hyperparathyroidism. Vitamin D should be given to prevent rickets.
4. Acidosis should be prevented by giving bicarbonate supplements.
5. Anaemia, caused by reduced production of erythropoietin, is addressed by supplementing iron and giving erythropoietin.
6. Improving growth. As well as nutritional intervention, growth hormone may be given to improve linear growth in children with CRF.

Dialysis and renal transplant are used to treat children in end-stage renal failure. Peritoneal dialysis is often tolerated better in younger children than haemodialysis. Automated overnight dialysis machines can help to facilitate school attendance. Approximately 80% of children with end-stage CRF survive for 10–15 years.

Hypertension

Hypertension is defined as repeatedly elevated systolic and/or diastolic blood pressure measurements over the 95th percentile. Normal blood pressure varies in children depending on gender, age and height. Renal causes account for approximately 80% of cases of hypertension before adolescence (see Key facts 40.1).

A good history should be taken, enquiring about UTI and hypertension or early stroke in relatives. Symptoms might be caused by the underlying cause or the hypertension itself. Physical examination might reveal a palpable renal mass, neurocutaneous markers or suggest essential hypertension if the patient is obese. All hypertensive children should be evaluated for organ damage and secondary causes of hypertension. Investigations should include urea and electrolytes, urine analysis and culture as well as renal ultrasound, DMSA and MAG3 scans and echocardiography. Complement, plasma renin/aldosterone and catecholamines are second-line investigations. A renal biopsy might be required to confirm glomerulonephritis.

Treatment of hypertension depends largely on the underlying cause and presence and severity of symptoms. The aim

---

ⓘ Key facts 40.1 Causes of hypertension

REDCAT:

R	Renal parenchymal disease (acute or chronic GN, HUS, polycystic kidneys, reflux nephropathy)
	Renovascular (renal artery stenosis, renal vein thrombosis)
E	Essential
D	Drugs (corticosteroids, ciclosporin)
C	Coarctation of aorta
A	Adrenogenital syndrome, hyperaldosteronism
T	Tumour (Wilms', phaeochromocytoma, neuroblastoma)

GN, glomerulonephritis; HUS, haemolytic-uraemic syndrome.

should be to reduce the blood pressure to below the 95th percentile. In essential hypertension a reduction of blood pressure can be achieved by exercise and weight reduction and a low-salt diet. Interventional procedures like angioplasty for renal artery stenosis or correction of coarctation of the aorta might be occasionally required. In a hypertensive emergency intravenous use of drugs like labetolol or sodium nitroprusside might be required. Correction of hypertension should be slow and controlled with a decrease of 25% in the first 8 hours and gradual normalisation over the next 48 hours. Drugs of choice for treatment of chronic hypertension are similar to drugs used in adult patients:

- ACE inhibitors;
- angiotensin receptor blockers;
- calcium channel inhibitors;
- beta-blockers;
- hydralazine;
- diuretics.

SUMMARY

Clinical case

Case investigations

After an infection screen was performed Connor was started on intravenous antibiotics. Urine microscopy showed over 100 WBC (white blood cells in a high-power field of view). Urine culture confirmed a significant growth of *E. coli*. Connor responded well to the antibiotics.

Connor presented to the local hospital with irritability, vomiting, poor weight gain and signs of sepsis. Although his symptoms were fairly unspecific given his age and sex, urinary tract infection should be considered. Urinary catheterisation was used as a method of obtaining urine so as not to delay antibiotic treatment. An ultrasound before discharge on day 3 showed left-sided hydronephrosis with a dilated renal pelvis and a normal right kidney. Connor was started on prophylactic antibiotics whilst further imaging was arranged. An MCUG a few weeks later confirmed unilateral vesicoureteric reflux (VUR). A DMSA scan at 5 months of age showed left-sided scarring with 32% function in the left kidney and 68% in the right kidney. Antibiotic prophylaxis was continued and Connor had regular follow-up.

Case conclusion

Despite having three further episodes of UTIs, imaging at 4 years of age showed resolution of his VUR and antibiotic prophylaxis was stopped. Connor will need to be followed up to monitor renal function and blood pressure.

Key learning points

- Renal and urinary problems, especially urinary tract infections, are common in childhood.
- Clinical features of renal and urinary problems are often non-specific.
- Appropriate investigations are key to successful management of diseases of the renal tract in children.

 Now visit **www.wileyessential.com/humandevelopment** to test yourself on this chapter.

CHAPTER 41

Dermatology

Rebecca Balfour

Case

Tom, a 4-year-old boy, presents to his GP with a rash and temperature. The temperature has been present for the past 4 days and the rash developed yesterday. He is miserable with red eyes and his mum reports that he has had reduced oral intake, complaining of pain in his throat. It is noted that he has not received any of his routine vaccinations as his mother had concerns about their side effects.

On examination he looks unwell; he has a temperature of 38.7°C, his heart rate is 120/min, respiratory rate of 25/min and oxygen saturations of 95%. His blood pressure is within normal limits for his age and his capillary refill time is 2 seconds. There is some cervical lymphadenopathy that is non-tender and less than 1 cm in size. His rash is a maculopapular, erythematous rash covering the majority of his body. He has red eyes, a red throat and some white spots on the inside of his cheeks although it is difficult to visualise as he is extremely upset when examined. He is sleepy and clinging onto his mother but he is able to nod and shake his head in response to your questions. He is able to walk to the toilet and drink some fluids from a cup. The rest of his examination is normal.

Learning outcomes

- You should be able to describe and identify common skin lesions in childhood, along with an understanding of what treatment (if any) they require.
- You should be able to distinguish different skin rashes in relation to systemic infection or underlying conditions.

Essential Human Development, First Edition. Edited by Samuel Webster, Geraint Morris and Euan Kevelighan
© 2018 John Wiley & Sons, Ltd. Published 2018 by John Wiley & Sons, Ltd.

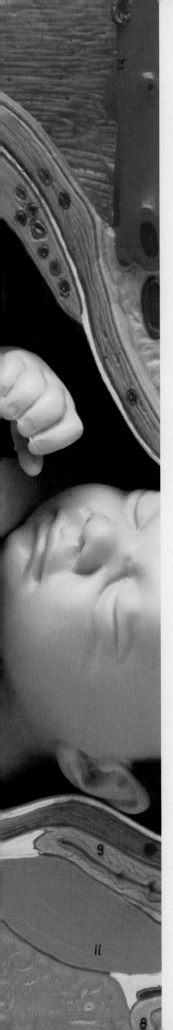

How to describe skin lesions

The best way to describe skin lesions is by looking at their distribution, location, morphology, shape, colour, consistency and texture. Other features to consider are associated lesions and the surrounding skin. Being able to describe and classify lesions makes it easier to make a diagnosis and communicate the appearance to others.

The following is a list of different skin lesions and how to define them:

- **Macule:** a non-palpable lesion, with a different pigmentation to the surrounding skin, flat to the skin with no elevations or depressions.
- **Papule:** a palpable, discrete lesion, <5 mm in diameter, which can be isolated or grouped.
- **Plaques:** superficial flat lesions, >5 mm in size; they can be a confluence of papules.
- **Nodules:** palpable, discrete lesions, >6 mm in size; these can be isolated or grouped.
- **Cysts:** enclosed cavities with a lining containing liquid or semisolid material.
- **Pustules:** small, circumscribed skin papules containing purulent material.
- **Vesicles:** small, circumscribed (<5 mm) skin papules containing serous material.
- **Bullae:** large (>6 mm) vesicles.
- **Petechiae:** small (1–2 mm) red/purple macules that are a result of minor haemorrhage.
- **Purpura:** larger (0.3–1 cm) red/purple macules secondary to vasculitis.

Dermatological conditions in infants and children

Skin rashes are a common reason for attendance in the primary care setting and therefore an understanding of the serious and significant rashes is important. Inflammation and infection are the most common causes of rashes in children.

Inflammatory skin conditions

Dermatitis

Atopic dermatitis (eczema)

Atopic dermatitis is a chronic inflammatory condition of the skin, leading to disruption of the skin surface, which is then more susceptible to irritants and infections. It causes crusting, weeping, excoriation and cracking (fissures). It is very common in childhood and affects 5–20% of children. Symptoms usually start before 5 years of age with more than half starting in the first 12 months of life.

The exact pathogenesis of atopic dermatitis is unknown. There may be a familial inheritance and it is often linked to asthma and hay fever. Atopic dermatitis can be further classified depending upon the age of symptom onset:

- **Infantile stage (up to 2 years)** – usually presents with red, scaly, itchy crusted lesions on the extensor surfaces, cheek or scalp. There is sparing of the nappy area. Lesions may be vesicular, with exudates and crusting.
- **Childhood (2–12 years)** – this tends to involve the flexural surfaces such as antecubital and popliteal fossae, wrists, ankles and neck. It is less exudative than infantile atopic dermatitis and can become lichenified plaques. Itching is usually a significant feature, which is worse at night.
- **Adult stage (>12 years)** – this is generally more localised, lichenified and in similar distribution to the childhood stage. Although it can be located just on the palms and soles of the feet (dyshidrotic eczema).

Treatment options for atopic dermatitis

Spontaneous remission is rare as most cases are chronic but the symptoms can be controlled by therapy. Therefore the goal of treatment is to improve symptoms while minimising exposure to potentially toxic drugs. The following treatment options are available for the management of atopic dermatitis:

- The first step is elimination of exacerbating factors. These include excessive bathing, low humidity, emotional stress, dry skin, overheating, exposure to solvents and detergents, and infection. Eliminating these will help to prevent acute flares and aid in long-term management.
- Maintaining skin hydration is essential as evaporation of water from the skin surface leads to dry skin. Thick creams with low water content or no water content are the ideal option (i.e. E45® cream, Oilatum® cream or shower emollient, paraffin ointment, Diprobase® cream or Doublebase® shower gel). They protect against the skin drying out but can be greasy. They are best applied immediately after bathing when the skin is well hydrated.
- Controlling pruritus is best done using antihistamines. Evidence is weak but sedating antihistamines are more effective for the sedating purpose (Piriton®) to help the child sleep at night. Non-sedating antihistamines (cetirizine) are especially helpful if there is an urticarial component.
- Wet dressings can help soothe skin, limit access, and reduce redness and itching.
- Treating inflammation is mainly done with topical corticosteroids. These can be low potency for mild atopic dermatitis (1% or 2.5% hydrocortisone) or moderate potency (e.g. Eumovate® or Betnovate®) if the disease is more severe or extensive. Very potent forms (Dermovate®) can be used for acute flare-ups for short periods but should be avoided on skin folds and the face. They can be used one or more times daily. In older children a short course of oral prednisolone can be considered for severe cases, although this is not recommended in younger children due to side effects.
- Another topical treatment option is topical tacrolimus ointment (a calcineurin inhibitor); unlike topical corticosteroids it does not cause skin atrophy or other steroid side effects. This makes it useful for dermatitis on the face, neck and skin folds. It is generally equal in strength

to mid-potency topical corticosteroids. Adverse effects are transient burning, erythema and pruritus. Currently it is only used in patients who are unresponsive or intolerant to other treatments.

- Other treatment options are ultraviolet light therapy, oral ciclosporin or oral tacrolimus. These last two options have associated side effects that need monitoring. Occasionally immunosuppressants such as methotrexate or azathioprine can be used in severe or resistant cases.
- If relapses are recurrent they can be prevented by continued intermittent use of low-dose topical steroid treatment.

Secondary infections with atopic dermatitis

Staphylococcus aureus bacteria frequently colonise the skin of children with atopic dermatitis. Signs of this infection include honey-coloured pustules or folliculitis. Treatment is mostly with topical antibiotics although oral antibiotics may be required if the infection is more extensive.

If infection is suspected and there is no improvement with antibiotics then eczema herpeticum, or infection with herpes simplex, should be considered as this needs treatment with an oral antiviral agent. Examination of the skin will show punched-out erosions, haemorrhagic crusts or vesicles. It can be itchy or painful. Rarely it can disseminate and cause a life-threatening infection; therefore severe cases should be treated with intravenous aciclovir.

Other types of dermatitis

Dyshidrotic dermatitis (pompholyx) is dermatitis in a palmo-plantar distribution. It is usually symmetrical with itchy, chronic and recurrent vesicular dermatitis. Due to the distribution it can interfere with activities of daily living. Treatment is with medium to potent topical steroids. Occasional light therapy or a short course of systemic corticosteroids are needed if resistant.

Irritant contact dermatitis is caused by chemicals penetrating the epidermal barrier. This is most commonly seen in the napkin area as a result of prolonged contact with urine or faeces. It is differentiated from candidiasis due to sparing of the skin fissures and lack of satellites lesions. Treatment is by careful cleaning, allowing the area to air dry fully, minimal use of soap and frequent nappy changes.

Allergic contact dermatitis usually presents as acute dermatitis with erythema, vesiculation and oozing. It occurs at the site of contact, for example beneath a metal necklace. Common causes are nickel, topical medications, cosmetics, soaps and perfumes. It can last up to 3 weeks even after the allergen is removed due to cell-mediated immunity. Treatment is with avoidance of the allergen and topical steroid ointments.

Seborrhoeic dermatitis can occur in the neonate and the adolescent. The cause is unknown and is usually self-limiting. There is chronic dermatitis (erythematous scale) and overproduction of sebum (yellowish scales) on the scalp, face, midchest or perineum. In infants this occurs between 3 weeks

and 12 months of age. Treatment is with ketoconazole (for 2 weeks) or hydrocortisone (for 1 week) and emollients. If it very widespread in a child who is failing to thrive and suffering from recurrent infections, an immunodeficiency disorder should be considered.

Acne vulgaris

This is the most prevalent skin condition in paediatrics (Figure 41.1). It occurs in newborns (see 'Neonatal skin conditions' below) and adolescents. It can have significant psychological effects. Scars in particular can be disfiguring and lifelong.

Acne vulgaris peaks in late adolescence and continues into the twenties. Eighty-five percent of adolescents will get acne to a varying degree. It affects the face, chest and back. It occurs as a result of increased sebum production, inflammation, *Propionibacterium acnes* colonisation and follicular hyperkeratinisation. Its peak in puberty is due to the sebaceous glands enlarging and increased sebum production.

Types of lesions

1. Closed comedones (white heads) – accumulation of sebum and keratinous material within the sebaceous gland.
2. Open comedones (black heads) – obstruction at the opened follicular orifice with continued distension.
3. Inflammatory lesions - once the follicles rupture they develop into inflammatory lesions, which may lead to papule or nodular formation.

If the lesions are cystic or there is severe inflammatory acne then scar formation and post-inflammatory hyperpigmentation is more common. An important differential diagnosis is

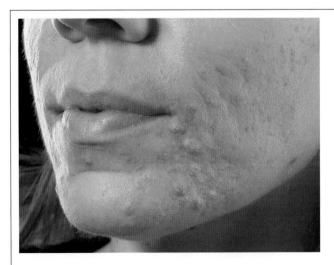

Figure 41.1 Acne vulgaris. (Source: R. Graham-Brown, K. Harman, G. Johnson (2016) *Lecture Notes: Dermatology*, 11th edn. Wiley-Blackwell. Reproduced with permission of John Wiley & Sons, Ltd.)

rosacea, which is distinguished by the absence of comedones and the presence of telangiectasia.

Treatment of acne vulgaris

- Treatment starts with trying to reduce exacerbating factors such as stress, medications, rubbing of face, picking skin and wearing tight clothing.
- Topical retinoids can be used as a monotherapy if there is comedonal acne. If there is inflammatory involvement then antimicrobials (benzoyl peroxide) or topical antibiotics (erythromycin or clindamycin) can be used. Retinoids can cause irritation and dry skin.
- Oral antibiotics (tetracycline or doxycycline) are used if there is moderate or severe inflammatory acne; this is usually for a prolonged period such as 3–6 months. These medications are associated with gastrointestinal upset, photosensitivity and damage to developing fetal teeth.
- The use of oral isotretinoin (a retinoid) is considered if there is extensive and severe acne, nodulocystic acne or acne that is resistant to other treatment options. It requires treatment for 4 months. It is teratogenic and therefore its use in girls of child-bearing age should be limited or the clinician must ensure that they are on adequate contraception.

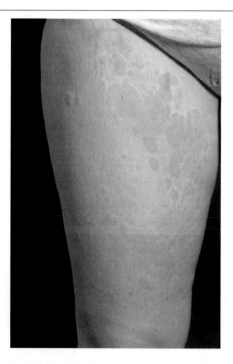

Figure 41.2 Urticaria. (Source: R. Graham-Brown, K. Harman, G. Johnson (2016) *Lecture Notes: Dermatology*, 11th edn. Wiley-Blackwell. Reproduced with permission of John Wiley & Sons, Ltd.)

Urticaria and angioedema

Urticaria is the skin presentation of a hypersensitivity reaction where there is histamine release and mast cell activation (Figure 41.2). It tends to occur in response to infections, bites, stings, drugs, foods and some systemic disorders. There is a sudden onset of wheals, which are lesions 2–15 mm in size with a raised, flat-topped, oedematous centre and an itchy red border. They are often multiple and can become confluent. These wheals can last for 20 minutes to 3 hours; with the whole episode lasting between 1 day and 3 weeks.

Angioedema is characterised by large, deep swellings with indistinct borders, affecting the eyelids, lips, hands and feet and usually occurring along with urticaria in a severe hypersensitivity reaction. This can progress to anaphylaxis, which is a life-threatening condition.

Most cases of urticaria will resolve spontaneously; however, acute treatment involves:

- Antihistamines, i.e. chlorphenamine or cetirizine.
- Systemic steroids can be added to the above, either i.m. or i.v., if there is a more severe reaction; these can be hydrocortisone or a brief course of oral prednisolone.
- Adrenaline is reserved for anaphylaxis or airway obstruction. Therefore parents may require training in the use of a portable injecting device (e.g. EpiPen®) in case of future events if a child has a severe allergic reaction.

Psoriasis

Psoriasis is a chronic condition and tends to increase in severity in adulthood. Onset can occur in childhood and is usually more associated with a family history of the illness. Biopsy shows inflammation associated with features of epidermal proliferation.

It is characterised by thick, silvery scales, in a specific distribution, with nail involvement. Areas affected are scalp, ears, eyebrows, elbows, knees, gluteal crease and genitalia. The involvement of palms and soles is rare in children. Nail involvement occurs in 15% of children; this includes pitting (multiple small pits on the surface of the nails), onycholysis (separation of the nail plate from the nail bed), thickening of the distal nail (distal keratosis) or destruction of the entire nail. Itching is variable. Only 1% of children with psoriasis develop arthritis. The scalp is involved in most children although hair loss does not tend occur.

Guttate psoriasis consists of multiple discrete papules leading to plaques. They are drop-like, usually seen on the trunk and the proximal extremities; this is more common in children than in adults.

Treatment of psoriasis involves three different options:

1. **Topical:** Steroids are the mainstay of treatment for children and these can be given in high doses topically. Topical vitamin D analogues or retinoids can also be used. Salicylic acid is good for softening scales on the scalp and can be used in conjunction with tar shampoo.

2. **Ultraviolet light:** Ultraviolet light therapy is an effective form of management. The use of PUVA (psoralen + UVA) is reserved for children who fail standard treatment regimes.
3. **Systemic therapy:** Systemic steroids are not given in childhood as psoriatic erythroderma (fever, low albumin and metabolic changes) can occur on withdrawal. Systemic therapy options include oral retinoids, ciclosporin and methotrexate; these are considered when other therapies are ineffective but they are not without side effects.

Remission can be achieved but this requires prolonged treatment of up to 4–8 weeks. Exacerbations are linked to times of emotional stress as well as trauma to the skin.

Bacterial skin infections

Impetigo

This is a highly contagious superficial bacterial infection. It occurs most commonly in children aged 2–5 years. It is usually caused by *Staph. aureus* or group A *Streptococcus*. It spreads easily in areas of humidity and overcrowding. The lesions start as papules and then progress into pustules before breaking down to form golden crusts (Figure 41.3). This whole process takes about a week. The lesions are well localised but can be multiple and usually occur on the face and extremities.

Microscopic breaks in the epidermal barrier from trauma or scratching allow entry of the bacteria into the skin layers. Treatment can be topical if there are a few lesions that are non-bullous, using fusidic acid. Oral antibiotics should be used if topical treatments are not appropriate or ineffective. Oral options are flucloxacillin, cefalexin or clindamycin, for 7 days. Handwashing is important to prevent spread. There have been reports of post-streptococcal glomerulonephritis and rheumatic fever after impetigo.

Cellulitis

Cellulitis is a localised or diffuse inflammation of dermal and subcutaneous skin layers with associated connective tissue inflammation. The area affected is tender, warm and red with poorly defined borders. Fever and regional lymphadenopathy are often associated. Penetrating trauma or puncture usually precedes the onset of symptoms. Cellulitis of certain areas has different complications; for example, if located over a joint then there may be extension into the joint space, especially in the knee, hip or shoulder.

Orbital cellulitis needs to be treated promptly because of clinical implications. The concern with orbital cellulitis is extension of the inflammation causing an orbital abscess, visual loss, cavernous sinus thrombophlebitis or a brain abscess. Prompt treatment with intravenous antibiotics and possible surgical drainage is required for these patients.

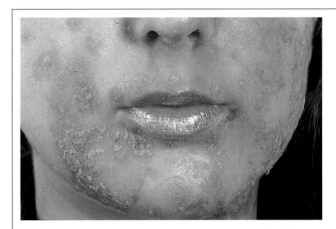

Figure 41.3 Impetigo. (Source: R. Graham-Brown, K. Harman, G. Johnson (2016) *Lecture Notes: Dermatology*, 11th edn. Wiley-Blackwell. Reproduced with permission of John Wiley & Sons, Ltd.)

Staphylococcal scaled skin syndrome (SSSS)

SSSS begins like impetigo and then progresses to form widespread fluid-filled blisters. It is caused by the release of exotoxins from the *Staph. aureus* bacteria. The blisters are thin-walled and rupture easily on rubbing resulting in desquamation of the skin (Nikolsky's sign). It commonly occurs in children under 5 years of age but in newborns it can occur as a severe form called Ritter's disease.

Treatment is supportive (i.e. fluid and pain management) as well as with parenteral antibiotics such as flucloxacillin, clindamycin or vancomycin. Prognosis is usually very good, with complete resolution after 10 days of treatment without significant scarring. The important differential diagnosis is toxic epidermal necrolysis, which is life threatening but usually involves the mucous membranes whereas SSSS does not.

Scarlet fever

Scarlet fever, also known as 'scarlatina', consists of a diffuse erythematous, blanching, 'sand paper' like rash with associated pharyngitis. It frequently affects children aged 2–10 years. It is a delayed-type skin hypersensitivity reaction, following previous exposure to *Streptococcus pyogenes*. The bacteria enter via the pharynx or a skin wound.

The rash consists of numerous small papules and usually starts on the head and neck; it is accompanied by a strawberry tongue (thick white coat over hypertrophied red papillae) with circumoral pallor. It then spreads to cover the extremities and trunk; eventually the rash desquamates. The rash is most prominent in skin folds, with a petechial quality in the antecubital fossae and axillary folds (Pastia's lines). Treatment is with penicillin or erythromycin for 10–14 days. If treated promptly this greatly reduces complications such as rheumatic fever, pneumonia and meningitis.

Viral skin infections

Hand-foot-and-mouth syndrome

This illness, caused by coxsackievirus, is characterised by fever, vesicles on the buccal mucosa and tongue, and tender cutaneous papules on the hands, feet (Figure 41.4), buttocks and, rarely, the genitalia. The lesions are usually few in number. It is contagious and there is an incubation period of 3–5 days. The illness usually resolves in 3 days so no treatment is required. In a very small proportion of patients there can be visceral involvement.

Molluscum contagiosum (MC)

This is caused by a poxvirus, is transmitted by direct skin-to-skin contact, and can spread anywhere over the body by self-inoculation. It can also spread between family members by sharing towels, clothing and so forth. The incubation period is about 1–6 weeks. The lesions are 1–6 mm in size, firm, dome-shaped, yellow-white papules with a central indentation or umbilication. They can occur anywhere on the body, but are typically found on the trunk, axillae, and the antecubital and popliteal fossae.

More lesions can be seen in children with atopic dermatitis. The lesions are extensive and large in HIV-infected and immunocompromised patients. If untreated MC can take months to years to resolve spontaneously. If the lesions persist for many years then removal may be performed using curettage or liquid nitrogen.

Warts (human papillomavirus)

These are caused by human papillomavirus (HPV). There are lots of different subtypes that affect different areas of the body. They are very common in children and young adults, and spread via skin-to-skin contact. The common wart (verruca vulgaris) is a solitary papule, with an irregular and rough surface (Figure 41.5). They can occur anywhere on the body but usually on the extremities. If treatment is required or requested then most simple plantar and palmar warts can be treated with salicylic acid or liquid nitrogen.

Skin manifestations of viral illnesses

Any cutaneous eruption associated with a viral infection is termed a viral exanthem. If the mucosa is involved then it is termed an enanthem. The most common exanthem seen in children is following enteroviral or adenoviral infections. See also Chapter 34.

Rubella

In childhood this is generally a mild illness with very little prodrome or complications. The exanthem is a faint pin-point pink maculopapular eruption that appears first on the face and then spreads to the trunk and extremities. Within 24 hours it becomes more generalised. The rash lasts between 2 and 8 days. Arthritis occasionally occurs as a complication of rubella.

If rubella infection occurs during the first trimester of pregnancy then it can result in a neonatal syndrome. More information can be found in Chapter 25.

Roseola (human herpesvirus 6)

In children an infection with human herpesvirus 6 presents as roseola infantum, also known as sixth disease. There is a prodromal fever for 3–5 days prior to the development of

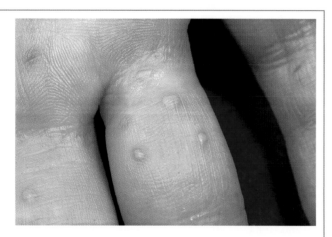

Figure 41.4 Hand-foot-and-mouth syndrome. (Source: R. Graham-Brown, K. Harman, G. Johnson (2016) *Lecture Notes: Dermatology*, 11th edn. Wiley-Blackwell. Reproduced with permission of John Wiley & Sons, Ltd.)

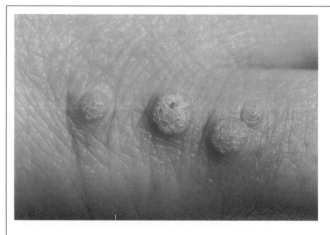

Figure 41.5 Warts. (Source: R. Graham-Brown, K. Harman, G. Johnson (2016) *Lecture Notes: Dermatology*, 11th edn. Wiley-Blackwell. Reproduced with permission of John Wiley & Sons, Ltd.)

a morbilliform, pink rash that disappears in 24 hours. It can be associated with febrile convulsions, cough and otitis media.

Human parvovirus B19 (erythema infectiosum)

Erythema infectiosum, also known as fifth disease, can occur as outbreaks in children. After non-specific prodromal symptoms there is an intense, confluent redness of both cheeks ('slapped cheek' appearance). It can also involve arms, legs, chest and abdomen with a lace-like reticulated rash. The eruption lasts 3–5 days.

Parvovirus can also present with a symmetrical arthritis that affects the hands, wrists, knees and feet. In those with chronic haemolytic anaemia it can cause an aplastic crisis and in pregnancy it can cause fetal death.

Herpes simplex (human herpesvirus 1 and 2)

These two viruses can cause infection in different areas and can occur as primary or recurrent infections. HSV-1 commonly causes gingivostomatitis or erosions within the oral cavity. It can also affect the eyes, cheeks and hands. Eye involvement can lead to corneal ulceration.

HSV-2 almost exclusively affects the genital area; it is contagious and sexually transmitted. It can also be transmitted to neonates of mothers with active lesions at the time of delivery. It carries a high morbidity and mortality if there is neonatal infection.

Zoster infection (shingles)

This is a recurrence of the varicella zoster virus infection. The lesions begin as chickenpox does with macules, then papules, then vesicles. They occur as groups of lesions within a dermatome (Figure 41.6) or adjacent dermatomes, commonly involving the thoracic segments. The rash may be preceded by dermatomal pain.

The illness usually lasts 7–10 days. Visceral involvement can occur in immunosuppressed patients, although they usually recover without long-term complications. Lesions located within the ear canal can result in geniculate ganglion involvement and facial palsy (Ramsay Hunt syndrome). Oral aciclovir should be given for treatment of Ramsay Hunt syndrome. Post-zoster neuralgia is rare in children.

Fungal skin infections

Dermatophytes are fungi that invade and proliferate in the outer layer of the epidermis. They can also affect the hair and nails. They are more common in hot, humid climates and in overcrowded situations.

Tinea capitis (scalp infection)

Tinea capitis is a dermatophyte infection of the scalp (Figure 41.7). It is seen commonly in prepubertal children. There is

scaling of the scalp with inflammation and associated hair loss. It is differentiated from alopecia areata because of the scalp changes and lymphadenopathy that occur in tinea capitis.

Diagnosis is usually confirmed using Wood's light (an ultraviolet black lamp), which will show yellow-green fluorescence of the thickened scalp hairs. Scalp scrapings of broken hairs can also be examined in KOH (potassium hydroxide) solution, which may show hyphae or spores in the hair shaft. Fungal culture of these scrapings is the most reliable test. Treatment is with oral griseofulvin for 6–12 weeks or terbinafine for 2–4 weeks; the latter has fewer associated side effects than griseofulvin.

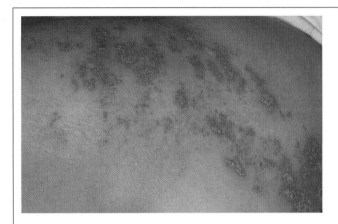

Figure 41.6 Shingles. (Source: R. Graham-Brown, K. Harman, G. Johnson (2016) *Lecture Notes: Dermatology*, 11th edn. Wiley-Blackwell. Reproduced with permission of John Wiley & Sons, Ltd.)

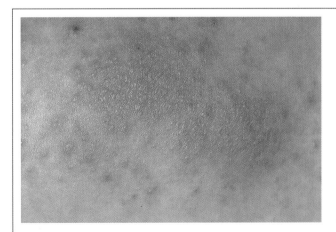

Figure 41.7 Tinea capitis. (Source: R. Graham-Brown, K. Harman, G. Johnson (2016) *Lecture Notes: Dermatology*, 11th edn. Wiley-Blackwell. Reproduced with permission of John Wiley & Sons, Ltd.)

Tinea corporis

This is dermatophyte infection of the skin only, consisting of one or several circular erythematous patches. They can be papular or scaly with an annular border and a clear centre. Other sites include the feet (tinea pedis), face (tinea faciei) and inner thighs (tinea cruris). They are all diagnosed clinically or using skin scrapings. Topical therapy is the usual treatment option, but this can take up to 2–4 weeks before the lesions clear. Rarely oral therapy is required.

Candidiasis

Candidiasis is due to invasion by the yeast *Candida albicans*.

Oropharyngeal thrush is common in young infants and older children who are immunodeficient or have been treated with antibiotics, steroids or chemotherapy. It appears as white plaques with a red base in the buccal mucosa, palate or tongue. It can cause difficulty in eating due to discomfort. Treatment involves topical antifungal agents such as nystatin suspension. Prolonged therapy of up to 2 weeks with oral fluconazole is recommended for immunocompromised children.

Nappy candidiasis is common in young infants. Classically it occurs in the inguinal region, with confluent erythema and discrete plaques, with superficial scales and 'satellite lesions'. Treatment is usually with topical antifungal creams.

Other *Candida* infections include vulvovaginitis and balanitis, as well as more invasive forms such as oesophagitis, meningitis and septicaemia. Treatment is usually with oral antifungals. For invasive candidiasis, which can occur in neonates, those on ITU and immunocompromised children, treatment will usually be with intravenous antifungal agents.

Skin infestations

Scabies

This is an infestation of the skin by the mite *Sarcoptes scabiei*. It results in intensely itchy papules. Symptoms occur 3–6 weeks after the primary infestation. The small, red papules are accompanied by pathognomonic burrows (which are thin grey-red lines about 2–15 mm in length). Scabies commonly affects the sides and webs of fingers, flexor aspect of the wrists, axillary folds, extensor aspects of the elbows, male genitalia, trunk and feet. Secondary infection with *Staph. aureus* can occur. Treatment is with topical permethrin cream, which has a 98% cure rate. Antihistamines can help with itching.

Head lice

Children are commonly affected by head lice; transfer occurs from hair-to-hair contact and sharing brushes, towels and so forth. The head lice are small, white, mobile insects about 3–4 mm in size. The eggs of the louse attach tightly to the hair shaft anywhere on the body, but most commonly on the scalp. The lice hatch and crawl up the hair to feed on the scalp.

Night-time itching can be severe. Diagnosis is usually by visualisation of the live lice. Treatment is with topical insecticides such as permethrin or malathion. Retreatment in 7 days is recommended.

Neonatal skin conditions

Cradle cap

Cradle cap is isolated seborrhoeic dermatitis of the scalp in infants. Most commonly it affects the frontal and vertex areas. It has a self-limiting course and resolves spontaneously in weeks to months. Treatment is usually conservative with olive oil, mild shampoos and removal of scales with a soft brush. If more extensive or persistent then a short course of topical steroids or ketoconazole cream or shampoo can be used.

Neonatal acne

Neonatal acne first appears as inflammatory papules at 2–4 weeks of age as a response to maternal androgens. It lasts until about 4–6 months of age. It commonly affects the face, upper chest and back. It will resolve spontaneously without intervention.

Erythema toxicum neonatorum

This occurs in up to 70% of full-term infants; the cause is unknown. It is characterised by multiple erythematous macules and papules (1–3 mm in size) that rapidly progress to pustules on an erythematous base. They are usually seen on the trunk and proximal extremities with sparing of the palms and soles. It typically starts at 24–48 hours of age, and resolves spontaneously by 7 days of age.

Milia

These are white papules caused by retention of keratin and sebaceous material in the pilaceous follicles. They are usually found on the nose and cheeks, and resolve spontaneously in the first few weeks of life.

Haemangiomas

Only 20% of haemangiomas are present at birth, the rest appear between 2 and 4 weeks of age. They affect females more than males and are more common in extremely premature babies. They are benign tumours of the capillary endothelium (Figure 41.8). Twenty percent of patients will have multiple lesions. They can be found anywhere but commonly they affect the head and neck. They can also be found on internal organs.

- Superficial haemangiomas are the most common type and present as bright-red papules or nodules. Previously they have been called strawberry or capillary haemangiomas.

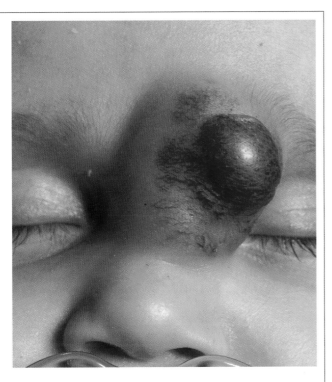

Figure 41.8 Haemangioma. (Source: R. Graham-Brown, K. Harman, G. Johnson (2016) *Lecture Notes: Dermatology*, 11th edn. Wiley-Blackwell. Reproduced with permission of John Wiley & Sons, Ltd.)

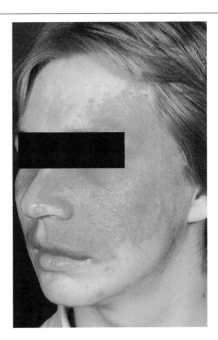

Figure 41.9 Port wine stain. (Source: R. Graham-Brown, K. Harman, G. Johnson (2016) *Lecture Notes: Dermatology*, 11th edn. Wiley-Blackwell. Reproduced with permission of John Wiley & Sons, Ltd.)

■ Deep haemangiomas are raised, skin-coloured nodules with a bluish hue or central telangiectases. They are also known as cavernous haemangiomas.

There is a rapid growth phase for the first few months for both types of haemangiomas, then a slower growth phase until about 12 months of age. Regression of the haemangioma starts to occur around the second year of life. Fifty percent will have reached maximal regression by 5 years of age and 90% by 9 years. There may be residual telangiectases or hypopigmentation after regression.

Haemangiomas can have associated complications such as ulceration, bleeding, obstruction of vital function (i.e. eyesight), high-output cardiac failure, and infection with *Staph. aureus* or *Pseudomonas*.

Treatment is reserved for those who are likely to have complications or for cosmetic reasons (i.e. located on the face). Beta-blockers are usually successful in causing regression of haemangiomas.

Port wine stain

Port wine stains are capillary malformations (Figure 41.9). The incidence is 3 in 1000 births. They present at birth as light pink macules that progress to the dark red colour over time. They do not regress but grow with the child and get darker; in adulthood they can become nodular. The cause is unknown although there are some heritable forms.

They can occur anywhere on the body although the face is a common site. On the face they follow the distribution of the trigeminal nerve branches. If the ophthalmic division is affected then Sturge–Weber syndrome should be considered. This condition is associated with central nervous system and ophthalmological abnormalities. Treatment of port wine stains is usually with laser therapy.

Hair disorders

There are three main causes of hair loss; these are alopecia areata, tinea capitis and traction alopecia. Hair pulling can result in alopecia – there will be broken hairs of different lengths with an irregular border to the hair loss. Scalp excoriations and follicular petechiae may also be seen. It can be associated with times of stress or an underlying psychiatric disorder and therefore treatment should be directed towards these.

Alopecia areata

Alopecia areata is characterised by complete or almost complete hair loss in a circumscribed area. There are usually no scalp changes. Up to 40% have a positive family history. In up to 40% of children there is also nail involvement, most commonly nail pitting. In most children there is spontaneous remission and hair regrowth within a year; in 30% alopecia will recur and in 10% there is chronic disease. It is likely to be caused by an autoimmune mechanism. There is no specific treatment as 95% have spontaneous regrowth.

Skin manifestations of systemic conditions

Erythema multiforme (EM)

EM is an acute immune-mediate condition characterised by target lesions. These are oval/round, fixed, red, symmetrical lesions that last between 1 and 3 weeks. There is a central area of duskiness, which looks like a 'target' with a surrounding ring of oedema. It commonly involves palms, soles of the feet, face, neck and flexor surfaces of extremities. There can be mucosal involvement and it can be difficult to distinguish from Stevens–Johnson syndrome or acute urticaria.

In the majority of children there is an association with herpes simplex; other associations are CMV (cytomegalovirus), EBV (Epstein–Barr virus), *Mycoplasma pneumoniae*, certain medications, malignancy, autoimmune conditions and immunisations. It usually affects 20–40-year-olds but can affect children.

Stevens–Johnson syndrome (SJS) and toxic epidermal necrolysis (TEN)

These two conditions are likely to be a continuum and therefore it is difficult to distinguish between them. The main differential is the percentage of total body surface area involved; in TEN greater than 30% of the body surface area is affected. For both conditions there is a prodrome as opposed to EM where this is absent. The prodrome may last up to 2 weeks, with fever, headache, sore throat and malaise. There is severe mucosal involvement of at least two mucosal surfaces, most commonly the eyes and oral mucosa.

The skin lesions are widely distributed red macules that progress to full-thickness epidermal necrosis, which appears like an extensive burn. It can be very painful, especially in the early stages. In children it tends to occur between 2 and 10 years of age. The most common trigger is medications (non-steroidal anti-inflammatory drugs, sulphonamides and anticonvulsants); other causes include systemic disease, infections and vaccinations.

Treatment involves removal of the possible trigger factors. The rest of treatment is generally supportive as for burns, that is wound care, fluid and electrolyte balance, nutritional support, eye care, pain control and treatment of secondary infections. There can be a high mortality rate (up to 35%) if there is extensive skin involvement. Other treatment options have conflicting evidence such as intravenous immunoglobulins and steroids.

Long-term complications include scarring, hair loss, abnormal regrowth of nails, corneal scarring and pulmonary involvement (bronchiolitis and bronchiectasis).

Erythema nodosum

Erythema nodosum is an abrupt onset of symmetrical, very tender, red nodules on the extensor surfaces of the extremities, most commonly the legs. These lesions last 2–6 weeks. It occurs most commonly in adolescents and young adults. Lesions resolve to leave a bruise discoloration.

They are associated with infections (streptococcal/TB/EBV), connective tissue disorders and inflammatory disorders. Circulating immune complexes cause perivascular inflammation, which leads to the skin changes. Treatment is with antihistamines and analgesia.

Kawasaki's disease

This is a vasculitis classically consisting of fever, conjunctival injection, lymphadenopathy, and oral and skin involvement. These changes include:

- Oral changes – erythema, fissures and crusting of the lips, redness of the oropharynx and strawberry tongue.
- Skin changes – oedema and induration of the hands and feet, erythema of palms and soles, desquamation beginning at the finger tips or a generalised erythematous rash.
- Lymphadenopathy – more than 1.5 cm in size, most commonly cervical.

Dermatomyositis

See Chapter 33.

Henoch–Schönlein purpura

See Chapter 40.

Bullous skin disorders

Epidermolysis bullosa (EB)

EB is a rare group of inherited disorders. Several genes code for the structural proteins in the basement membrane zone of the skin and mucosa, and mutations of these genes can cause EB. It is characterised by mechanical fragility of epithelial tissues, which results in blistering and erosions following minor trauma. There are four major types, which vary in severity. EB can involve the hair, nails, eyes, oral cavity, gastrointestinal and genitourinary tract.

Clinical case

Case investigations

Children often present to their GPs with rashes and temperatures and it is important to make sure that serious conditions are not missed. From the history this is likely to be an enanthem. The fact that this child is unvaccinated means that uncommon conditions need to be considered. He appears to be systemically unwell with a high temperature and reduced oral intake. It is important to make sure that these children drink well, and that they are passing adequate urine. Oral intake can be helped by giving adequate analgesia and drinking small amounts frequently as this is better tolerated.

His observations show that he has a fever, but with a normal HR and RR making it unlikely that he is dehydrated or in shock. The rash is characteristic of a viral infection, with the lack of serious features such as non-blanching petechiae. There is also mucosal involvement with conjunctivitis and oral inflammation. The white spots within the oral mucosa may be Koplik spots as these would fit with the viral enanthem. Neurologically the child has no overtly concerning features, and although he is clingy and sleepy, which is usual for a child with a febrile illness, he is rousable and able to respond to questions.

The most likely diagnosis in view of all the above findings is measles, and the lack of vaccinations makes this diagnosis much more likely than in a child who has received the full UK vaccination schedule. The Koplik spots are also classical of measles although sometimes these can be missed in an upset and non-compliant child. Children with measles look miserable and can have a very high fever but it is not usually life threatening. The more serious acute problems they can exhibit are pulmonary involvement, otitis media or neurological sequelae. These may require hospital admission for treatment. Otherwise children should be managed conservatively at home to avoid the spread of the infection as it is highly contagious and spreads via droplets.

Case conclusion

The diagnosis is measles. This is a notifiable disease and public health should be informed. Pregnant women, children under 6 months of age and immunosuppressed children will be particularly at risk and may require immunoglobulins. Unvaccinated children over 12 months old who have been exposed to measles should receive the vaccination as soon as possible, as they will develop some immunity within 3 days of the vaccination.

Key learning points

- In children skin lesions and rashes are most commonly due to an inflammatory or infectious cause.
- Skin manifestations may be the first or most visible indicator of an infection or underlying conditions.
- Examining mucosal membranes, hair and nails may help when diagnosing dermatological problems.

 Now visit **www.wileyessential.com/humandevelopment** to test yourself on this chapter.

CHAPTER 42
Rheumatology and orthopaedics

Rebecca Balfour

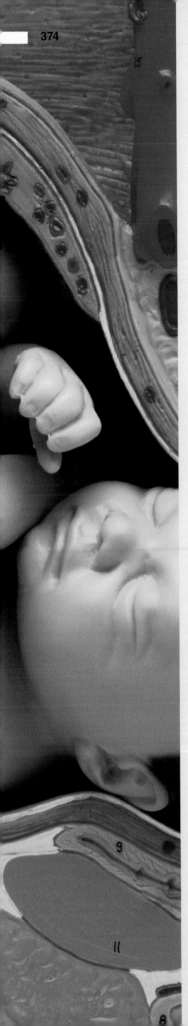

Case

An 8-year-old girl is referred to the paediatric unit with a 7-week history of persistent swelling and redness of her right knee. There is no history of trauma or recent foreign travel; she has been feeling weak, but has not had a fever, weight loss or other constitutional symptoms. On further questioning she has had pain recurring every month for the past 4 months, lasting about a week each time. There is no family history of note. Her general examination is unremarkable. She walks with an antalgic gait, and her right knee is red and swollen with restricted movements and a small joint effusion. There is no leg length discrepancy. Investigations show a normal full blood count, C-reactive protein, liver function tests, bone profile and immunoglobulins. Also her ANA (anti-nuclear antibodies) and rheumatoid factor (RF) tests are negative. Her knee X-ray shows evidence of soft tissue swelling.

Learning outcomes

- You should be able to recognise the signs and symptoms of childhood rheumatological and orthopaedic conditions and briefly describe their typical causes.

- You should be able to describe how to examine a child with musculoskeletal pain or deformity and outline the management or treatment of their condition.

Essential Human Development, First Edition. Edited by Samuel Webster, Geraint Morris and Euan Kevelighan

Introduction

Bone structure and anatomy

Bone has a structural function for locomotion, respiration and protection of internal organs as well as a role in calcium, phosphorus and carbonate metabolism. Long bones such as the femur and tibia consist of three different components. The main shaft is called a diaphysis, with an epiphysis at either end. These two components are separated by a cartilaginous area of growth called an epiphyseal plate; this area is very sensitive to insults and therefore if affected overall growth can be affected. Once skeletal maturity is reached, growth will stop and this cartilage will be converted to bone.

Principally there are two different types of bone that have different functions. Firstly there is the dense and compact cortical bone, which forms the outer layer of all bones. Its main function is to provide strength. The second type of bone is trabecular or spongy bone, which is found only in long bones, the pelvis and vertebral bodies; this also has a structural function but is more involved in the metabolism of calcium and phosphate.

Within all bones there are several different types of cells with different roles. Osteoblasts come from mesenchymal stem cells; they make a protein called osteoid, which mineralises to become bone. They also produce alkaline phosphatase (ALP), which is involved in bone mineralisation. Osteocytes develop from osteoblasts. These become trapped within the bone matrix and occupy spaces called lacunae; their function is to form bone, maintain the matrix and also participate in calcium homeostasis. Osteoclasts are responsible for bone resorption.

Variations of normal bone anatomy

Examples of these include:

- Genu valgum (knock knees): deformity where the knees point towards the midline.
- Genu varum (bow legs): deformity where the knees point away from the midline.
- Out-toeing: where the feet or toes point away from the midline when walking.
- In-toeing: where the feet or toes point towards the midline when walking.

In normal development there is a degree of varus as children are learning to walk. By 2 years of age there should be a neutral alignment followed by valgus alignment until about 4 years of age, when there will again be neutral alignment. Both in-toeing and out-toeing are usually a variation of normal and resolve spontaneously. In-toeing is most apparent at around 5–6 years of age.

In the majority of cases knock knees are physiological and improve without any intervention. These children generally present with clumsiness, recurrent falls and flat feet. Pathological causes include fractures, rickets (younger than 18 months), skeletal dysplasias, mucopolysaccharidoses and neoplasms.

These tend to worsen once the child is over 4 years of age. Investigations with X-rays are not recommended in children less than 3 years. Bow legs are most commonly physiological, but pathological causes include nutritional rickets (if older than 18 months), metabolic bone disease, skeletal dysplasias (i.e. achondroplasia) and asymmetrical growth (trauma, infection and neoplasia).

The majority of varus and valgus deformities can be managed conservatively as they will spontaneously resolve. Other treatment options depend on the cause of the deformity, and for most treating the underlying condition may give a resolution. Surgery may be required if there is severe pain or significant deformity, and this is usually performed after 10 years of age. Long-term complications include pain, meniscal tears and increased risk of osteoarthritis.

Paediatric orthopaedic and rheumatology conditions

Children often present to acute services with several different signs and symptoms that can be due to rheumatological or orthopaedic conditions. The following sections cover common presentations such as a limp or pain, and rheumatological and orthopaedic symptoms as part of a systemic disorder or chronic disorder.

The limping child

Limping is a common paediatric presentation and it is therefore important to be able to differentiate the most likely cause and treat appropriately to avoid long-term damage to the joint. Most cases are, however, due to trauma or a self-limiting condition.

Common causes can be grouped depending on the age of the child:

1–3 years: trauma, inflammation, infection, paralysis.
3–10 years: trauma, infection, Perthes disease, JIA (juvenile idiopathic arthritis).
>10 years: SCFE (slipped capital femoral epiphysis), trauma, pain syndromes.

When taking a history it is important to differentiate between an acute onset of a limp, which is most likely due to trauma or infection, and a chronic limp, which is more likely to be due to Perthes disease, SCFE or systemic illness. Pain characteristics can also be used to differentiate the diagnosis; for example, if the child wakes at night with pain then then this is a worrying feature and requires further investigation to rule out malignant conditions. Associated symptoms can help point to the diagnosis such as morning stiffness, neurological symptoms and recent infections.

Other conditions that can cause a limp that are not covered in this section are septic arthritis, osteomyelitis, psoas abscesses, retroperitoneal abscesses, skeletal tuberculosis, meningitis, abdominal pathology such as appendicitis or testicular torsion, juvenile idiopathic arthritis (JIA), systemic illnesses and neuromuscular conditions.

obesity is the main risk factor; others include renal failure, a history of radiotherapy, hypothyroidism, growth hormone deficiency and Down syndrome.

Hip conditions

Irritable hip (transient synovitis)

This is the most common cause of non-traumatic hip pain in children. Usually it presents in children aged 3–8 years, affecting boys more than girls. For most children there is a preceding viral upper respiratory tract infection (URTI). Over a few days they will then have progression of pain, a limp or refusal to weight bear without fever. When examined they will hold the hip in abduction and externally rotated.

Investigations will show normal bloods, and a hip ultrasound may show a mild effusion. This diagnosis is generally a diagnosis of exclusion. Most will have spontaneous resolution of symptoms over 1–4 weeks and therefore treatment is conservative with the use of NSAIDs (non-steroidal anti-inflammatory drugs) for pain relief. It can recur in 15% of children. The most common differential diagnoses are JIA or Perthes disease.

Perthes (Legg–Calvé–Perthes) disease

This occurs when there is avascular necrosis of the femoral head. It occurs in children aged 3–12 years, affecting boys more than girls, and in 15% of children it is bilateral. In most cases the cause is unknown although in a small proportion it is familial. They present with a limp, and pain is mild or referred to the knee. There will be limitation of internal rotation and abduction of the hip on examination.

Diagnosis is usually made clinically, and X-rays will be normal or show changes consistent with the diagnosis such as widening of the medial joint space, irregularity of the epiphyseal plate, or crescent sign (subchondral fracture). MRI and bone scans may also be helpful. Treatment is with bed rest to reduce weight bearing and further damage. Surgery or splints will then be used to keep the femoral head within the acetabulum. Long-term outcome is variable and depends on the degree of involvement and the age at disease onset.

Slipped capital femoral epiphysis (SCFE)

Slipped capital femoral epiphysis is characterised by displacement of the femoral head from the femoral neck through the epiphyseal plate. It occurs in adolescents aged between 10 and 15 years, affecting males more than females. In 25% of cases it can be bilateral. Slipping usually occurs over months and therefore the joint is more stable than if it occurs acutely. Acute slipping occurs when the symptoms are present for less than 3 weeks; it can be associated with trauma and usually there is more severe pain. The cause of SCFE is unknown although

Leg pain

Growing pains

Growing pains are recurrent, self-limiting extremity pains; they are benign and usually resolve within 2 years of the onset of symptoms. They are not related to times of rapid growth and affect children aged 2–12 years, with girls affected more often than boys.

The pain is very variable in both intensity and timing, and there can be long periods of time between episodes. It usually occurs in the lower extremities, bilaterally and deep within the muscles. It can interrupt sleep overnight but is commonly present in the evenings. There will be no limitation in activity and examination will be normal. There may be associated abdominal pain and headaches. Blood tests and X-rays will be normal and can help to rule out serious causes of leg pains. Treatment is mainly with education, and the pain can be relieved by massage, heat and mild analgesics.

Shin splints

Shin splints consist of anterior lower leg pain that occurs at the start of exercise and then persists after exercise has ceased. It occurs in puberty as a result of repeated mechanical stress on the calf from jumping or excessive running. There will be tenderness on palpation of the medial margin of the anterior tibia. Treatment is generally conservative with reduction in activity, but if severe NSAIDs and physiotherapy may be required.

Hypermobility

Hypermobility is classified as painless movement of joints beyond the normal range of movement. It can affect any joint and is thought to be due to a collagen defect that results in reduced strength and increased fragility of the tissues. Often children will present with a history of being clumsy or having poor coordination.

It is assessed using the Beighton score: this involves performing several manoeuvres such as opposition of the thumb to forearm, hyperextension of fingers, hyperextension of elbows, hyperextension of the knees, and the ability to place palms on the floor when flexing the spine. A score greater than 4 (9 available in total) implies generalised hypermobility.

If there is pain associated with hypermobility then it is classified as joint hypermobility syndrome. However, it is associated with lax upper eyelids, weakness in abdominal and pelvic floor muscles leading to herniation, reflux and urinary dysfunction as well as back pain from joint laxity, carpal tunnel syndrome, and temporomandibular joint (TMJ) pain.

In Marfan syndrome there is hypermobility as well as increased arm span-to-height ratio, arachnodactyly of fingers and toes, kyphosis, eye symptoms and dilatation of proximal aorta and dissection. Ehlers–Danlos syndrome is associated with hyperelasticity and fragility of the skin with joint hypermobility. It is a group of disorders and one of the subtypes is associated with spontaneous rupture of large and medium-sized arteries without dissection. The skin is usually atrophic. Diagnosis can be made with skin biopsy or genetic testing.

Management of hypermobility is usually conservative, with education, physiotherapy to improve muscle strength, and occupational therapy input to improve function and reduce pain. Braces or orthotics may be required for certain joints. Analgesia may be required with anti-inflammatories.

Osgood–Schlatter disease

Osgood–Schlatter disease is tendonitis of the distal insertion of the infrapatellar tendon, with or without a small avulsion fracture at the epiphysis of the upper tibia. This is a condition that affects children aged 9–14 years, caused by overuse in sports such football or gymnastics. It affects boys more than girls and can be bilateral in up to 50% of cases.

Patients present with anterior knee pain that is exacerbated by movement, kneeling and jumping, and relieved by rest. Examination shows localised tenderness, with possible soft tissue or bony swelling.

Treatment is usually conservative with NSAIDS, and reduction in activity but not stopping exercise completely. Rarely physiotherapy, steroid injections or surgery may be required. It is usually a self-limiting condition that stops when the tibial growth plate closes.

Complex regional pain syndrome (CRPS; reflex sympathetic dystrophy, or RSD)

This is a disorder of the extremities where children present with pain, swelling, limited range of movement, vasomotor instability and skin changes. The aetiology is unknown although there is often a psychological stress or a psychological disorder in these patients. It most commonly affects girls aged 12–14 years although it is much more common in adults.

The classic presentation is with leg pain that is out of proportion to the history and physical findings. The pain usually improves with activity, but can be severe to light touch (allodynia). There is also episodic mottling, cyanosis, and increased sweating or a difference in temperature between the affected and unaffected limb. It can interrupt sleep and the patient may have incongruent affect (i.e. cheerful while reporting severe pain). Investigations are generally normal but will help to rule out other causes of pain. There may be mild changes on isotope bone scans and MRIs.

The aim of management is to reduce pain and improve function. It requires a multidisciplinary approach involving physiotherapy, occupational therapists, psychologists (for relaxation techniques and stress management) and analgesia. The effectiveness of medications remains uncertain. Pain-reducing procedures such as TENS (transcutaneous electrical nerve stimulation), regional sympathetic block or epidurals may be used in extreme cases but have no trial data to support their usage. The majority of patients will have a complete resolution, but a few will relapse within 6 months. Relapse is more likely to occur if there are psychological concerns at presentation.

Back pain

The most common causes of back pain are trauma or benign musculoskeletal disease. Muscular pains tend to be localised to the paraspinal muscles in the thoracic or lumbar area and are usually related to overuse or following an acute injury. It may worsen on twisting or lifting. Usually it resolves with few long-term consequences.

Ankylosing spondylitis

This is an inflammatory disease of the spine and pelvis associated with psoriatic arthritis or inflammatory bowel disease. Often there is a family history or HLA-B27 positivity. Clinically there will be morning stiffness, with limited mobility improving with activity and returning after periods of inactivity. The pain is usually mild and not severe in nature. Tenderness will be felt over the sacroiliac joint and pain on movement of this joint. MRI scans are good at detecting early disease although changes may be seen on X-ray. Treatment is similar to that of other types of JIA (juvenile idiopathic arthritis), which is covered later in this chapter.

Scoliosis

Scoliosis is abnormal lateral curvature of the spine with accompanying rotation. Most cases are idiopathic but other causes include congenital spinal anomalies, muscular spasm, paralysis, infection or tumours. It can be associated with some syndromes such as Marfan, osteogenesis imperfecta and neurofibromatosis. It affects males and females equally. It is generally painless, therefore severe pain would require the ruling out of other causes of back pain.

It is usually detected incidentally because of spinal asymmetry. Examination should look for leg length discrepancy as this may cause compensatory scoliosis or associated features such as skin lesions in neurofibromatosis. Neuromuscular causes may be considered if there are also high-arched feet or claw toes.

When examining the degree of scoliosis, the patient will be asked to bend forwards to look for any asymmetry. A scoliometer can be used for screening to measure the angle of trunk rotation. If this suggests scoliosis then X-rays are required, which will give the degree of curvature, using the Cobb angle. If this angle is greater than 10° then scoliosis is confirmed. If there is a suggestion of intraspinal pathology then an MRI is required.

The curvature will continue to progress until there is skeletal maturity; this progression is variable and therefore requires regular monitoring. Treatment is dependent on the degree of curvature and the rate of progression. Those with a Cobb angle of less than 20° require observation only. Bracing can be used to prevent worsening of the curvature but it does not correct it. Corrective surgery or spinal fusion is reserved for those with a Cobb angle greater than 50° at skeletal maturity or greater than 40° when skeletally immature.

Fractures in non-accidental injury (NAI)

Fractures are the second most common presentation of NAI. The majority of these occur in infants and young children. Common sites are the femur, humerus and skull, although these are also common areas for accidental injuries, and the developmental age of the child, the history and the type of fracture will help to decide if this is likely to be a NAI. Other suspicious injuries include fractures of ribs or sternum, bilateral long bone fractures and multiple fractures in different stages of healing.

Children with chronic renal disease, osteogenesis imperfecta or rickets are more likely to sustain a fracture from a minor incident and this needs to be taken into consideration. General treatment is with plaster casts or splints. If there is physeal or articular involvement then surgical intervention may be required. There is a good prognosis for these fractures as children of this age have rapid healing and remodel well. Further investigations and management of NAI are covered in Chapter 32.

Juvenile idiopathic arthritis (JIA)

Juvenile idiopathic arthritis is a chronic idiopathic inflammatory disorder that is a diagnosis of exclusion. This was previously known as juvenile rheumatoid arthritis. The most recent classification is that of the ILAR (International League of Associations for Rheumatology). JIA occurs in children aged under 16 years who have had arthritis in one or more joints persisting for more than 6 weeks, and for which no other cause is found. It is an autoimmune condition and therefore the cause is likely to be multifactorial.

The classification consists of the following:
1. Oligoarticular.
2. Polyarticular.
3. Systemic disease.
4. Enthesitis related.
5. Psoriatic.
6. Undifferentiated.

Oligoarticular arthritis

Oligoarthritis is more common than polyarthritis, affecting girls more than boys, with a peak in early childhood (2–5 years). It accounts for around 50% of cases of JIA. It is further divided into persistent and extended types. Persistent is when four or fewer joints are affected throughout the disease process. Extended means that during the first 6 months four or fewer joints are involved but with further joint involvement after 6 months.

Clinically it affects large joints (knees, ankles, wrists and elbows) with pain, and morning stiffness that lasts for more than 30 minutes, which is worse with prolonged immobility and improves on physical activity. Rarely there will be some constitutional symptoms. On examination the joints are swollen, tender and warm. Investigations will usually show ANA positivity, but only a mildly elevated ESR (erythrocyte sedimentation rate), WBC (white blood cells) and platelets indicating little systemic inflammation.

Complications are uveitis and leg length discrepancy.

Polyarticular arthritis

In polyarthritis there are five or more joints involved during the first 6 months from the onset of symptoms. This can then be further divided depending on whether rheumatoid factor (RF) testing is positive or negative. Those who are RF positive are more likely to be older at the time of presentation, have rheumatoid nodules and articular erosions. If they are RF positive then they tend to have a worse prognosis, with symptoms continuing into adulthood and similar findings to adult rheumatoid arthritis. Polyarticular JIA accounts for 20–30% of cases of JIA, and it occurs more often in females than males. There are two peaks in age at onset at 2–5 years and then 10–14 years.

The disease usually progresses slowly in younger children, with periods of improvement followed by relapses. They get symmetrical involvement of the knees, wrists and ankles. Uveitis is rare. In older children the disease tends to progress more quickly, often affecting the small joints of their hands as well as the elbows, cervical spine and hips.

Investigations will show an elevated ESR and anaemia. They may be RF positive, and possibly ANA positive. If ANA positive then this is not related to the severity of the disease but increases the likelihood of uveitis.

Treatment involves physiotherapy, and NSAIDs to control inflammation. Second-line treatment is with intra-articular steroids or disease-modifying anti-rheumatic drugs (DMARDs).

Complications of the disease can result in weakness, reduced mobility, synovitis, osteopenia and reduced growth. TMJ involvement can lead to micrognathia. In later life they may require joint replacement. For children with polyarticular arthritis complete resolution is very unlikely despite treatment.

Systemic disease (previously Still's disease)

Children with systemic disease can present at any age (although to be classified as JIA symptoms must start before

16 years of age). There is a similar male to female incidence, it can begin as early as 2 years of age and accounts for 10–20% of cases of JIA.

Clinically they present with arthritis and fever, with one or more of the following: rash (a salmon-pink macular rash primarily in the axillae and around the waist), lymphadenopathy, hepatosplenomegaly and serositis. The fever tends to be intermittent in nature and needs to be present for 2 weeks (>38.5°C). The arthritis is usually oligoarticular at the start but progresses to polyarticular. It most commonly involves the knees, wrists and ankles. It can also involve the cervical spine, hips, TMJ and the small joints of the hands.

Investigations show evidence of systemic inflammation with elevated WBC, CRP and an ESR over a 100, with thrombocytosis and anaemia. In view of the findings differential diagnoses can include acute infection. Rarely they will have an elevated ANA or RF. Treatment is similar to that of other types of JIA, using NSAIDs as the first-line treatment and then as a second line short courses of systemic steroids or DMARDs such as methotrexate.

Complications include disability from reduced function and amyloidosis in adulthood. They may also have growth retardation from the disease or treatment, and osteoporosis. Extra-articular complications are more common in this form than other forms of JIA. These include pericarditis or pericardial effusions (usually these are small and insignificant), pulmonary interstitial disease, and renal and endocrine complications. Prognosis is variable, and usually about 50% of children will have almost complete resolution of symptoms. The other half will have recurrent episodes or progressive disease with increasing involvement of more joints.

Enthesis-related arthritis

Children with enthesis-related arthritis either have enthesitis (pain at site of tendon insertion) and arthritis, or arthritis plus two of the following: sacroiliac joint involvement, HLA-B27 antigen positivity, onset at more than 6 years in a male, acute anterior uveitis or a first-degree relative with HLA-B27-related disease. These children can have associated inflammatory bowel disease, erythema nodosum and pyoderma gangrenosum. There is usually a good prognosis for peripheral joint involvement but permanent changes in the hips and spine occur frequently. They may have anterior uveitis.

Psoriatic arthritis

Psoriatic arthritis can be diagnosed in children with arthritis and psoriasis or arthritis plus two of the following: dactylitis, nail pitting/onycholysis or psoriasis in a first-degree relative. There is an equal male to female involvement.

Usually skin changes tend to occur before the arthritis is apparent. The arthritis can be oligo or polyarticular, usually it is asymmetrical, and it can involve the DIP (distal interphalangeal) joints and the spine. In its most severe form

(arthritis mutilans) there is destructive arthritis and deformity. Other clinical findings include psoriasis, nail changes, pitting oedema of the hands and feet, and occasionally eye involvement.

Nail changes include:

- Dactylitis: diffuse swelling of an entire finger or toe, due to inflammation of the soft tissues.
- Nail pitting: depressions in the nail plate, caused by shedding of the nail plate.
- Onycholysis: separation of the nail from its bed.

Blood tests will show an elevated WBC count and ESR. Rarely they will have a positive RF, ANA or anti dsDNA antibodies. X-rays show erosive changes and new bone formation. MRI scans may also be helpful. Complications include osteoporosis and increased risk of fractures. The severe forms result in disability and reduced function. Prognosis is variable and depends upon the subtype.

Undifferentiated arthritis

The classification of undifferentiated arthritis is used for any JIA that does not fit the criteria for any of the above categories. It is also used if the arthritis fulfils the criteria for two or more of the categories.

Treatment of JIA

Many children with chronic arthritis go into remission and this should be the main aim of treatment. Further treatment is directed towards controlling pain, preserving joint function, and facilitating normal growth and psychological development. Pharmacological treatment should start with the safest measures and escalate depending upon disease progression and response to medications.

NSAIDs are recommended as the first-line treatment because rapidly controlling inflammation can reduce permanent sequelae. With NSAIDs gastroprotective medication may need to be considered. Clinical response to these medications can be variable and can take as long as 4 weeks to see any improvement in symptoms.

Intra-articular glucocorticoid injections are indicated in oligoarthritis or polyarticular arthritis when one or a few joints have not responded to adequate anti-inflammatory treatment. Repeat injections may be required. This will usually involve a general anaesthetic for children under 7 years and if the hip joint is being injected. It is associated with some rare side effects such as subcutaneous atrophy, cutaneous depigmentation, and increased pain for a few days.

If NSAIDs are not effective or the symptoms are severe then steroids or DMARDs are to be considered. Second-line therapy is usually with methotrexate, and this can be used in conjunction with intra-articular steroid injections. Methotrexate is recommended because of the rapid onset of action and acceptable side effects. For most children there will be improvement within 3 months although it can take up to 12 months, and treatment is usually continued until there is 2 years of disease control, when the dose can be reduced slowly, which may result in a flare-up of the disease.

Other medications that can be used are systemic corticosteroids; these should be kept to a minimum dose and given in short courses to reduce the long-term side effects. Newer biological agents are now being used, including tumour necrosis factor (TNF) inhibitors such as etanercept and infliximab, and these give rapid control of severe arthritis but are associated with an increased risk of infections and malignancy.

Bone tumours

Benign bone tumours

Most benign tumours are asymptomatic and therefore detected incidentally. If any symptoms are present then they will usually include localised pain, swelling, deformity or pathological fractures. Most present in the teenage years, with short-lived easy to manage pain. Plain X-rays are usually the best way to visualise the lesions.

Malignant tumours of the bone

Primary malignant tumours are Ewing's sarcoma, or osteogenic sarcomas. Symptoms are usually vague to begin with. Malignant tumours should be considered if there is bone pain, especially at night or at rest in non-articular locations. Commonly they occur in the distal femur and the proximal tibia.

X-rays will help differentiate between benign and malignant tumours; the latter are rapidly growing and have poorly defined borders, periosteal reactions and destruction of the surrounding areas with extension in the soft tissues. See Chapter 35 for more details on treatment and prognosis.

Other malignancies causing a limp or pain include metastatic disease, leukaemia, lymphoma, and soft tissue, spine and brain tumours.

Infections

Osteomyelitis

The incidence of osteomyelitis (infection of bone) is 1 in 5000 children, commonly affecting children less than 5 years of age. It occurs as a result of haematogenous spread or direct extension from soft tissues. There is increased risk in those with sickle cell anaemia or reduced immunity.

Haematogenous spread usually only affects one site, and multifocal involvement is seen more commonly in unwell neonates or those children with methicillin-resistant *Staphylococcus aureus* (MRSA). Spread is usually to areas of good blood flow such as growing metaphyses in the long bones, that is femur, tibia and fibula. If left untreated the infection can spread to the bone cortex causing bone necrosis; if it is chronic then an abscess may form.

Acute osteomyelitis

Acute osteomyelitis presents with fever, localised pain and decreased mobility, and may result in a limp and refusal to weight bear. Around 2% of limping children will have osteomyelitis. The onset of symptoms usually occurs over 7 days, initially with non-specific symptoms before the localising signs and symptoms occur. Rarely there is spread to the surrounding tissues. In 50% of cases the causative organism is *Staphylococcus aureus*.

Investigations show an elevated ESR, CRP and WBC. In suspected cases two blood cultures should be taken prior to starting antibiotic therapy in order to direct appropriate treatment. X-rays rarely confirm osteomyelitis before 7–10 days after the onset of the infection, but can be useful earlier to rule out other causes of the symptoms. Other investigations include isotope bone scans, which can be positive as early as 24 hours into the illness; MRI scans can also provide extra information such as the extent of involvement. Joint aspiration is useful although 50% of cultures will be negative.

Antibiotics are directed towards the common causative organisms, such as *Staph. aureus*. Other causative bacteria in those under 3 years are *Kingella kingae* and *Streptococcus pneumoniae*. In those with sickle cell anaemia, *Salmonella* and *Escherichia coli* should be considered. The treatment course is usually prolonged. Those with positive cultures should have 4 weeks of appropriate antibiotics, usually intravenously for 7–10 days and then orally. If cultures are negative then sometimes treatment can be stopped, usually after a repeat X-ray. If, however, there is strong clinical suspicion and clinical improvement with treatment then empirical antibiotics should be continued for 4 weeks. If treatment fails then *Mycobacterium tuberculosis*, cat scratch disease and fungi should be considered.

Other treatment options include immobilisation to reduce pain. Surgical treatment may be required to drain abscesses or remove devitalised bone. Response to treatment can be monitored by a reduction in CRP/ESR with no progression of the disease on X-rays; however, it can take months for radiographical abnormalities to resolve. Complications include venous thrombosis, septic emboli, damage to growth plates and therefore abnormal bone growth, pathological fractures and chronic osteomyelitis. Without treatment osteomyelitis has a high mortality rate. After successful treatment most children will have complete resolution.

Neonatal osteomyelitis

Initial findings can be quite non-specific in the neonates. They are usually afebrile but irritable, with vomiting. Initially there will be decreased movement of a limb followed by swelling and erythema of the surrounding skin and soft tissues. Generally it is the unwell neonates who get haematogenous osteomyelitis often following a systemic infection. Other risk factors include prematurity, skin infections, complicated delivery and central venous catheter insertions. Common causative organisms are GBS (group B *Streptococcus*) and Gram-negative organisms.

Chronic osteomyelitis

Osteomyelitis is classified as chronic if the symptoms have been present for at least 2 weeks and there is radiological evidence of bone involvement. It is uncommon and often occurs as a result of inadequate therapy. It may be caused by major trauma or follow surgical procedures. It can present as an abscess or a draining sinus. Treatment is with long-term antibiotics, surgical debridement and bone grafting.

Septic arthritis

Generally children with septic arthritis present with fever and appear unwell, but neonates and infants may present with irritability and pseudoparalysis of the affected limb, with or without fever. In the older child it can present with a limp or lack of use of a limb in a previously mobile child. Clinically there will be joint effusions, warmth, tenderness and severe pain on movement. Most commonly it affects the knee or hip and usually only affects one joint.

The most common causative organism is *Staph. aureus* in infants and children, and other causes include *Haemophilus influenzae* (less common since vaccination introduction) and *Kingella kingae*. In neonates GBS and *Neisseria gonorrhoeae* are the common causative organisms. The bacteria cause a synovial reaction, with oedema that leads to accumulation of purulent material; this increases articular pressure and leads to destruction of the articular cartilage. Joint subluxation and dislocation can also be seen.

Blood investigations will show an elevated CRP (this is the best indicator of septic arthritis), ESR and WBC count. X-rays will show subtle signs of joint effusion (widening of the joint space), soft tissue swelling and loss of normal fat planes. Definitive diagnosis is usually with aspiration of synovial fluid. Normal synovial fluid is viscous, clear and acellular, with a protein concentration one-third that of plasma and a glucose content similar to that of plasma. If septic then there will be very elevated synovial WBC with or without a growth of bacteria. Treatment is with antibiotics and surgical drainage. If cultures are negative then *N. gonorrhoeae*, *Mycobacterium tuberculosis* and fungi should be considered.

Neonatal problems

Developmental dysplasia of the hip (DDH)

Developmental dysplasia of the hip is abnormal development of the acetabulum and proximal femur creating mechanical instability of the hip joint. The cause is usually idiopathic but it can also be associated with Ehlers–Danlos syndrome, Down syndrome, arthrogryposis and neuromuscular hip dysplasias such as spina bifida or cerebral palsy.

All newborns in the UK should undergo screening for DDH at birth and again at 6–8 weeks of age. The earlier DDH is detected the better the outcome, and risk factors include breech delivery, a family history and female sex. Its incidence is higher in first-born infants and in those with oligohydramnios. If DDH is not detected at newborn screening then it may present when the child begins to walk. This will be with a limp, limited abduction or obvious limb shortening.

If there is bilateral DDH (occurs in 20% of patients) then this can be detected at less than 3 months using Ortolani and Barlow manoeuvres (see Chapter 22). However, as patients get older the hip will be irreducible and stable, therefore it will be more difficult to detect. If DDH is left untreated there is rarely any pain and children will still manage to achieve developmental milestones appropriately. In later years there will be pain, loss of function, compensatory scoliosis and degeneration of the hip joint.

Classification of DDH is as follows:

1. **Dislocated:** there is no contact between the femoral head and the acetabulum; the Galeazzi test will show a leg length discrepancy, the Barlow test may be normal, and if the hip is reducible then this will be observed on the Ortolani manoeuvre.
2. **Dislocatable:** the femoral head will sit within the hip joint at rest but will become dislocated on the Barlow manoeuvre. The Galeazzi test will usually be normal and with the Ortolani manoeuvre you should feel the hip relocate back into the joint. This is an unstable joint.
3. **Subluxable:** the femoral head is in the joint at rest, but can be partially dislocated with manoeuvres. This gives mild hip instability.
4. **Dysplasia:** the hip joint has an abnormal shape.

DDH is best detected using ultrasound in infants up to 6 months of age, and the diagnosis is made using the Graf system, which measures specific angles. If there are risk factors for DDH then according to local guidelines these neonates undergo screening with an ultrasound scan. In those over 6 months old X-rays are more useful, as are MRI and CT scans.

Treatment is usually to position the femoral head appropriately within the acetabulum to allow for growth and reshaping. The first-line treatment option in those under 6 months is a splint, that is a Pavlik harness, which holds the hips flexed and abducted. It needs to be worn for 23 hours a day for 6 weeks, at which time the hip should be stabilised. The harness can then be used overnight only until 3 months of age. Complications of the harness include avascular necrosis of the femoral head and femoral nerve palsy. Surgery may be required in those children in whom the harness has failed or if DDH is detected at older than 6 months of age. Following surgery spica casting will be needed to maintain position.

Prognosis depends on the severity and timing of treatment. In those less than 6 months the Pavlik harness will provide correct positioning of the hip in 95% of patients. If there is any residual dysplasia then there is an increased risk of osteoarthritis in later years.

Talipes

Talipes has a prevalence of 1–3/1000 live births, affecting males more often than females, and in up to 60% of affected neonates it occurs bilaterally. The majority of cases are idiopathic although 10% are associated with other abnormalities.

Positional talipes

These cases are a result of positioning within the uterus and are not fixed but flexible, and can be moved into the neutral position gently. They can be associated with oligohydramnios and uterine abnormalities (fibroids or amniotic bands), breech presentation or multiple gestations. Generally physiotherapy is the mainstay of treatment, and very few result in any long-term complications. If physiotherapy is not effective then casting and bracing may be required. It can be associated with DDH as there are similar risk factors. Positional talipes is usually detected at birth.

Club foot (talipes equinovarus)

This is a fixed developmental deformity of the feet, where one or both feet are held plantarflexed, with the sole facing inwards (Figure 42.1). It is usually detected antenatally on ultrasound scanning. Along with the bony deformity there are also fibrous and shortened tendons, with underdeveloped perineal muscles. This limb will be shorter than the unaffected leg. It can be associated with chromosomal or genetic abnormalities,

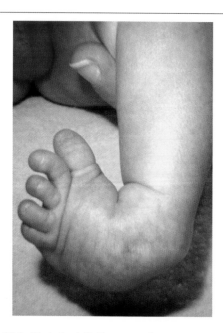

Figure 42.1 Club foot (talipes equinovarus). (Source: U.S. Centers for Disease Control and Prevention. Photo Credit: James W. Hanson, MD)

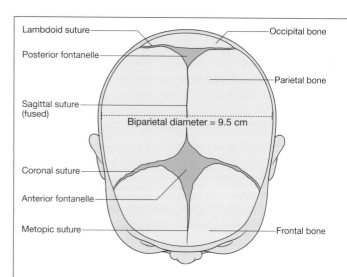

Figure 42.2 Craniosynostosis and the neonatal cranial sutures.

including spina bifida, Down syndrome and Edward's syndrome. Treatment involves manipulation of the foot to bring it into the midline if fixed, then plaster casting and bracing may be needed (this is known as the Ponseti method).

Craniosynostosis

Craniosynostosis is a premature fusion of one or more cranial sutures (Figure 42.2), affecting 1 in 2000 births. With this fusion there is restriction of growth at the affected suture, and continued growth on the unaffected side with brain development leading to skull deformity.

In utero the skull comprises skull plates that can slide over each other during delivery. There are four major sutures: metopic, coronal, sagittal and lambdoid. The first three meet together at the anterior fontanelle. The posterior fontanelle is where the sagittal and lambdoid sutures meet. At 2 months of age the posterior fontanelle closes, although the anterior one can take up to 2 years to close. The metopic suture closes at 2 years of age, and the other sutures close in adulthood once growth is completed.

Torticollis/sternocleidomastoid tumour

Torticollis is a twisted or rotated neck, which can be congenital or acquired. If it is congenital then there is often associated facial asymmetry.

Congenital torticollis

Muscular torticollis is the most common form of congenital torticollis. It is thought that malposition in utero or injury leads to fibrosis of the sternocleidomastoid muscle (SCM). The incidence is increased in breech delivery. The infant presents at around 2–4 weeks of age holding their head tilted to one side. Examination shows restricted neck movements, and a shortened SCM with rotation of the chin to the opposite side. A mass may be palpable in the inferior third of the SCM; this is well circumscribed and often described as a tumour. Associations include hip dysplasia, club foot and subluxation of C1-2 vertebral joints.

Diagnosis is usually clinical although sometimes ultrasound may be required to confirm that the mass in the SCM is muscular. Treatment is best commenced early with passive stretching and positioning to encourage the infant to move the head towards the midline. This prevents plagiocephaly and facial asymmetr, which if present may require surgical myotomy to release and lengthen the muscle at around 6–12 months of age, with good results.

Acquired torticollis

There are many different causes of acquired torticollis, and these include:

- Acute infections, such as pharyngitis, retropharyngeal abscess or viral URTI leading to muscle spasm or referred pain.
- SCM and trapezius muscle injury or inflammation.
- Cervical muscle spasm or cervical nerve irritation (from cranial pathology such as brain tumours).
- Ocular torticollis occurring when a child tilts their head to compensate for ocular misalignment such as in a squint to prevent double vision.
- Dystonic reaction from antiepileptic medications causing acute spasms.
- Sandifer syndrome, which is when gastro-oesophageal reflux causes torsion spasms of the neck and abnormal posturing. Treatment of reflux will resolve the symptoms.

Investigations include plain X-rays if there is trauma, or persistent or severe pain. CT and MRI scans will also be helpful. Treatment depends on the cause, and for most cases treating the cause will resolve the torticollis, otherwise NSAIDs or muscle relaxants may be helpful.

Arthrogryposis

Arthrogryposis is a non-progressive disorder that presents at birth with multiple joint contractures as a result of fibrosis of the affected soft tissue and muscles in the extremities. It is a very rare condition and has a multifactorial aetiology. There are rarely any other associations and intelligence is normal. Treatment is conservative along with correction of any contractures and deformities. They may need surgical release or bony reconstructive procedures.

Inherited disorders

Achondroplasia

Achondroplasia is the most common form of the skeletal dysplasias. Ninety percent occur as sporadic mutations, and the rest are inherited in an autosomal dominant pattern. It is a rhizomelic disorder where the proximal long bones are shorter than the distal bones. Clinical findings include short-limbed dwarfism, bowing of the lower extremities (genu varum), lumbar lordosis, a narrowed cervical and lumbar spinal canal with possible spinal canal stenosis and spinal cord impingement. Usually lifespan and cognitive ability are unaffected.

Osteogenesis imperfecta ('brittle bone disease')

This can be inherited in an autosomal recessive or dominant pattern as a result of a mutation in type 1 collagen genes that affects collagen maturation. As a result there is primitive woven bone formation that does not progress to stronger osteonal bone. This leads to fragility and fractures from minor stresses. It is estimated to affect 1 in 20 000 births and has nine different subtypes with varying severity.

Management generally involves reducing the fracture rate, improving function and treating complications. Prognosis depends upon the type, and the more severe forms will have an increased risk of premature death from immobility and thoracic deformities leading to pulmonary infections and loss of function.

Clinical case

Case investigations

This child presents with a long history of swelling in her knee. This will exclude more acute conditions such as trauma or infection. This is further supported by the lack of other symptoms such as fever. Recurring pain in an intermittent pattern points to a chronic condition.

The examination findings are consistent with joint inflammation, with pain, swelling, redness and a small joint effusion. The lack of leg length discrepancy excludes a chronic hip condition causing the limp. It is therefore likely that this patient has arthritis of her hip.

As the symptoms have been present for more than 6 weeks and the child is under 16 years of age then juvenile idiopathic arthritis is a diagnosis of exclusion in this case. This can be further classified by looking at the investigations and findings. All the blood investigations are normal and there are no systemic features and only one joint is involved, so this will rule out polyarticular arthritis and systemic arthritis. There are no other features to suggest psoriatic and enthesis-related arthritis. Although there is a negative ANA the most likely diagnosis is oligoarticular arthritis.

SUMMARY

Case conclusion

The diagnosis is therefore oligoarticular juvenile idiopathic arthritis. She is treated with an NSAID but the symptoms in her knee do not improve over the 6-week treatment course. This is followed by a series of intra-articular steroid injections into the knee with methotrexate, and her pain and swelling are reduced during the first 6 months. The treatment continues for 12 months with steroid and 24 months with methotrexate. No other recurring, significant joint pain develops during this time.

Key learning points

- Children often present to acute services with several different signs and symptoms that can be due to rheumatological or orthopaedic conditions, and it is therefore important to be able to differentiate the most likely cause and treat appropriately to avoid long-term damage to the joint, to recognise non-accidental injuries, and fractures related to another condition that has resulted in a weakened bone. Most cases are due to trauma or a self-limiting condition.
- Congenital and inherited musculoskeletal disorders are likely to manifest at an early age, or be expected by parental medical history, and may be recognised in the neonate.

 Now visit **www.wileyessential.com/humandevelopment** to test yourself on this chapter.

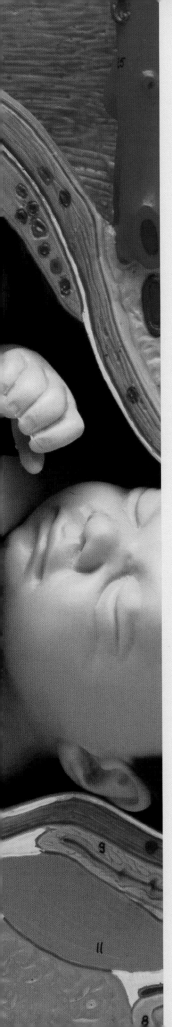

CHAPTER 43
Paediatric surgery

Toni Williams

Case

A 5-week-old baby, Adam, presents with frequent vomiting, poor weight gain and lethargy. The frequency of vomiting has increased in the last week, occurring with nearly every feed. Adam is hungry and eager to feed, and the vomit appears to be clear of blood and bile. Adam's mother thinks that the force with which Adam vomits is increasing, and she is concerned and upset. She worries that Adam is intolerant of breast milk.

Learning outcomes

- You should be able to recognise the signs and symptoms of common paediatric gastrointestinal and genitourinary conditions.

- You should be able to recommend further investigations and relevant surgical or other treatment options for common paediatric gastrointestinal and genitourinary conditions where appropriate.

Essential Human Development, First Edition. Edited by Samuel Webster, Geraint Morris and Euan Kevelighan
© 2018 John Wiley & Sons, Ltd. Published 2018 by John Wiley & Sons, Ltd.

Gastrointestinal conditions

Neonatal conditions

Malrotation and volvulus

Malrotation occurs when the gut fails to rotate completely during embryological development (see Chapter 7). As a result there is abnormal positioning of the gastrointestinal system. Most commonly there is incomplete rotation around the axis of the superior mesenteric artery, resulting in the caecum lying in the mid upper abdomen. The mesentery is on a narrow stalk predisposing the bowel to twist on itself causing a midgut volvulus, leading to obstruction and ischaemia of the small bowel. Malrotation may be associated with Ladd's bands – bands of peritoneum that can cause extrinsic compression and duodenal obstruction (Figure 43.1). Up to three-quarters of patients with malrotation present in the neonatal period with bilious vomiting secondary to volvulus. Presentation can occur later with bilious vomiting, abdominal distension and bloody stools. Rarely malrotation can remain asymptomatic until adolescence or adulthood. It is therefore important to treat bilious vomiting seriously at any age. An upper GI contrast study will confirm malrotation with abnormal position of the duodenal-jejunal flexure and corkscrew duodenum in the presence of volvulus. Malrotation requires surgical correction in all patients due to the risk of volvulus.

Oesophageal atresia and tracheo-oesophageal fistula

Oesophageal atresia is a congenital abnormality affecting the development of the oesophagus. Incidence is 1 in 3000 live births. There are several different types (Figure 43.2) and there is usually an associated tracheo-oesophageal fistula. Oesophageal atresia is associated with polyhydramnios antenatally secondary to the fetus being unable to swallow. At birth, there are frothy oral secretions with choking and cyanotic episodes. Babies with an H-type fistula without an associated atresia are symptomatic on feeding with coughing and choking as milk is aspirated into the lungs. In up to half of infants there can be other associated anomalies with VACTERL (Vertebral, Anal, Cardiac, Tracheo-oEsophageal, Renal and Limb abnormalities) and VATER (Vertebral, Anal, Tracheo-oEsophageal, Renal or Radial abnormalities) associations. Management is with surgical correction.

Atresia of the GI tract

Congenital atresias can occur during embryological development resulting in interruption of the GI tract. They can occur at any part, but are most common in the jejunum or ileum. Diagnosis can be made on antenatal scans suggested by polyhydramnios, a dilated loop of bowel or hyperechoic bowel. Babies with intestinal atresias will present within the first 48 hours of life with bilious vomiting and abdominal distension. An abdominal X-ray will show evidence of intestinal obstruction with dilated loops of bowel proximal to the atresia, air-fluid levels and absence of gas in the rectum. Intestinal atresias require surgical resection.

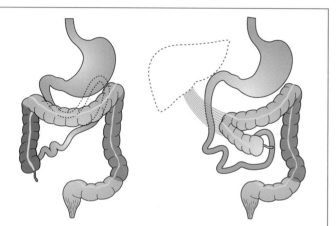

Figure 43.1 Ladd's bands can cause malrotation of the gastrointestinal tract.

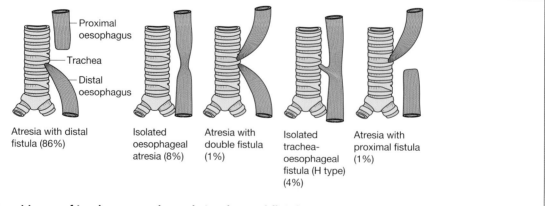

Figure 43.2 Different types of tracheo-oesophageal atresias and fistulas.

Congenital diaphragmatic hernia

Congenital diaphragmatic hernia (CDH) is a congenital defect of the diaphragm. The majority of these hernias (90%) are left-sided (Figure 43.3), known as a Bochdalek type; the rest are right-sided or occur through the oesophageal hiatus. Incidence is approximately 1 in 2200. As a result of the defect, there is herniation of the abdominal contents into the thorax resulting in cardiac displacement to the right and poor development of the lungs (pulmonary hypoplasia). CDH can be diagnosed on antenatal ultrasound. In babies without an antenatal diagnosis, presentation is with severe respiratory distress, a scaphoid abdomen and displacement of the cardiac apex to the right. The defect requires surgical correction but there are often ongoing respiratory difficulties secondary to the pulmonary hypoplasia.

Gastroschisis and exomphalos

Gastroschisis and exomphalos (or omphalocoele) are congenital conditions that are often diagnosed antenatally. In gastroschisis there is a defect of the abdominal wall adjacent to the umbilicus. As a result the bowel and occasionally other organs are outside the abdomen at birth (Figure 43.4). There is no overlying peritoneal covering and there is a large risk of fluid and protein loss. The bowel may be scarred or have adhesions resulting in stenosis, strictures and atresias. At birth, the baby is likely to require ventilator support with good fluid management and ongoing nutritional support. Smaller defects can be repaired with primary closure of the abdomen whilst in larger defects the bowel is covered with a silicone sac and gradually returned to the peritoneal cavity. Complications of gastroschisis include short bowel syndrome and failure to thrive. Over recent years the incidence of gastroschisis has been increasing, with current incidence in the UK of 4 per 10 000 live births, with an overall survival rate of over 90%.

In exomphalos there is herniation of the bowel through the umbilicus (see Figure 43.4). The defect is covered by peritoneum. Exomphalos has an incidence of 1 in 5000. The condition is often associated with other congenital abnormalities such as renal malformations, and with chromosomal anomalies such as trisomy 13 and trisomy 18. As with gastroschisis, repair can be either primary closure of small defects or a staged approach in more complex cases.

Hirschsprung's disease

Hirschsprung's disease is a congenital condition where there is failure of migration of ganglion cells to the submucosal and myenteric plexuses of the large bowel. This results in an aganglionic segment, which is narrow and contracted, extending from the anus proximally for a variable length of bowel. Hirschsprung's disease has an incidence of 1 in 5000 and is more common in males. Infants with Hirschsprung's disease can present with delayed passage of meconium (i.e. not passing meconium in the first 24–48 hours of life) and intestinal obstruction with abdominal distension, followed by bilious vomiting. Enterocolitis is a life-threatening complication of Hirschsprung's disease where there is infection and inflammation of the bowel, which can progress to perforation and septicaemia. Hirschsprung's disease can present later in life with a history of chronic severe constipation from birth. Diagnosis is made with a suction rectal biopsy, which shows an absence of ganglion cells. Surgical resection

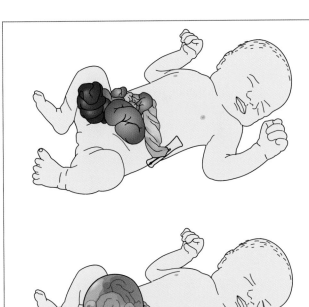

Figure 43.4 Gastroschisis herniation of the abdominal contents through the abdominal wall near the umbilicus (left) and exomphalos herniation of the bowel within the umbilicus (right).

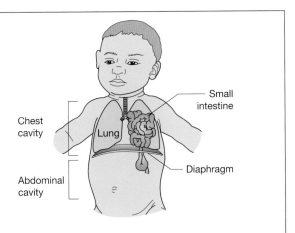

Figure 43.3 Congenital diaphragmatic hernia.

of the affected segment of bowel is required. In short segment Hirschsprung's this can be a one-stage procedure but if a larger segment is involved, a colostomy may be required to relieve the obstruction followed by a pull-through procedure where the normally innervated bowel is anastomosed to the anus.

Infants/older children

Intussusception

Intussusception occurs when one segment of bowel telescopes into an adjacent segment leading to an obstruction. This most commonly occurs proximal to the ileocaecal valve. As a result the blood supply is compromised and the bowel can quickly become necrotic. Intussusception is the most common cause of intestinal obstruction in children aged 5 months to 3 years and is most frequent from 5 to 10 months of age. In the UK the incidence is reported as 1.6–4 per 1000 live births and is more common in males than females.

The vast majority of intussusceptions are idiopathic where the aetiology is unclear. In 2–12% a lead point can be identified such as an intestinal polyp or Meckel's diverticulum. The classical presentation is a triad of abdominal pain, vomiting and passage of blood per rectum ('redcurrant jelly stools' – a mixture of mucus, sloughed mucosa and blood). However, redcurrant jelly stools are in fact a rare and late sign. Intussusception should be considered in an infant presenting with colicky abdominal pain, vomiting and lethargy with intermittent episodes of screaming associated with marked pallor (secondary to vagal stimulation). Examination may reveal a sausage-shaped mass within the right hypochondrium. Abdominal X-ray is abnormal in 60% of cases, showing signs of small bowel obstruction and paucity of air in the right iliac fossa. Abdominal ultrasound has a high specificity and sensitivity for diagnosing intussusception, showing a target-shaped mass. A contrast enema (air or barium) can be therapeutic as well as diagnostic, by hydrostatically reducing the intussusceptions and is successful in up to 75% of cases. Surgical intervention with manual reduction or resection is used in those where enema reductions fail or are contraindicated.

Appendicitis

Acute appendicitis occurs when the blind-ending appendix becomes obstructed and inflamed. It can occur throughout childhood but is commonest between 10 and 19 years. The classical presentation of acute appendicitis is central abdominal pain that migrates to the right iliac fossa, vomiting, anorexia and low-grade fever. However, this occurs in less than 60% of children and diagnosis can be difficult especially in the very young. On examination there is tenderness and guarding secondary to peritonitis. If the appendix is in an abnormal position, such as retro-caecal or pelvic, then the typical signs may not be present. Diagnosis is made based on clinical assessment but blood tests may show neutrophilia, and an abdominal ultrasound scan may (but not always) demonstrate an inflamed appendix. In those in whom the diagnosis is unclear, urine analysis is useful to exclude

a urinary tract infection and care should be taken to exclude a pneumonia. Management is with appendicectomy. Complications include perforation, appendix abscess and appendix mass.

Meckel's diverticulum

This is a remnant of the vitellointestinal tract and may contain gastric or pancreatic tissue. Meckel's diverticulum occurs in around 2% of the population. The diverticulum is approximately 5 cm long and can be found 60 cm from the ileo-caecal valve. People with a Meckel's diverticulum are often asymptomatic but the condition should be considered in patients with rectal bleeding, intussusception, volvulus or acute appendicitis. A technetium scan can be used to identify a Meckel's diverticulum due to increased uptake by the gastric mucosa. Surgical resection is required.

Pyloric stenosis

In this condition, which develops in the first few weeks of life, there is hyperplasia and hypertrophy of the muscular layers of the pylorus and the whole pylorus becomes thickened. Pyloric stenosis is the most common cause of intestinal obstruction in infancy with an incidence of 2–4 per 1000 live births, and is more common in males than females (4:1), with 30% of affected infants being first-born males. Aetiology is multifactorial with both genetic and environmental factors.

Pyloric stenosis presents in the first few weeks of life (usually between 3 and 12 weeks of life) with non-bilious vomiting, which becomes projectile in 70% of cases. The baby often remains hungry following the vomit. The infant may have poor weight gain or weight loss.

During a 'test feed' a firm, non-tender, 'olive-shaped', 1–2 cm mass (the thickened pylorus) can be palpated in the right upper quadrant at the lateral edge of the rectus abdominis muscle in 60–80% of patients. Gastric peristalsis may be observed just prior to vomiting.

The classical acid–base disturbance seen in pyloric stenosis is a hypochloraemic, hypokalaemic metabolic alkalosis. This is due to the loss of gastric fluids containing hydrochloric acid and the retention in the kidney of hydrogen ions in favour of potassium ions. The classical clinical and laboratory picture is becoming less common now that diagnosis tends to be made earlier.

An ultrasound scan will demonstrate the thickened pylorus with a target lesion on transverse images. Initial management involves rehydration and correction of electrolyte disturbances. Definitive management is corrective surgery, with the Ramstedt pyloromyotomy being the procedure of choice.

Urological conditions

Hypospadias

Hypospadias is a congenital malformation seen in boys where the urethral meatus is in an abnormal position (Figure 43.5). This is a relatively common finding in boys, affecting approximately 1 in 250, usually with milder forms.

Hypospadias can be associated with chordee, a ventral curvature of the penis, and an abnormal foreskin due to incomplete closure around the glans causing a hooded prepuce. The site of the meatus can vary from the ventral surface of the glans just proximal to its usual position, to more severe forms with the opening on the penile shaft, penoscrotal junction or perineum. The different forms of hypospadias are outlined in Figure 43.5. Severity is graded according to the distance of the urethral opening from its usual position and the degree of curvature.

Hypospadias can be associated with cryptorchidism and inguinal hernias. Infants with hypospadias should be assessed for the need for surgical correction. Milder forms may not need surgery but males with moderate and severe hypospadias may have problems with urinary stream and erectile dysfunction. Timing of surgery is important and in most centres is performed in the second year of life. Circumcision should be avoided prior to surgery since the foreskin may be used during the repair.

Phimosis

Phimosis describes a condition in which the foreskin of the penis is adherent to the glans penis. Before 3 years of age, a non-retractile foreskin is a normal finding. In older boys, phimosis is most commonly secondary to scarring of the tip, known as lichen sclerosus et atrophicus – balanitis xerotica et obliterans (BXO, when it affects the penis) or posthitis (PXO, when it affects the foreskin). Milder degrees of phimosis can be managed conservatively with good hygiene to reduce the risk of inflammatory phimosis and occasional gentle retraction in a warm bath. In more severe cases and in BXO/PXO circumcision may be required. A paraphimosis occurs when the foreskin is retracted beyond the coronal sulcus and cannot be reduced. This restricts the venous and lymphatic drainage of the distal penis and urgent reduction is required.

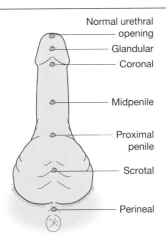

Figure 43.5 Sites of hypospadias urethral openings.

Circumcision

Circumcision is the surgical removal of the foreskin and is most commonly performed for religious reasons. The medical indications for circumcision are:

- Recurrent urinary tract infections, particularly if associated with renal abnormalities or renal damage.
- Recurrent balanitis.
- Phimosis, in older boys as a result of scarring.

Testicular torsion

Testicular torsion occurs when the testicle twists on the spermatic cord, thereby restricting blood supply. Although this can occur at any age, it is more common in adolescence. Males with testicular torsion develop sudden-onset pain to the scrotum, groin or lower abdomen associated with swelling. Without urgent surgical correction, the testis will be irreparably damaged within 6–12 hours. At the time of surgical exploration, both testes are fixed in case of an anatomical abnormality predisposing to torsion. The main differential diagnosis of testicular torsion is epididymo-orchitis secondary to viral or bacterial infection. Surgical exploration of these patients may be necessary to confirm the diagnosis and exclude testicular torsion.

Hydrocele

A hydrocele is a common finding in infancy especially after birth. They occur when peritoneal fluids move down into the scrotum through a narrow patent processus vaginalis. They present as a fluctuant scrotal swelling, which transilluminates with a torch. Most will resolve spontaneously over time, but large, persistent hydroceles can be treated with surgical ligation of the processus vaginalis.

Undescended testes (cryptorchidism)

The testes develop intra-abdominally in utero and descend through the inguinal canal in the third trimester. Cryptorchidism is therefore commoner in preterm infants. Approximately 3.5% of boys have unilateral or bilateral undescended testes at birth (Figure 43.6). In some cases, further testicular descent can occur after birth, with 1.5% of boys at 3 months of age having undescended testes. After 9 months of age, the testes rarely descend spontaneously.

Examination may reveal that the testis(es) is/are:

- Retractile (testis can be massaged down into the scrotum but retracts into the inguinal canal).
- Palpable or impalpable.
- Incompletely descended but in the normal line of descent.
- Ectopic (testis is located away from the normal line of descent).

It is important to distinguish the retractile testis from the ectopic or undescended testis, and orchidoplexy should be considered for impalpable or maldescended testes. Further

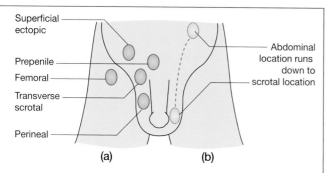

Figure 43.6 Route of the testes'descent. (a) Possible ectopic locations and (b) normal descent. (Source: S. Webster and R. de Wreede (2012) *Embryology at a Glance*. Reproduced with permission of John Wiley & Sons, Ltd.)

investigations such as karyotyping and evaluation for possible congenital adrenal hyperplasia must be considered in the case of bilateral undescended testes.

Orchidoplexy

Undescended testes have an increased risk of malignancy, torsion and subfertility and therefore surgical correction (orchidoplexy) is performed between 1 and 2 years of age. This can be a one- or two-stage procedure and the testis is surgically placed into the scrotum. Intra-abdominal testes that cannot be brought into the scrotum should be removed (orchidectomy) due to the risk of malignant change.

Inguinal hernias

In children, inguinal hernias are usually indirect and a result of a patent processus vaginalis. They are more common in males and in infants born prematurely. Presentation is with a swelling in the groin or scrotum, which enlarges with crying or straining. The spermatic cord will be palpable within the scrotum. Inguinal hernias can become irreducible, identifiable as a hard, tender lump. The child may be unwell with vomiting and irritability. The irreducible hernia can be reduced with sustained pressure to the swelling. All inguinal hernias should be repaired due to the risk of becoming strangulated..

SUMMARY

Clinical case

Case investigations

Adam's birthweight was 3.2 kg, and at 3 weeks he weighed 4.3 kg. At this visit he weighs 4 kg. On examination Adam is dehydrated, with serum sodium of 128 mEq/L, serum potassium of 2.8 mEq/L and serum chloride of 76 mEq/L. Abdominal examination finds a small mass in Adam's epigastrium.

Ultrasonography is used to examine the pylorus of his stomach and measures the muscle wall in this region at 6 mm thick for a length of 18 mm. Adam has hypertrophic pyloric stenosis.

Case conclusion

Adam's electrolyte levels and fluids are restored to normal over a 36-hour period in hospital, and a pyloromyotomy is planned.

Adam is placed under general anaesthetic and the surgeon finds the pylorus of the stomach by laparoscopy. She makes a longitudinal incision in the hypertrophied muscle of the pylorus to the depth of the mucosa, which is left intact. The mucosa bulges into the cut space, giving room for expansion of the internal canal between the stomach and duodenum.

After the operation Adam recovers well and is able to feed 6 hours after surgery. He then feeds regularly every 2 to 3 hours in small and slowly increasing volumes but shows no signs of abnormal emesis. Over the subsequent 8 weeks Adam's weight and length gain are restored to the expected curve on his growth chart.

Key learning points

- Many paediatric gastrointestinal conditions require surgical intervention to treat and manage. Congenital urological issues, particularly in boys, also need surgery to repair effectively.

- Recognising these neonatal issues and understanding the methods, risks and advantages of surgery is helpful when speaking to the family and when discussing options with the surgical team.

 Now visit **www.wileyessential.com/humandevelopment** to test yourself on this chapter.

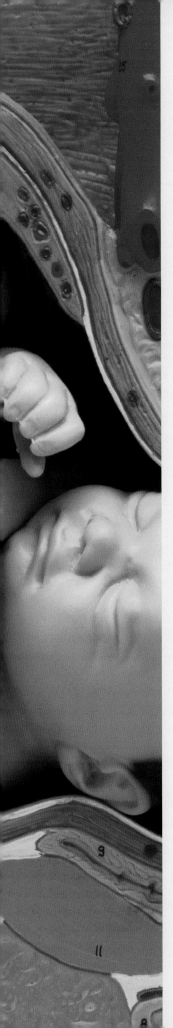

CHAPTER 44

Paediatric pharmacology

Lakshmipriya Selvarajan

Case

A 7-year-old boy, Andy, is presented to primary care by his mother. She describes his development of a cough and sometimes wheezy breathing over the last year, particularly at football training and when riding his bicycle. The symptoms appear and disappear, and seem to be worse during the autumn and winter, and he sometimes coughs and wakes during the night. His last cough was treated with antibiotics and cough suppressant syrups 8 months ago, but the cough returned soon after.

Learning outcomes

- You should be able to calculate drug doses for paediatric patients.
- You should be able to describe the considerations that must be made when prescribing in neonates and children.

Essential Human Development, First Edition. Edited by Samuel Webster, Geraint Morris and Euan Kevelighan.
© 2018 John Wiley & Sons, Ltd. Published 2018 by John Wiley & Sons, Ltd.

Introduction

It is important to recognise that children are not 'mini-adults' and hence we must be cautious in extrapolating adult data into paediatric practice. Most paediatric doses are calculated based on bodyweight and by body surface area (Table 44.1).

Children have been termed 'therapeutic orphans' as only a small range of drugs and/or formulations are licensed for use in children. There is information available in the British National Formulary for Children under individual drug entries to inform prescribers when indications or products are off-label or unlicensed.

Off-label use can be for a variety of reasons:

- Different age, e.g. diazepam rectal solution <1 year, fluticasone <4 years.
- Different indication, e.g. aspirin for Kawasaki disease.
- Different route, e.g. rectal lorazepam injection.
- Different frequency, e.g. 4-hourly salbutamol.
- Modifying the formulation by crushing or preparing a suspension.

Pharmacokinetics

The developmental changes that occur throughout childhood affect the response to drugs and the dose required to achieve a therapeutic effect without causing toxicity. Often standard doses (e.g. expressed in mg/kg) are useful to initiate treatment but must then be adjusted according to the individual child based on developmental differences and response.

Absorption and administration

The oral route is most commonly used. It is easy, safe and cheap. The drawbacks are that certain medications are unpalatable and tablets need to be crushed. The intravenous route is reliable and effective but requires venepuncture.

Intramuscular injections can be useful for stat injections or if the intravenous route is temporarily unavailable, but in general they are avoided if at all possible, even in older children.

The per rectal route is used in emergencies. Diazepam and paracetamol can be given this way.

Mucosal administration via the buccal or nasal route helps to bypass the hepatic first-pass metabolism and hence is rapidly absorbed. The bioavailability has been found to be greater compared to adults, for example with buccal midazolam.

As regards the percutaneous (topical) route, children have a far greater surface area to weight ratio than adults meaning that any systemic absorption will give higher plasma concentrations relative to adults. Topical administration is not commonly used in children, with the exception of hyoscine patches for hypersalivation.

Intraosseous administration is an infusion into the bone marrow, which can be used as an alternative to intravenous access as young children still have very soft bones. Most drugs are suitable to be given by this route, and administration has a rapid onset of action.

Distribution

When a baby is born, he or she contains around 80% water until day 3 or 4 of life when there is a large diuresis. Even after this, neonates and infants have greater total body water and relatively large extracellular fluid compartments compared with adults.

The determinants of drug distribution can largely be classified in terms of **drug** factors and **patient** factors.

Drug factors

Highly lipid-soluble and small non-ionised molecules will easily cross membranes such as the blood–brain barrier. A further drug factor that is extremely important is protein binding. The greater the protein binding of a drug, the less 'active' free drug is available to cross cell membranes and have a pharmacological effect.

A drug with high protein binding will therefore have a lower volume of distribution. Protein binding for a particular drug is altered in the neonate and is discussed below.

Patient factors

There are differences between adults and children in terms of drug distribution; body composition and protein binding are responsible for many of these differences. Both premature and full-term neonates have a much greater proportion of their bodyweight in the form of water compared to older children (Table 44.2).

Note the overall total body water is as high as 85% in the premature neonate compared to 60% at 1 year. The percentage of extracellular water reduces in the first few months of life, while the intracellular value increases. The 1-year-old is very similar to an adult in terms of water composition and distribution.

Most water-soluble drugs, for example most antibiotics, require a larger initial dose in neonates, because they have the greatest amount of total body water. The larger volume also means delayed excretion so doses are less frequent.

Table 44.1 Body surface area (BSA) at different ages.

Age	Weight (kg)	BSA (m²)
Newborn	3.5	0.25
6 months	7.7	0.40
1 year	10	0.50
5 years	18	0.75
12 years	36	1.25
Adult	70	1.80

Table 44.2 The developmental changes in body water composition.

Age	Preterm neonate	Neonate	1-year-old	Adult
Total body water (%)	85	80	60	60
Intracellular water (%)	25	35	35	40
Extracellular water (%)	60	45	25	20

Metabolism and excretion

In preterm neonates the kidney is still undergoing development; therefore renal function at birth is dependent on gestation. The glomerular filtration rate (GFR) increases dramatically during the first 2 weeks of life. Renal tubular secretion increases more slowly, but by 8–12 months both glomerular and tubular function are close to adult values.

This is why the dose frequency of renally excreted drugs (e.g. penicillin) increases over the first month of life. Care must be taken to individualise dose regimens of narrow therapeutic index drugs (e.g. gentamicin) to prevent accumulation. Conversely, patients with cystic fibrosis generally have high GFRs, which means that they require higher doses of renally excreted drugs.

Pharmacodynamics

At present very little is known about the difference in pharmacodynamics between age groups, therefore simply observe the usual considerations (e.g. vancomycin causing renal impairment, antiepileptics causing enzyme induction, etc.).

Intravenous fluids

As with all medicines in children, maintenance fluid requirements should be calculated based on the child's weight. The 24-hour fluid requirement for children over 1 month of age is calculated using:

First 10 kg	100 mL/kg
Second 10 kg (i.e. 10–20 kg)	+50 mL/kg
Every kg over 20 kg	+20 mL/kg

So, for example, a 23 kg child would require:

$100 \times 10 = 1000$ mL
$+ 50 \times 10 = 500$ mL
$+ 3 \times 20 = 60$ mL
Total = 1560 mL per 24-hour period
1560 mL/24 = 65 mL/hour

Maximum volumes are 2000 mL/day for girls and 2500 mL/day for boys.

The usual maintenance fluid is 0.9% normal saline with 5% dextrose, and the resuscitation fluid is 0.9% normal saline.

Calculating the deficit in dehydration

This is based on a child's weight and percent dehydration. *Calculation for fluid deficit for %dehydration:*

= (%dehydration/100) × weight (kg) × 1000 mL.

This can be simplified to:

%dehydration × weight × 10 = total fluid deficit (mL).

This should be replaced over 24 hours in case of gastroenteritis, and over 48 hours in case of diabetic ketoacidosis. This represents the **extra** fluid that is needed, so it should be added to the total maintenance requirements.

NPSA Alert (National Patient Safety Agency)

Hyponatraemia may develop as the result of any fluid regimen, due to a dilutional effect. Symptomatic hyponatraemia is a medical emergency and there have been numerous reports of neurological injury or even death following inappropriate fluid treatment.

The NPSA therefore published a Patient Safety Alert ('Reducing the risk of hyponatraemia when administering intravenous infusions to children'), which should be read in full. There is also an interactive case history available from BMJ Learning (http://learning.bmj.com).

Clinical case

Case investigations

On examination Andy is found to have an expiratory wheeze, and is diagnosed with asthma. His examination is otherwise normal. He is prescribed a Salbutamol inhaler, to be taken as two puffs of 100 µg each when needed, no more than four times per day, as recommended by the British National Formulary for Children guidance.

Case conclusions

Andy's symptoms responded to the Salbutamol inhaler when playing sports, removing the wheeze and preventing the development of a cough.

In this case the dosage recommendations of the inhaled short-acting β_2-agonist, Salbutamol, for children over 5 years of age and adults are the same, and Andy is

SUMMARY

unlikely to need his dosage to be adapted as he grows. If Andy experiences a worsening of symptoms and requires further treatment careful consideration of appropriate drugs and their dosage will need to be made depending upon the severity of his illness and his age.

Key learning points

- Oral administration is more acceptable to children.
- A number of pharmacokinetic and pharmacodynamic differences exist between children and adults, and change as a child grows.
- Care is needed with premature and term neonate pharmacology to avoid errors.
- Hepatic metabolism of drugs changes as hepatic enzyme systems and blood flow develops.
- The effects of a drug upon a young child can be difficult to predict, and children should be carefully monitored and dosage adjusted in response.

 Now visit **www.wileyessential.com/humandevelopment** to test yourself on this chapter.

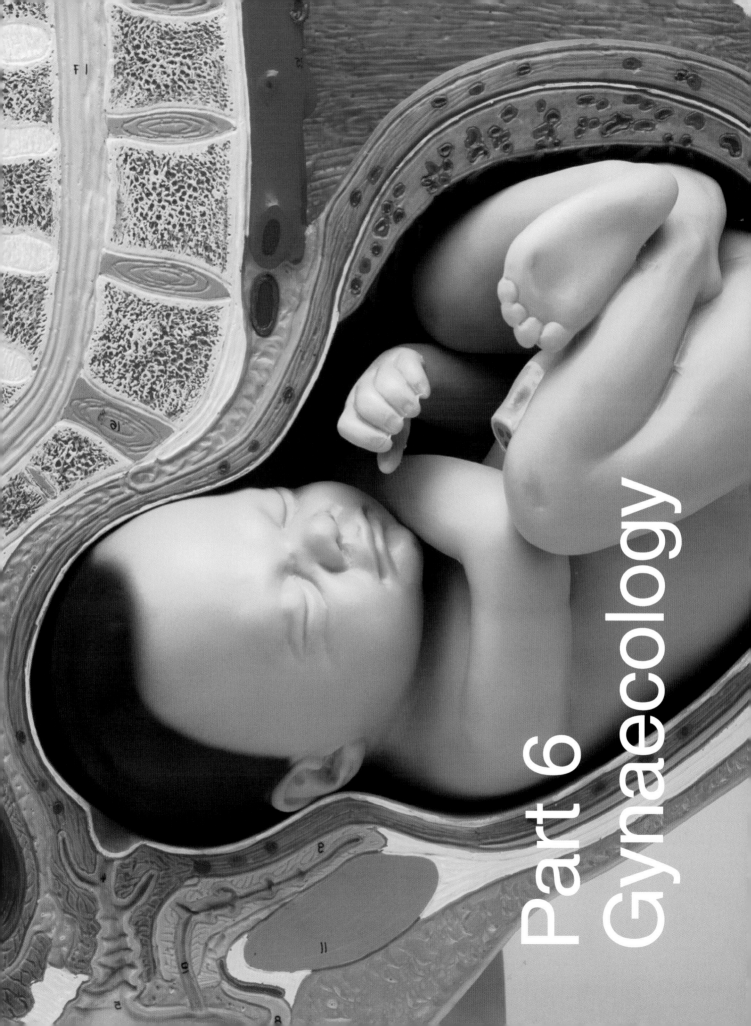

Part 6
Gynaecology

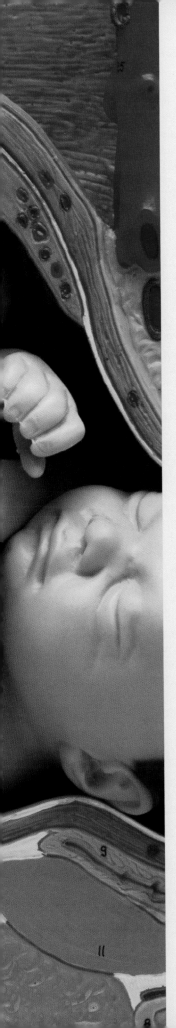

CHAPTER 45
Problems in early pregnancy

Manju Nair

Case

Mrs A is referred by her GP to the Early Pregnancy Assessment Unit with symptoms of pain and bleeding. She gives a history of 8 weeks of amenorrhoea and a positive pregnancy test. On examination, she is haemodynamically stable, there is no abdominal tenderness and the cervical os is closed with a small amount of bleeding.

An ultrasound scan shows a fetus with no heartbeat. This is her third miscarriage.

All her previous pregnancies have been complicated. Her first pregnancy was complicated with severe pre-eclampsia at 28 weeks and she was delivered by emergency caesarean section. This child is now 5 years old and doing well. In her second pregnancy she passed the products of conception at home and after investigations was told by her doctor that she had a complete miscarriage. In her third pregnancy she had an early scan at 10 weeks confirming a live fetus but subsequently she presented at 12 weeks with bleeding. She had medical management for an incomplete miscarriage.

Learning outcomes

- You should be able to list the common complications encountered in early pregnancy.
- You should be able to link the relevant embryology, anatomy, physiology and pharmacology to problems of early pregnancy.
- You should be able to describe the causes of bleeding and pain in early pregnancy.
- You should be able to diagnose and treat cases of miscarriage, ectopic pregnancy and molar pregnancy.
- You should be able to investigate and treat severe nausea and vomiting in pregnancy.

Essential Human Development, First Edition. Edited by Samuel Webster, Geraint Morris and Euan Kevelighan

Introduction

Early pregnancy is defined as gestational age up to 12 weeks. Some of the common symptoms encountered in this period are bleeding, pain, nausea and vomiting. The most important conditions contributing to these symptoms are miscarriage, ectopic pregnancy, gestational trophoblastic disease and hyperemesis gravidarum. These conditions are important as prompt diagnosis and treatment may save a mother's life.

In order to provide quick access to specialist care and to improve the standard of the care to these women, it is recommended that hospitals should provide an early pregnancy assessment unit. In the UK, all hospitals have a designated early pregnancy unit with scanning provision with a specialist team of nurses and doctors.

Embryology

Awareness of the stages of development prior to birth is important to understand the pathogenesis of most of these conditions, and is also useful when counselling (Table 45.1).

Cleavage stage

First the fertilised ovum completes the second phase of meiotic division. This is followed by a series of rapid mitotic cell divisions when the fertilised ovum is converted from the diploid stage to the 16-cell (morula) stage, followed by the formation of the blastocyst and implantation into the uterine wall (see also Chapter 5).

Embryonic period

During the embryonic period the cells of the inner cell mass differentiate and proliferate to form the systems of the body (see also Chapters 5 and 7), supported by the cells of the outer cell mass, which merge with structures of the uterus and form the surrounding sacs and placenta.

Development of placenta and membranes

In response to the circulating progesterone and the blastocyst there is decidualisation of the endometrium, which involves increased vascularisation and enlargement of the endometrial stromal cells with glycogen. There are three distinct areas at the site of implantation – the decidua basalis, which underlies the embryo; decidua capsularis (overlying the embryo); and the decidua parietalis (remainder of the decidua).

The maternal component of the placenta consists of the decidua basalis. The maternal surface is characterised by cotyledons. The fetal component consists of tertiary villi derived from the trophoblast and extra-embryonic mesoderm.

In early pregnancy the placenta mainly consists of cytotrophoblast and syncytiotrophoblast. In later pregnancy the former is replaced by connective tissue with fetal blood vessels.

Relevant endocrinology

There are two hormones that play an important role in early pregnancy. Understanding their roles will be useful in the management of some of the conditions.

Human chorionic gonadotrophin (HCG)

This is a glycoprotein with alpha and beta subunits. The beta subunit has a larger carbohydrate and protein component and its unique structure allows the production of highly specific antibodies and specific immunological assays. It is secreted by the syncytiotrophoblast cells and its main function is to support the corpus luteum. Beta-HCG (BHCG) can first be detected in the maternal blood 8 days after ovulation, about 1 day after implantation. The levels range from 100 IU/L at the time of a missed period to 100 000 IU/L at around 8–10 weeks. It reduces to 10 000–20 000 IU/L at around 18–20 weeks and remains at that level until term.

Clinical applications

Discriminatory zone of HCG

This is the level at which there is visualisation of the gestation sac in ultrasound scans (USS). The minimum levels of HCG in maternal blood required for visualisation are more than 1500 IU/L by transvaginal scan and 6500 IU/L by the transabdominal ultrasound scan.

It is useful in the monitoring of ectopic pregnancy. During the first 6 weeks of a normal pregnancy the HCG level follows a linear pattern of doubling every 48 h until reaching a level of around 10 000 IU/L, when it starts to follow a non-linear pattern. There can be deviations to this norm, and some normal pregnancies (10%) can have an abnormal pattern.

Trophoblastic disease

These cases have a high level of BHCG and show a slow regression curve after the resolution of pregnancy.

- High levels are related to hyperemesis gravidarum. Hence the higher incidence of hyperemesis in multiple pregnancy and molar pregnancy.
- Due to this hormone's structural similarity to thyroid-stimulating hormone, high levels of HCG can be associated with hyperthyroidism. Hence it is vital to assess thyroid function in cases of hyperemesis gravidarum.

Table 45.1 Three key stages of development.	
Cleavage stage	1st week following fertilisation This includes mitosis of fertilised ovum, morula formation, appearance of blastocyst and implantation
Embryonic period	2nd to 8th week
Fetal period	9th week to birth

Progesterone

This is produced by the corpus luteum until the 10th week of gestation.

Clinical application

Viable pregnancy

Progesterone prepares the endometrium and makes it ready for implantation. Levels less than 5 ng/mL are mostly associated with a non-viable pregnancy. However, on their own the values are not useful in making a diagnosis. It is more useful when combined with the results of the HCG levels and ultrasound results.

Progesterone also suppresses the maternal immunological response to the fetal antigens thus preventing maternal rejection of the trophoblast (see also Chapter 8 for effects of progesterone).

Miscarriage

Definition

Miscarriage is defined as the spontaneous loss of pregnancy from the time of conception until viability (approximately 24 weeks; see Table 45.2). The World Health Organization (WHO) defines miscarriage as the expulsion of an embryo or fetus weighing 500 g or less.

The term abortion should be avoided when referring to spontaneous miscarriage. In the UK it generally refers to termination of pregnancy.

Incidence

Spontaneous miscarriage will occur in 8 to 20% of pregnancies at less than 20 weeks gestation, and 80% of these occur in the first 12 weeks of gestation. Recurrent miscarriage affects 1% of couples.

Classification

The terminologies in Table 45.3 are helpful in classifying the different types of miscarriage.

Risk factors

- **Previous miscarriage:** The risk of miscarriage in a future pregnancy is approximately 20% after one miscarriage, 28% after two consecutive miscarriages, and 43% after three or more consecutive miscarriages.
- **Environmental factors:** Excess alcohol and smoking in a dose-dependent manner.
- **Maternal age:** This is due to a decline in the number and quality of the oocytes.
- **Obesity.**
- **Genetic factors.**
- **Chromosomal abnormalities:** Parental chromosomal rearrangements – one of the parents may have a balanced translocation or an abnormality in the chromosome arrangement but usually with a normal phenotype. Embryonic chromosomal abnormalities may also be a factor.
- **Structural causes:**
  - congenital or acquired uterine abnormalities (e.g. uterine septum, submucosal leiomyoma, intrauterine adhesions);
  - cervical incompetence.
- **Endocrinological factors:**
  - uncontrolled diabetes;
  - antithyroid antibodies;
  - polycystic ovary syndrome with hyperinsulinaemia.
- **Acute maternal infection** causing significant bacteraemia or viraemia.
- **Antiphospholipid antibody syndrome:** This is characterised by the presence of antiphospholipid antibodies and adverse pregnancy outcomes like three or more consecutive miscarriages before 10 weeks gestation, one or more morphologically normal fetal losses after the 10th week of gestation, or one or more preterm births before the 34th week of gestation owing to placental disease.
- **Thrombophilia:** This group includes activated protein C resistance, hyperhomocysteinaemia, factor V Leiden mutation, deficiencies of protein C/S and antithrombin III, and prothrombin gene mutation. This causes increased placental vascular thrombosis and impaired uteroplacental blood flow.

Symptoms

The symptoms of miscarriage include bleeding, lower abdominal pain, usually intermittent and crampy, and history of passing products of conception.

Signs

The patient can present in a state of shock in cases of severe haemorrhage. The vital signs may be normal or abnormal based on the extent of the bleeding.

Investigations for bleeding in early pregnancy

- **Full blood count:** To assess degree of anaemia secondary to haemorrhage
- **Estimate blood group and antibody status:** At less than 12 weeks gestation, anti-D Ig prophylaxis is indicated only

Table 45.2 Classification of miscarriage based on gestation.	
First trimester	Less than 12 weeks
Mid-trimester/second trimester/late miscarriage	Between 12 and 23 weeks

Table 45.3 Further miscarriage classifications.

Classification	Symptoms and clinical signs	Ultrasound findings
Complete miscarriage	History of passing products of conception. Bleeding then settles and the cervical os is closed	Midline echo or blood clot
Incomplete	History of passing some tissue. Bleeding continues	Heterogeneous tissue in the uterus with or without gestational sac. No fetal cardiac activity
Inevitable	Cervical os is dilated and products of conception may be seen	Gestation sac or fetal pole noted
Missed	Minimal brownish loss. Cervical os closed	CRL >7 mm, no cardiac activity, or no change in 7 days. Gestational sac >25 mm, no embryonic pole or yolk sac, or if less than 25 mm, no change in size
Recurrent	Three or more consecutive miscarriages	
Threatened	Bleeding that settles. Cervical os closed	Live pregnancy continues
Septic miscarriage	Complication of any of the above with sepsis. Characterised by fever, tachycardia, tachypnoea, abnormal bleeding or discharge with uterine tenderness	Retained products of conception serving as a focus of infection
Anembryonic pregnancy	USS diagnosis	CRL >7 mm, no cardiac activity, or no change in 7 days. Gestational sac >25 mm, no embryonic pole or yolk sac, or if less than 25 mm, no change in size
Pregnancy of unknown location	Diagnosis based on investigations. Increasing incidence due to very early presentation with symptoms of pain and bleeding	Positive pregnancy test and HCG levels less than discriminatory zone. No evidence of intrauterine or extrauterine pregnancy on USS
Pregnancy of uncertain viability		Intrauterine gestational sac with no embryonic heartbeat (and no findings of definite pregnancy failure)

CRL, crown–rump length; HCG, human chorionic gonadotrophin; USS, ultrasound scan.

in cases of ectopic pregnancy, molar pregnancy, termination of pregnancy, and heavy and persistent uterine bleeding. It should be administered in all cases after 12 weeks gestation. At less than 20 weeks, a minimum dose of 250 IU should be administered within 72 h of the event. After 20 weeks the dose increases to 500 IU, followed by a test for feto-maternal haemorrhage to determine if an additional dose is required.

- **Ultrasound scan (transvaginal or transabdominal):** Following is the chronology of appearance of structures seen on ultrasound scan in a normally developing early pregnancy: gestational sac appears around 5 weeks, followed by yolk sac at 5–6 weeks, fetal pole at 6 weeks and double decidual sign at 7 weeks. The 'double decidual sign'

refers to the sonological appearance of two concentric rings surrounding an anechoic area. The two rings represent the outer decidua parietalis lining the uterine cavity and the decidua capsularis surrounding the gestation sac.

Poor prognostic features on a scan are an irregular gestational sac, an abnormal yolk sac, a subchorionic haematoma and a slow fetal heart rate.

- **HCG:** Serum HCG level on its own is not useful in diagnosing miscarriage. It is useful in cases of pregnancy of unknown location (PUL). This term is used in cases where the urine pregnancy test is positive but neither an intrauterine nor an extrauterine pregnancy can be identified on transvaginal ultrasound (TVS). This could either be an early intrauterine pregnancy or an ectopic pregnancy.

- Two serum HCG levels taken 48 h apart may be useful in distinguishing between a viable intrauterine pregnancy or an ectopic pregnancy. A rise in the HCG level by more than 63% in 48 h is suggestive of a viable intra uterine pregnancy. An ultrasound scan should be offered in 7–14 days or earlier if the levels are greater than or equal to 1500 IU/L.
- If the HCG level plateaus or rises by less than 50% at 48 hours it is more likely to be a failing pregnancy. A urine pregnancy test should be repeated in 14 days. It is important to explain to the woman that diagnosis is not confirmatory and an ectopic pregnancy cannot be completely excluded.

    If the rise in the HCG value over 48 h is between 50 and 63% it could be an ectopic pregnancy.
- In all cases of PUL it is vital to assess the clinical signs and symptoms at all stages and provide the woman with information about contacting the emergency services in case she feels unwell or experiences symptoms of increased bleeding or pain.

Management

Miscarriage may be managed expectantly, medically or surgically (Table 45.4 and Figure 45.1).

- Mifepristone is an antiprogesterone agent that binds to and blocks the progesterone receptor thus inhibiting the action of progesterone. It also softens and dilates the cervix, causes decidual necrosis, increases prostaglandin release, increases uterine contractions, and enhances uterine sensitivity to administered prostaglandin.
- Misoprostol, a prostaglandin E1 analogue, binds to myometrial cells to cause strong myometrial contractions. This agent also causes cervical ripening with softening and dilation of the cervix.

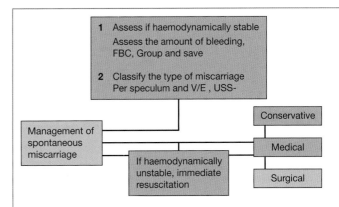

Figure 45.1 Management of spontaneous miscarriage. FBC, full blood count; V/E, vaginal examination; USS, ultrasound scan.

Recurrent miscarriage

Recurrent miscarriage may occur for a number of reasons, some of which remain unknown (Table 45.5).

Ectopic pregnancy

Definition

Ectopic pregnancy (EP) is defined as a pregnancy located outside the uterine cavity (Table 45.6 and Figure 45.2). The reported incidence of ectopic pregnancy is 1 in 90. Recently there has been a rise in the incidence of ectopic pregnancy, due to a combination of increased diagnosis and an increase in risk factors like pelvic infection and assisted conception techniques.

Heterotopic pregnancy is the term used for combined intrauterine pregnancy and extrauterine pregnancy. It has an

Table 45.4 Management of miscarriage.			
Type of management	**Method**	**Advantages**	**Disadvantages**
Expectant	No intervention Serial follow-up weekly Can convert at any time to medical/surgical	Non-invasive: • Natural • More successful if incomplete miscarriage	Prolonged follow-up More patient anxiety
Medical	Mifepristone and misoprostol (prostaglandin E1)	Success rates of 84–94% Cheap and safe	Risk of haemorrhage and infection due to retained products Prolonged follow-up
Surgical	Suction evacuation	One-stop management Less chance of failure Indicated in cases of heavy bleeding, haemodynamically unstable patient and molar pregnancy	Risks of anaesthesia Perforation and visceral injury Infection Haemorrhage Cervical damage Asherman's syndrome (intrauterine adhesions)

Table 45.5 Known causes of recurrent miscarriage and treatment methods.

Causes	Investigations	Treatment
Chromosomal disorders Parental chromosomal rearrangements (2–5%) Chromosomal abnormalities of the embryo (30–57%)	Cytogenetic analysis of products of conception Parental karyotyping should be performed if products of conception reports an unbalanced structural chromosomal abnormality	Referral for genetic counselling. Options include prenatal diagnostic tests, preimplantation genetic screening, gamete donation or adoption
Uterine anomalies (1.8–37%)	Ultrasound scan	
Antiphospholipid antibody syndrome (APLA; 15% incidence)	Screening for APLA antibodies	Low-dose aspirin plus heparin
Thrombophilia	Thrombophilia screening	Heparin therapy
Cervical incompetence	History of second-trimester miscarriage preceded by spontaneous rupture of membranes or painless uterine activity	Cervical cerclage in case of a strong history of cervical incompetence and if the cervical length is <25 mm before 24 weeks gestation

Table 45.6 Incidence of sites of ectopic pregnancy.

Classification according to the site of implantation	Incidence
Fallopian tube:	
Ampullary segment	80%
Isthmic segment	12%
Fimbrial end	5%
Cornual and interstitial	2%
Abdominal	1.4%
Ovarian	0.2%
Cervical	0.2%

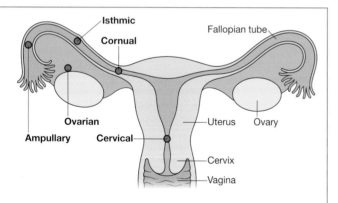

Figure 45.2 Anatomical sites of extrauterine implantation.

incidence of 1 in 30 000. However, the incidence can be as high as 1 in 100 after assisted conception.

Clinical significance

If undiagnosed patients may present in a state of shock due to a rupturing ectopic pregnancy. Ruptured ectopic pregnancy is the major cause of pregnancy-related maternal mortality in the first trimester.

One of the most important advances in recent times is the increasing accuracy with which ectopic pregnancy can be diagnosed and the availability of the various treatment modalities. Hence with adequate knowledge and expertise many of these deaths can be prevented.

Aetiology

Risk factors for an ectopic pregnancy are usually present in 25–50% of patients presenting with symptoms. Common associations include:

- previous ectopic pregnancy;
- tubal surgery;
- sterilisation;
- infertility;
- history of *Chlamydia* infection;
- intrauterine contraceptive device in situ;
- failed contraception with progestogen-only pill;
- age greater than 40 years;
- smoking;
- endometriosis.

Symptoms

- Over 50% of women are **asymptomatic** before tubal rupture.
- **History of amenorrhoea:** Usual presentation is around 6–8 weeks but it can be as early as 4 weeks.
- **Pain:** Pelvic or generalised lower abdominal pain. They may also present with shoulder tip pain due to diaphragmatic irritation from intraperitoneal bleeding. The diaphragm and tip of shoulder are innervated by the phrenic nerve (C5).
- **Bleeding:** This is usually light. Lack of adequate hormonal support leads to shedding of the decidua. This can take the

shape of the uterine cavity and is referred to as the decidual cast (see also Chapter 8).

- **Syncopial attack.**
- **Diarrhoea or tenesmus** (pain during defecation) due to peritoneal irritation from the haemoperitoneum.

Clinical assessment

Due to the potential complications of an undiagnosed ectopic pregnancy it is advisable to have a low index of suspicion for any woman in the reproductive age group with a positive pregnancy test who has any of the above symptoms.

Systemic examination

These patients can present in a state of shock due to a ruptured ectopic.

Abdominal examination

Localised abdominal tenderness, signs of haemoperitoneum with shifting dullness, guarding and rigidity may be noted.

Pelvic examination

There is minimal bleeding, and the cervical os is usually closed. Movement of the cervix will usually cause pain, a commonly noted sign of positive cervical excitation. It can also be positive in cases of pelvic inflammatory disease, uterine infection or endometritis. There may be an adnexal mass or tenderness.

Investigations

Investigations aid in the diagnosis and in the specific treatment.

- **Full blood count:** This helps in assessing the volume of blood loss in case of a ruptured ectopic and also in determining if blood transfusion is required.
- **HCG:** On its own may not be useful but together with an ultrasound scan has an increased sensitivity and specificity. The mean doubling time for the hormone ranges from 1.4 to 2.1 days in early pregnancy. In 85% of viable intrauterine pregnancies, the HCG concentration rises by at least 66% every 48 hours during the first 40 days of pregnancy; only 15% of viable pregnancies have a rate of rise less than this threshold.
- **Progesterone:** Levels <25 mmol/L are associated with a non-viable pregnancy. Levels >60 mmol/L are strongly associated with viable pregnancy.
- **Blood group:** Evaluate the need for anti-D in cases of surgical management irrespective of the gestation. Also required for cross-matching the blood if blood transfusion needed.
- **USS:** Transvaginal scan (TVS) has a higher specificity than transabdominal scan (TAS) in diagnosing an ectopic pregnancy. The TVS can detect an intrauterine pregnancy at a BHCG level of 1500 IU/L while levels of 6500 IU/L and above are usually required before detection by TAS.
- USS features suggestive of an ectopic pregnancy include:
  - absence of intrauterine gestation sac;
  - free fluid in pouch of Douglas;
  - gestation sac outside the uterus.

A pseudosac is present in 15% of cases due to the decidualisation of the endometrium. It is usually centrally located with a single echogenic rim compared to the healthy gestational sac, which is eccentrically located.

Management

If left untreated, an ectopic pregnancy in the fallopian tube can progress to a tubal abortion or tubal rupture, or it may regress spontaneously. It is important to assess whether the patient is haemodynamically stable or not.

Expectant management

This is an option for a clinically stable asymptomatic woman with no signs of rupture or intraperitoneal bleeding. The success rate for a spontaneous resolution is 88% when the initial HCG level is less than 2000 IU/L but only 25% at levels greater than 2000 IU/L. The risk of rupture in a woman with an ectopic exists until the HCG level has fallen to less than 20 IU/L. The patient should be appropriately counselled about the possibility of prolonged follow-up and to be alert for symptoms suggestive of rupture, such as increasing abdominal pain.

Criteria for expectant management
- Only for tubal ectopic.
- Titre of HCG <2000 IU/L.
- Size of the ectopic should be no more than 4 cm.
- No haemoperitoneum or haemodynamic instability.

Medical management

Methotrexate is a folic acid antagonist that inhibits DNA synthesis. The drug stops the pregnancy developing any further and the pregnancy is gradually reabsorbed. There is 90% success with a single-dose regime.

Criteria for medical management
- Hemodynamically stable without active bleeding or signs of haemoperitoneum.
- Patient desires future fertility.
- General anaesthesia poses significant risk.
- Patient able to return for follow-up care.
- Patient has no contraindications to methotrexate.
- Unruptured adnexal mass <3.5 cm at greatest dimension.
- BHCG that does not exceed 5000 IU/L.

Contraindications
- Hepatic, renal or haematological disease.
- Active pulmonary disease.

- Peptic ulcer disease.
- Immunodeficiency.
- Chronic liver disease, alcoholism, alcoholic liver disease.
- Blood dyscrasias: thrombocytopenia, leucopenia, significant anaemia, bone marrow hypoplasia.

Protocol for methotrexate administration

- Dose: 50 mg/m^2 single dose i.m. injection.
- Follow-up with HCG assays on day 4 and day 7 and weekly until normal.
- If the HCG level fails to drop by at least 15% a second dose of methotrexate can be administered, or consider surgery.
- Recurrent ectopic pregnancy rate is 10–20%.

Adverse effects of methotrexate

- Nausea and vomiting.
- Stomatitis.
- Gastrointestinal upset.
- Deranged liver function.
- Dizziness.
- Severe neutropenia (rare).
- Reversible alopecia (rare).
- Pneumonitis.

Surgical management

Surgical management can involve either salpingectomy or salpingostomy.

The route of entry can be via either a laparoscopy or laparotomy. A laparoscopic approach is preferable to an open approach. However, in the presence of haemodynamic instability entry should be by the most rapid method and this is nearly always via laparotomy

Laparoscopic salpingostomy should be considered as the primary treatment in the presence of contralateral tubal disease and the desire for future fertility. There is a 15% risk of persistent trophoblastic tissue; hence follow-up with BHCG is essential.

Hyperemesis gravidarum

Definition

About 50–90% of all pregnancies are accompanied by nausea and vomiting. The condition is usually self-limiting and usually disappears by 20 weeks.

Hyperemesis gravidarum occurs in 0.5–3% of pregnancies and is defined as severe vomiting associated with weight loss of more than 5% of pre-pregnancy weight, dehydration, electrolyte imbalances, ketosis and the need for admission to hospital for treatment.

Aetiology

Several theories have been postulated to explain the cause of nausea and vomiting in pregnancy. The hormonal theory suggests that there is linear relation with levels of HCG. This explains the higher incidence of hyperemesis in multiple pregnancy and trophoblastic diseases.

Thyroid function may be physiologically altered during pregnancy due to the structural homology between HCG, thyroid-stimulating hormone and their receptors. The degree of hyperthyroidism and HCG concentrations correlate with the severity of vomiting; in most women thyroid dysfunction is self-limiting.

Some studies have suggested a deficiency in vitamin B$_6$. Other possible causes are hyperacuity of the olfactory system due to an oestrogen effect, and delayed gastric emptying in pregnancy due to progesterone stimulus. Being seropositive for *Helicobacter pylori* is also associated with an increased risk of hyperemesis gravidarum.

The evolutionary adaptation theory suggests that nausea and vomiting are a mechanism to prevent the woman eating potentially harmful foods. It has also been postulated that it is an abnormal response to stress or negative feelings about the pregnancy. However, it is more likely that the psychological symptoms may be a result, rather than a cause, of nausea and vomiting in pregnancy.

Clinical significance

If untreated severe vomiting can lead to dehydration and electrolyte imbalance.

Other complications include depression, Mallory–Weiss tears of the oesophagus, Wernicke's encephalopathy due to vitamin B$_1$ deficiency, and an increased risk of venous thromboembolism due to dehydration, prolonged immobilisation and increased coagulopathy related to pregnancy. Fetal complications include fetal growth restriction.

Management

Hospitalisation may be required at the initial presentation in order to stabilise the patient. Outpatient management in dedicated settings with specialised personnel is another option based on the clinical assessment.

- Examine for signs of dehydration (e.g. tachycardia, postural hypotension).
- Urinalysis for ketones, urinary tract infection.
- Laboratory investigations such as full blood count, urea and electrolytes, liver function tests and thyroid function tests.
- Assess for any signs of depression due to the psychological impact.
- Ultrasonography to identify predisposing factors (e.g. multiple or molar pregnancy).
- Exclude any other causes.

Specific management

Hydration

Normal saline (0.9%; 150 mmol/L sodium) or Hartmann's solution are appropriate fluid replacement choices. Rapid correction can cause central pontine myelinolysis. Wernicke's encephalopathy may be precipitated by intravenous dextrose, hence this should be avoided.

Vitamins

In order to prevent Wernicke's encephalopathy, a thiamine (vitamin B_1) supplement should be given routinely to all women with hyperemesis. This can be administered as thiamine hydrochloride tablets 25–50 mg t.d.s. The intravenous regime consists of 100 mg thiamine diluted in 100 mL of normal saline infused over 30–60 minutes weekly. Pyridoxine supplements (20 mg t.d.s.) may also be considered if there is evidence of deficiency such as anaemia and peripheral neuropathy.

Alternative therapies, such as herbal treatments, homeopathy, hypnosis, hypnotherapy and psychotherapy, have also been tried with limited success.

Proton pump inhibitors and H_2 blockers

These are useful in women who also have dyspepsia.

Antiemetics

Antiemetics can be safely administered to women with hyperemesis gravidarum (Table 45.7). There is no evidence that this is associated with an increased incidence of congenital abnormalities compared to the general population.

Corticosteroids

Prednisolone 40–60 mg p.o. reducing by half every 3 days, or hydrocortisone 100 mg i.v. b.i.d. is an alternative if there is no response with routine antiemetic treatment.

Enteral feeding with nasogastric tube

In severe cases not responding to any of the above treatments, total parenteral nutrition (TPN) may be required. The complications of TPN are infection, thrombosis and metabolic problems.

Gestational trophoblastic disease

Definitions

Gestational trophoblastic disease (GTD) comprises a group of disorders caused by abnormal proliferation of trophoblastic tissue. It includes the benign group of complete and partial molar pregnancy and malignant conditions like invasive mole, choriocarcinoma and placental site trophoblastic tumour (PSTT).

Gestational trophoblastic neoplasia forms the subgroup that requires chemotherapy and includes the invasive mole, choriocarcinoma and PSTT.

The term hydatidiform mole is derived from the Greek word *hydatis*, which means drop of water, and the Latin word *mola*, which means a mass.

An invasive mole is a tumour invading the myometrium with trophoblastic hyperplasia. It usually follows a complete hydatidiform mole. It may regress spontaneously but rarely metastasises.

Choriocarcinoma is a carcinoma arising from the trophoblastic epithelium and can follow normal pregnancy, miscarriage, ectopic pregnancy and/or a molar pregnancy.

Table 45.7 Antiemetic regimes that may be used to treat hyperemesis gravidarum.

Drug	Dose	Side effects
Cyclizine	50 mg p.o./i.v./i.m. t.d.s.	Drowsiness
Promethazine	25 mg p.o./i.m.	Less common side effects: headache, psychomotor impairment, and antimuscarinic effects, such as urinary retention, dry mouth, blurred vision and gastrointestinal disturbances
Metoclopramide	10 mg p.o./i.v./i.m. t.d.s.	Acute dystonic reactions involving facial and skeletal muscle spasms and oculogyric crises. These are more common in the younger age group (<20 years). This usually occurs within a few days of starting treatment and disappears within 24 h of cessation. Procyclidine 5–10 mg i.v. can be used for treatment of a dystonic attack. Other adverse effects include drowsiness, restlessness and diarrhoea
Prochlorperazine	10 mg p.o./i.m. 8-hourly or 25 mg rectal suppository 12-hourly or buccal tablets 3–6 mg b.i.d.	Drowsiness, anticholinergic side effects, transient side effects like acute dystonia
Ondansetron	4 mg t.d.s. or 8 mg p.o./i.v. b.i.d.	Constipation, headache and flushing. Less common adverse effects include hiccups, hypotension, bradycardia, chest pain, QT prolongation, arrhythmias, movement disorders and seizures

Clinical significance

There is a 10–20% risk of choriocarcinoma following a complete molar pregnancy, and a 0.5–3% risk after partial mole.

Incidence

The incidence in the UK is 1 in 3000, but in the east Asian population it is as high as 1 in 300.

Pathology

It is caused by trophoblastic proliferation of both the cytotrophoblast and syncytiotrophoblast. There is no embryo in a complete mole. A partial mole has an embryo, which usually dies early. It happens following fertilisation of an egg that has lost its nucleus. The partial hydatidiform mole is triploid (XXX) with one maternal and two paternal chromosomes.

Risk factors

- Age >40 years.
- High incidence in Asia, parts of Africa and central America.
- Previous molar pregnancy.

Symptoms

- Irregular vaginal bleeding.
- Hyperemesis.
- Excessive uterine enlargement.
- First trimester miscarriage.
- Passage of hydropic vesicles (grape-like material).
- Rarer presentations include hyperthyroidism, early onset pre-eclampsia or abdominal distension due to theca lutein cysts, or neurological symptoms such as seizures due to metastatic disease.

Diagnosis

- **Ultrasound:** Snowstorm appearance is a classical diagnostic sign of a molar pregnancy. Multiple sonolucent spaces are noted in the uterine cavity. No embryonic tissue is noted in a complete mole. In a partial mole in addition to the finding of silent miscarriage there may be multiple sonolucent areas in the amniotic cavity.
- **Definitive diagnosis** is by histology of the products of conception.

Management

- Suction evacuation of the uterus.
- Anti-D prophylaxis – for all RhD-negative women.
- Medical evacuation of complete molar pregnancies should be avoided due to a risk of embolisation with oxytocic agents.
- All women diagnosed with GTD should be referred for follow-up to a trophoblastic screening centre. There are three centres in the UK – in Sheffield, at Charing Cross Hospital in London and at Ninewells Hospital in Dundee. If HCG has reverted to normal within 56 days of the pregnancy event then follow-up will be for 6 months from the date of uterine evacuation. If HCG has not normalised within 56 days the follow-up should be for 6 months from normalisation of the HCG level. The barrier method of contraception is advised until the normalisation of HCG levels is achieved. Use of the combined pill during this period increases the risk of developing GTD, and intrauterine contraceptive devices increase the risk of uterine perforation.

Management of subsequent pregnancies

There is a 1 in 100 risk of developing a repeat molar pregnancy. Therefore, ultrasound should be obtained in the late first trimester of subsequent pregnancies to confirm normal fetal development. Additionally, the HCG level should be obtained 6 weeks after completion of subsequent pregnancies to rule out occult choriocarcinoma. The products of conception should be sent for histological examination following any pregnancy loss.

Predictors of development of GTN requiring treatment

- HCG level >100 000 IU/L.
- Theca lutein cysts >6 cm in diameter.
- Plateau in the serum HCG concentration over 3 weeks after evacuation of uterus (in this situation it is important to exclude a new pregnancy).
- Persistence of detectable serum HCG for more than 6 months after molar evacuation.

Summary of approach to common problems in early pregnancy

Key facts 45.1 to 45.3 and Table 45.8 provide useful algorithms for the diagnosis and management of commonly encountered problems in early pregnancy.

ⓘ Key facts 45.1 Differential diagnosis of bleeding in early pregnancy

- Physiological relating to implantation in case of mild spotting
- Miscarriage including threatened miscarriage
- Ectopic pregnancy
- Gestational trophoblastic disease
- Cervical, vaginal, or uterine pathology

ⓘ Key facts 45.2 Differential diagnosis of pain in early pregnancy

- Ectopic pregnancy
- Ruptured ovarian cyst
- Haemorrhagic ovarian cyst
- Haemorrhagic corpus luteum
- Miscarriage
- Pelvic Inflammatory disease
- Diverticulitis
- Appendicitis

ⓘ Key facts 45.3 Causes of nausea and vomiting in pregnancy

- Physiological
- Hyperemesis gravidarum
- Genitourinary conditions, e.g. urinary tract infection, pyelonephritis and ovarian torsion
- Metabolic disorders and endocrine conditions, e.g. hypercalcaemia, thyrotoxicosis, diabetic ketoacidosis, Addison's disease
- Gastrointestinal conditions, e.g. peptic ulcer, pancreatitis, bowel obstruction, hepatitis, cholelithiasis, appendicitis
- Neurological disorders, e.g. vestibular disease, migraine
- Eating disorders, e.g. anorexia nervosa and bulimia
- Drug-induced vomiting

Table 45.8 Algorithm for management of pain and bleeding in early pregnancy.

History	Examination	Investigations	Treatment
LMP	General	FBC, G&S	Expectant
Risk factors	Abdominal	Urine: pregnancy test, microscopy	Medical
Symptoms	Speculum	culture and sensitivity	Surgical
	Bimanual pelvic examination	HCG	
		Progesterone	
		USS: TVS, TAS	

FBC, full blood count; G&S, group and saving of serum; LMP, last menstrual period; TAS, transabdominal scan; TVS, transvaginal scan; USS, ultrasound scan.

Clinical case

Case investigations

Mrs A has a diagnosis of missed miscarriage in view of the light bleeding and USS showing an embryonic pregnancy. She opted to have surgical management by suction evacuation under general anaesthesia.

Since this is her third miscarriage possible causes for recurrent miscarriage need to be evaluated. She had parental chromosome analysis, and the products of conception were sent for cytogenetic analysis to exclude chromosome defects. Other investigations included ultrasound scan (normal), thrombophilia screening (normal) and APL (antiphospholipid antibody) screening, which was positive.

Case conclusions

A diagnosis of antiphospholipid antibody syndrome was made. For her next pregnancy she will be offered treatment with aspirin and low molecular weight heparin.

Summary

Key learning points

- Main causes of bleeding in early pregnancy are miscarriage, ectopic pregnancy, physiological (related to implantation of the pregnancy) or local causes like cervical or vaginal pathology.
- It is important to exclude an ectopic pregnancy, since a ruptured ectopic pregnancy can result in maternal morbidity and mortality.
- Ultrasonography (mainly transvaginal) is a useful diagnostic tool in early pregnancy. However, the role of clinical examination cannot be ignored in reaching a diagnosis and to plan appropriate management.
- Evaluate the need for anti-D in rhesus-negative women (see the section on 'Miscarriage' above for indications of anti-D prophylaxis).

 Now visit **www.wileyessential.com/humandevelopment** to test yourself on this chapter.

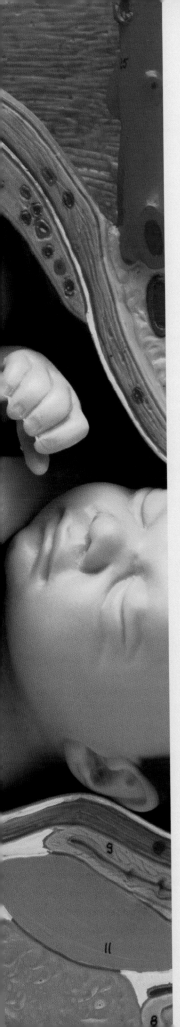

CHAPTER 46
Subfertility

Gurpreet Singh Kalra

Case

A 37-year-old female, Mrs X, has been trying for a pregnancy for 4 years. She has a history of chronic pelvic pain and irregular periods. Her partner, Mr Y, is a 46-year-old male. Neither have pregnancies in the past. Both have a normal BMI, are non-smokers and have minimal alcohol intake. Neither has ever had an STI or any surgery. They are both fit and have healthy diets. Mrs X is taking folic acid.

Learning outcomes

- You should be able to list and describe known causes of subfertility, and be able to recommend lifestyle changes that may improve fertility, and identify factors associated with subfertility.

- You should be able to recommend further investigation options for a patient with subfertility.

- With investigation results and medical histories you should be able to recommend appropriate treatment options or management plans for a couple with history of subfertility.

Essential Human Development, First Edition. Edited by Samuel Webster, Geraint Morris and Euan Kevelighan
© 2018 John Wiley & Sons, Ltd. Published 2018 by John Wiley & Sons, Ltd.

Introduction

Subfertility is defined as the inability of a couple to achieve pregnancy after 2 years of regular unprotected sexual intercourse, where the female is of fertile age and is non-lactating. Male age is increasingly being considered relevant and there is evidence that increasing male age has a negative impact on chances of fertility. Subfertility is defined as primary or secondary depending upon whether the couple have ever achieved a pregnancy together. Most often there is more than one cause for a couple's subfertility, which may involve both partners. It is therefore considered as a couple problem rather than a condition affecting an individual. Management of subfertility focuses on identifying the cause and helping the couple conceive. The aim is to achieve a live birth of a healthy child.

History of assisted reproduction

In 1678 one of the first microscopists, Anton van Leeuwenhoek (1632–1723), made original observations of spermatozoa in male semen and described them as minute tadpole-like creatures made of transparent substance with very brisk movements called at that time 'animalcules or spermatick worms'. The history of the oocyte is older and probably starts in 1555 when 'Vesalius' made the first authoritative observation of an ovarian follicle. But it wasn't until 1852 that fertilisation was first recorded, when Henry Nelson directly observed an *Ascaris* (nematode worm) sperm penetrate a transparent ovum. Yanagimachi and Chang reported the first successful in vitro fertilisation (IVF) in animals in 1963 using in vitro capacitated sperm. Later the collaboration of Patrick Steptoe, a gynaecological laparoscopist, and Robert Edwards, an embryologist, and three centuries of history, philosophy and science of reproduction culminated in the birth of Louise Brown in July 1978 at Oldham General hospital – the first 'test tube' baby

Changing reproductive behaviour

Over the last 50 years a significant change has happened in the reproductive behaviour of human society. The way people think about reproduction has changed. It has become more a matter of choice rather than a natural outcome of marriage and sexuality. This change has in turn had an important impact on the problem of infertility. The trend for women to become more educated and participate fully in the labour force has entailed more demands on their time and effort from their professional life. There have been increasing moves towards choosing to delay having children, to not have children at all, to decrease the number of children per couple, and to extend the intervals between children. The increased incidence of divorce has added to this. Another factor facilitating this change was the introduction of safe and reliable methods of contraception in the 1960s, which made it easy to plan childbirth.

The age at which women have their first child has gone up across Europe. In The Netherlands in 1970 the average age at which women had their first child was 24.6 years. This had gone up to 29.1 years in 1999 (see also www.cbs.nl).

Prevalence

Approximately one out of every six to seven couples will need help with fertility. For demographic studies a 5-year exposure period of unprotected sexual intercourse is used to define subfertility, with live birth as the outcome rather than clinical pregnancy.

A World Health Organization (WHO) systematic analysis of 277 surveys from 190 countries from 1990 to 2010 suggested that among women aged 20–44 years exposed to risk of pregnancy, 1.9% were unable to achieve a live birth or had primary subfertility. Amongst women who had at least one live birth, 10.5% were unable to achieve a further live birth or had secondary subfertility. No statistically significant change in prevalence of subfertility has been noted for most world regions over the period from 1990 to 2010.

A recent publication from the UK Office of National Statistics suggests that the prevalence of childlessness amongst women born in 1967 and reaching the end of their fertile age (45 years) by 2012 is 19%, while amongst women born in 1940 childlessness by the end of their fertile age was 11%. There seems therefore to be a fall in fecundity in women in the UK. This fall is likely to be related to change in female reproductive behaviour whereby childbearing is delayed or abandoned for the aforementioned reasons. A fall in sperm count has also been proposed, which seems to be related to environmental factors such as oestrogenic pollutants. There also seems to be an increasing incidence of testicular tumours, cryptorchidism and hypospadias, postulated to have similar causes.

The hypothalamo-pituitary-gonadal axis

In order to be able to understand reproductive physiology, it is essential to have a good understanding of the hypothalamo-pituitary-gonadal axis. The hypothalamo-pituitary-ovarian axis forms the basis of the physiology of ovulation (see also Chapters 2 and 8). An understanding of this will not only enhance your knowledge regarding managing ovulatory subfertility but also your understanding of various aspects of ovarian stimulation used during different types of assisted reproduction. The hypothalamo-pituitary-testicular axis regulates spermatogenesis as well as male sexual function.

The secretion of gonadotrophin-releasing hormone (GnRH) is pulsatile, peaking about every 2 hours. It leads to a pulsatile pattern of secretion of luteinising hormone (LH) and follicle-stimulating hormone (FSH) from the anterior pituitary gland. LH and FSH are produced by the same cells (gonadotrophs) in the anterior pituitary but under different types of stimuli from varying frequency or amplitude of the GnRH pulses.

The female hypothalamo-pituitary-ovarian axis

Figures 46.1 and 46.2 are graphic representations of the flow of hormones and the processes or changes they lead to in the ovary during the follicular and luteal phases of menstrual cycle.

Key effects in females

- In females the hypothalamo-pituitary-gonadal (H-P-G) axis is cyclical, going through the same cycle every month.
- Oestrogen is the main controlling factor during the follicular phase while progesterone predominates during the luteal phase.
- Both oestrogen and progesterone influence GnRH, LH and FSH by their positive and negative feedback to both the anterior pituitary and hypothalamus.
- In turn the influence of GnRH on LH/FSH and eventually upon oestrogen and progesterone synthesis occurs due to a specific frequency and amplitude of the GnRH pulses, which are different for the follicular and luteal phases.

- Oestrogen at low levels has a negative feedback effect on FSH/LH, which is rapid, but at very high levels it has a positive feedback effect on LH/FSH leading to the pre-ovulatory surge. This is a slow action, taking about 48 hours.
- Progesterone has a direct negative feedback effect on LH/FSH and also blocks the effect of rising levels of oestrogen in the luteal phase to stimulate a rise in LH/FSH.
- Inhibin plays a key role by exerting a negative feedback effect on FSH.
- Oestrogen decreases the GnRH pulse amplitude while progesterone decreases the GnRH pulse frequency. Hence the pulsatile secretion of GnRH is of high frequency and low amplitude in the follicular phase while it is of low frequency and high amplitude in the luteal phase.

The hypothalamo-pituitary-testicular axis

The basic principles of the H-P-G axis in males are similar to those in females, where pulsatile secretion of GnRH from the hypothalamus causes pulsatile secretion of LH and FSH

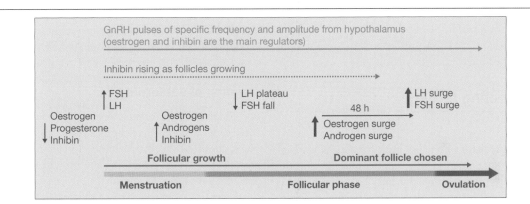

Figure 46.1 Hypothalamic-pituitary-ovarian interaction during the follicular phase. FSH, follicle-stimulating hormone; GnRH, gonadotrophin-releasing hormone; LH, luteinising hormone.

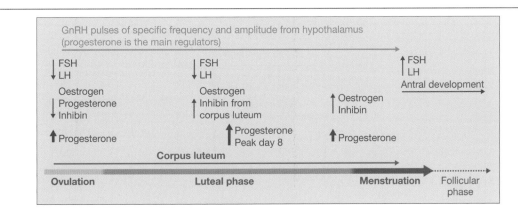

Figure 46.2 Hypothalamic-pituitary-ovarian interaction during the luteal phase. FSH, follicle-stimulating hormone; GnRH, gonadotrophin-releasing hormone; LH, luteinising hormone.

from the anterior pituitary. The gonadotrophins act on different groups of cells in the testes and lead to the production of sex steroids – mainly testosterone but also other hormones including inhibin (Figure 46.3).

Key effects in males

- In males the H-P-G axis is not cyclical and hence fertility is constant rather than cyclical.
- Testosterone and inhibin are the main hormones regulating the H-P-G axis in males although they work in different compartments.
- Testosterone and inhibin work only by negative feedback.
- GnRH is pulsatile leading to pulsatile secretion of LH and FSH, which in turn influence production of androgens, inhibin, other hormones and spermatogenesis.
- LH is mainly responsible for stimulating testosterone production from Leydig cells while FSH mainly acts on Sertoli cells to regulate spermatogenesis.
- Testosterone at all levels exerts a negative feedback effect on the hypothalamus and anterior pituitary gland, contrary to oestrogen. It has negative feedback control of LH but possibly to a lesser degree also of FSH.
- Inhibin, like in females, plays a key role with a negative feedback effect on FSH. But unlike testosterone, inhibin acts only at the anterior pituitary level.

Factors affecting fertility

Age

Age is a strong predictor of fertility both for natural conception and assisted reproduction. The number of follicles in the ovary is genetically predetermined for each individual and this finite pool of follicles is already produced by the end of the fetal stage of development. From a maximum number of about 6–7 000 000 follicles by mid-gestation of the female fetus, there is a constant fall in follicle number up to menopause.

After the age of about 37.5 years there is an accelerated loss. The total number of follicles left in the ovaries, amongst other factors, decides the age of menopause in women, at which point only a few hundred or about a thousand remain. The age of optimal fertility in a human female is considered to be between 18 and 30 years, after which there is a decline in ovarian function leading to the final event of menopause through stages of subfertility, sterility and cycle irregularity.

The occurrence of a higher rate of oocyte aneuploidy and increasing rates of miscarriages with age has been extensively studied. There is a significant increase in the incidence of trisomy 21 with age, which is much higher after 40 years of age. These findings suggest that the best oocytes are probably recruited first, leaving poorer quality oocytes with advancing age of the human female. There seems therefore to be a direct relationship between the number of oocytes left in the ovary and the quality of oocytes at any age. Thus ovarian ageing or the age-dependent loss of female fertility is considered to be a combination of decline in quantity and quality of oocytes. The success of IVF has been seen clearly to be dependent on female age, and declines significantly after 40 years of age.

There is increasing evidence suggesting that male fertility also declines with age although to a lesser extent. The decline is not linear and is more profound after 35 years.

Duration of subfertility

For couples having regular sexual intercourse about two to three times a week where the age of the female is less than 40 years, about 80–90% will achieve pregnancy in the first 12 months. Half of the remaining couples will achieve pregnancy over the following 12 months. Only a small proportion of those remaining will succeed in the next 12 months. Couples waiting longer than 3 years are significantly less likely to conceive. A duration of subfertility longer than 3 years is therefore a negative predictor.

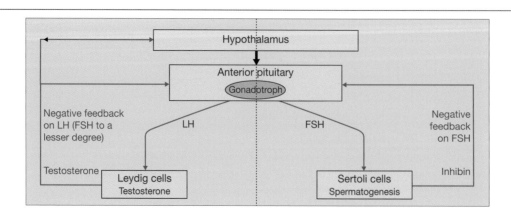

Figure 46.3 Hypothalamic-pituitary-ovarian axis in males. FSH, follicle-stimulating hormone; LH, luteinising hormone.

Obesity

Women with a body mass index (BMI) over 30 kg/m² take longer to conceive, and weight loss seems to improve their chances of fertility. There is an increased risk of aneuploidy in obese women, which may in turn be responsible for an increased risk of miscarriage in obese women. In males, increased numbers of abnormal spermatozoa and increased DNA fragmentation are associated with a BMI over 25 kg/m².

Low body weight

A weight loss of around 15% can cause menstrual irregularity while a weight loss of around 30% can cause secondary amenorrhoea. A BMI of less than 19 kg/m² has been reported to cause delay in conception. Low body weight is known to cause hypogonadotrophic (hypo-oestrogenic) hypogonadism. Weight gain in these cases can restore ovulation and hence fertility.

Smoking

Cigarette smoking delays fertility significantly, and there is good evidence that it impacts male as well as female fertility. Women who smoke are about 35% less likely to conceive in the first year of trying compared to non-smokers. Even passive smoking seems to have a negative impact on fertility. There also seems to be an association between cigarette smoking and semen quality but the link is not as strong as with female fertility.

Occupation

Certain occupational agents have a deleterious effect on fertility and it may involve some types of working patterns. There is good evidence that the following common exposures can reduce fertility:

- Shift work or physically intensive work can prolong time to pregnancy in females.
- Exposure to nitrous oxide and other anaesthetic gases can reduce fertility in occupations like anaesthetists, theatre nurses and dental nurses.
- Certain types of pesticides (dibromochloropropane, polychlorinated biphenyls) are known to cause abnormal sperm parameters in agricultural workers.
- Exposure to vibrations in engine drivers or operators of machinery such as diggers can cause oligospermia or asthenozoospermia.
- Exposure to prolonged heat leading to raised scrotal temperature is known to cause abnormal sperm parameters amongst welders, bakers and drivers.
- Exposure to X-rays amongst radiographers is known to cause abnormal sperm parameters.

Recreational drugs

Marijuana is known to prevent ovulation, while cocaine use in females is known to cause tubal factor infertility by an unknown aetiology. Cocaine and androgenic anabolic steroids are known to cause poor sperm quality.

Alcohol

Excessive alcohol intake may be deleterious to semen quality but the effect seems to be reversible. While the evidence regarding excessive alcohol intake on female subfertility is lacking there is strong evidence regarding harmful effects of alcohol on the fetus.

Types of subfertility

One out of every six to seven couples will need help with achieving fertility. Aetiology is multifactorial in the majority of cases. The prevalence of subfertility at any given time varies globally, depending upon the region of the world, ethnicity and local environmental, social and cultural factors. It is estimated that in the UK at any given time about 10% of the population may be subfertile, which includes primary and secondary subfertility. The different types of subfertility and their estimated prevalence in the UK include:

- ovulatory disorders 21–32%;
- tubal factors 14–26%;
- endometriosis 5–6%;
- uterine disorders 3–5%;
- male factor 19–57%;
- coital problems 2–6%;
- unexplained subfertility 15–30%

About 30% of couples are estimated to have combined subfertility with both male and female factors contributing to it.

Ovulatory disorders

Failure of ovulation or infrequent ovulation can delay time to conception and is one of the commonest causes of subfertility. Fortunately ovulatory subfertility has a high successful treatment rate. Couples with purely ovulatory subfertility can achieve almost normal fertility, but this comes at the expense of increased risk of multiple pregnancies. Age is a strong predictor of subfertility in females, and there is a linear fall in follicle numbers with age. The rate of fall in number of follicles is accelerated from about 35–38 years of age. With women choosing to have children later in life, ovulatory subfertility is more likely to occur.

Ovulatory subfertility can be further subdivided into subtypes.

Hypogonadotrophic hypogonadism

Low serum oestradiol levels (<40 ng/mL or <110 pmol/mL) and lack of bleeding after progesterone withdrawal is typical of this condition. These women are usually amenorrhoeic. The levels of FSH and LH are also usually low. It constitutes 5–10% of all ovulatory subfertility.

The condition may be congenital where there is a defect of gonadotrophin synthesis associated with olfactory sensory defect (Kallmann's syndrome). Or it may be acquired as classically seen in anorexia nervosa, underweight women or women doing regular strenuous exercise as athletes. A critical amount of fat is required as a proportion of a female's body weight in order to have regular cycling of hormones and to maintain reproduction. Low body weight may therefore lead to anovulation and amenorrhoea. Hypo-oestrogenic hypogonadism may also be secondary to acute or chronic extreme emotional stress. Non-functioning pituitary adenomas or hypothalamic tumours, including craniopharyngiomas, can also lead to this condition. Acute ischaemia and necrosis of the pituitary gland, for example during massive postpartum haemorrhage (Sheehan's syndrome), are also known causes.

Diagnosis
- Low BMI, <19.
- Low serum oestradiol levels.
- Serum FSH and LH will usually be low.
- Specific tests depending upon the condition suspected, e.g. MRI for brain tumours, pituitary adenomas or acute ischaemic lesions.

Treatment
- Controlled ovarian hyperstimulation with gonadotrophins and timed sexual intercourse.
- Controlled ovarian hyperstimulation with intrauterine insemination.
- IVF.

Normogonadotrophic hypogonadism

Women with normogonadotrophic anovulation have normal levels of oestrogen as well as normal levels of FSH and LH. They do therefore experience bleeding on progesterone withdrawal. About 70–85% of all ovulatory subfertility is caused by this condition. The aetiology of anovulation seems to be a disturbance in the pattern of pulsatile GnRH secretion from the hypothalamus.

Polycystic ovaries

The largest contributor to this group is polycystic ovarian syndrome (PCOS), which largely manifests as oligo-ovulatory subfertility, menstrual irregularities, hirsutism and acne. PCOS is a heterogeneous group of disorders characterised by androgen excess, hyperinsulinaemia, glucose intolerance and low sex hormone-binding globulin, apart from a characteristic ultrasound appearance of ovaries with multiple peripheral small follicles of 2–10 mm in a 'string of beads' appearance, with 12 or more on each side (Figure 46.4). These are seen in about 80% of women with PCOS. Androgen excess, however, may also be caused by conditions like congenital adrenal hyperplasia and ovarian or adrenal tumours, which also cause

normogonadotrophic anovulation. The hyperandrogenism in conditions other than PCOS is much more marked.

Excess body weight or a high BMI is also known to be an independent risk factor for ovulatory dysfunction. More than 50% of patients with PCOS also tend to be obese. Disorders involving either an overactive or underactive thyroid gland are known to cause ovulatory dysfunction, and stabilising thyroid function establishes ovulation in the majority of cases.

Diagnosis
- Baseline bloods including serum FSH, LH and prolactin. LH levels are raised and are almost double the FSH levels.
- Free testosterone, sex hormone-binding globulin (serum SHBG).
- Transvaginal ultrasound scan showing typical multiple peripheral small follicles.
- Serum C peptide and insulin levels to check for insulin resistance.

Treatment
- Lifestyle advice if obese (weight loss).
- Metformin – evidence of benefit in women with insulin resistance.
- Clomiphene citrate with or without metformin. Metformin on its own seems to cause ovulation in about 80% of cases. This improves further if clomiphene citrate is given while the patient is on metformin. Alternatively aromatase inhibitors like letrozole can be used for ovulation induction.
- Ovarian drilling in clomiphene-resistant cases.
- Intrauterine insemination with controlled ovarian hyperstimulation for ovulation induction. Better success rates are reported with gonadotrophins as compared to clomiphene citrate.
- IVF.

Hypergonadotrophic hypogonadism

When the ovaries are depleted of follicles or are resistant to gonadotrophins, this leads to low oestrogen levels with high levels of gonadotrophins, particularly FSH. The following conditions are typical:
- Premature ovarian failure, occult as well as those related to autoimmune conditions and fragile X syndrome.
- Chemotherapy or radiotherapy.
- Turner syndrome.
- Gonadal dysgenesis.

Diagnosis
- Serum FSH and LH.
- Serum anti-Müllerian hormone or antral follicle count if available as these are better tests of ovarian reserve and response as compared to FSH.
- Serum oestradiol.
- Chromosome analysis for karyotype to check for Turner syndrome or other X chromosome abnormalities including very rare translocations of X chromosome material to autosomes.

- Molecular genetics for fragile X or *FMR1* (fragile X mental retardation protein) premutation.
- Autoimmune screen including antithyroid peroxidase antibody and serum adrenal antibodies.

Treatment

- Hormone replacement therapy to prevent consequences of oestrogen deficiency like osteoporosis, vasomotor flushes and diminished sexual wellbeing including vaginal dryness.
- Oocyte donation. There is a small potential for spontaneous ovulation but the rate of spontaneous conception remains very low. Oocyte donation and IVF therefore offers the best success rates as the same or better than that of IVF with own eggs at the given age.

Hyperprolactinaemia and drugs

Prolactin-secreting adenomas are the main cause of high prolactin levels resulting in disruption of ovulation. Prolactin seems to disrupt ovulation by affecting follicular maturation as well as inhibiting steroidogenesis.

Primary hypothyroidism, if untreated, can lead to ovulatory subfertility but apart from that can also lead to raised prolactin in some, as thyrotrophin-releasing hormone (TRH) has a prolactin-stimulating action. PCOS can also show a relatively modest rise in prolactin levels.

Some antidepressants – e.g. some selective serotonin reuptake inhibitors (SSRIs), monoamine oxidase inhibitors (MAOIs) and tricyclics – as well as antipsychotics (e.g. risperidone) can raise prolactin levels and interrupt ovulation.

Diagnosis

- Serum prolactin, FSH and LH.
- Serum thyroxine and TSH.
- MRI of the brain.

Treatment

- Consider change of medication if hyperprolactinaemia is drug induced.
- Dopamine agonists bromocriptine and cabergoline are drugs of choice for hyperprolactinaemia. Cabergoline has lesser side effects while bromocriptine has a better and well-established safety profile with regard to teratogenesis.
- Treat hypothyroidism if underactive.
- Ovulation induction with clomiphene or gonadotrophins.

Tubal factor subfertility

Fallopian tubes are not only the conduits required for the male and female gametes to come together. They are very specialised organs aiding the ovum to be picked up by fimbriae on its journey to meet the sperm. Part of the process of sperm capacitation takes place in the tube. The critical step of fertilisation takes place in the tube as well, and the early developing embryo is nourished in the tube.

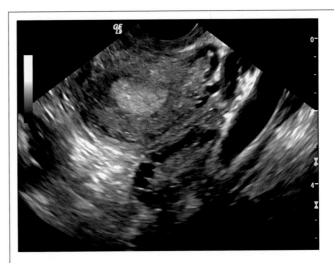

Figure 46.4 Ultrasound scan of polycystic ovaries.

Partial or complete blockage of the tubes is known to cause 14–26% of subfertility in developed countries while in developing countries the proportion can be up to 80% of all subfertility. A population-based study of the epidemiology of subfertility in Bristol and Avon in 1985 suggested the incidence to be 14%.

Common causes of tubal disease

- Pelvic inflammatory disease. About 60% of all tubal factor infertility in the developed world is caused by *Chlamydia trachomatis*. About 1% of all women infected with *C. trachomatis* will develop tubal factor infertility. *Chlamydia* is asymptomatic in about 60–70% of women. Gonorrhoea also contributes but in a much smaller proportion.
- Genital tuberculosis is the largest contributor in developing countries.
- Endometriosis can lead to adhesions around tubes and cause tubal blockages.
- Adhesions around tubes after previous pelvic or abdominal surgery.
- Appendicitis.
- Inflammatory bowel disease.

Diagnosis

- **Hysterosalpingogram (HSG):** The traditional non-invasive test of tubal patency. The catheter is passed through the cervical canal into the uterine cavity and contrast is insufflated while a series of radiographs are taken to assess the uterine cavity as well as the passage through the tubes. The procedure has high sensitivity and specificity for tubal patency for distal tubal blocks. The drawbacks are the exposure to radiation as well as significant discomfort.
- **Hysterosalpingo-contrast sonography (HyCoSy):** This is the non-invasive tubal patency test that involves an ultrasound scan of the uterus while a contrast medium is

insufflated through a catheter placed in the uterine cavity. The accompanying ultrasound scan imaging of the pelvis can show any ovarian cysts, fibroids, polyps or endometriomas. Neither HyCoSy nor HSG can diagnose mild grades of endometriosis or peritubal adhesions.

HyCoSy has a negative predictive value for tubal block of about 85–95% with a positive predictive value of about 44–60%. There is good concordance between HyCoSy and HSG for sensitivity and specificity for tubal patency as compared to laparoscopy and dye test. The pain and discomfort with HyCoSy are less compared to HSG and there is no exposure to radiation.

- **Laparoscopy and dye test**: This is the gold standard as it gives maximum information. It involves a laparoscopy under general anaesthetic, usually as a day case. Blue dye is insufflated through the cervical canal and the passage of dye is assessed through the tubes to ascertain patency. This procedure also gives an opportunity to visualise the uterus and both ovaries for any relevant pathology including peritubal adhesions and endometriosis. Another advantage is the opportunity to treat the pathology and therefore optimise fertility. These benefits come at the cost of surgical risks as well as the risks of general anaesthetic.

Treatment

The treatment for tubal factor infertility is either tubal surgery or IVF depending upon the grade of tubal damage.

Tubal surgery

The pregnancy and live birth rates after tubal surgery are higher in low grades of tubal damage while the ectopic pregnancy rate is higher with a high grade of tubal damage.

- Distal tubal block is more suitable for tubal surgery than proximal tubal block. Surgery may involve adhesiolysis, fimbrioplasty and neosalpingostomy.
- Opening of proximal tubal blockage can be attempted by hysteroscopic cornual catheter or by selective salpingography under radiographic guidance.
- Presence of unilateral or bilateral hydrosalpinges is known to lower the pregnancy and live birth rates after IVF. Surgical removal of hydrosalpinx is therefore recommended.
- The success rate for tubal reanastomosis for reversal of sterilisation depends on age, time since sterilisation and method of sterilisation. The success rate can vary between 46 and 73% for ages 20–49 years. The success rates are highest for clip or ring sterilisation and lowest for diathermy.

Assisted reproduction for tubal disease

IVF has a higher success rate in women with severe tubal disease than compared to tubal surgery although each IVF cycle gives only one chance. The success rate of IVF compared to tubal surgery is also higher in older women and women with bilateral hydrosalpinges. The recommendation in case of hydrosalpinges however is that these patients should have salpingectomy prior to IVF.

Endometriosis

Endometriosis can be seen in up to 40% of all women of fertile age. And it causes subfertility in up to 5% of all women. It is described in more detail in Chapter 50.

Management of subfertility

About 5–6% of subfertility is caused by endometriosis, and removal of all grades of endometriosis improves rates of spontaneous conception. The results seem to be better after surgical excision than with diathermy or laser ablation.

The success rate of IVF treatment is reduced in the presence of all grades of endometriosis and surgical removal seems to improve the success rate. However, there may not be a significant benefit to removal of unilateral endometriomas more than 3 cm in size prior to IVF treatment.

Suppression of endometriosis with GnRH analogues alone or as an adjunct to surgical excision pre- or post-operatively does not seem to confer a significant benefit on pregnancy rates via natural conception. There is some evidence suggesting benefit of a 3–6-month suppression of the ovaries with GnRH analogues post-surgical excision but prior to treatment in IVF cycles.

Uterine factor infertility

Müllerian anomalies

A small proportion of subfertility, about 3–5%, may be due to factors local to uterine and cervical anatomy. Uterine factors seem to increase the rate of miscarriage rather than decreasing fertility.

Congenital anomalies (Müllerian defects) like uterine septum (Figure 46.5), bicornuate uterus or uterus didelphys are the commonest.

The cervix may be affected by a cervical septum (or two cervices), and the vagina may have a vaginal septum in its upper third portion. A uterine septum with an arcuate uterus

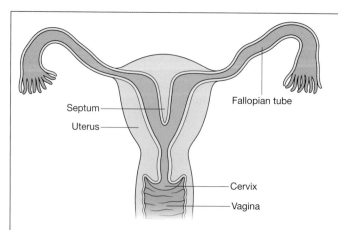

Figure 46.5 A uterine septum is a congenital defect that affects fertility.

(heart-shaped cavity) accounts for 90% of the Müllerian vertical fusion defects. There is evidence that pregnancy and live birth rates improve after surgical resection of intrauterine septa.

Anomalies of kidneys and urinary tracts are found in 20–30% of cases of Müllerian abnormalities.

Unexplained subfertility

Unexplained subfertility is delay in achieving pregnancy in heterosexual couples after having regular sexual intercourse when all other causes have been ruled out.

The duration is arbitrarily taken as a couple having tried to conceive for 12 months. However, if the female age is more than 35 years the duration is taken as 6 months in order to avoid delays in treatment, as there is a risk of declining ovarian reserve influencing any treatment outcomes.

The aetiology of unexplained subfertility is unclear but various factors are implicated, some of which may be:
- subtle decline in ovarian reserve;
- subtle decline in semen parameters;
- cervical factors;
- problems with endometrial receptivity and implantation failure.

About 15–30% of subfertility is thought to be of unexplained origin.

Management

There is a 1–3% chance of a woman who is trying to conceive becoming pregnant at each menstrual cycle with no treatment for these couples; this possibility can be enhanced by education about lifestyle changes to benefit reproduction. There is evidence that trying to conceive for 3 years without success is a negative predictor for achieving natural conception. Few couples will be keen to wait longer or keep trying.

Ovulation induction does not improve the conception rate in couples with unexplained subfertility unless used in conjunction with intrauterine insemination (IUI). IUI should be offered for up to six cycles followed by IVF.

Male factor subfertility

The overall incidence of male factor subfertility, including both purely male causes and in combination with female causes, may approach 50%, while solely male factors may be the cause in up to 30% of cases. There is increasing evidence that male fertility declines with age, especially after 45 years of age. The evidence is, however, weaker in the case of assisted reproduction treatments. There is evidence that semen quality has deteriorated over the last 50 years, along with a higher incidence of genitourinary abnormalities including testicular cancer, cryptorchidism, hypospadias, and so forth.

Idiopathic male factors

Up to 50% of male subfertility factors will fall into this idiopathic group where semen parameters are normal. This group is difficult to differentiate from unexplained subfertility.

Congenital causes

- Hypogonadotrophism with anosmia (Kallmann's syndrome).
- Cryptorchidism or undescended testes.
- Y chromosome microdeletions.
- Klinefelter's syndrome (XXY and other variants).
- 5-Alpha reductase deficiency.
- Androgen insensitivity syndromes.
- Absence (unilateral or bilateral) of vas deferens (cystic fibrosis mutation).

Acquired causes

- Chronic illness including chronic renal insufficiency, hepatic cirrhosis, diabetes mellitus.
- Obesity.
- Exposure to high-temperature environments (e.g. welders, bakers).
- Androgen excess – exogenous (anabolic steroids) or endogenous (congenital adrenal hyperplasia, adrenal tumours).
- Pituitary or hypothalamic tumours, hypogonadotrophism.
- Hyperprolactinaemia.
- Drugs (psychotropic drugs, opioids, antiandrogens).
- Epididymo-orchitis (*Chlamydia*, gonorrhoea, mumps virus).
- Trauma/testicular torsion.
- Ionising radiations.
- Male sterilisation.

Management

Treatment of male infertility should be based on identifying and dealing with the specific cause. Improving lifestyle and general health including weight loss, education regarding occupational hazards and stopping smoking seems to benefit outcomes.

Hypothalamic-pituitary causes of hypogonadism can be treated with a pulsatile GnRH agonist on an infusion pump. Alternatively LH and FSH injections can help induce spermatogenesis over a period of time.

Surgical repair of obstructive azoospermia caused by an epididymal block can be attempted if expertise is available. However, surgical sperm retrieval with intracytoplasmic sperm injection (ICSI) has a higher conception success rate. Varicocele repair does not make a significant difference to sperm quality and is no longer recommended.

In a large number of cases, including advanced conditions with moderate to severe abnormalities in sperm parameters and idiopathic cases, the most effective treatment will be assisted reproduction in the form of ICSI with or without surgical sperm retrieval or using donor sperm. Mild male factors can be remediated by using intrauterine insemination.

Clinical case

Case investigations

Initial investigations show that Mrs X and Mr Y both have normal BMI measurement, healthy lifestyles, are non-smokers and have minimal alcohol intake. Mrs X has irregular periods. Her serum FSH is 12 IU/L and LH is 9 IU/L. Mr Y's semen analysis shows a volume of 2 mL, density 14 million/mL, motility 40% and a normal morphology of 15%.

Both Mrs X and Mr Y are at high risk of declining fertility due to their ages. Mrs Y's ovarian reserve test serum FSH in the early follicular phase is 12 (<10 is normal). A raised value suggests low ovarian reserve. Serum anti-Müllerian hormone or antral follicle count by ultrasound scan is likely to have a better predictive value. Her serum progesterone in mid-luteal phase is 16 (>30 is normal), which is low and suggests no ovulation in this cycle.

Semen analysis for Mr Y shows marginal volume, low count and low motility.

Mrs X and Mr Y have been trying to conceive for 4 years, hence their chances of natural conception are diminishing.

A pelvic ultrasound scan on Mrs X showed normal findings other than a 4 cm echogenic cyst on the right ovary. A laparoscopy and dye test performed on Mrs X found endometriotic spots on both uterosacral ligaments as well as both ovaries, along with an endometriotic cyst of 4 cm on her right ovary. Both uterine tubes looked normal and were patent. Most of the endometriosis was surgically either excised or ablated with bipolar diathermy. The ovarian endometriotic cystectomy was performed. She was consented for potential endometriosis surgery and for risk of loss of the ovary. Endometriosis is likely to have contributed to their primary subfertility.

Mr Y was suggested to take zinc and selenium supplements along with some lifestyle advice, followed by a repeated semen analysis 3 months later.

Mrs X was offered ovulation induction for six cycles. A further trial of natural conception was not suggested due to the couple's advancing ages although their chances might have improved following the removal of endometriosis.

Case conclusions

Mrs X became pregnant after three cycles of treatment with clomiphene citrate and had a live birth of an infant at term.

Other management options would have been intrauterine insemination and IVF. She was recommended medical management of endometriosis for pain control if her pain relapsed.

Key learning points

- Subfertility affects one in every six to seven couples, and causes include ovulatory disorders, tubal disease, male factors, uterine factors or a combination of these. Up to one in three couples have unexplained subfertility.

- Ovulatory disorders may respond to ovulation induction, tubal disease to surgery or IVF, and male factors to donor sperm or ICSI if some sperm are present.

Now visit **www.wileyessential.com/humandevelopment** to test yourself on this chapter.

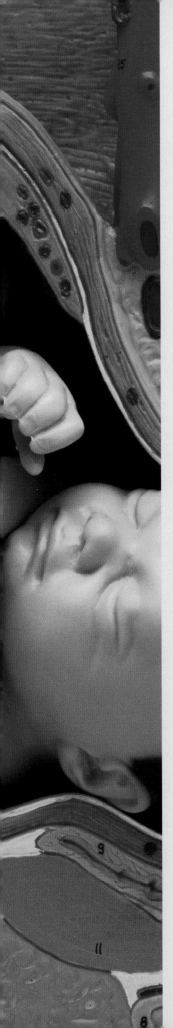

CHAPTER 47
Vaginal discharge, pelvic pain and endometriosis

Aisling Carroll-Downey and Euan Kevelighan

Case

A 28-year-old woman, Anna, attends your clinic seeking advice regarding abdominal pain and subfertility. She and her husband have been trying to conceive for almost 2½ years with no success, and she is worried that they might not be able to have children.

You discover from the history that she has had regular menstruation from the age of 13. She was using Depo-Provera® for contraception, but stopped it 2½ years ago when she and her husband started trying to conceive. She tells you that her periods are heavy and painful especially on days 1 to 3, and that she sometimes needs to take a day or two off work during menstruation. She has a regular 28-day cycle with 5 days of bleeding. She takes ibuprofen, which her GP prescribed for pain relief to some effect. She mentions to you that she sometimes finds intercourse painful. She met her husband in secondary school, and has never had any other sexual partner. She has never been pregnant. There is no other past medical history of note. Her BMI is normal at 24.

Learning outcomes

- You should be able to identify symptoms and signs associated with endometriosis and know how to manage this common condition.

- You should be able to distinguish normal from abnormal vaginal discharge, and investigate and treat appropriately.

Essential Human Development, First Edition. Edited by Samuel Webster, Geraint Morris and Euan Kevelighan
© 2018 John Wiley & Sons, Ltd. Published 2018 by John Wiley & Sons, Ltd.

Vaginal discharge

Physiological discharge

It is normal for women to experience some degree of vaginal discharge during their reproductive life. Normal physiological discharge is usually clear or white, and changes in volume and consistency during the course of the menstrual cycle in women of childbearing age. This mainly reflects the effects of cyclical hormones on cervical mucus. Early in the menstrual cycle oestrogen levels are low, and cervical mucus is relatively viscous. Around the time of ovulation there is more circulating oestrogen, and cervical mucus becomes clearer, less viscous, and presents less of a barrier to semen. Cervical mucus becomes progressively thicker again following ovulation. After the menopause there is a reduction in circulating oestrogen and a reduction in vaginal discharge secondary to this. Other constituents of physiological discharge include secretions from various glands that lubricate and protect the vaginal mucosa.

Rarely vaginal discharge can occur in newborn infants due to high levels of maternal oestrogen. This is characterised by a small volume of discharge, sometimes containing blood, which usually resolves within 2 weeks.

Infective causes of vaginal discharge

Non-sexually transmitted diseases

Vulvovaginal candidiasis

Vulvovaginal candidiasis ('candida' or 'thrush') is a yeast infection caused most commonly by the organism *Candida albicans*, although sometimes other species of *Candida* can be implicated such as *C. glabrata* or *C. krusei*. *C. albicans* is a constituent of the normal body flora and does not normally cause any problems; however, under certain circumstances it can overgrow causing symptomatic disease. Women can become predisposed to infection for a number of reasons. Organic or iatrogenic immunocompromise can promote the overgrowth of *C. albicans*, for example in cases of bone marrow failure or suppression, HIV infection and chemotherapy. Diabetes can predispose to vulvovaginal candidiasis, particularly if it is poorly controlled. Pregnant women and women using combined oral contraceptives are at higher risk of infection. Courses of antibiotics can disturb the normal flora of the vagina and facilitate the overgrowth of *C. albicans*. Other risk factors include wearing tight-fitting synthetic underwear/clothes, and the use of perfumed soaps.

Vulvovaginal infection typically presents with a non-offensive, white 'cottage cheese' discharge and local pruritus and/or discomfort. Patients may also complain of superficial dyspareunia, and dysuria. On examination, the characteristic discharge may be seen, as well as signs of local erythema and irritation. There may be fissuring and signs of excoriation. It is recommended that a diagnosis be made on the basis of sample microscopy and culture. Swabs for analysis should be taken from the anterior fornix upon speculum examination. This facilitates exclusion of other potential pathology that may mimic vulvovaginal candidiasis, such as dermatitis, and can help detect the presence of a species other than *C. albicans* that may be resistant to commonly used antifungal agents. In practice, however, this condition is often diagnosed clinically, without formal microbiological identification of the causative organism.

Treatment for uncomplicated vulvovaginal candidiasis is with imidazole antifungal agents. These can be given orally or topically depending on patient preference and other factors such as drug history.

- Clotrimazole 1% cream, 2% cream, pessaries – *pessaries are safe in pregnancy. The patient should be warned to insert the pessary only as far as is comfortable.*
- Clotrimazole and hydrocortisone cream.
- Miconazole cream/ointment.
- Miconazole and hydrocortisone cream/ointment.
- Oral fluconazole 150 mg given as a single dose – *care must be taken with regard to other medications as fluconazole is an inhibitor of CYP450 enzymes, and may affect drugs such as warfarin. Contraindicated in pregnancy and breastfeeding.*

In addition, patients should be advised to avoid tight-fitting synthetic underwear/clothing, and perfumed soaps when washing. Most of the above treatments are available over the counter in the UK.

Vulvovaginal candidiasis is not a sexually transmitted infection, and as such no partner notification is required. The partner may be the source of reinfection. If he is symptomatic then he should be treated also.

Bacterial vaginosis

Bacterial vaginosis is the most common cause of pathological vaginal discharge in women of childbearing age. In the healthy vagina, lactic acid-producing lactobacilli predominate and maintain a normal local pH of 4.5. Bacterial vaginosis is caused by an imbalance in the normal vaginal flora, characterised by the overgrowth of anaerobic and facultative anaerobic bacteria, which gives rise to an increase in the vaginal pH to between 4.5 and 6.0. Some of the most frequently implicated bacteria are listed in Key facts 47.1.

Risk factors for bacterial vaginosis include smoking, vaginal douching, black race, and a recent change of sexual partner. It presents typically as a 'fishy', thin, white-grey discharge that does not tend to be associated with any local irritation, inflammation or itchiness. There are several sets of diagnostic criteria used to confirm bacterial vaginosis. Amsel's criteria are a widely used example, and are outlined in Key facts 47.2.

ⓘ Key facts 47.1 Causative organisms in bacterial vaginosis

- *Gardnerella vaginalis* (most common)
- *Prevotella* spp.
- *Mycoplasma hominis*
- *Mobiluncus* spp.

> ### ⓘ Key facts 47.2 Amsel's criteria for the diagnosis of bacterial vaginosis
>
> - Characteristic discharge
> - pH >4.5
> - Clue cells on microscopy
> - Positive whiff test - fishy odour on addition of potassium hydroxide

The mainstay of treatment is oral metronidazole 400 mg t.d.s. for 5 to 7 days. There is a 70–80% initial cure rate in bacterial vaginosis; however, relapses are frequent (over 50% in 3 months).

Bacterial vaginosis in pregnancy can give rise to an increased risk of mid-trimester miscarriage, premature rupture of membranes, low birthweight, preterm labour and delivery and postpartum endometritis. It is therefore important to recognise and treat it in pregnancy also. Oral metronidazole is safe in pregnancy.

Though bacterial vaginosis occurs almost exclusively in sexually active women, it is not considered a sexually transmitted disease. Therefore, notification and treatment of the woman's sexual partner is unnecessary.

Foreign body

Foreign bodies within the vagina can arise for a number of reasons across a wide age range. Their significance and complications can be serious; therefore it is a diagnosis worth keeping in mind when a female patient presents with pathological vaginal discharge. Typically the discharge associated with a foreign body is offensive and purulent, and may be bloodstained. There may also be associated pain or discomfort. Vaginal foreign bodies can give rise to complications, which can also be reflected in the presenting symptoms/signs:

- infection +/– abscess formation;
- toxic shock syndrome/sepsis;
- pressure ischaemia +/– fistula;
- intrapelvic migration +/– infection.

In adult females, foreign bodies that can be found within the vagina include:

- tampon;
- condom or fragment of a broken condom;
- pessary;
- surgical item – e.g. swab.

It may be that the object was simply forgotten, has become irretrievable, or the patient may not be aware of it. In some instances the patient may not be able to communicate to those caring for them that there is an object such as a tampon or pessary within the vagina. This can arise, for example, in an unconscious or sedated patient, or in some cases of psychiatric illness.

Management may be as simple as removal of the foreign body and local irrigation with an antiseptic fluid. Antibiotics may be required to treat associated local or systemic infection.

Sexually transmitted diseases

Chlamydia

Chlamydia trachomatis is an obligate intracellular pathogen that can infect the epithelial cells of the endocervix as well as the urethra, rectum and conjunctiva. Infection with *C. trachomatis* can lead to local fibrosis and scarring, especially with repeated episodes. In the context of the genital tract, *C. trachomatis* can cause ascending infection from the endocervix to the uterus, fallopian tubes and the pelvic peritoneum, and can lead to pelvic inflammatory disease, ectopic pregnancy and infertility. Unfortunately *Chlamydia* infection is frequently asymptomatic (in as many as 70% of cases), and this facilitates its ongoing transmission in the community and makes it difficult to ascertain the prevalence of the disease. This is why patients may not present at the time of initial infection, but later with the complications of long-standing disease. *Chlamydia* is primarily transmitted during penetrative sexual intercourse. Risk factors include young age, new sexual partner, multiple sexual partners and inconsistent use of condoms.

Symptomatic disease can present in a variety of ways depending on the anatomical location affected. Cervicitis can present with pathological vaginal discharge as a result of mucopurulent secretions from the cervix. Upon speculum examination, cervical discharge may be visible, as well as areas of ectopy, and the cervix may be bleeding spontaneously, or bleed easily upon contact. Abnormal vaginal bleeding may signify that the endometrium has become infected. Infection of the fallopian tubes is often silent and not detected until it causes an ectopic pregnancy or infertility. If the woman has concurrent infection of the urethra, she may complain of dysuria, frequency and pyuria (dysuria-frequency syndrome). *Chlamydia* should be kept in mind when any young, sexually active woman presents with right upper quadrant pain, nausea, vomiting and/or fever.

Culturing this organism is technically difficult and time consuming, and a nucleic acid amplification technique (NAAT) is used to confirm the diagnosis. This has been proven to be highly sensitive for both endocervical and vulvovaginal swabs and first-catch urine specimens.

Patient education has an important role in the management of *Chlamydia*. Patients must be made aware that it is a sexually transmitted infection, and that there can be serious long-term sequelae. Patients should be encouraged to have a full sexually transmitted infection screen upon diagnosis to detect any concomitant infection. Partner notification and treatment are required. Standard treatment is usually with 1 g azithromycin stat., or 100 mg doxycycline b.i.d. for 7 days. Patients are asked to abstain from penetrative and/or oral intercourse for the duration of treatment and/or the treatment of their partner (or for 7 days after treatment with azithromycin). There is currently a *Chlamydia* screening programme in the UK for women under the age of 25.

It is important to recognise and treat *Chlamydia* in pregnancy. *Chlamydia* can be transmitted to the neonate during delivery and can lead to early-onset sepsis, pneumonia and conjunctivitis. Pregnant (or breastfeeding) women can be treated with 1 g azithromycin stat., or amoxicillin 500 mg t.d.s. for 7 days, or erythromycin 500 mg q.d.s. for 7 days.

Trichomonas vaginalis

Trichomonas vaginalis is a flagellated protozoan that is a common parasite found on both women and men. It is mainly a sexually transmitted infection; however, it is possible to become infected due to the presence of fomites such as towels or bathing wear. *T. vaginalis* gives rise to a superficial vaginal infection with a characteristic yellow-green, frothy, offensive discharge, vulvovaginal pruritus, lower abdominal pain and/or dysuria (when the urethra is affected). On speculum examination, there may be the characteristic 'strawberry cervix', visible discharge and signs of vulvovaginal inflammation. Some patients are asymptomatic, with normal examination.

Swabs are taken from the posterior fornix at the time of speculum examination, or the patient can swab the vagina themselves. Direct microscopy of a wet mount or acridine orange-stained sample can be used to identify the presence of a motile, flagellated organism. The preferred method, however, is culture of *T. vaginalis*. Patient education plays an important role in management, as does partner notification and treatment. Standard medical treatment is with metronidazole, either a 2 g stat. dose, or 400–500 mg b.d.s. for 5–7 days. A 2 g stat. dose can be helpful when compliance may be an issue; however, it is associated with a higher failure rate. Patients are advised to abstain from penetrative and/or oral sexual intercourse during their and/or their partner's treatment.

T. vaginalis infection in pregnancy is associated with premature delivery and low birthweight babies. Metronidazole has been found to be safe in pregnancy and breastfeeding, though it is advised that high doses are avoided in these instances.

Gonorrhoea

Neisseria gonorrhoeae in a Gram-negative diplococcus that is an intracellular pathogen. The clinical picture in *N. gonorrhoeae* infection is similar to that of *Chlamydia*, and it should always be a differential diagnosis when *Chlamydia* is suspected, and vice versa (patients should be tested for both in such circumstances when possible). Increased or altered vaginal discharge is the most frequently reported symptom in female patients (50%), with similar characteristics on examination to *Chlamydia*. However, gonorrhoea tends to have a more abrupt onset of symptoms if present, and can disseminate leading to bacteraemia, endocarditis and/or meningitis in some cases. It can also lead to a syndrome of arthritis, tenosynovitis and/or dermatitis (acute arthritis-dermatitis syndrome). It is a sexually transmitted infection, and the endocervix is the primary site of urogenital infection.

Vaginal and endocervical swabs are used to obtain samples for diagnostic purposes. NAAT is considered preferable as it is more sensitive than culture, and concomitant *C. trachomatis* infection can be picked up using this method. Patient education on the nature and complications of gonorrhoea is important in the management of infection, as is partner notification and treatment. Standard medical management for uncomplicated infection is 500 mg ceftriaxone stat. by deep intramuscular injection, with 1 g azithromycin stat. orally. *N. gonorrhoeae* has become increasingly resistant to antibiotics over time, and an extended-spectrum cephalosporin in conjunction with azithromycin is given to overcome this and to delay eventual resistance to ceftriaxone. Patients are advised to abstain from penetrative and/or oral sexual intercourse for the duration of their treatment and/or their partner's treatment (abstain for 7 days after azithromycin).

Gonorrhoea can have serious implications in pregnancy. It predisposes to spontaneous abortion, premature rupture of membranes, premature delivery and acute chorioamnionitis. It can also be transmitted to the neonate during delivery, leading to ophthalmic and pharyngeal infection in some cases. Pregnant or breastfeeding women should be treated with a regime similar to that for the non-pregnant population.

Pelvic inflammatory disease (PID)

Pelvic inflammatory disease (PID) is usually caused by an ascending infection of the genital tract. Both *C. trachomatis* and *N. gonorrhoeae* are frequently implicated in PID, as are the organisms associated with bacterial vaginosis and a condition known as aerobic vaginosis (similar to bacterial vaginosis, but causative organisms are aerobic, often including *Escherichia coli*, group B streptococci, and/or enterococci). Rarely, PID can arise from infection spread via the bloodstream or lymphatics such as tuberculosis.

PID may be silent, or present with symptoms such as lower abdominal pain, post-coital bleeding and abnormal discharge. On examination, there may be visible signs of genital tract infection, cervical excitation, adnexal tenderness or an adnexal mass. The long-term sequelae of PID include intrapelvic/abdominal adhesions, ectopic pregnancy and infertility due to the progressive scarring of the fallopian tubes, and it may be that the patient presents with these complications rather than symptoms of initial infection. It is for this reason that it is important to have a high index of suspicion for PID and the infections that may cause it.

The US Centers for Disease Control and Prevention outline diagnostic criteria for PID (Key facts 47.3). A diagnosis of PID is made once other causes of lower abdominal pain have been excluded such as ectopic pregnancy and acute appendicitis.

The mainstay of treatment for PID is oral broad-spectrum antibiotics. The likely causative organisms must be weighed up in the choice of antibiotic regime. It is advisable to cover *C. trachomatis* and *N. gonorrhoeae* infection, and to consider the use of additional metronidazole when anaerobic involvement is suspected. PID can be managed in the outpatient setting for the most part. However, there are some circumstances when admission for parenteral antibiotics is indicated, for

> **(!) Key facts 47.3 Centers for Disease Control and Prevention diagnostic criteria for diagnosis of pelvic inflammatory disease (PID)**
>
> **Minimum criteria**
> - Lower abdominal/pelvic pain plus:
> - Cervical excitation or
> - Uterine tenderness or
>
> Additional criteria (making correct diagnosis more likely in addition to the minimum criteria):
> - Oral temperature >38.3°C
> - Abnormal vaginal/cervical discharge
> - Abundant WBC on saline microscopy of vaginal secretions
> - Raised ESR
> - Raised CRP
> - Laboratory documentation of cervical infection with *C. trachomatis* or *N. gonorrhoeae*
> - Adnexal tenderness
>
> **Definitive criteria**
> - Endometrial biopsy with histopathologic evidence of endometritis
> - Transvaginal sonography or magnetic resonance imaging techniques showing thickened, fluid-filled tubes with or without free pelvic fluid or tubo-ovarian complex, or Doppler studies suggesting pelvic infection (e.g. tubal hyperaemia) or
> - Laparoscopic abnormalities consistent with PID
>
> CRP, C-reactive protein; ESR, erythrocyte sedimentation rate; WBC, white blood cells.

example if the patient is severely unwell or pregnant, or other acute abdominal pathology cannot be ruled out.

Malignant causes of vaginal discharge

Pathological vaginal discharge can be associated with malignancy, especially in an older, postmenopausal patient. It can occur with any of the gynaecological cancers to varying degrees and frequencies, and it may take the presence/absence of other symptoms and signs to narrow down the potential diagnosis. It may be useful to ascertain whether the patient has had any recent weight loss, swollen lymph nodes, or a family/past history of gynaecological cancer.

Fistulae

Occasionally, the presence of a vaginal discharge can reflect an abnormal communication between the genital tract and the urinary or gastrointestinal tract, or both (Table 47.1).

The aetiology of fistulae can broadly be divided into congenital and acquired causes. Congenital fistulae can arise due to the failure of normal embryological development, whereas an acquired fistula can arise due to obstetric trauma. During even a straightforward delivery, there is the potential for trauma to the genital tract, particularly tears in the posterior vaginal wall and the rectum. Iatrogenic damage can occur to the local structures during an instrumental or caesarean delivery. Prolonged obstructed labour can give rise to pressure ischaemia as the presenting part of the fetus compresses the

soft tissue structures of the pelvis against the pelvic bones and/or the sacral promontory. In such cases, the devitalised tissue sloughs away between days 3 to 10 of the puerperium leading to fistulae and incontinence (this is the leading cause of urogenital fistulae in the developing world). Other iatrogenic causes include pelvic radiotherapy and accidental trauma during surgery, particularly hysterectomy. Malignancy can cause fistulae to form, especially cancer of the vagina, cervix and rectum. Inflammatory bowel disease and diverticular disease can also cause fistulae, especially Crohn's disease (inflammatory bowel disease is the most common cause of intestinogenital fistulae in the UK).

Fistulae can present as incontinence and frank passing of urine or faeces per vagina, or more subtly as a watery or offensive discharge. The history may give some reason to suspect the diagnosis. Inspection of the vagina with a Sim's speculum may show an obvious communicating defect, although very small fistulae may be difficult or impossible to visualise. Other investigations such as endoscopy, barium studies or CT may be necessary to confirm the diagnosis.

Table 47.1 Sites where fistulae may form between the urogenital and gastrointestinal tracts.

Genital tract	Urinary tract	Gastrointestinal tract
• Vagina	• Bladder	• Rectum
• Cervix	• Urethra	• Colon
• Uterus	• Ureter	• Small bowel
		• Anal canal

In some circumstances, fistulae will heal with conservative measures. In most cases, however, they will require surgical repair for definitive management.

Other causes of vaginal discharge

- Postoperative discharge.
- Postpartum discharge - lochia.
- Cervical ectropion.
- Vulval dermatitis.
- Atrophic changes.

Endometriosis

Endometriosis is the presence of functioning endometrial tissue outside the uterus. Most commonly, endometriotic tissue is associated with the pelvic organs and peritoneum, although it can occur at other sites such as the bladder, bowel and lungs. Like the normal endometrium, endometriotic tissue responds to cyclical oestrogen and progesterone, and bleeding occurs during the time of menstruation. This accounts for some of the characteristic symptoms associated with the condition such as dysmenorrhoea and menorrhagia. However, the presentation can vary for a number of reasons including the severity, location and complications of the disease. Some women may be asymptomatic, and endometriotic tissue may be an incidental finding during the investigation or treatment of another condition. This in part makes the exact incidence difficult to determine, but it is estimated that 8–10% of women have endometriosis. Endometriosis can affect women at any time from menarche to menopause, but is most common between 25 and 35 years of age.

Pathology, histology and aetiology

Characteristic of endometriosis is the presence of ectopic endometrial deposits outside the uterus. Such deposits have been found to occur almost anywhere within the female body; however, they are found most commonly within the pelvic cavity. The most frequently affected structures are the ovaries, the pouch of Douglas and the uterosacral ligament. Table 47.2 lists some of the other structures that can be similarly affected.

Endometriosis can arise within the smooth muscle of the uterus, a condition known as adenomyosis. It can also be manifest in a cyst-like mass known as an endometrioma or 'chocolate cyst'.

The mechanism by which these deposits come to exist and persevere remains unclear. A number of theories have been postulated. It is thought that the most likely aetiology relates to retrograde menstruation, which is the passage of menstrual debris via the fallopian tubes into the peritoneal cavity. Retrograde menstruation occurs in up to 90% of women, and in the majority of cases the errant endometrial tissue is cleared by phagocytosis or apoptosis. In endometriosis, however, it is postulated that underlying immune dysfunction or deficiency undermines this clearing process, and endometriotic tissue can become implanted ectopically and grow. The presence of disease in more distal sites has a number of potential explanations. Endometriotic tissue may disseminate via the lymph, blood and by mechanical means (e.g. at the time of surgery). It is also thought that in some cases it arises from metaplasia of otherwise differentiated cells to endometrial-type cells. Some evidence exists that there is a genetic predisposition underlying the development of endometriosis.

Secondary to the presence of endometriotic tissue, scarring of the underlying peritoneum and adhesions can occur. The most common complication of endometriosis is infertility, and this can be the most significant aspect of the disease from the patient's point of view. Whether the presence of ectopic endometriotic tissue directly leads to infertility or whether infertility simply coexists in predisposed individuals remains unclear.

Though endometriotic tissue usually comprises the same glandular and stromal cell types as normal endometrium, their histological appearances are rarely the same. An orderly arrangement of glands and stroma is characteristic of normal endometrial tissue, whilst endometriotic tissue is more disordered, and the proportions of glandular and stromal cells can differ. The appearance of a network of arterioles or focal stromal haemorrhage can also indicate endometriotic tissue.

Presentation (history and examination)

The classical presentation is a history of dysmenorrhoea, dyspareunia, menorrhagia and subfertility (Key facts 47.4).

There may be generalised tenderness on abdominal examination, and no lymphadenopathy. Speculum examination may

Table 47.2 Structures that may be affected by ectopic endometrial deposits.

Intrapelvic structures	Extrapelvic structures
• Serosal surface of the uterus	• Gastrointestinal tract
• Fallopian tubes	• Ureters
• Round ligament	• Umbilicus
• Sigmoid colon	• Lungs
• Rectum	• Vagina
• Bladder	• Cervix
	• Perineum
	• Surgical scars

① Key facts 47.4 Symptoms of endometriosis

- Chronic pelvic pain
- Ovulation pain
- Cyclical or premenstrual symptoms relating to the site of disease, e.g. haematuria
- Chronic fatigue
- Dyschezia

be completely unremarkable, except if there are endometriotic deposits within the vagina, which may appear as blue-black areas. Bimanual examination may reveal some generalised tenderness. The uterus may be in a fixed retroverted position due to adhesions within the pelvis. It may be possible to palpate deposits on the uterosacral ligaments or an endometrioma in the adnexae of the pelvis

Investigation and diagnosis

If an adnexal mass is palpated on vaginal examination, then an ultrasound scan may suggest whether a cyst is likely to be endometrioma or other, for example a simple or complex ovarian cyst. The gold standard for the diagnosis of endometriosis is diagnostic laparoscopy and visualisation and staging of the lesions. A number of tools are used to stage endometriosis; however, these have been found to over- or under-stage the disease and usually the diagnosing clinician makes a judgement on the severity of disease from experience, and photos or a DVD of the findings are documented in the medical notes rather than using a formal staging tool. The severity of endometriosis is not correlated with the severity of pain.

Management

The management of endometriosis differs from case to case but should be based on:

- reason for treatment, i.e. pain or fertility;
- side effects of medications;
- cost-effectiveness of medications.

Medical treatment for pain

Symptom control can be achieved using simple analgesia or hormonal therapies that aim to interrupt the cyclical stimulation of endometriotic tissue (Table 47.3).

It is reasonable to trial analgesics, combined oral contraceptive pill (COCP) or progestagen treatment for symptom control on clinical suspicion of endometriosis. It is important to consider the possibility of other pathology if a woman does not respond to treatment for endometriosis.

Analgesia

Non-steroidal anti-inflammatory drugs (NSAIDs) can be used to treat the pain associated with endometriosis. There is no evidence that one particular NSAID is superior to another in the management of endometriosis. This may be an appropriate option for women who do not wish to use hormonal or surgical treatments. All women taking NSAIDs should be counselled on the potential side effects such as peptic ulceration, nausea, vomiting, headaches and drowsiness.

Hormonal treatment

The aim of hormonal treatment is to prevent the cyclical stimulation of endometriotic tissue with endogenous oestrogen and progesterone. A number of drugs may be used including the combined contraceptive pill, progestogens and gonadotrophin-releasing hormone (GnRH) agonists. These treatments usually provide good symptom control. There are some potential drawbacks as all of these drugs delay fertility and can have unacceptable adverse effects. As hormonal treatments do not treat the underlying mechanism of disease, there is a high rate of symptom recurrence, and some women do not achieve complete symptom control.

Combined oral contraceptive pill

The combined oral contraceptive pill (COCP) prevents cyclical stimulation of endometriosis by suppressing ovulation. This may be more effective if the monthly withdrawal bleed is omitted and packs are taken tricyclically. One of the main advantages of COCP is that it can be used long-term, though its contraceptive effects may be undesirable if the woman is

Table 47.3 Medical treatment for endometriosis.

Drug	Duration	Mechanism of action	Side effects
NSAIDs, e.g. ibuprofen, diclofenac	Take during episode of pain only	Cyclo-oxygenase inhibitor	Gastrointestinal upset, e.g. nausea, diarrhoea and bleeding
COCP	21 days with 7-day break or tricyclic Long term	Inhibits ovulation and ovarian suppression	Nausea, diarrhoea and vomiting, headaches, very rarely stroke
Progestagens, e.g. MPA	Continuous long-term	Ovarian suppression	Weight gain, irregular bleeding Acne, depression
GnRH analogue	6 months (longer if add-back HRT used)	Ovarian suppression	Hot flushes, vaginal dryness, osteoporosis (reversible)
Levonorgestrel releasing IUS	Long-term – change after 5 years	Endometrial suppression	Irregular bleeding for 3–4 months

COCP, combined oral contraceptive pill; GnRH, gonadotrophin-releasing hormone; MPA, medroxyprogesterone acetate; NSAIDs, non-steroidal anti-inflammatory drugs; IUS, intrauterine system.

planning to become pregnant. The COCP is contraindicated in those with a history of thromboembolic disease and migraine due to the oestrogen component.

Progestagens

A number of progestagens have been used in the treatment of endometriosis such as medroxyprogesterone, levonorgestrel and norethisterone. These also produce ovarian suppression and thereby inhibit the cyclical stimulation of endometriotic tissue.

GnRH agonists

GnRH agonists such as leuprorelin and goserelin can be used to suppress pituitary release of gonadotrophins. When given continuously GnRH agonists at first stimulate the release of luteinising hormone and follicle-stimulating hormone and then inhibit it, leading to reduced ovarian production of oestrogen and progesterone. The use of GnRH agonists in the treatment of endometriosis is limited to 6 months unless add-back hormone replacement therapy (HRT) is given, for example tibolone 2.5 mg daily. One of the adverse effects is loss of bone mineral density. Using 'add-back' HRT with a GnRH agonist from the outset can prevent bone mineral density loss and ameliorate menopausal side effects. Add-back HRT does not affect the efficacy of GnRH agonists in endometriosis.

Surgical treatment for pain

The ideal treatment for endometriosis is ablation of endometriotic tissue at the time of laparoscopic diagnosis. Skin lesions such as endometriotic tissue in surgical scars can be excised. If a woman has completed her family, and has severe refractory dysmenorrhoea despite adequate medical treatment, hysterectomy and bilateral salpingo-oophorectomy can be performed. Endometriotic tissue should be ablated concurrently. This produces a surgical menopause and add-back HRT may be required to counteract symptoms of hot flushes and to protect against premature osteoporosis.

Medical treatment for subfertility

NSAIDs may inhibit ovulation when taken mid-cyclically. This may be due to suppression of prostaglandin production. Fortunately, most women have severe pain just prior to and during menstruation.

Hormonal treatment does not improve the chances of a subsequent successful pregnancy. Also hormonal manipulation delays ovulation.

Surgical treatment for subfertility

In cases of minimal to mild endometriosis ablation of endometriotic deposits likely improves fertility rates. In moderate to severe disease the benefits are not proven. Any endometriomas greater than 3 cm in diameter should be removed.

In moderate to severe endometriosis IVF is often the best option to achieve a successful outcome.

Support

Dealing with the symptoms and complications of endometriosis, particularly infertility, can be very distressing for a woman. Many find it beneficial to express their experiences of endometriosis and find solace among others in a similar situation to themselves. There are numerous endometriosis support organisations across the UK to which women can turn for information, advice and support.

Prognosis

Those with mildly symptomatic disease may manage well with analgesia and/or hormonal therapy. Hormonal treatments can lead to symptom control, but there is a high recurrence rate. Surgery can eradicate the disease in most cases; however, there are a proportion of women for whom symptoms will persist, at times because not all the endometriotic tissue was destroyed. Almost all cases of endometriosis will resolve naturally with the menopause.

SUMMARY

Clinical case

Case investigations

Abdominal examination and inspection of the vulva and vaginal orifice is normal. There is no abnormality on speculum examination, and you take endocervical and high vaginal swabs. Anna has generalised tenderness on bimanual examination, and the uterus is fixed in a retroverted position. No uterosacral nodules are palpated. You arrange a full blood count and LH and FSH, day 21 serum progesterone, semen analysis and rubella immunity. She returns to outpatients in 2 months. The results are as follows:

- Swabs for *Chlamydia* and gonorrhoea negative.
- Serum LH and FSH in normal range.
- Haemoglobin is 95 g/L (normal 105–140 g/L).
- Day 21 serum progesterone 42 (normal >30 nmol/L).
- Semen analysis: volume = 2.5 mL (normal >1.5 mL), sperm concentration 26 million spermatozoa/mL (normal >15 million).
- Rubella immunity >10 IU/L (normal >10).

Anna and her husband have been trying to conceive for 30 months. Her periods are regular, which is highly suggestive of regular ovulation. Day 21 serum progesterone confirms ovulation. Semen analysis from husband is within normal parameters. The pelvic pain suggests endometriosis.

She has no other medical issues, and she is of normal weight, so it is unlikely that pituitary dysfunction is the underlying pathology. She has no hirsutism or oligomenorrhoea making polycystic ovarian syndrome (PCOS) very unlikely. She is over 25, denies any sexual partners other than her husband, endocervical swabs are negative for *Chlamydia* and gonorrhoea, making PID a very unlikely diagnosis. A fixed, retroverted uterus could be due to adhesions within the pelvis, which could be caused by either PID or endometriosis. The symptoms, however, of dysmenorrhoea, menorrhagia and deep dyspareunia point more towards a diagnosis of endometriosis.

Case conclusions

A diagnostic laparoscopy reveals moderate endometriosis. The deposits are removed by ablation with diathermy. Postoperatively she is not given medical treatment as this does not improve pregnancy rates. Six months later she conceives and following an uneventful pregnancy has a vaginal delivery of a healthy girl of 3.8 kg.

Key learning points

- Common causes of abnormal vaginal discharge include *Candida*, bacterial vaginosis and sexually transmitted infections, the commonest in UK being *Chlamydia*.

- Endometriosis is an oestrogen-dependent condition associated with subfertility and pain (frequently chronic pelvic pain) although some patients have widespread pelvic endometriosis and are asymptomatic.

 Now visit **www.wileyessential.com/humandevelopment** to test yourself on this chapter.

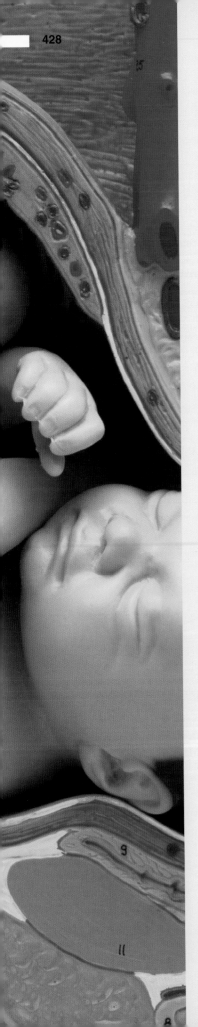

CHAPTER 48
Termination of pregnancy

Sophie Walker and Jennifer Davies-Oliveira

Case

Miss A, an 18-year-old female whose LMP was 3/12 ago, presents with a positive pregnancy test. Her boyfriend broke up with her when she told him she was pregnant, and she feels she is not able to continue with the pregnancy.

Learning outcomes

- You should be able to discuss the ethical and legal issues surrounding termination of pregnancy.
- You should be able to describe the indications for termination of pregnancy.
- You should be able to state the methods used for termination of pregnancy.
- You should be able to consider the physical and psychological sequelae of termination of pregnancy.

Essential Human Development, First Edition. Edited by Samuel Webster, Geraint Morris and Euan Kevelighan
© 2018 John Wiley & Sons, Ltd. Published 2018 by John Wiley & Sons, Ltd.

Introduction

In the UK abortion is common. The number of abortions carried out per year is around 190 000 and approximately 96% of these are funded by the NHS. One in three women in the UK will have had a termination before the age of 45. Whilst terminations have been performed for many years under UK case law, it was not until 1967 that the Abortion Act clarified the law and the position of the medical practitioner with regards to termination of pregnancy. This Act of Parliament gave medical practitioners a legal defence for carrying out terminations and legalised the woman's right to a safe, regulated and lawful termination of pregnancy.

Legal considerations

In 1990 the Human Fertilisation and Embryology Act became law; this updated and amended the Abortion Act of 1967. First of all, it lowered the gestational age at which terminations could take place from 28 to 24 weeks, but also stated that a pregnancy of any gestation could be terminated due to serious fetal anomaly. There are five conditions under which termination is permissible in the UK (see Box 49.1). A medical emergency is the exception to this, when a single medical practitioner may perform a termination if the woman's life is in immediate danger. All terminations are performed in the interests of the mother, as a fetus has no legal rights until it is born.

In the UK almost all terminations are carried out under Section C, which states that 'the pregnancy has NOT exceeded its 24th week and that the continuance of the pregnancy would involve risk, greater than if the pregnancy were terminated, of injury to the physical or mental health of the pregnant woman'. Most medical professionals agree that the psychological and medical problems associated with pregnancy are greater than those associated with the termination of the pregnancy. Two medical practitioners must agree and certify the abortion under one or more of the grounds as stated in the Act and complete the required documentation. Usually, it is the woman's GP who signs the first part of the certificate and the gynaecologist performing the abortion signs the second. The termination must take place in an NHS or NHS-approved facility, and it is then the responsibility of the clinician performing the procedure to inform the Chief Medical Officer of the termination, within 14 days. This is how abortions are controlled and regulated in the UK.

Ethical considerations

Termination of pregnancy is surrounded by ethical issues and is a cause of much controversy. Many healthcare practitioners, for a variety of personal, cultural and religious reasons, are uncomfortable taking part in the termination of a viable pregnancy. For this reason, the Abortion Act has a conscientious objection clause, which enables doctors to refuse to take part in termination of pregnancy unless it is a medical emergency and the woman's life is in danger. Parliament clarified that only the medical practitioner performing the procedure is allowed to refuse to partake under this clause. The British Medical Association, the trade union and professional association of doctors, acknowledges that General Practitioners signing the form for the termination are morally involved in the procedure so allows conscientious objection in this case. However, in this instance, there must be another doctor who is able to offer the necessary information, support and referral for termination of pregnancy without delay. The roles of other members of the team, for example, the medical secretary and junior doctors doing the preoperative clerking, are not deemed to be directly involved in the procedure and therefore cannot refuse to partake under this clause.

Termination for fetal abnormalities

Pregnancies can be terminated at any gestation under ground E of the Abortion Act. A very small percentage (1%) of

---

Box 48.1 Grounds for abortion in the UK

In the UK, Section 37 of the Human Fertilisation and Embryology Act 1990 Act amends the Abortion Act 1967. Abortion may be granted under one of the following circumstances:

- A – The continuance of the pregnancy would involve risk to the life of the pregnant woman greater than if the pregnancy were terminated.
- B – The termination is necessary to prevent grave permanent injury to the physical or mental health of the pregnant woman.
- C – The pregnancy has NOT exceeded its 24th week and that the continuance of the pregnancy would involve risk, greater than if the pregnancy were terminated, of injury to the physical or mental health of the pregnant woman.
- D – The pregnancy has NOT exceeded its 24th week and that the continuance of the pregnancy would involve risk, greater than if the pregnancy were terminated, of injury to the physical or mental health of any existing child(ren) of the family of the pregnant woman.
- E – There is a substantial risk that if the child were born it would suffer from such physical or mental abnormalities as to be seriously handicapped.

terminations are performed under ground E, and structural abnormalities account for half of these. Termination for chromosomal abnormalities is also applied under ground E, with trisomy 21 (Down syndrome) being the chromosomal abnormality most commonly reported.

As the law stands, where there is a substantial risk that if a fetus is born it would be severely handicapped due to physical and mental abnormalities, that fetus can be terminated at any gestation. What constitutes a 'substantial risk' and a 'severe handicap' is a controversial issue. Neither are defined by law so the decision lies with the doctors involved to advise on the severity of the abnormalities the child is likely to suffer. The pregnant woman and medical staff face difficult decisions on whether the pregnancy should continue. Despite no universal consensus on what types and degree of impairment are included in this category, only fetuses likely to be severely handicapped with significant suffering or long-term impairment should be considered for termination under this ground. This scenario is very difficult for pregnant women, and all cases of late termination for fetal abnormalities need to be treated with special care and consideration.

Termination of pregnancy: the global view

In 2008 the rate of abortions in developed countries was 24/1000 women, and 29/1000 women in the developing world. The rate of induced abortions is not lower in those countries with restrictive abortion laws. Generally, abortion laws are much more restrictive in the developing world and the facilities less suitable and therefore a much higher proportion of abortions were deemed unsafe. Having more liberal abortion laws does not increase the number of abortions that take place, but does make it safer and protects the women involved.

Unsafe abortions, defined by the World Health Organization (WHO) as a procedure for termination of an unintended pregnancy done either by people lacking the necessary skills or in an environment that does not conform to minimum medical standards, or both, are a significant cause of maternal mortality and morbidity. WHO states that abortions that are done illegally are more likely to be unsafe, as they are usually performed by unskilled practitioners in inappropriate environments.

Indications for termination of pregnancy

The indications for terminating a pregnancy are set out by the Abortion Act 1967 and updated by the Human Fertilisation and Embryology Act 1990. The indications are given in Box 48.1.

As discussed previously a medical emergency where the pregnant woman's life is at risk is an absolute indication for termination of pregnancy if clinically indicated.

The process for termination of pregnancy

Considerate and sensitive communication is key in dealing with cases of termination of pregnancy.

Pre-abortion management

The pregnancy should be confirmed with a thorough history and a urinary pregnancy test. It is important to explore the degree of certainty that the pregnant woman has regarding her decision to terminate the pregnancy and her understanding of the implications.

In the assessment it is important to determine:
- Woman's history including family history.
- Rhesus blood status – anti-D IgG should be given, by injection into the deltoid muscle, to all non-sensitised RhD-negative women within 72 hours following abortion.
- Blood group with screening for red cell antibodies, haemoglobin and haemoglobinopathies including sickle cell disease or trait if not previously tested with a positive family history or in at-risk ethnic groups.
- Venous thromboembolism (VTE) risk assessment.
- Cervical cytology screening – if indicated.
- Discussion of methods of contraception.
- Screen for *Chlamydia trachomatis* and risk assess +/- screen for other STIs including HIV, gonorrhoea and syphilis.

The gestational age is calculated with the date of the last menstrual period (LMP). Ultrasound scanning is often used in determining gestational age. However, this is only indicated if women are uncertain of the date of their last menstrual period, there are clinical reasons to suspect wrong dates, or the woman is obese or difficult to examine.

After determining gestation, give relevant information regarding the different methods of termination of pregnancy including potential adverse effects and complications (Tables 48.1 and 48.2).

Complications of medical and surgical termination of pregnancy

The Royal College of Obstetricians and Gynaecologists (RCOG) recommends that women should be informed that abortion is a safe procedure for which major complications and mortality are rare at all gestations. In 2011 the UK had a rate of complication after termination of pregnancy of 1 in every 700 procedures.

A recent Cochrane Systematic Review showed no difference in complication rates between medical and surgical abortion in the first trimester. However, those having a medical termination of pregnancy at more than13 weeks gestation have been shown in small studies to have a higher all-cause adverse effect rate than surgical terminations at the same gestation.

Table 48.1 Medical termination of pregnancy.

Gestation (weeks)	Less than 9	9–24
Method	**<49 days – mifepristone 200 mg** orally and 24–48 hours later one dose of misoprostol 400 µg **<63 days – mifepristone 200 mg** and 24–48 hours later one dose of misoprostol 800 µg (vaginal, buccal or sublingual)	**9–13 weeks – mifepristone 200 mg** orally followed 36–48 hours later by 800 µg vaginally with a maximum of four further doses of 400 µg at 3-hourly intervals (vaginally or orally) **13–24 weeks** – as above but if abortion does not occur mifepristone can be repeated at 3 hours and 12 hours
Follow-up	Aspirate exam for presence of gestational sac Serum human chorionic gonadotrophin	
Other information	Safe to complete at home with a robust follow-up strategy and support	

Table 48.2 Surgical termination of pregnancy.

Gestation (weeks)	Less than 7	7–14	14–16	13–24
Method	Vacuum aspiration	Electric or manual vacuum aspiration	Vacuum aspiration (large-bore cannula)	Dilatation and evacuation (vacuum aspiration and forceps) with ultrasound guidance
Cervical preparation	Misoprostol 400 µg vaginally or sublingually 3 hours prior to surgery	Misoprostol 400 µg vaginally or sublingually 3 hours prior to surgery	1) Osmotic dilators 2) Up to 18 weeks, misoprostol 400 µg vaginally or sublingually 3 hours prior to surgery	
Follow-up	1) Aspirate inspection for presence of gestational sac 2) Serum human chorionic gonadotrophin			
Other information	Local anaesthesia is recommended for surgical termination of pregnancy Sedation – i.v. opioids (fentanyl) and sedative (midazolam or propofol) Offer pain relief, e.g. NSAID			

Common physical symptoms after termination of pregnancy (TOP)

- Pain.
- Bleeding from the genital tract (more common in a medical TOP).
- Gastrointestinal symptoms (especially in a medical TOP).

Complications of TOP

Most common

- Infection.
- Cervical trauma (surgical) – damage to cervical external os 1/100.

Uncommon complications

- Haemorrhage: requiring transfusion <1/1000, rising to 4/1000 beyond 20 weeks gestation.

- Uterine perforation (surgical) 1–4/1000.
- Incomplete abortion (medical): <5% requiring further surgical intervention.
- Failure to end the pregnancy <1/100.
- Thromboembolic disease.
- Psychiatric morbidity.
- Uterine rupture. In medical abortion at later gestations the risk is <1/1000. Previous caesarean section is a risk factor.
- Death.

Focus on infection

Ten percent of women undergoing induced abortion develop a genital tract infection, including pelvic inflammatory disease. This is usually caused by pre-existing infection, for example *C. trachomatis*, *Neisseria gonorrhoeae* and bacterial vaginosis. Post-abortion infection causes immediate morbidity but may also lead to tubal subfertility and an increased risk of ectopic pregnancy. The use of prophylactic antibiotics and bacterial screening reduces these risks.

Current guidelines are as follows:

1. Azithromycin 1 g orally on day of abortion plus metronidazole 1 g rectally or 800 mg orally.

OR

2. Doxycycline 100 mg orally b.i.d. for 7 days plus metronidazole 1 g rectally or 800 mg orally.

Psychological sequelae of termination of pregnancy

A range of emotional responses are commonly experienced during and following a termination of pregnancy, including relief, sadness, anger, guilt and regret. It is important to reiterate that these feelings are a normal response to a termination of pregnancy. For some, recurring thoughts can be triggered by life events such as subsequent pregnancy difficulties and birthdays.

The emotions experienced during and after a termination of pregnancy are influenced by the circumstances that lead to the unplanned pregnancy, how women are supported when faced with indecision and how they are enabled to make the right choice.

Those who need additional support and counselling should be identified. Those who are more likely to need counselling are young women, women with mental health problems, women with poor social support and evidence of coercion.

SUMMARY

Clinical case

Case investigations and management

After taking a full history and performing a urinary pregnancy test to confirm pregnancy, Miss A is referred to the abortion clinic.

At the clinic Miss A is asked regarding her certainty to terminate the pregnancy and her understanding of the implications. A thorough history including a family history and LMP is undertaken. She is blood group AB and her rhesus blood group is positive. A VTE risk assessment is done and shows that she is at low risk. Future methods of contraception are discussed. Miss A is offered an STI screening, which is also carried out.

The gestational age is calculated to be 12 weeks from Miss A's LMP date, this is confirmed via ultrasound scan. Information is given regarding medical and surgical termination of pregnancy with a discussion of any potential adverse effects and complications that may ensue.

Case conclusion

Miss A opts for a medical termination as she then can go home after taking the treatment. She is then given mifepristone 200 mg orally and returns home. She returns 2 days later and has 800 mg mifepristone vaginally. She then takes 400 mg 3 hours later orally. She passes fetes and products of conception a few hours later and is discharged home on same day. Miss A experiences abdominal pain for a few days and bleeding per vagina for a week. There are no other complications and her beta-human chorionic gonadotrophin (BHCG) level returns to normal.

Key learning points

- The law in many countries clearly defines whether or not termination of pregnancy is legal, and in what situations it may be applied. The ethical arguments surrounding this issue should also be considered by healthcare professionals.
- Counselling before termination and assessment of the certainty of the patient to proceed should be carried out.

- Counselling after termination may also be required, and patients requiring further support should be identified.
- Termination of pregnancy may exacerbate a pre-existing genital tract infection.
- Termination of pregnancy may be performed medically or surgically.

 Now visit **www.wileyessential.com/humandevelopment** to test yourself on this chapter.

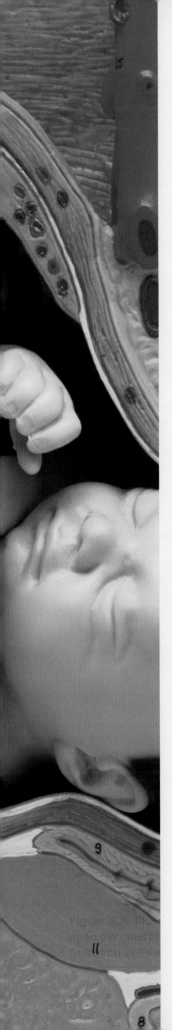

CHAPTER 49
Contraception

Ruth Frazer

Case

Kylie is a 16-year-old with a chaotic lifestyle who does not think she ever wants children after having had a recent termination. She is not in a long-term relationship and is likely to have multiple sexual partners. She meets with you to discuss family planning options.

Learning outcomes

- You should be able to describe contraceptive methods and options, and make recommendations based upon a patient's lifestyle, family planning and medical history.

- You should be able to explain how contraceptive methods work, their limitations, risks and probability of failure.

Essential Human Development, First Edition. Edited by Samuel Webster, Geraint Morris and Euan Kevelighan
© 2018 John Wiley & Sons, Ltd. Published 2018 by John Wiley & Sons, Ltd.

Natural family planning (or 'rhythm methods')

The basis of natural family planning (NFP) methods is to not have sex when there is a chance of a pregnancy occurring (or alternatively to ensure that sex does occur at this time if a pregnancy is wanted). There are various methods for ensuring that there is minimal chance of sperm and ovum meeting.

Withdrawal method

Whilst it can be argued that withdrawing the penis just before the moment of ejaculation is not 'natural', if used well this method reduces the number of sperm in the vagina. Unfortunately there are sperm in the pre-ejaculate, so whilst this reduces the sperm load from around 20 million to as many as a hundred thousand, there is still a small possibility of fertilisation.

Counting days

NFP is based around the fact that sperm live 3–6 days in the female genital tract, and ova, once released, last a maximum of 48 hours. Ovulation occurs usually about 14 days **before** the start of the next period of menstruation, meaning that in a 28-day cycle ovulation occurs on about day 14 (in a 35-day cycle ovulation occurs on about day 21). This means that in a regular 28-day cycle fertilisation may be low risk on days 1 to 6 or 7, and after day 16 or 17. Unfortunately the woman needs a very regular cycle to have any hope of efficiently using this method, making it less suitable for the older woman who might be most interested in trying this. This method also fails when ovulation occurs later or earlier than usual. It also requires either abstinence or use of a barrier method for 10 days or so mid-cycle.

Temperature chart

This method requires the temperature to be taken at the same time each day (preferably first thing in the morning). It is based around the fact that on the day of ovulation the body's basal temperature rises (by about 0.4°C) and under the influence of progesterone it stays at this higher level until menstruation starts, when it reverts to the normal lower level. This method fails if sex has occurred in the 7 days before the temperature change, so requires temperature charts to be made for a few months until the ovulation increase can be predicted to occur at a regular day of the month.

Mucus method

This is based around the changes in cervical mucus under the influence of different hormones. Normally in the early cycle mucus is thick and sticky and it stays like this until the oestrogen levels increase, when it becomes much slimier and thinner (known as spinnbarkeit). After the egg has died the mucus thickens again. This method requires the woman to insert her finger into the vagina and examine the mucus by stretching it between her thumb and finger. The more stretchy the mucus the more fertile she is likely to be.

Advantages and disadvantages

The advantages of natural family planning are:
- no hormones;
- no side effects.
 The disadvantages are:
- regular menstrual cycle needed for effective use;
- need to abstain from intercourse for 9+ days each month.

Barrier methods

Male and female condoms

Condoms are not only contraceptives but also give protection against infection. They are usually made of latex, or silicone for those sensitive to latex. The male condoms are lubricated with a non-spermicidal gel since it was found some years ago that the normal spermicide nonoxynol-9 made the area hyperaemic and led to an increase in the risk of transmission of HIV. The female condoms often have nonoxynol-9. It is important that the condoms are fitted before any genital contact occurs.

When teaching male condom use, it is important to stress checking that the condom has a kite or CE mark in Europe, or a similar quality testing mark in other parts of the world. The expiry date must also be checked, and that the packet is intact and undamaged. The condom should then be removed from the packet and the teat (small 'hat') if present should be squeezed to expel the air before it is put on the erect penis. Once the male has ejaculated, the penis with condom must be withdrawn from the vagina whilst still erect. The condom should be removed carefully and checked to ensure there is no breakage or leakage. It should then be disposed of. There must be no further genital contact unless a new condom is put on.

Many couples may be too embarrassed to ask their partner to use a condom, and may in fact not understand proper condom use. It is often regarded as 'washing up with rubber gloves on' as it can reduce sexual sensitivity, particularly for the man, although it can be helpful for those men who are over-sensitive and may have premature ejaculation. Condoms also mean that sex stops as soon as the man ejaculates, which can leave the woman unsatisfied.

Lubricants can be used with condoms but must be water based, as oil-based lubricants can destroy condoms very quickly.

Female condoms are very similar but are inserted into the vagina, and this can be done before the male becomes erect. They can be fairly noisy as they move with the friction of intercourse. They also protect to a certain extent against sexually transmitted infections.

Caps and diaphragms

Caps and diaphragms are made of latex or silicone, and are designed to fit over the cervix (Figure 49.1). They need to be used

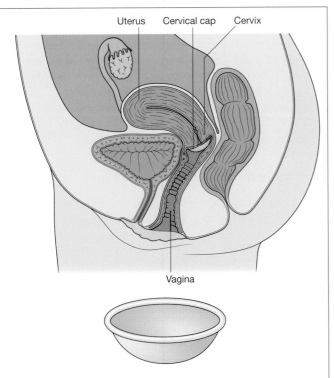

Figure 49.1 A contraceptive cap and its anatomical location for use.

with spermicide as they are largely vehicles to keep spermicide against the cervix. They have to be fitted by an expert to ensure the correct size is used, and the woman is then taught how to insert and remove their own device. Caps and diaphragms have an advantage over the condom in that they can be inserted up to 2 hours before sex (or immediately before), but must be kept in situ for a minimum of 6 hours after sex. It should not interfere with sensitivity of either partner. The woman has to be confident and able to insert her fingers into herself, and she needs to have a suitable anatomy. Lax vaginal muscles or a prolapse can make using a cap impossible. Unfortunately it is a rather messy method with significant leakage of sperm and spermicide from the vagina after sex, but as a non-hormonal method it may be chosen by those who find themselves unable to tolerate hormonal side effects.

Advantages and disadvantages

The advantages of barrier methods are:
- No hormones or hormonal side effects.
  The disadvantages are:
- Male condoms need to be put on when the penis is erect. Some loss of sensitivity.
- Female condoms must be inserted by the woman.
- Women must have a suitable anatomy for diaphragms and caps.

Combined oral methods

Oestrogen and progesterone can be used daily to stop ovulation, thicken the cervical mucus and to stop endometrial thickening. These preparations can be taken daily as pills, weekly as stick-on skin patches, or monthly as a vaginal ring.

The original idea when these contraceptive methods were first introduced was to mimic the body's hormonal cycle by taking the combined oral pill for 21 days and then have 7 days hormone free during which time the body would have a 'period'. In fact this is not a typical menstrual period as such, and is instead a hormonal withdrawal bleed. The combined methods are the only methods in which the woman has control of when she bleeds and can manipulate her withdrawal bleed to suit her lifestyle. It is now being suggested that these methods can, or even should be, used for significantly longer than 21 days without a break because they might reduce the risk of some cancers and can also stop pregnancy with pill failures due to not restarting.

There are many different preparations of these pills and together with the Evra® patch and the NuvaRing®, they all contain between 15 and 35 µg of oestrogen and progestogens.

Second generation progestogens (norethisterone and levonorgestrel) are androgenic and can give androgenic side effects (acne, greasy hair, mood changes and headaches; see Table 49.1). They are, however, regarded as slightly safer in regards to cardiovascular episodes.

Third generation progestogens (gestodene, desogestrel, etc.) are much more potent progestogenically and side effects tend to be better tolerated. There seems to be some evidence that they may be less safe in terms of cardiovascular side effects.

Usually one pill must be taken daily, but can be taken up to almost 24 hours late. If one pill is missed the efficacy is still thought to be good, but if two or more are missed altogether then there is an increased risk of pregnancy if alternative contraception is not used for the next seven pill-taking days.

There are 'UK medical eligibility' criteria for various reversible contraceptive methods in general, which quickly identify levels of contraindications for each method based upon the patient's medical history. The categories are:

UKMec 4: absolute contraindication (an unacceptable risk if the contraceptive method is used).

UKMec 3: relative contraindication (not really safe but safer than the woman getting pregnant if no other method

Table 49.1 Hormonal side effects from combined contraceptive pills.

Oestrogenic side effects	Progestogenic side effects
• Headache	• Mood changes
• Nausea	• Bloating and weight changes
• Dizziness	• Acne and greasy hair
• Breast symptoms	• Breast tenderness
• Increased vaginal secretions	• Vaginal dryness

suitable. The risks outweigh the advantages of using the contraceptive method).

UkMec 2: some interactions (the advantages outweigh the risks of using the contraceptive method).

UkMec 1: no interactions (no restrictions on using the contraceptive method).

For example, oestrogen is contraindicated (UKMec 4) in women who have high blood pressure, have focal migraines, are smokers over 35 years old, or have a history of clotting problems.

It is advisable not to give a UKMec 3 item to a woman with a body mass index (BMI) over 35 or a first-degree relative with a history of venous thromboembolism under the age of 45, or if the patient suffers migraine with aura.

UKMec 2 items include smoking, a BMI over 30 and a history of cholestasis in pregnancy.

Advantages and disadvantages

The advantages of combined oral contraception methods are:
- Menstrual cycle control.
- Reduced bleeding.
- Control of dysmenorrhoea.
  The disadvantages are:
- The daily pill requires good compliance. Methods exist to help remembering to take the daily pill.
- Hormonal side effects.

Progesterone-only pills

As the name suggests, progesterone-only pills (POP) contain only progesterone and must be taken daily.

The original POPs worked primarily by making the mucus in the cervical canal too thick for sperm to penetrate. Newer desogestrel pills work like the combined pills by stopping ovulation, and by affecting the cervical mucus and endometrium. They need to be taken once daily within a few hours of the chosen time (3 hours for the older POPS and 12 hours for the new pills). If taken later than this the woman should not rely on the pills for 48 hours after restarting/taking the late pill. The contraindications to taking these are much less as they are thought to have minimal effect on the blood and give much less, if any, risk of clots forming. In fact, they can be given to women who are on anticoagulation treatment for repeated venous thromboembolism.

Advantages and disadvantages

The advantages of progesterone-only pills are:
- under the woman's control;
- can be stopped quickly.
  The disadvantages are:
- the daily pill requires very good compliance;
- need to be taken every day;
- no cycle control;
- hormonal side effects.

Long-acting reversible contraception (larc)

Long-acting reversible contraception comprises a group of contraceptive methods including the coils (copper, and copper with progesterone such as IUS/Mirena®) and implants. Depo-Provera® ('the pill injection') is also included at present but this method is typically considered a medium-acting reversible contraception.

Injection contraception

Depo-Provera is a 3-monthly intramuscular injection of medroxyprogesterone that works at the hypothalamic/pituitary level to stop the hormonal cycle. Most women end up amenorrhoeic. There is also a subcutaneous preparation that should be suitable for self-injection.

Noristerat® is another injectable contraceptive that is given every 2 months, but should only be given twice; it is rarely used in the UK.

Due to the fact that this method works at the cerebral level it has some effects on other pituitary hormones and it may reduce bone mineral density by up to 5% over the first 2 years of use. This is reversible when the preparation is stopped, but care must be taken when giving it to those under 18 (who have not yet reached peak bone density) and those approaching the menopause, as it is important that these women go into the menopause with peak density.

The progesterone level is fairly high with this method meaning that most women find they have almost no menstrual bleeding; however, they can get significant progesterone side effects (e.g. acne, greasy hair, increased appetite leading to weight gain, breast tenderness and mood problems). Although each injection lasts 14 weeks (licensed for 12 but known to last 14), in some women the progesterone level is enough to stop fertility for an average of a year, meaning the side effects can also last this long.

Advantages and disadvantages

The advantages of injection contraception are:
- three-monthly injection;
- reduced or stopped menstrual bleeding.
  The disadvantages are:
- side effects may be long lasting;
- repeated injections every 12 to 14 weeks.

Implants

Nexplanon® is a small rod impregnated with etonogestrel, a progestogen. It is injected subdermally into the arm and works extremely well (better than sterilisation) as a contraceptive for at least 3 years. The rod has to be fitted and removed by a trained health professional. It works by increasing cervical mucus, stopping endometrial thickening and usually stopping ovulation.

As with other progesterone methods Nexplanon can cause side effects including acne, depression, increased appetite and breast tenderness. It also has an unpredictable effect on bleeding, and this is the main reason why women request removal as it can cause almost continuous menstrual bleeding. This may be managed by adding contraceptive pills – a combined oral contraceptive (COC) if suitable, Depo-Provera, or a potentially less effective POP or doxycycline can be used to try to stabilise the endometrium.

Advantages and disadvantages

The advantages of progestogen implants are:
- Extremely effective contraception for 3 years with no input from patient after insertion.
  The disadvantages are:
- Irregular bleeding.
- Progesterone side effects.
- Contraception is not under the woman's control.

Coils

Coils are contraceptive devices that have to be fitted by medical professionals into the uterine cavity.

Copper coils

Copper coils are fitted into the uterus (Figure 49.2). They work because copper is intensely spermicidal. The copper also gives rise to immune complexes in the uterine walls, which encourage the failure of any fertilised egg to implant, and promote endometrial shedding. They have no hormones so there are no hormonal side effects, but they do increase menstrual loss and discomfort.

Copper coils last between 5 and 10 years. The gold standard coil, the T-Safe® 380, lasts 10 years due to the copper bands on the horizontal arms. This arrangement not only ensures good copper levels around the tubal orifices, but also that the copper does not disintegrate in the same way that the copper wire on the vertical axis does.

Copper coils can be fitted to any woman, including nulliparous young women and women approaching the menopause. They can also be used as emergency contraception due to their action of stopping implantation.

Once removed, fertility is immediately resumed, with no long-term effects. If fitted after the woman's 40th birthday the coil can be left as contraception until the menopause.

Advantages and disadvantages
The advantages of copper coils are:
- no hormonal side effects;
- effective contraception for up to 10 years.
  The disadvantages are:
- fitting must be done by an expert;
- pain on fitting;

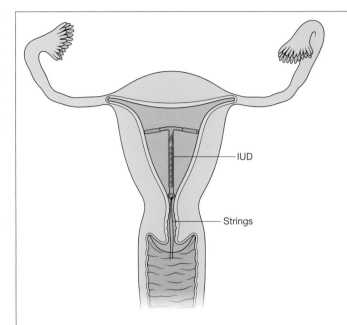

Figure 49.2 A copper contraceptive coil fitted within the uterus.

- increased menstrual blood loss;
- increased menstrual pain.

Intrauterine system (IUS) and Mirena® coils

The intrauterine system and Mirena coils incorporate a source of progesterone around the vertical stem. They work by stopping endometrial buildup and also by making cervical mucus thick and impenetrable. In some women they may also have some effect on ovulation but most continue to ovulate.

These coils are very useful in reducing menstrual flow and also menstrual pain, particularly in those who have endometriosis and adenomyosis. Their action is via progesterone so they may cause side effects such as irregular bleeding (usually fairly light and may just be spotting but can be frequent and prolonged for the first year), and the hormonal side effects of acne, depression and increased appetite. These side effects should be minimal because the level in the blood of progesterone from the IUS is about 25% of that when taking the POP itself, but it can be a nuisance in a few women.

The IUS cannot be used as an emergency contraceptive.

If fitted after the woman's 45th birthday the IUS can be left in until it is no longer needed, although if the woman has coil amenorrhoea this can be difficult to ascertain.

Advantages and disadvantages
The advantages of an IUS coil are:
- reduced menstrual bleeding and pain.
  The disadvantages are:
- must be fitted by an expert;

- pain on fitting;
- hormonal side effects (progesterone);
- nuisance bleeding.

Emergency/postcoital contraception

Emergency contraception methods are used after unprotected sex.

Levonelle® (levonorgestrel 5 mg) works by delaying ovulation. Levonelle is licensed for use up to 72 hours after sex, but probably works best in the first 48 hours (95–85%). Levonelle fails to be effective once the surge of luteinising hormone (LH) starts at about day 12 of a 28-day cycle (see Chapter 2).

ellaOne® (ulipristal) works as an antiprogesterone and stops ovulation. It works up to 5 days after sex, is about 85% effective, but is significantly less effective around ovulation.

Copper coils work up to 5 days after ovulation by stopping implantation, and this method is almost 100% effective. The coil can subsequently be removed once menstruation begins, or it can be left in situ for up to 10 years.

Sterilisation

Male sterilisation (vasectomy) is more efficient than female methods and involves a small operation under local anaesthetic to cut the ductus (vas) deferens (see Chapter 3). Because it is done under local anaesthetic it is safer than female sterilisation, which usually requires a general anaesthetic. Ejaculate is evaluated for spermatozoa to confirm successful sterilisation.

Female sterilisation can be done laparoscopically where the uterine tubes are either cut, clipped or cauterised. This works contraceptively as soon as the woman has a period (ensuring that no ovum had been released before the operation). There is a very small chance that the clips may come loose, or are not placed correctly, but this method is generally considered to have a lifetime failure rate of about 1 in 200.

Essure® is a method of female sterilisation that can be done via the hysteroscope. Small metal implants are inserted into the uterine ends of the uterine tubes. Over the following 2 or 3 months a tissue response occludes the tubes at the ostia. This method requires a further test some months after the operation to ensure that it has worked to occlude the tubes. This form of sterilisation is completely irreversible.

Clinical case

Case investigations

Kylie is likely to have multiple sexual partners and would like a reliable method of contraception that she has control of. You discuss a number of options and the advantages and disadvantages in her case.

Kylie does not think that natural family planning methods would work, as she would not reliably abstain during her fertile period and would not be confident in her planning. She is aware of the advantages of using condoms to protect against STIs but does not feel that she can always rely on that method. She does not like the idea of caps or female condoms, partly because she would need to carry them when out, and because she does not feel confident in fitting them herself.

The combined oral contraceptive (COC) pill might be suitable if she can be organised, but a tablet needs taking every day. Contraceptive patches can be dislodged or peel off, and Kylie comments that it would be difficult to hide the patch. The vaginal ring could be suitable if she is organised enough to remove it monthly and if she is willing to put it in and remove it. Progesterone-only pills (POPs) are probably not suitable for Kylie as they would need to be taken more regularly with more accurate timings than the COC. The POP is usually only used for those who cannot tolerate supplemental oestrogen.

With regards to a contraceptive implant such as Depo-Provera, Kylie is under 18 so effects on her bone development need to be considered, alongside whether she will return for repeat implant placements, but otherwise this is potentially a good option.

A coil could be used, but Kylie's chaotic lifestyle and previous termination of pregnancy (TOP) suggest her risk of STIs is increased, and this leads to a significant risk of PID if she is infected within the first 3 weeks of insertion before the mucus plug recovers.

Sterilisation is not suitable for a 16-year-old no matter what she may say or feel at this stage in her life, and she has no regular partner so vasectomy is not an option.

Case conclusion

Kylie decided that her options were the COC pill, injection or implant, and after suitable counselling decided on the COC pill, which she decided to keep in her makeup bag, which went with her when she stayed with her boyfriend, or went to stay with her grandmother, or when she was at home. She liked the idea that she could manipulate her bleeding pattern to suit her lifestyle and decided that she was organised enough to remember to take one daily with an application on her mobile phone to remind her.

Key learning points

- There are a range of methods of contraception, and different methods have a number of advantages and disadvantages. Knowledge of these methods can be aligned with a patient's needs and medical history when recommending appropriate options.

- Sterilisation is a surgical method of contraception that should be considered permanent.

 Now visit **www.wileyessential.com/humandevelopment** to test yourself on this chapter.

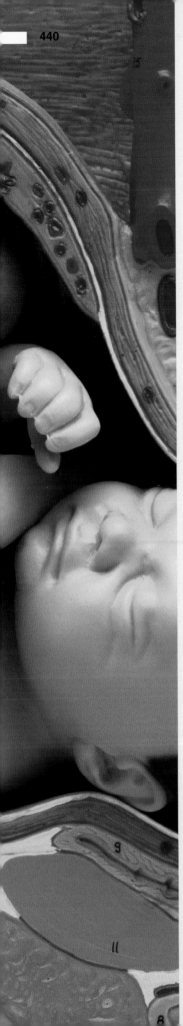

CHAPTER 50
Obstetric and gynaecological operations

Nisha Kadwadkar and Euan Kevelighan

Case

A 25-year-old primigravida is admitted for induction of labour at 42 weeks gestation. On examination the cervix is unfavourable and two doses of prostaglandins (Prostin® 3 mg tablets) are administered vaginally 6 hours apart. The next morning the woman is re-examined and the cervix is favourable, i.e. an artificial rupture of membranes (ARM) can easily be performed. She is transferred to the labour ward and following ARM an oxytocin infusion is commenced intravenously. An epidural was sited for pain relief 4 hours later. She labours slowly and 12 hours later the cervix is fully dilated. One hour later she commences pushing. The cardiotocogragh (CTG) remains normal throughout labour.

Three hours following full dilatation she is re-examined and the findings are as follows: cervix fully dilated; position right occipito-lateral, caput 2+, moulding 1+, station +2 (cm below the ischial spines). The woman is exhausted. The CTG remains normal and liquor is clear.

Learning outcomes

- You should be able to understand the principles of common surgical procedures in obstetrics and gynaecology.
- You should be able to use the information in this chapter to enable you to understand in more detail and ask deeper questions when you witness the operations described. It will also make assisting at these procedures more meaningful.

Essential Human Development, First Edition. Edited by Samuel Webster, Geraint Morris and Euan Kevelighan
© 2018 John Wiley & Sons, Ltd. Published 2018 by John Wiley & Sons, Ltd.

Episiotomy

Definition

An episiotomy is an incision through the perineum made to enlarge the diameter of the vulval outlet and assist childbirth.

Prevalence

In the UK, rates of episiotomy are approximately 10%, in keeping with the World Health Organization's recommendation. However, there is considerable international variation (rates are 50% in the USA and 99% in Eastern Europe).

Technique

During antenatal care the possibility of episiotomy should be explained to women. During the period of fetal head crowning informed verbal consent should be obtained prior to performing episiotomy.

Episiotomy is performed in the second stage, usually when the perineum is being stretched and the procedure is deemed necessary. Adequate analgesia is required – either a good epidural block or infiltration with local anaesthetic.

The incision can be midline (common in the USA) or at an angle from the posterior fourchette (mediolateral episiotomy; see Figure 50.1). Mediolateral episiotomy (popular in the UK) should start at the posterior fourchette, move laterally downwards at an angle of 45° to the posterior fourchette on one side, so that any extension will avoid damaging the anal sphincter. Most episiotomies are right mediolateral as the majority of practitioners are right-handed.

A mediolateral episiotomy is usually preferred in the UK. A midline episiotomy has an advantage of being an incision through a comparatively avascular area and results in less bleeding, quicker healing and less pain; however, there is an increased risk of extension to involve the anal sphincter (third/fourth-degree tear).

Complications

Complications include haemorrhage, infection (prophylactic antibiotics may be indicated if contamination is suspected), extension to anal sphincter (third/fourth-degree tears) and dyspareunia.

Operative or assisted vaginal delivery

Definition

Operative vaginal delivery refers to any operative procedure designed to expedite vaginal delivery, and includes forceps delivery and vacuum extraction.

There is no proven benefit of one instrument over another. The choice of which instrument to use is dependent largely on the clinician's preference and experience.

Indications

The **maternal indications** include:
- Maternal exhaustion.
- Prolonged second stage of labour:
    - Nulliparous: 3 hours with regional analgesia or 2 hours without regional analgesia.
    - Multiparous: 2 hours with regional analgesia or 1 hour without regional analgesia.
- Medical indications (need to avoid maternal expulsive efforts):
    - Cardiac disease (myocardial infarction, reduced ejection fraction).
    - CNS conditions (intracranial aneurisms).
    - Spinal cord injury.
    - Myasthenia gravis.

The **fetal indications** are:
- Suspected fetal distress.

The commonest reasons to perform instrumental delivery are prolonged second stage of labour, presumed fetal distress (abnormal CTG) and maternal exhaustion.

Contraindications

Relative contraindications are prematurity and suspected fetal coagulation disorder.

Prerequisites for operative vaginal delivery

Maternal criteria

1. Adequate analgesia.
2. Fetal head not palpable abdominally.
3. Verbal and/or written consent (written consent is required for procedure in theatre).
4. Lithotomy position.
5. Bladder empty.

Uteroplacental criteria

1. Cervix fully dilated.
2. Membranes ruptured.
3. No placenta praevia.

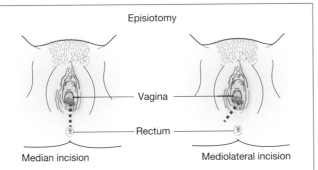

Figure 50.1 Episiotomy incisions.

Fetal criteria

1. Vertex presentation.
2. Station at or below spines (0 or +1).
3. Position, caput and moulding is known.

Other criteria

1. An experienced operator.
2. Capability to perform an emergency caesarean delivery if required.

Forceps delivery

Instruments

Forceps can be classified into three categories:
1. Classical forceps (such as Neville–Barnes/Simpson forceps), which have a pelvic curvature, a cephalic curvature and locking handles (Figure 50.2).
2. Rotational forceps (such as Kielland forceps), which lack a pelvic curvature and have a sliding lock.
3. Forceps designed to assist breech deliveries (such as Piper forceps), which lack a pelvic curve and have long handles on which to place the body of the breech while delivering the head.

A classification of forceps deliveries by type of procedure is given in Table 50.1.

Technique

By convention, the left blade is inserted before the right with the accoucher's hand protecting the vaginal wall from direct trauma. With proper placement of the forceps blades, they come to lie parallel to the axis of the fetal head and between the fetal head and the pelvic wall. The operator then locks the blades, checking their application before applying traction.

Table 50.1 Classification of forceps deliveries.

Type of procedure	Criteria
Outlet forceps	Fetal head is at or on the perineum, scalp is visible at the introitus without separating the labia, sagittal suture is in the anteroposterior diameter or right or left occiput anterior or posterior position, rotation is ≤45°
Low forceps	Leading point of the fetal skull is at ≥+2 cm rotation may be: a) ≤45° or b) >45°
Mid-forceps	Station <+2 cm but head engaged
High forceps	Not included in classification

Traction should be synchronised with the uterine contractions and maternal expulsive efforts. Traction should follow the pelvic curve by using Pajot's manoeuvre. There are two separate components to this – the dominant hand (usually the right hand) holding the forceps blades applies traction while the other hand presses downwards on the shanks of the forceps. The force applied by the left hand is important – too much force increases the risk of perineal trauma and too little results in increased likelihood of failure to deliver. As the head begins to crown, the blades are directed towards the vertical and the head is delivered gently, whilst guarding the perineum.

Episiotomy is recommended whenever an instrumental vaginal delivery is performed (see Table 50.1). This is not based on any robust evidence. Perineal trauma will occur in most nulliparous women undergoing instrumental vaginal delivery, and episiotomy should be considered in these women in order to limit multiple lacerations.

Complications

- Maternal perineal injury, especially with rotational forceps.
- Common fetal injuries are facial or scalp bruising and/or laceration. Facial nerve palsy, skull fractures, cervical spine injuries and intracranial haemorrhage are rare.

Ventouse delivery

Types of ventouse cup

The most widely used metal cups are the 'Bird-modification' types. They have a central traction chain and a separate vacuum pipe. The anterior cups are used for the occipito-anterior position and are in 4, 5 and 6 cm sizes. The posterior cup is designed to be inserted higher up in the vagina to allow the correct placement over the occiput when the head is deflexed in the occipito-posterior position.

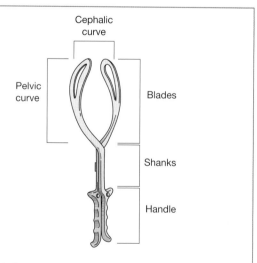

Figure 50.2 Delivery forceps design.

More recently a number of soft cups have been developed, one example of which is the silicone-rubber cup. The Kiwi® cup is another example of a ventouse cup (Figure 50.3), which is widely used for lift-out delivery when the fetal head is low.

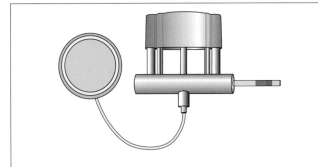

Figure 50.3 Kiwi® ventouse cup.

Prerequisites

- Full dilatation of cervix and full engagement of the head.
- Cooperation of the patient.
- Good contractions should be present.

Indications

Indications for ventouse delivery are the same as for forceps delivery.

Contraindications

The contraindications for ventouse delivery include:
- Face presentation.
- Gestation less than 34 weeks.
- Maternal infections (e.g. HIV, syphilis).
- Maternal bleeding disorders (e.g. low platelets, haemophilia).

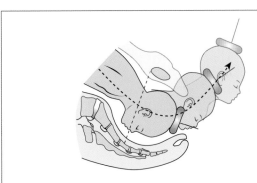

Figure 50.4 The angle of traction with ventouse delivery

Technique

The appropriate cup should be chosen. It should be connected to the pump and a check should be made for leakages prior to commencing the delivery.

The vacuum cup is then gently inserted into the vagina with one hand whilst the other hand parts the labia. The pressure of $0.8\ kg/cm^2$ is achieved, following which traction is given with the next contraction.

Traction should be along the pelvic axis (downwards at 45°) for the duration of the contraction (Figure 50.4).

One hand should rest on the cup whilst the other applies traction. The hand on the cup detects any early detachment and also indicates whether the head moves downwards with each pull. The fingers on the head can promote flexion and can help to guide the head under the arch of the pubis by using the space in front of the sacrum. As the head crowns the angle of traction changes upwards through an arc of over 90°. At this point an episiotomy is performed if required and perineum is supported with the hand that was on the cup.

Rules for ventouse delivery

- The delivery should be completed within 10 minutes of application.
- The head, not just the scalp, should descend with each pull.
- The cup should be reapplied no more than twice.
- If failure with the ventouse occurs despite good traction the forceps should not be tried as well.

Increased risks of failure

- Incorrect placement of cup.
- Excessive caput.
- Poor maternal effort.
- Traction in wrong direction.

Complications

Maternal complications include:
- Trauma to the genital tract.
- Unrecognised injury of the cervix.
  Fetal complications include:
- Chignon (oedematous skin bump) at the site of cup application.
- Cephalohaematoma (subperiosteal bleed).
- Intracranial injuries – rare, and usually occur if multiple attempts at delivery are made.

Caesarean section

Definition

Caesarean section is a procedure to deliver the fetus through the abdomen. Abdominal skin incision is usually Pfannenstiel, or less commonly midline or upper transverse. A Pfannenstiel incision is a transverse incision two finger breadths above the pubic symphysis. The midline abdominal incision is used in a woman who may require a classical caesarean section. Indications for classical caesarean section are shown in Box 50.1. The upper transverse is an incision used in high BMI women in order to get better access; the skin incision is transverse but above the pannus.

The most common uterine incision is a transverse incision in the lower segment of the uterus (Figure 50.5). A midline uterine incision is called a classical incision. An inverted T-incision is occasionally required to achieve better access for difficult deliveries, for example to deliver the after-coming head during a breech delivery by caesarean section.

Preparation

The patient should be in the left lateral position with a wedge under the right buttock (to prevent aorta-caval compression with supine hypotension and fetal distress). Premedication

---

Box 50.1 Indications for caesarean section

- Obstructed labour, malpresentation, malposition, multiple gestation
- Fetal distress/prolapsed cord
- Maternal medical conditions requiring urgent/controlled delivery
- Obstetric complications, e.g. placenta praevia
- Previous caesarean section

Indications for classical caesarean section:
- Preterm delivery with poorly formed lower segment
- Placenta praevia/abruption with large vessels in lower segment
- Premature rupture of membranes, poor lower segment and transverse lie
- Transverse lie with back inferior
- Large cervical fibroid
- Severe adhesions in lower segment reducing accessibility
- Postmortem caesarean section

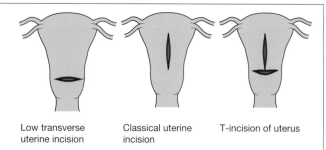

Low transverse uterine incision

Classical uterine incision

T-incision of uterus

Figure 50.5 Uterine incision methods during caesarean delivery.

with antacid is standard. In theatre, the operating table must also be kept in left lateral tilt position until after the delivery. Thrombo-prophylaxis should be considered for all patients and prophylactic antibiotics should be administered.

Operative procedure

Double gloving reduces the likelihood of needle puncture, and use of a clear plastic shield reduces exposure of the face. A transverse suprapubic skin incision is made. The bladder is reflected inferiorly before incising the uterus. Care needs to be taken whilst incising the uterus or the baby may experience a scalpel injury. The placenta is delivered with controlled continuous cord traction to avoid uterine inversion. Both angles of uterine incision should be secured first to reduce the bleeding. The peritoneum does not require suturing. The uterus is usually closed in two layers with Vicryl® (absorbable suture). The skin can be closed with continuous absorbable suture, such as Monocryl®, Prolene® (needs removal in a few days) or staples (also require removal a few days post-op).

Postmortem caesarean section

If a pregnant woman has a cardiac arrest, a postmortem caesarean section should be carried out within 4 minutes. This is performed at the site of resuscitation, via midline skin and uterine (classical) incisions. The purpose of this is not only to try to save the baby's life, but mainly to facilitate resuscitation of the mother (improves the ventilation and venous return).

Complications

The risks of both early and long-term complications are increased in women delivered by caesarean section, when compared with the outcomes after normal vaginal delivery. The risks are surgical and anaesthetic. The main problems are thrombo-embolism, infection and haemorrhage, which can be minimised by appropriate prophylaxis and surgical skill.

Hysteroscopy

Definition

Hysteroscopy is a procedure that passes a small diameter telescope, either flexible or rigid, through the cervix to directly inspect the uterine cavity (Figure 50.6). A flexible hysteroscope is used as an outpatient procedure and uses saline or carbon dioxide as a distension medium. Rigid instruments use fluids and therefore can be used even if there is bleeding during the procedure.

Indications

Any abnormal bleeding from the uterus can be investigated by hysteroscopy including:

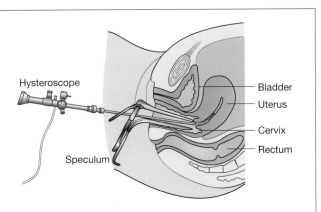

Figure 50.6 Hysteroscopic access to the uterus.

- Postmenopausal bleeding.
- Irregular menstruation, intermenstrual bleeding and post-coital bleeding.
- Persistent menorrhagia.
- Persistent discharge.
  It can also be used to:
- Investigate suspected uterine malformations.
- Investigate suspected Asherman's syndrome.
- Perform procedures like resection of polyps and fibroids.

Complications

- Perforation of uterus.
- Cervical damage if cervical dilatation is necessary.
- Ascent of any coexisting infection.

Laparoscopy

Definition

Laparoscopy is a procedure that allows visualisation of the peritoneal cavity. This involves insertion of a needle, called a Veress needle, through an incision in the umbilicus. This allows insufflation of the peritoneal cavity with carbon dioxide so that a larger instrument can be inserted. The majority of instruments used for diagnostic laparoscopy are 5 mm in diameter, while 10-mm instruments are used for operative laparoscopy.

Indications for operative laparoscopy

- Suspected ectopic pregnancy.
- Undiagnosed pelvic pain.
- Tubal patency testing.
- Sterilisation.
- Ovarian cystectomy.
- Oophorectomy.
- Endometriosis treatment with diathermy or laser.

- Reversal of sterilisation.
- Hysterectomy.

Complications

Complications are uncommon but include damage to intra-abdominal structures including bowel and major blood vessels. The bladder is emptied prior to the procedure to avoid bladder injury. Incisional hernia may occur from the port sites. Another rare complication is gas embolism.

Abdominal and vaginal hysterectomy

Definition

Vaginal hysterectomy is a procedure that involves removal of the uterus through the vaginal passage. Abdominal hysterectomy involves removal of the uterus through an abdominal incision.

Vaginal hysterectomy is associated with a quicker recovery than abdominal hysterectomy, due to lack of an abdominal incision and is therefore preferred. However, when there is malignancy an abdominal approach is usually preferred as the ovaries often need to be removed and lymph nodes examined and sampled. If the uterus is larger than that of a 12-week pregnancy then usually an abdominal hysterectomy is performed.

Procedure

Most abdominal hysterectomies are performed through a Pfannenstiel incision, which is a low (bikini line) suprapubic transverse incision. Patients recover more quickly from this incision and the cosmetic result is more acceptable than from a midline incision. However, for larger masses and malignancies a midline incision is usually preferred to gain adequate access.

Although a complete description of abdominal hysterectomy is outside the scope of this chapter, the procedure involves taking three or four pedicles:
- The infundibulo-pelvic ligament, which contains the ovarian vessels.
- The uterine artery.
- The angles of the vault of the vagina, which contain vessels ascending from the vagina.
- The ligaments to support the uterus can be taken with this pedicle or separately.
In vaginal hysterectomy the same steps are taken but in the reverse order.

Indications for abdominal hysterectomy

- Uterine, ovarian, cervical and fallopian tube carcinoma.
- Pelvic pain from chronic endometriosis or chronic pelvic inflammatory disease where the pelvis is frozen and vaginal hysterectomy is impossible.
- Symptomatic fibroid uterus greater than 12-week size.

Indications for vaginal hysterectomy

- Menstrual disorders with a uterus less than 12 weeks in size.
- Microinvasive cervical carcinoma.
- Uterovaginal prolapse.

Complications

Specific complications of hysterectomy include:
- Haemorrhage – major blood vessel injury.
- Ureteric injury.
- Bladder and bowel injury.

Surgical prolapse procedure

Anterior repair

Anterior repair (anterior colpoperineorrhaphy) is the commonest performed surgical procedure for the anatomical correction of cystourethrocele. An anterior vaginal wall incision is made and the fascial defect allowing the bladder to herniate through is identified and closed. With the bladder position restored any redundant vaginal epithelium is excised and the incision closed.

Posterior repair

Posterior repair (posterior colpoperineorrhaphy) is the commonest procedure performed to repair rectocele. A posterior vaginal wall incision is made and the fascial defect allowing the rectum to herniate through is identified and closed. With the rectal position restored any redundant vaginal epithelium is excised and the incision closed.

For an enterocele the surgical procedure is similar to posterior repair but the peritoneal sac containing the small bowel is excised. In addition, the pouch of Douglas is closed by approximating the peritoneum and/or the uterosacral ligaments.

Uterovaginal prolapse surgeries

If the woman does not wish to conserve her uterus for fertility or other reasons then a vaginal hysterectomy with support of the vault to the uterosacrals is sufficient. If uterine conservation is required then the sacrocolpopexy or Manchester operation are alternatives.

The Manchester operation involves partial amputation of the cervix and approximation of the cardinal ligaments below the retained cervix remnant.

In sacrocolpopexy the inverted vaginal vault is attached to the sacrum using a mesh.

Sacrospinous ligament fixation is a procedure where the vault is sutured to one or other sacrospinous ligaments. This is performed vaginally so does not involve opening the abdomen. The vaginal vault is secured to one of the sacrospinous ligaments. Although this results in the vagina being angulated it does not interfere with sexual function.

Surgery for stress incontinence

The aims of surgery are:
1. Restoration of the proximal urethra and bladder neck to the zone of intra-abdominal pressure transmission.
2. To increase urethral resistance.
3. A combination of both.

Tension-free vaginal tape (TVT)

The aim of this operation is to provide suburethral support. This involves insertion of a Prolene® (polypropylene) tape underneath the mid-urethra. The insertion is through a very small vaginal incision with two tiny abdominal incisions. The tape is self-retaining and does not require fixation. Early and medium-term results (up to 10 years) are very encouraging with cure rates of approximately 85%. Operation time is short and the procedure can be performed under local anaesthetic.

Trans-obturater tape (TVT-O)

This involves insertion of the tape underneath the urethra, which passes through the obturater foramen on either side. This procedure requires regional or general anaesthesia. Success rates are similar to TVT, and the main advantage is that bladder injury is significantly less with TVT-O compared with conventional TVT. The main disadvantage is the risk of groin pain – approximately 9%.

Colposuspension operation

Abdominal colposuspension involves elevation and alignment of the bladder neck with the symphysis pubis.

Open abdominal colposuspension is associated with success rates of over 95% at one year, falling to 78% at 15-year follow-up. Laparoscopic colposuspension is gaining popularity but is associated with lower success rates than the traditional procedure. Colposuspension was the gold standard operation for stress urinary incontinence until the advent of tension-free vaginal tapes.

Other surgeries

Other surgeries for stress incontinence include artificial sphincter and periurethral injections. Artificial sphincter is a major procedure performed only in tertiary referral centres because of the level of expertise required.

A range of materials may be used for periurethral injections. These include collagen, subcutaneous fat and microparticulate silicone. The principle is to inject the agents into the periurethral tissues at the level of the bladder neck aiming for bladder neck coaptation. Early success at 3-month follow-up ranges from 80 to 90%, but there is a time-dependent decline to approximately 50% at 3–4 years. Complications are uncommon and minor – dysuria, urinary tract infection and retention requiring overnight catheterisation are occasionally encountered.

Clinical case

Case management

The woman is exhausted, has been pushing for 2 hours and fully dilated for 3 hours. She requires delivery. She can either be delivered instrumentally (by forceps or ventouse) or by caesarean section. The criteria required for instrumental delivery are:

- Adequate analgesia (she has a working epidural).
- Cervix fully dilated.
- Position of fetal head is ROA – mid-cavity forceps can be used for positions ROA, direct OA and LOA, ventouse can be used for all fetal head positions.
- The station of the fetal head is 2 cm below the ischial spines so it is safe to undertake instrumental delivery.
- Membranes are ruptured.

There is significant caput 2+ and some moulding 1+. The woman is exhausted so forceps would be more likely to secure a safe delivery than ventouse. The ventouse is more likely to fail if the patient is unable to push and caput is present as the vacuum seal is less adherent with caput.

Caesarean section is not indicated as a safe instrumental delivery is very likely.

The woman is counselled and consents verbally for forceps delivery in the room. There is no need to take her to theatre as delivery is likely to be straightforward

On re-examination the findings are identical to those described above. Neville–Barnes forceps are applied, first the left blade followed by the right blade, and they lock together as described above under forceps technique. The blades are parallel but at a slight angle as the fetal head is in the right occipito-anterior position. The practitioner ensures no vaginal wall or cervix is trapped and with the next contraction traction using Pajot's manoeuvre is applied. As the head crowns a right mediolateral episiotomy is performed.

The baby is delivered, cries at birth and is placed on the patient's abdomen. One minute later the umbilical cord is clamped. An intramuscular injection of Syntometrine® is given to the woman by the midwife when the baby is delivered. This facilitates the third stage of labour. Following signs of placental separation (see Chapter 18) the placenta is delivered via controlled cord traction. The episiotomy is repaired in three layers with absorbable sutures (e.g. Vicryl®), and vaginal and rectal examinations performed. Swabs and needles are checked with the midwife and found to be correct. The patient is informed regarding the procedure and the importance of keeping the episiotomy area clean to reduce the risk of infection. Finally the indications, procedure and postoperative plan are documented in the patient's notes.

Key learning points

- The main obstetric operations are episiotomy, forceps and ventouse delivery, and caesarean section.
- The common gynaecological procedures are hysteroscopy, laparoscopy, pelvic floor repair (anterior and/or posterior repair), vaginal or abdominal hysterectomy.

- The most popular operation for stress urinary incontinence is tension-free vaginal tape – either TVT or TVT-O.
- Understanding the principles of the procedures described above will enhance your learning when you actually witness or assist at these operations.

 Now visit **www.wileyessential.com/humandevelopment** to test yourself on this chapter.

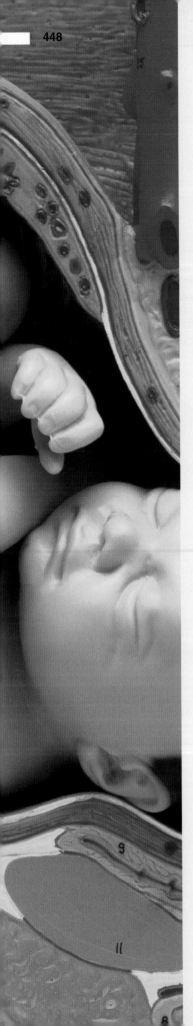

CHAPTER 51
The menopause

Kinza Younas

Case

A 49-year-old woman was referred by her GP to the gynaecology department with a history of no menstrual periods for the last 14 months following removal of the levonorgestrel (LNG) intrauterine system (IUS) (Mirena® coil). She complains of hot flushes and night sweats and mood disturbances, which interfere her daily routine. Her menarche occurred at age 14, her periods were irregular and heavy so a LNG-IUS was used to control the heavy menstrual bleeding. Previously she used the combined oral contraceptive pill for contraception. She is a non-smoker with a normal body mass index and takes no regular medications.

Learning outcomes

- You should be able to recognise signs and symptoms of perimenopause and menopause both natural or iatrogenic.

- You should be able to describe the causes of premature or iatrogenic menopause and suggest investigations, interpret results and outline appropriate management.

Essential Human Development, First Edition. Edited by Samuel Webster, Geraint Morris and Euan Kevelighan
© 2018 John Wiley & Sons, Ltd. Published 2018 by John Wiley & Sons, Ltd.

Introduction

The menopause is defined as the permanent cessation of menstruation following the loss of ovarian follicular activity. Menopause is recognised if 12 consecutive months of amenorrhoea occurs when no other pathological or physiological cause is present. It is a natural process that represents the termination of fertility. The ovaries become unresponsive to hypothalamic influx resulting in decreased production of oestrogen and progesterone. The menopause may be induced iatrogenically by surgery (bilateral oophorectomy), radiation to the ovaries or from chemotherapy.

The average age of menopause in Caucasian women is 51 years but this varies in different ethnic groups. Women respond to this change differently, some feel relieved they no longer need to worry about pregnancy, but some present with anxiety and low energy. The physical symptoms of decreased oestrogen are hot flushes, mood swings, night sweats, vaginal dryness and emotional symptoms that may disrupt sleep, result in low energy, and trigger anxiety and a feeling of sadness. Skin changes, osteoporosis and hair loss may also occur. These symptoms may start a year or two before the actual menopause, this is known as the perimenopause. The ovaries may stop working prematurely (usually before age 40), known as premature ovarian failure (POF), or iatrogenically, for example when ovaries are removed surgically, and the woman develops menopausal symptoms.

History taking

A detailed history in relation to the following is informative:

- insomnia, night sweats, hot flushes;
- emotional stress;
- mother's and sister's gynaecological history;
- family history of genetic disorder;
- weight loss;
- sexual activity;
- chronic systemic diseases, radiotherapy or chemotherapy.

Investigations

A serum follicle-stimulating hormone (FSH) level of more than 30 mIU/mL on two occasions 4–6 weeks apart is a useful parameter, plus low oestradiol levels.

Diagnosis

In women over 45 years of age amenorrhoea of more than 12 months in the presence of classical symptoms of menopause is sufficient to make a diagnosis of menopause (NICE, 2015).

FSH should not be used as a diagnostic criterion in women using combined contraceptive pills or high-dose progesterone as the true level of FSH will be masked by exogenous hormone use (NICE, 2015).

Premature ovarian failure (POF)

Premature ovarian failure is associated with elevated FSH, low oestrogen and cessation of menstruation before the age of 40. It affects 1–5% of women. If POF occurs in women younger than 30 years of age a karyotype should be requested to exclude sex chromosome translocations, short arm deletions or the presence of occult Y chromosome. POF is more common in women with autoimmune abnormalities, for example autoimmune thyroiditis, insulin-dependent diabetes mellitus, myasthenia gravis and parathyroid disease, compared to healthy women. Although no therapy for infertile patients with autoimmune ovarian failure has been proven effective, oestrogen and progesterone treatment to promote and maintain secondary sexual characteristics and reduce the risk of developing osteoporosis is recommended. Gonadotrophin levels may fluctuate in POF. Some ovarian follicles remain in ovaries with POF, which may result in spontaneous ovulation. Pregnancy may occasionally occur even in women taking exogenous oestrogens with or without progesterone.

Resistant ovarian syndrome

This rare condition presents with the same signs and symptoms as premature ovarian failure. Resistant ovaries result from functional disturbances of gonadotrophin receptors in ovarian follicles, and are resistant to exogenous gonadotrophin stimulation. The patient karyotype is 46XX, secondary sexual characteristics are normal, and FSH and LH are elevated. Ultrasound reveals a normal appearance of the ovarian follicles in contrast to premature ovarian failure. Occasionally, spontaneous ovulation occurs with oestrogen therapy.

Assessment of women for hormone replacement therapy (HRT)

In women with iatrogenic menopause and premature ovarian failure, HRT provides the sex hormones that the ovaries would normally produce. HRT use is sensible in these patients in the absence of risk factors up until the average age of menopause (approximately age 51).

Women should be assessed for increased cardiovascular risk factors (e.g. diabetes, raised blood pressure and cholesterol), irregular menstrual bleeding (intermenstrual bleeding, postcoital bleeding or postmenopausal bleeding), personal or family history of thromboembolism, and a high risk of breast cancer. In such cases consider lipid profile, mammography and thrombobophilia screening before starting HRT.

These patients require exogenous HRT to treat troublesome menopausal symptoms. The commonest presentation in menopause is vasomotor symptoms (hot flushes and night sweats), occurring in 75% of women, with 25% of cases judged severe (NICE, 2015). These symptoms may last from 2 to 7 years. Women with menopausal symptoms should be provided with adequate written and verbal information concerning HRT to make an informed choice as to whether to commence it or not. HRT is available in the form of tablets, gel, patches, nasal spray, pessaries or rings for local vaginal use.

Patients with a uterus need both oestrogen and progesterone to protect the uterus from the unopposed effects of oestrogen. In patients with a uterus two types of HRT are available depending on the woman's circumstances:

1. Cyclical (sequential).
2. Continuous combined HRT.

Cyclical/sequential HRT

This is used for menopausal symptoms in women who still have their periods or are within 1 year of their last menstrual period. There are two types of cyclical HRT:

- **Monthly HRT** – where oestrogen is used every day and progesterone added in for the last 12–14 days of the cycle. These women will have a withdrawal bleed (period) at the beginning of the next cycle when they recommence oestrogen-only HRT.
- **Three monthly HRT** – where oestrogen is used every day and progesterone for 12–14 days every 13 weeks to induce menstrual bleeding. It is usually prescribed for women experiencing abnormal or heavy periods or who want to 'bleed' every 3 months rather than every month.

Continuous combined HRT (no bleed HRT)

Oestrogen and a progestogen is taken every day without a break so no withdrawal bleeding (menstruation) occurs. It is recommended for postmenopausal women who are more than 1 year post-menopause or those women on sequential HRT who are aged 54 years or older. It ensures that the endometrium remains very thin so the patient remains amenorrhoeic – the 'no-bleed' HRT.

Oestrogen-only HRT (unopposed oestrogen)

This is recommended for women who have had a hysterectomy. These patients do not require progesterone to protect against the effect of oestrogen on the endometrium. Oestrogen-only HRT is also useful in women who have a levonorgestrel IUS in situ – the levonorgestrel protects the endometrium.

Other HRT options

In low-risk perimenopausal women the HRT choice would be a cyclical (sequential) monthly or 3-monthly bleed according to each woman's choice. In postmenopausal women with low libido tibolone may help. This is a synthetic combination of oestrogen, progestogen and androgen and is a type of 'no-bleed' HRT.

Once on HRT women should have an annual review to discuss the pros and cons of continuing therapy. In women

in whom HRT started at a younger age, for example for POF or iatrogenically induced menopause, once they reach age 50 a discussion about weaning off/stopping/continuing HRT should take place. In some women vasomotor symptoms persist after weaning off HRT.

Side effects of HRT

The side effects are usually transient with HRT use and take a few months to resolve. Side effects include oestrogen- and progesterone-related fluid retention, bloating, breast tenderness, nausea, headaches, leg cramps, vaginal bleeding and especially progesterone-related acne, lower abdominal pain and mood swings. Women should be encouraged to report any unusual symptoms or signs; unscheduled vaginal bleeding especially should be thoroughly investigated. There is no direct association with weight gain and HRT use.

HRT is commenced at a low dose and adjusted according to symptoms in menopausal women (to reduce side effects). A higher-dose oestrogen is often required in younger patients. HRT can be used in conditions like chronic renal failure, obesity, smoking, thyroid disease, controlled hypertension, diabetes, multiple sclerosis, sickle cell anaemia and depression. There are relevant contraindications where specialist advice is needed, for example active liver and cardiac disease, previous breast cancer, systematic lupus erythematosus, previous ovarian and endometrial cancer, and personal and family history of venous thromboembolism (VTE).

Obese women and smokers are at increased risk of VTE. The dose and delivery route may also add to the risks associated with HRT, especially for VTE. Transdermal application (patches, or gel) of HRT poses less risk compared to oral administration. In women with a history of migraine, controlled hypertension, obesity, smoking, hyperlipidaemia or previous VTE, transdermal preparations of HRT should be considered.

The benefits of using HRT include a reduction/abolition of vasomotor symptoms, protection against bone and connective tissue loss, and a reduction in bowel cancer; moreover, there is some evidence of improvement in neurocognitive functions. The maximum neuroprotection is seen in young, healthy postmenopausal women.

There has been a decline in the use of HRT over the last decade due to some controversial results published from large studies. The results of the HERS (Heart and Estrogen/Progestin Replacement Study) and the WHI (Women's Health Initiative) and Million Women studies have influenced national policies and recommendations (Table 51.1).

The Women's Health Initiative (WHI) was a large study looking at 161 000 postmenopausal women ranging from age 50 to 79 years. Women were randomised into groups. One group comprised hysterectomised women who were given conjugated equine oestrogen (CEE) or placebo, whereas women with intact uterus were randomised to CEE and medroxy

Table 51.1 Effects of hormone replacement therapy (HRT) observed in the Heart and Estrogen/Progestin Replacement Study (HERS), the Women's Health Initiative (WHI) study and the Million Women study.

Parameter	Study			
	HERS (I and II)	WHI oestrogen arm	WHI combined arm	Million Women study
Average age	66.7 years	50–79 years	50–79 years	50–64 years
Coronary vascular disease (CVD)	↑	↓ modest	↑ modest	↑
Venous thromboembolism (VTE)	↑	↑	↑	↑
Stroke	↑	↑	↑	↑
Ca. Breast	↑	Possible ↓	↑	↑
Hyperlipidaemia	↑	↑	↑	↑
Ca. Ovary	–	–	–	Small ↑
Ca. Endometrium	–	–	↓	–
Bone fractures	↓	↓	↓	↓
Bowel cancer	↓	↔	↓	↓
Dementia	–	↔	↔	↔
Alzheimer's	↔	↔	↔	↔

Ca., carcinoma.

progesterone acetate or placebo. After 5 years the HRT arm had more heart attacks, stroke, blood clots and breast cancer but fewer fractures and colon cancer than those in the placebo arm. The Million Women study considered those aged 50–64 years in the UK attending breast screening clinics. There was a significantly increased risk of breast cancer for women on combined HRT and less on oestrogen-only and tibolone (Beral, 2003). Later in 2012 a Cochrane systematic review concluded that HRT is not indicated for prevention of dementia, CVD or cognitive dysfunction although it has significant benefit for menopausal osteoporosis where other treatments are unsuitable (Marjoribanks *et al.*, 2012).

Problems with these studies

The WHI study investigated cardiovascular risks in women (average age of 63 years) while most women commencing on HRT do so around age 50 years, that is symptomatic younger women. Also women with known breast cancer were not excluded in the Million Women study, and in HERS some women already had established CVD.

The results of the WHI study were reanalysed in 2007. This demonstrated that HRT use in women within 10 years of menopause has fewer risks and does not increase CVD, while using HRT for more than 20 years post-menopause was associated with harm. The benefits of using HRT can be maximised by using it during the early phase of menopause, usually known as the 'window of opportunity'.

Conclusions about HRT

Not everybody needs HRT. Approximately 30% of women don't have any symptoms, 30% have mild symptoms while only 25% suffer with severe symptoms that require HRT. Flushes rarely last longer than a few years, and 3–5 years of HRT is usually all that is required. If HRT is used for a longer period, for example after surgical hysterectomy and bilateral salpingo-oophorectomy in women who are in their 30s or 40s or in premature ovarian failure, then it should be tapered off slowly before stopping it altogether at the average age of menopause if there are no other risk factors. HRT should always be tapered before stopping it altogether even when used for 3–5 years.

In conclusion the short-term use of HRT during the 'window of opportunity' is beneficial to women. In women with iatrogenic menopause or premature menopause HRT can be safely used until the average age of the menopause. Long-term use (>20 years since menopause) is associated with harm in postmenopausal women (Rossouw *et al.*, 2007).

The oestrogen-only HRT has a very small risk of breast cancer compared to combined oestrogen and progesterone, and any increased risk also reduces after stopping the HRT. In women with CVD HRT does not increase CVD risk and death when started before the age of 60 (NICE, 2015). In cases of hormone-dependent cancers in young women, specialist advice should be requested to improve the woman's quality of life.

Alternative therapies

There are some alternatives to hormone replacement for menopausal symptoms where women are not willing to use hormones. These include antidepressants like selective serotonin reuptake inhibitors (SSRIs – e.g. paroxetine, fluoxetine, citalopram and serotonin) and selective noradrenaline reuptake inhibitors (SNRI – e.g. venlafaxine). How these help to alleviate hot flushes is not clear, and they do not help in all cases. The side effects include nausea and decreased libido. Gabapentin is a drug usually used for epilepsy and neuropathic pain but sometimes relieves menopausal symptoms. These alternative therapies have a poor evidence base and are much less effective than HRT.

For vaginal dryness vaginal lubricants and moisturisers can be used as an alternative to HRT. Oestrogen creams work very well and systemic absorption is negligible.

Alternatives for bone health include regular weight-bearing exercises, food intake that is rich in calcium and vitamin D, supplements of calcium and vitamin D, stopping smoking and cutting down on alcohol intake. Bisphosphonates including alendronate, risedronate and etidronate are used to treat osteoporosis. These drugs work at the cellular level, promoting the manufacture of new bone cells, restoring some bone loss and helping to prevent fractures. HRT can be used in selected cases for a limited period of time.

Contraception and pregnancy with HRT

The oestrogen used in HRT formulations is different in strength than that used in contraceptive pills. It is possible that women can become pregnant when they are perimenopausal and using HRT. Women may be fertile for 2 years after the last menstrual period if they are less than 50 years old, or for 1 year if they are more than 50. Contraception is recommended in such cases – either barrier methods or an intrauterine contraceptive device, for example a copper coil or levonorgestrel intrauterine system (Lev-IUS). A levonorgestrel IUS is licensed for both contraception and heavy menstrual bleeding and can be used instead of the progestogen part of HRT.

SUMMARY

Clinical case

Case discussion

This woman is postmenopausal, and diagnosis is made on the presentation of symptoms without relying on laboratory results. She had heavy menstrual periods and an irregular cycle that was managed with LNG-IUS, and since taking out the IUS she has had no bleeding. She has no health issues, a normal BMI and is a non-smoker. She requires counselling to help her make an informed choice about available options of HRT and alternative therapies. She has no risk factors for CVD , thromboembolism or gynaecological cancers. Suitable HRT options include continuous combined low-dose oestrogen and progesterone patch or tablets according to her preference ('no bleed' HRT). She has had more than 12 months of amenorrhoea so likely will not experience breakthrough bleeding with the 'no bleed' option. Most women in the UK prefer to have no 'periods' when on HRT. Another suitable option is an oestrogen-only patch and protection of the endometrium with a LNG-IUS. One advantage of this is a very low dose of progestogen circulating as only 20 µg of LNG is released per day. A final option would be to offer conventional cyclical combined HRT (oestrogen every day and progestogen for the final 10–14 days per month). Should she choose this option it is likely she will have a 'withdrawal' bleed every month, similar to a period. She requires HRT for a couple of years to treat the vasomotor symptoms. If she wishes to use HRT in the long term, further discussion with the patient regarding the risks/benefits of HRT should occur to enable the patient to make an informed choice.

Key learning points

- Menopause is a common presentation as life expectancy is increasing.
- It is important to differentiate the natural menopause from premature ovarian failure and iatrogenic menopause in order to plan appropriate management.
- Women over 45 years of age with vasomotor symptoms can be treated with HRT without relying on laboratory results.
- In high-risk patients HRT use should be limited with careful selection of patients and duration of use.

 Now visit **www.wileyessential.com/humandevelopment** to test yourself on this chapter.

FURTHER READING

HRT guidance. British Menopause Society (https://thebms.org.uk/).

References

Beral, V. (2003) Breast cancer and hormone-replacement therapy in the Million Women Study. *Lancet* **362**: 419–427.

Marjoribanks, J., Farquhar, C., Roberts, H. and Lethaby, A. (2012) Long term hormone therapy for perimenopausal and postmenopausal women. *Cochrane Database of Systematic Reviews* 7 (Art. No.: CD004143). doi: 10.1002/14651858.CD004143.pub4.

NICE and National Collaborating Centre for Women's and Children's Health (2015) Menopause: full guideline (draft for consultation). National Collaborating Centre for Women's and Children's Health. Available at: https://www.nice.org.uk/guidance/ng23/documents/menopause-full-guideline2

Rossouw, J.E., Prentice, R.L., Manson, J.E., Wu, L., Barad, D., Barnabei, V.M., *et al.* (2007) Postmenopausal hormone therapy and risk of cardiovascular disease by age and years since menopause. *JAMA* **297**: 1465–1477.

Index

Page numbers in *italic* refer to figures. Page numbers in **bold** refer to tables.

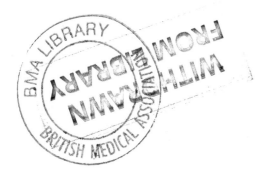